Medical Laboratory Science Review

SIXTH EDITION

Medical Laboratory Science Review

SIXTH EDITION

Patricia M. Tille, PhD, MLS(ASCP), AHI(AMT), FACSc
Professor, Graduate Program Director, Interim Department Chair
Clinical and Health Information Sciences Department
University of Cincinnati
Cincinnati, Ohio

Robert R. Harr, MS, MLS^{CM}(ASCP)
Adjunct Associate Professor
Bowling Green State University
Bowling Green, Ohio
Rush University
Chicago, Illinois

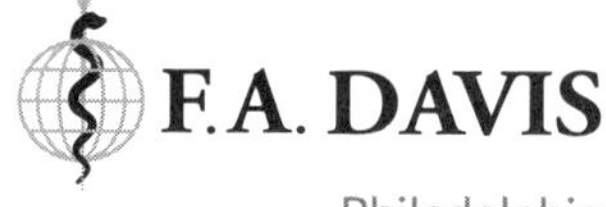

Philadelphia

F. A. Davis Company
1915 Arch Street
Philadelphia, PA 19103
www.fadavis.com

Printed in the United States of America

Last digit indicates print number: 10 9 8 7 6 5 4 3 2 1

Publisher: Christa Fratantoro
Manager of Content Development: George W. Lang
Content Project Manager: Megan Suermann
Design and Illustrations Manager: Carolyn O'Brien

Library of Congress Cataloging-in-Publication Data is available upon request.

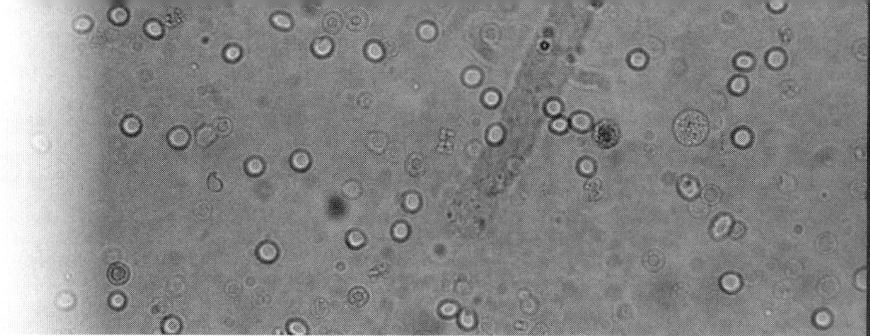

Preface

The primary purpose of the *Medical Laboratory Science (MLS) Review* is to assist candidates in the preparation for certification or licensure examinations. This review can also be used as a tool for practicing professionals to update their knowledge of medical laboratory science and renew their theoretical skills. In addition, educators in medical laboratory science and medical laboratory technician (MLT) programs may wish to recommend this review as a study guide as their students progress through the curriculum or as a resource in a programmatic review course within the curriculum.

The *MLS Review* is designed to facilitate learning. Unlike other review books, the questions create a progression of related content. Explanations accompanying each question expand on the content. The Sixth Edition includes more than 2,150 multiple-choice questions grouped into core content areas. Questions appear together with answers, explanations, and taxonomy levels. The questions in each section provide a thorough review of the discipline and are ordered to facilitate the coherent understanding of the subject. The book also contains a photomicrograph-based section. The review text begins with the Introduction section, which includes information on the design of the questions, use of the book to prepare for an examination, and test-taking tips. The introductory section is followed by questions arranged according to content area. Each area contains a list of references, which are also recommended for further review. An online resource that includes hundreds of additional questions is available at no charge to purchasers of the book. Davis Edge, an online progressive testing platform, allows users to prepare customized examinations to assist further in assessment of their strengths and weaknesses. The materials in the *MLS Review* were prepared by educators and clinical experts who have national recognition for their accomplishments in medical laboratory science. Materials from recent developments in practice as well as major textbooks were used in formulating the questions. The *MLS Review* is designed as an individual guidebook for measuring an individual's knowledge and test-taking skills. It is a valuable tool to support the student in preparation for a national certification examination, course examination, or licensure and for the practitioner updating theoretical skills.

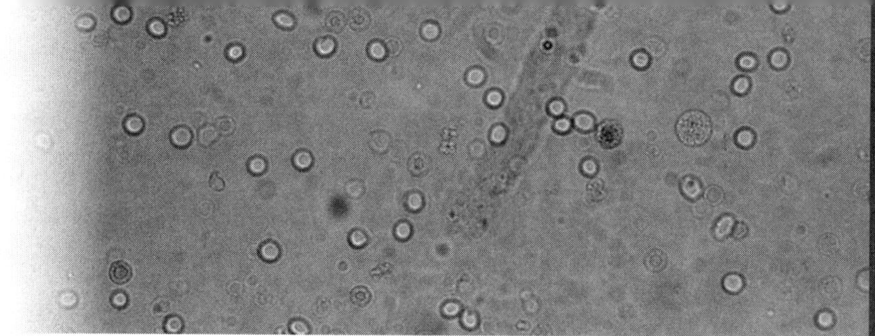

Contributors

DEMETRA CASTILLO, M.AD.ED., MLS(ASCP)^{CM}, AHI(AMT)
Associate Professor-Educator
Department of Clinical Health and Information Sciences
University of Cincinnati
Mount Prospect, Illinois

STEPHANIE L. JACOBSON, DCLS, MLS(ASCP)^{CM}, AHI(AMT)
Professor-Educator
MLS Graduate Faculty
University of Cincinnati
Hermosa, South Dakota

LEAH L. NARANS, MBA, MLS(ASCP), AHI(AMT)
Laboratory Program Director, SSM Health
Faculty Emeritus, Madison Area Technical College
Madison, Wisconsin

MILES TOMPKINS, MLT(ASCP)^{CM}, PBT^{CM}, QLS^{CM}
Technical Staffing Specialist
Diagnostic Laboratory of Oklahoma
Clinical Adjunct Faculty
Medical Laboratory Technology
Rose State College
Oklahoma City, Oklahoma

ELIZABETH WARNING, MS, MLS(ASCP)^{CM}, AHI(AMT)
Associate Professor-Educator
Department of Clinical and Health Information Sciences
University of Cincinnati
Cincinnati, Ohio

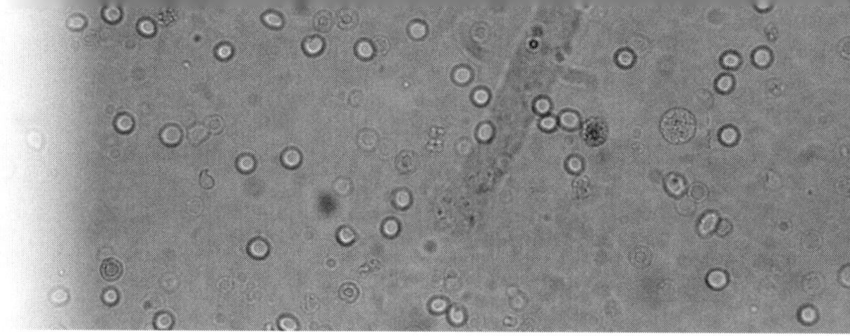

Contents

Preface *v*

Contributors *vii*

Introduction *xi*

Design of Questions *xi*

Preparing for a Certification Examination *xii*

Test-Taking Tips *xii*

CHAPTER *1* Laboratory Operations *1*

1.1 *Laboratory Calculations 3*

1.2 *Quality Control 8*

1.3 *Laboratory Statistics 15*

CHAPTER *2* Education and Management *23*

2.1 *Education Theory and Practice 25*

2.2 *Management Theory and Practice 28*

2.3 *Laws and Regulations 33*

2.4 *Laboratory Economics 38*

2.5 *Laboratory Safety 40*

CHAPTER *3* Immunology *43*

3.1 *Basic Principles of Immunology 45*

3.2 *Immunologic Techniques 51*

3.3 *Infectious Disease Methods 57*

3.4 *Autoimmune Disorders 69*

3.5 *Hypersensitivity 73*

3.6 *Immunodeficiency, Immunoglobulins, Complement, and Cellular Testing 75*

3.7 *Tumors, Transplantation, and Genetics 78*

CHAPTER *4* Molecular Diagnostics *83*

4.1 *Nucleic Acid Chemistry 85*

4.2 *Basic Concepts 87*

4.3 *Biochemical Reagents 88*

4.4 *Genetics 91*

4.5 *Molecular Techniques 94*

4.6 *Molecular Laboratory Practices 108*

CHAPTER *5* Urinalysis and Body Fluids *111*

5.1 *Routine Urinalysis 113*

5.2 *Urine Microscopy and Clinical Correlations 128*

5.3 *Cerebrospinal, Serous, and Synovial Fluids 139*

5.4 *Amniotic, Gastrointestinal, Seminal Fluids, and Blood Specimens 150*

CHAPTER *6* Clinical Chemistry *159*

6.1 *Instrumentation and Methodology 161*

6.2 *Blood Gases, pH, Electrolytes, and Vitamins 177*

6.3 *Carbohydrates, Hemoglobin, Iron, and Bilirubin 189*

6.4 *Creatinine, Uric Acid, BUN, and Ammonia 201*

6.5 *Proteins, Electrophoresis, and Lipids 207*

6.6 *Enzymes and Cardiac Markers 219*

6.7 *Clinical Endocrinology 233*

6.8 *Toxicology, Therapeutic Drug Monitoring, and Trace Metals 243*

6.9 *Tumor Markers 251*

CHAPTER *7* Hematology *257*

7.1 *Blood Physiology 259*
7.2 *Normocytic Normochromic Anemia 261*
7.3 *Microcytic Hypochromic Anemia 265*
7.4 *Macrocytic Normochromic Anemia 268*
7.5 *Laboratory Evaluation of Anemia 270*
7.6 *Qualitative and Quantitative Nonmalignant Leukocyte Disorders 280*
7.7 *Myelodysplastic Syndromes 285*
7.8 *Lymphoproliferative and Myeloproliferative Neoplasms 287*
7.9 *Acute Leukemia 293*
7.10 *Laboratory Evaluation of Leukocyte Disorders 296*

CHAPTER *8* Hemostasis and Coagulation *299*

8.1 *Coagulation Physiology 301*
8.2 *Primary Hemostasis Disorders: Platelet and Vascular Disorders 304*
8.3 *Secondary Hemostasis Disorders: Factor Deficiencies and Hemorrhagic Coagulation Disorders 310*
8.4 *Thrombosis Risk, Thrombotic Disorders, and Anticoagulant Therapies 314*
8.5 *Evaluation of Coagulopathies 319*

CHAPTER *9* Microbiology *323*

9.1 *Basic Concepts and Microscopy 325*
9.2 *Preanalytical Procedures 328*
9.3 *Antimicrobials and Susceptibility Methods 334*
9.4 *Enterobacterales 336*
9.5 *Nonfermentative Bacilli 349*
9.6 *Miscellaneous and Fastidious Gram-Negative Rods 355*
9.7 *Gram-Positive and Gram-Negative Cocci 366*
9.8 *Aerobic Gram-Positive Rods, Spirochetes, Mycoplasmas, Ureaplasmas, and Chlamydia 380*
9.9 *Anaerobic Bacteria 387*
9.10 *Mycobacteria 393*
9.11 *Mycology 399*
9.12 *Virology 411*
9.13 *Parasitology 419*

CHAPTER *10* Immunohematology *433*

10.1 *Genetics of Blood Groups 435*
10.2 *Immunology of Blood Groups 437*
10.3 *ABO Blood Group System 438*
10.4 *Rh Blood Group System 442*
10.5 *Testing for Antibodies 446*
10.6 *Compatibility Testing 452*
10.7 *Transfusion Reactions 456*
10.8 *Components 460*
10.9 *Donors 465*
10.10 *Hemolytic Disease of the Fetus and Newborn 469*
10.11 *Serological Testing of Blood Products 473*
10.12 *Transfusion Practice 475*

CHAPTER *11* Photomicrographs and Color Plate Examination *481*

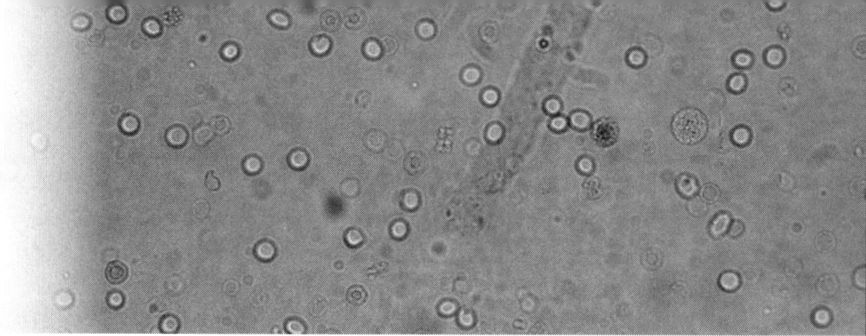

Introduction

The *Medical Laboratory Science (MLS) Review* is designed to provide a challenging individualized assessment of practical and theoretical knowledge needed by medical laboratory scientists and technicians. The *MLS Review* will assist the individual in identifying strengths, weaknesses, and gaps in their knowledge base. Because taxonomy level is a part of the assessment, individuals can concentrate on the type of questions that are the most difficult. The suggested approach to maximizing use of the MLS Review is to read the explanation that follows each question thoroughly, regardless of whether it was answered correctly or not. Highlight the content that was unfamiliar or confusing, and study it until committed to memory.

This *MLS Review* is a tool that can be used to facilitate both self-assessment and new learning. The units are arranged in a logical sequence corresponding to the organization of a typical laboratory science curriculum. The questions within a unit are related and can be used by individuals, students, and practicing professionals as they progress through the laboratory science curriculum or review to improve understanding. The sections are comprehensive, and the majority are suitable for all certification levels, although some questions may be more appropriate for one certification level than for another. The *MLS Review* is intended to supplement courses in the curriculum and assist anyone who is re-entering the laboratory after stepping out of the field. In addition, it is designed to improve performance on generalist, categorical, and specialist certification examinations.

Design of Questions

Test questions used in certification examinations are multiple choice. Each consists of a question, incomplete statement, or problem-solving/critical-thinking exercise called the *stem* and four alternative responses. One of the alternatives is the correct response and the remaining three are incorrect (these may be wrong, incomplete, partially correct, or less correct than the most appropriate response). Incorrect alternatives that appear plausible are called *distractors*. The difficulty of a question is determined by how close the distractors are to the correct response. Some questions were written for assessment of knowledge and others for learning. All multiple-choice questions have a *single best answer*. If a question contains two of the responses that appear true, then the correct response must be the response that provides the best outcome for patient care according to the standard of practice in laboratory science. Questions involving combinations of statements (multiple, multiple choice) are not used on certification examinations or in this text.

Each question is followed by the test item classification. Alongside each question is the correct answer and an explanation. The test item classification consists of the subject category and taxonomy level of the question. For example, a question in blood banking asking for an interpretation of an ABO problem may have the test item classification "Blood bank/ABO discrepancy/3." The test item classification places the question in the major category of blood banking; the subcategory is ABO discrepancy; and the taxonomy level classifies the question as problem solving. Some questions will have more than one subcategory that indicates the question can be classified as applicable to different areas or knowledge within the laboratory. Taxonomy level 1 questions address recall of information. Taxonomy 2 questions require calculation, application, correlation, comprehension, or relation. Taxonomy 3 questions require problem solving, critical thinking, analysis, interpretation, or decision making. Because the answers and explanations appear on the same page as the questions, it is recommended that the perforated flap be removed and used as a blocker to cover the answers while reviewing the questions. After reviewing the question and identifying the answer, slide the blocker down the page to reveal the correct response and explanation. The blocker is printed with a compilation of reference ranges for common analytes that can be used to answer questions.

It is also important to note that, to keep the textbook within a manageable length, the content is not fully comprehensive in all areas of the clinical laboratory. The online Davis Edge question bank includes a substantially larger text bank. Each purchase of the print textbook comes with a complimentary access to the Davis Edge for individuals to utilize online quizzes to improve their performance and enhance their knowledge.

Preparing for a Certification Examination

Ideally, an examination score should reflect an individual's knowledge of the content without the influence of other variables. However, a number of variables, such as stress, wellness, self-confidence, emotional state, and alertness, all influence performance. In addition, examination skills often factor into examination scores and can be decisive. A single question answered correctly can make the difference between passing and failing, the only two meaningful scores for a certification examination.

Certification examinations are usually delivered by computer. There are two major types of examinations: traditional and adaptive. Traditional examinations have a fixed length and content. Therefore, everyone taking the examination receives the same set of questions. If the exam is completed in a written format, the order of questions and responses are also identical for all participants and the exam is administered to everyone simultaneously. If the exam is delivered via a computer or technology based, it may be completed at the same time for all participants (synchronously) or at different times (asynchronously). In either case, the questions may be randomized, the answers for the same questions may be in a randomized order, or the questions themselves may vary but focus on equivalent content areas and taxonomy levels for all participants.

A computer adaptive examination may be fixed or variable in length, but every examination is different because the difficulty of the next question is determined by whether the participant answers the current question correctly. If a participant can answer a level 1 question in the content area correctly, the exam will provide a more difficult question. This continues until the participant reaches a question that is answered incorrectly. The exam will "adapt" to the user and drop to a lower question or a different content area. Although every examinee's question set may be different, similar to the randomized traditional exam, all questions come from a common database, and therefore, there is some overlap between the questions used.

The examination is constructed such that the number of questions in each category (e.g., hematology) is within the specifications published for the examination; however, the distribution of questions and the order of questions will vary significantly. Certification examinations are criterion referenced. This means that examination performance is scored passing or failing independently of the performance of other candidates taking the examination. The minimum passing score for certification examinations is normalized to minimize the variance between examinations. However, the minimum passing score often correlates with a range of 65% to 70% correct responses. A score below 65% on any content area in the *MLS Review* is a strong indicator that an individual has not mastered the material in this area and that further study is required.

Preparation for a certification examination requires a study plan. Begin with a review of the examination content outline available by the certification agency. For example, if 20% of the examination is microbiology but only 2% of the examination is laboratory management, the individual should spend significantly more time studying the former. Each content area also includes subcategories (e.g., bacteriology and parasitology under microbiology). If 60% of the microbiology content is bacteriology and only 10% is parasitology, then the individual should devote significantly more time to studying the former.

Allow sufficient time prior to the examination to review each content area. Use this review text to test the knowledge of the respective content area. Devote time to reading the explanation for each question, regardless of whether a question was answered correctly or not. The explanation may provide additional material that can be beneficial to the understanding of related questions. Highlight or make note of the information that may be new or expands upon the information that can be applied to more complex questions. Rarely will any of the same questions appear on a certification examination; however, variants of the questions or the content are likely to be included. Repeat the content areas in each chapter or specific levels of questions in the *MLS Review* based on each individual's comprehensive evaluation. Additional questions are available online in the F.A. Davis companion website, Edge. For instructions and password needed to access online content, see the inside front cover of the text. The online questions are all different from those in the text, and provide the user with an opportunity to utilize many more question variations and interpretations of photomicrographs.

Test-Taking Tips

Before the Examination

First, make a study plan such as the one suggested earlier. It is unrealistic to review all of this material in only a few days. Allow at least 1 month to study all areas completely and carefully. Set aside an allotted time period each day to review materials.

Assemble all study materials before beginning the review. Choose a quiet, comfortable area for review. Find a place that is free from distractions. After some review, utilize the text to simulate taking a test. Pick a section of the text and go through the questions, writing down the correct response. The practice should be timed, uninterrupted, and designed to observe realistic testing practices.

A few days before the examination, be sure to again read through the instructions provided by the certification agency. Some types of calculators (e.g., graphing or programmable calculators) may be prohibited by the certification agency.

On Examination Day

Make sure to bring the required identification documents or examination confirmation required by the certification agency. Do not bring notes, books, or any unnecessary materials as they are generally not permitted in the testing area.

During the Examination

Read all the instructions on how to complete the examination. Read the questions carefully, and note the key words. Accept the question as written and do not read other information into the question, and do not look for hidden meanings. Consider what the best response is regarding patient care and accuracy of testing.

Quickly look at all the answers. Next, carefully read all the choices. Often two responses will be correct, but one is more correct than the other. Pick items that are more specific or detailed than the others. Answer all questions. There is no penalty for guessing on certification examinations. A computer-adapted examination selects the next question based on the previous answer.

Do not overlook such words as *not*, *never*, *always*, *most*, *least*, *best*, *worst*, and *except*. Statements that contain unqualified absolutes (*always*, *never*) are usually incorrect. In contrast, alternatives that are worded to contain exceptions (*usually*, *generally*) may be true. Work steadily and do not spend too much time on any question; keep an eye on the time.

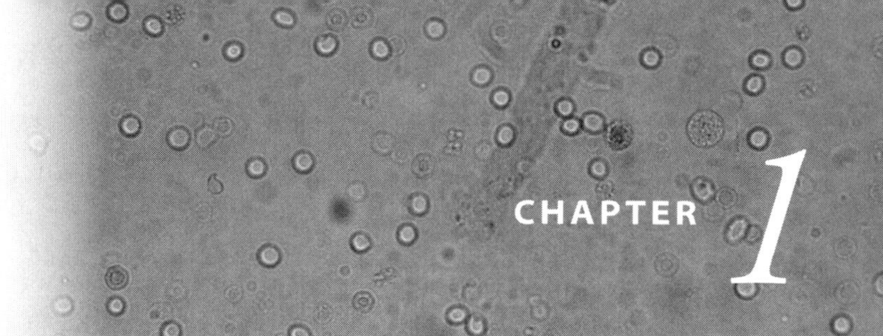

Laboratory Operations

1.1 *Laboratory Calculations*

1.2 *Quality Control*

1.3 *Laboratory Statistics*

1.1 Laboratory Calculations

1. **How many grams of sodium hydroxide (NaOH) are required to prepare 150.0 mL of a 5.0% weight/volume (w/v) solution?**
   A. 1.5 g
   B. 4.0 g
   C. 7.5 g
   D. 15.0 g
   Laboratory operations/Calculations/2

2. **How many milliliters of glacial acetic acid are needed to prepare 2.0 L of 10.0% v/v acetic acid?**
   A. 10.0 mL
   B. 20.0 mL
   C. 100.0 mL
   D. 200.0 mL
   Laboratory operations/Calculations/2

3. **A biuret reagent requires preparation of a stock solution containing 9.6 g of copper II sulfate ($CuSO_4$) per liter. How many grams of $CuSO_4 \cdot 5H_2O$ are needed to prepare 1.0 L of the stock solution?**

   Atomic weights: H = 1.0; Cu = 63.6; O = 16.0; S = 32.1

   A. 5.4 g
   B. 6.1 g
   C. 15.0 g
   D. 17.0 g
   Laboratory operations/Calculations/2

Answers to Questions 1–3

1. C A percent solution expressed in w/v refers to grams of solute per 100.0 mL of solution. To calculate, multiply the percentage (as grams) by the volume needed (mL), and then divide by 100.0 (mL).

$(5.0\,g \times 150.0\,mL) \div 100.0\,mL = 7.5\,g$

To prepare the solution, weigh 7.5 g of NaOH pellets, and add to a 150.0 mL volumetric flask. Add sufficient deionized H_2O to dissolve the NaOH. After the solution cools, add deionized H_2O to the 150.0 mL line on the flask, and mix again.

2. D The expression percent v/v refers to the volume of one liquid in milliliters present in 100.0 mL of solution. To calculate, multiply the percentage (as mL) by the volume required (mL), then divide by 100 (mL).

$(10.0\,mL \times 2{,}000.0\,mL) \div 100.0\,mL = 200.0\,mL$

To prepare 2.0 L of a 10.0% v/v solution of acetic acid, add approximately 1.0 L of deionized H_2O to a 2.0 L volumetric flask. Add 200.0 mL of glacial acetic acid, and mix. Then, add sufficient deionized H_2O to bring the meniscus to the 2.0 L line, and mix again.

3. C Determine the mass of $CuSO_4 \cdot 5H_2O$ containing 9.6 g of anhydrous $CuSO_4$. First, calculate the percentage of $CuSO_4$ in the hydrate, and then divide the amount needed (9.6 g) by the percentage.

$\%\,CuSO_4 = \text{molecular weight (MW) } CuSO_4 \div \text{MW } CuSO_4 \cdot 5H_2O \times 100$

$= (159.7 \div 249.7) \times 100 = 63.96\%$

$\text{Grams } CuSO_4 \cdot 5H_2O = 9.6\,g \div 0.6396 = 15.0\,g$

A convenient formula to use is:

g hydrate = (MW hydrate ÷ MW anhydrous salt) × g anhydrous salt

4. How many milliliters of nitric acid (HNO_3) (purity 68.0%, specific gravity 1.42) are needed to prepare 1.0 L of a 2.0 N solution?

Atomic weights: H = 1.0; N = 14.0; O = 16.0

A. 89.5 mL
B. 126.0 mL
C. 130.5 mL
D. 180.0 mL

Laboratory operations/Calculations/2

5. Convert 10.0 milligrams per deciliter (mg/dL) calcium (atomic weight = 40.1) to the International System of Units (SI).

A. 0.25
B. 0.40
C. 2.5
D. 0.4

Laboratory operations/Calculations/2

6. Convert 2.0 milliequivalents per liter (mEq/L) magnesium (atomic weight = 24.3) to mg/dL.

A. 0.8 mg/dL
B. 1.2 mg/dL
C. 2.4 mg/dL
D. 4.9 mg/dL

Laboratory operations/Calculations/2

7. How many milliliters of a 2,000.0 mg/dL glucose stock solution are needed to prepare 100.0 mL of a 150.0 mg/dL glucose working standard?

A. 1.5 mL
B. 7.5 mL
C. 15.0 mL
D. 25.0 mL

Laboratory operations/Calculations/2

Answers to Questions 4–7

4. C The MW of HNO_3 is 63.0 g. Because the valance of the acid is 1 (1 mole of hydrogen is produced per mole of acid), the equivalent weight is also 63.0 g. The mass needed is calculated by multiplying the normality (2.0 N) by the equivalent weight (63.0 g) and volume (1.0 L); therefore, 126.0 g of acid are required.

Because the purity is 68.0% and the specific gravity 1.42, the amount of HNO_3 in grams per milliliter is 0.68 × 1.42 g/mL, or 0.9656 g/mL. The volume required is calculated by dividing the mass needed (126.0 g) by the grams per milliliter.

$$mL\ HNO_3 = 126.0\,g \div 0.9656\,g/mL = 126.0\,g \div 1.0\,mL/0.9656\,g = 130.5\,mL$$

5. C The SI unit is the recommended method of reporting clinical laboratory results. The SI unit for all electrolytes is millimoles per liter (mmol/L). To convert from mg/dL to mmol/L, multiply by 10 to convert to milligrams per liter, then divide by the atomic mass expressed in milligrams.

$$10.0\,mg/dL \times 10.0\,dL/1.0\,L = 100.0\,mg/L$$

$$100.0\,mg/L \times 1.0\,mmol/40.1\,mg = 2.5\,mmol/L$$

6. C To convert from mEq/L to mg/dL, first calculate the milliequivalent weight (equivalent weight expressed in milligrams), which is the atomic mass divided by the valence. Because magnesium is divalent, each mole has the charge equivalent of 2 moles of hydrogen. Then, multiply the mEq/L by the milliequivalent weight to convert to milligrams per liter (mg/L). Next, divide by 10 to convert mg/L to mg/dL.

$$\text{Milliequivalent weight Mg} = 24.3 \div 2 = 12.15\,mg/mEq$$

$$2.0\,mEq/L \times 12.15\,mg/mEq = 24.3\,mg/L$$

$$24.3\,mg/L \times 1.0\,L/10.0\,dL = 2.4\,mg/dL$$

7. B To calculate the volume of stock solution, divide the concentration of working standard by the concentration of stock standard, and then multiply by the volume of working standard that is needed.

$C_1 \times V_1 = C_2 \times V_2$,

where C_1 = concentration of stock standard

V_1 = volume of stock standard

C_2 = concentration of working standard

V_2 = volume of working standard

$$2{,}000.0\,mg/dL \times V_1 = 150.0\,mg/dL \times 100.0\,mL$$

$$V_1 = (150.0 \div 2{,}000.0) \times 100.0\,mL$$

$$V_1 = 7.5\,mL$$

8. What is the pH of a solution of HNO_3 if the hydrogen ion (H^+) concentration is 2.5×10^{-2} molar (M)?

A. 1.0
B. 1.6
C. 2.5
D. 2.8

Laboratory operations/Calculations/1

9. Calculate the pH of a solution of 1.5×10^{-5} M ammonium hydroxide (NH_4OH).

A. 4.2
B. 7.2
C. 9.2
D. 11.2

Laboratory operations/Calculations/1

10. How many significant figures should be reported when the pH of a 0.060 M solution of HNO_3 is calculated?

A. 1
B. 2
C. 3
D. 4

Laboratory operations/Calculations/1

11. What is the pH of a 0.05 M solution of acetic acid?

Dissociation constant (K_a) = 1.75×10^{-5}, $pK_a = 4.76$

A. 1.7
B. 3.0
C. 4.3
D. 4.6

Laboratory operations/Calculations/2

Answers to Questions 8–11

8. B For a strong acid, the pH is equal to the negative logarithm of the H^+ concentration.

$pH = -Log\,[H^+]$

$pH = -Log\,0.025$

$pH = 1.6$

9. C First, calculate the pOH of the solution.

$pOH = -Log\,[OH^-]$

$pOH = -Log\,1.5 \times 10^{-5} = 4.82$

Then, solve for pH.

$pH = 14 - pOH$

$pH = 14 - 4.8 = 9.2$

10. B When zeros appear by themselves to the left of the decimal point, they are not significant. When they are to the left of the decimal point and are preceded or followed by a number, they are significant. Zeros after the decimal point preceding a number are not significant. However, they are significant if they follow another number (either before or after the decimal point) or are between two numbers. Therefore, 0.060 M has only two significant figures (the underlined digits). In laboratory practice, most analytes are reported with two significant figures. Routine analytes that are exceptions are pH, which includes three significant figures, and analytes with whole numbers above 100, such as sodium, cholesterol, triglycerides, and glucose.

11. B Weak acids do not completely ionize, and pH must be calculated from the dissociation constant of the acid (in this case, 1.75×10^{-5}).

$$K_a = \frac{[H^+] \times [Ac^-]}{[HAc]}$$

$$1.75 \times 10^{-5} = \frac{[H^+] \times [Ac^-]}{5.0 \times 10^{-2}}$$

Since $[H^+] = [Ac^-]$

$X^2 = (1.75 \times 10^{-5}) \times (5.0 \times 10^{-2}) = 8.75 \times 10^{-7}$

$x = \sqrt{8.75 \times 10^{-7}} = [H^+] = 9.35 \times 10^{-4}\,M$

$pH = -Log\,9.35 \times 10^{-4}\,M = 3.0$

Alternatively, $pH = \frac{1}{2}(pK_a - Log\,HA)$

$pH = \frac{1}{2}(4.76 - Log\,5.0 \times 10^{-2})$

$= \frac{1}{2}(4.76 + 1.30)$

$= 3.0$

12. What is the pH of a buffer containing 40.0 mmol/L $NaHC_2O_4$ and 4.0 mmol/L $H_2C_2O_4$?

$pK_a = 1.25$

A. 1.35
B. 2.25
C. 5.75
D. 6.12

Laboratory operations/Calculations/2

13. A solvent needed for high-performance liquid chromatography (HPLC) requires a 20.0 mmol/L phosphoric acid buffer, pH 3.50, made by mixing potassium dihydrogen phosphate (KH_2PO_4) and phosphoric acid (H_3PO_4). How many grams of KH_2PO_4 are required to make 1.0 L of this buffer?

Formula weights: $KH_2PO_4 = 136.1$; $H_3PO_4 = 98.0$; pK_a $H_3PO_4 = 2.12$

A. 1.96 g
B. 2.61 g
C. 2.72 g
D. 19.2 g

Laboratory operations/Calculations/3

14. A procedure for cholesterol is calibrated with a serum-based cholesterol standard (200 mg/dL) determined by the Abell-Kendall method. Assuming equal volumes of sample and reagent are used, calculate the cholesterol concentration in the patient's sample from the following results:

Standard Concentration	Absorbance of Reagent Blank	Absorbance of Standard	Absorbance of Patient Serum
200 mg/dL	0.00	0.860	0.740

A. 123 mg/dL
B. 172 mg/dL
C. 232 mg/dL
D. 314 mg/dL

Laboratory operations/Calculations/3

Answers to Questions 12–14

12. B The Henderson-Hasselbalch equation can be used to determine the pH of a buffer containing a weak acid and salt of the acid.

$$pH = pK_a + \frac{\log salt}{acid}$$

$$= 1.25 + \log \frac{40.0 \text{ mmol/L}}{4.0 \text{ mmol/L}}$$

$$= 1.25 + \log 10$$

$$= 2.25$$

13. B The Henderson-Hasselbalch equation is used to calculate the ratio of salt to acid needed to give a pH of 3.50.

$$pH = pK_a + \log (salt/acid)$$

$$3.50 = 2.12 + \log (KH_2PO_4/H_3PO_4)$$

$$1.38 = \log (KH_2PO_4/H_3PO_4)$$

$$Antilog\ 1.38 = KH_2PO_4/H_3PO_4$$

$$23.99 = KH_2PO_4/H_3\,PO_4$$

Rearranging gives $KH_2PO_4 = 23.99 \times H_3PO_4$. Because the phosphate in the buffer is 20.0 mmol/L, then $H_3PO_4 + KH_2PO_4$ must equal 20. Because $KH_2PO_4 = 23.99 \times H_3PO_4$, then:

$$H_3PO_4 + (23.99 \times H_3PO_4) = 20.0 \text{ mmol/L}$$

$$24.99 \times H_3PO_4 = 20.0 \text{ mmol/L}$$

$$H_3PO_4 = 20.0/24.99 = 0.800 \text{ mmol/L}$$

$$KH_2PO_4 = 20.0 - 0.800 = 19.2 \text{ mmol/L } (0.0192\ M)$$

To determine the grams required, multiply the moles of KH_2PO_4 by the formula weight.

$$0.0192 \text{ mol/L} \times 136.1 \text{ g/mol} = 2.613 \text{ g}$$

14. B Applying the Beer-Lambert Law, $C_u = A_u/A_s \times C_s$, where C_u = concentration of unknown, A_u = absorbance of unknown, A_s = absorbance of standard, and C_s = concentration of standard.

$$C_u = 0.740/0.860 \times 200 \text{ mg/dL}$$

$$= 172 \text{ mg/dL}$$

15. **A glycerol kinase method for triglyceride calls for a serum blank in which lipase is absent from the reagent to measure endogenous glycerol. Given the following results, and assuming equal volumes of sample and reagent are used for each test, calculate the triglyceride concentration in the patient's sample.**

Standard Concentration	Absorbance of Reagent Blank	Absorbance of Standard	Absorbance of Patient Serum	Absorbance of Serum Blank
200 mg/dL	0.000	0.62	0.750	0.100

A. 119 mg/dL
B. 131 mg/dL
C. 156 mg/dL
D. 180 mg/dL

Laboratory operations/Calculations/3

16. **A procedure for aspartate aminotransferase (AST) is performed manually because of a repeating error code for nonlinearity obtained on the laboratory's automated chemistry analyzer; 0.05 mL of serum and 1.0 mL of substrate are used. The reaction rate is measured at 30°C at 340 nm using a 1.0 cM light path, and the delta absorbance (–ΔA) per minute is determined to be 0.382. Based on a molar absorptivity coefficient for nicotinamide adenine dinucleotide (NADH) at 340 nm of $6.22 \times 10^3\ M^{-1}\ cM^{-1}\ L^{-1}$, calculate the enzyme activity in international units (IUs) per liter.**
A. 26 IU/L
B. 326 IU/L
C. 1,228 IU/L
D. 1,290 IU/L

Laboratory operations/Calculations/3

Answers to Questions 15–16

15. **B** The serum blank absorbance is subtracted from the result for the patient's serum before applying the ratiometric formula to calculate concentration.

$C_u = [(A_u - A_{SB})/A_s] \times C_s$

where

A_{SB} = *absorbance of serum blank*

$= (0.750 - 0.100)/0.620 \times 125\ mg/dL$

$= 131\ mg/dL$

16. **D** The international unit (IU) is defined as 1 µmol (micromole) of substrate consumed or product produced per minute. The micromoles of NADH consumed in this reaction are determined by dividing the change in absorbance per minute by the absorbance of 1 µmol of NADH. Because 1 mol/L/cm would have an absorbance of 6.22×10^3 absorbance units, then 1 µmol/mL/cm would produce an absorbance of 6.22. Therefore, dividing the ΔA per minute by 6.22 gives the micromoles of NADH consumed in the reaction. This is multiplied by the dilution of serum to determine the micromoles per minute per milliliter and multiplied by 1,000 to convert to liters.

$$IU/L = \frac{\Delta A/min \times TV(mL) \times 1{,}000\ mL/L}{6.22(A/\mu mol/mL/cM) \times 1\ cm \times SV(mL)}$$

where TV is total volume and SV is sample volume

$$= \frac{\Delta A/min \times 1.05 \times 1{,}000}{6.22 \times 0.05}$$

$$= \Delta A/min \times \frac{1{,}050}{0.311}$$

$$= \Delta A/min \times 3{,}376$$

$$= 0.382 \times 3376 = 1{,}290\ IU/L$$

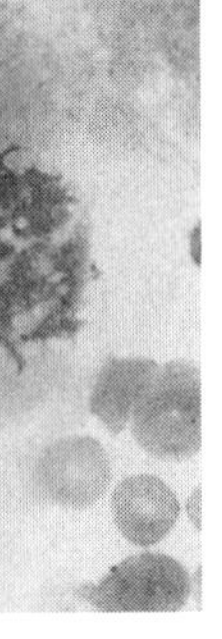

1.2 Quality Control

1. **When referring to conventional quality control (QC) results, what parameter *usually* determines the acceptable range?**
   A. The range that includes 75% of the results
   B. The 95% confidence interval for the mean
   C. The central 68% of results
   D. The range encompassed by ±2.5 standard deviations (s)

   Laboratory operations/Quality control/1

2. **Which of the following QC rules would be broken one out of 20 times by chance alone?**
   A. 1_{2s}
   B. 2_{2s}
   C. 1_{3s}
   D. 1_{4s}

   Laboratory operations/Quality control/1

3. **Using conventional QC rules, which of the following conditions requires the rejection of an analytical run?**
   A. Two consecutive controls greater than 2s above or below the mean
   B. Three consecutive controls greater than 1s above the mean
   C. Four controls steadily increasing in value but less than ±1s from the mean
   D. One control above +1s and the other below −1s from the mean

   Laboratory operations/Quality control/1

4. **One of two controls within a run is above +2s and the other control is below −2s from the mean. What do these results indicate?**
   A. Poor precision has led to random error (RE)
   B. A systematic error (SE) is present
   C. Proportional error is present
   D. QC material is contaminated

   Laboratory operations/Quality control/1

Answers to Questions 1–4

1. B The acceptable range for QC results is often set at the 95% confidence interval. This is defined as the range between −1.96s and +1.96s. This means that we can expect a QC result to fall within this range 95 out of 100 times. For practical purposes, this is the same as ±2s (95.4 out of 100 results should fall within ±2s of the mean based on chance). However, this limit will result in a high rate of false rejections (rejecting satisfactory results) when the assay has a low bias and coefficient of variation (CV) (in other words, performs significantly better than the allowable error limit for the test).

2. A The notation 1_{2s} means that one control is outside ±2 standard deviation units. QC results follow the bell-shaped curve called the *Gaussian (normal) distribution*. If a control is assayed 100 times, 68 out of 100 results would fall within +1s and −1s of the mean. Ninety-five (95.4) out of 100 results would fall within +2s and −2s. This leaves only 5 out of 100 results (1:20) that fall outside the ±2s limit. Also, 99.7 out of 100 results fall within ±3s of the mean.

3. A Rejecting a run when three consecutive controls fall between 1s and 2s or when a trend of four increasing or decreasing control results occurs would lead to frequent rejection of valid analytical runs. Appropriate control limits are four consecutive controls above or below 1s (4_{1s}) to detect a significant shift, and a cumulative sum control chart (CUSUM) result exceeding the ±2.7s limit to detect a significant shift or trend. When controls deviate in opposite directions, the difference should exceed 4s before the run is rejected.

4. A When control results deviate from the mean in the opposite direction, the run is affected by RE, which results from imprecision. An analytical run is rejected when two controls within the same run have an algebraic difference more than 4s (R_{4s}). The R_{4s} rule is applied to the controls within a run (level 1–level 2), never across runs or days.

5. Two consecutive controls are beyond –2s from the mean. How frequently would this occur based on chance alone?

A. 1:100
B. 5:100
C. 1:400
D. 1:1,600

Laboratory operations/Quality control/2

6. The term R_{4s} is used when:

A. Four consecutive controls are greater than ±1 standard deviation from the mean
B. Two controls in the same run are greater than 4s units apart
C. Two consecutive controls in the same run are each greater than ±4s from the mean
D. There is a shift above the mean for four consecutive controls

Laboratory operations/Quality control/1

7. A trend in QC results is most likely caused by:

A. Deterioration of the reagent
B. Miscalibration of the instrument
C. Improper dilution of standards
D. Electronic noise

Laboratory operations/Quality control/2

8. In most circumstances, when two controls within a run are both greater than ±2s from the mean, what action should be taken first?

A. Recalibrate, and then repeat controls followed by selected patient samples if QC is acceptable
B. Repeat the controls before taking any corrective action
C. Change the reagent lot, and then recalibrate
D. Prepare fresh standards, and recalibrate

Laboratory operations/Quality control/2

9. When establishing a QC acceptable range, which of the following practices is *inappropriate*?

A. Using last month's QC data to determine current target limits
B. Exclusion of any QC results greater than ±2s from the mean
C. Using control results from all shifts on which the assay is performed
D. Using limits determined by reference laboratories using the same method

Laboratory operations/Quality control/2

Answers to Questions 5–9

5. D QC results follow a Gaussian or normal distribution. Ninety-five percent of the results fall within ±2s of the mean; therefore, 2.5 out of 100 (1:40) are above +2s and 2.5 out of 100 are below –2s. The probability of two consecutive controls being beyond –2s is the product of their individual probabilities. 1/40 × 1/40 = 1/1,600 trials by chance.

6. B The R_{4s} rule is applied to two control levels within the same run. The rule is violated when the algebraic difference between them (level 1–level 2) exceeds 4s. The rule is never applied across different runs. The R_{4s} rule detects RE (error caused by lack of precision).

7. A A trend occurs when six or more consecutive QC results either increase or decrease in the same direction; however, this is not cause for rejection until a multirule is broken. Trends are SEs (affecting accuracy) linked to an unstable reagent, calibrator, or instrument condition. For example, loss of volatile acid from a reagent causes a steady pH increase, preventing separation of analyte from protein. This results in lower QC results each day.

8. A When the 2_{2S} rule is broken, this usually means that excessive SE is present and corrective action is required (repeating just the QC will not correct the problem). If recalibration yields acceptable QC results, both sets of QC results and the corrective action taken are documented in the QC log. If the magnitude of the error is large enough to be medically significant, then all patient samples since the last previously acceptable QC must be repeated. If in question, the magnitude of the error can be evaluated by repeating abnormal patient samples. If the average difference between results before and after recalibration is greater than 2s or error limit, then all samples should be repeated since the last acceptable QC.

9. B Data between ±2s and ±3s must be included in calculations of the next month's acceptable range. Elimination of these values would continuously reduce the distribution of QC results, making "out of control" situations a frequent occurrence. Generally, QC results greater than 3s are not used to calculate the next month's mean.

10. Which of the following assays has the poorest precision?

	Analyte	Mean (mmol/L)	Standard Deviation
A.	Calcium (Ca)	2.5	0.3
B.	Potassium (K)	4.0	0.4
C.	Sodium (Na)	140	4.0
D.	Chloride (Cl)	100	2.5

Laboratory operations/Quality control/2

11. Given the following data, calculate the coefficient of variation for glucose:

Analyte	Mean	Standard Deviation
Glucose	76 mg/dL	2.3

A. 3.0%
B. 4.6%
C. 7.6%
D. 33.0%

Laboratory operations/Quality control/2

12. Which of the following plots is *best* for detecting all types of QC errors?
A. Levey-Jennings
B. Tonks-Youden
C. CUSUM
D. Linear regression

Laboratory operations/Quality control/1

13. Which of the following plots is *best* for comparison of precision and accuracy among laboratories?
A. Levey-Jennings
B. Tonks-Youden
C. CUSUM
D. Linear regression

Laboratory operations/Quality control/1

14. Which plot will give the earliest indication of a shift or trend?
A. Levey-Jennings
B. Tonks-Youden
C. CUSUM
D. Histogram

Laboratory operations/Quality control/1

Answers to Questions 10–14

10. A Although calcium has the lowest s, it represents the assay with poorest precision. Relative precision between different analytes or different levels of the same analyte must be evaluated by the CV because standard deviation is dependent on sample concentrations. CV = (s × 100)/Mean. This normalizes standard deviation to a mean of 100. The CV for calcium in the example is 12.0%.

11. A The CV is calculated by dividing the standard deviation by the mean and multiplying by 100.

$$\% CV = \frac{s}{X} \times 100$$

$$= \frac{2.3}{76} \times 100 = 3.0\%$$

CV is the most appropriate statistic to use when comparing the precision of samples that have different means. For example, when comparing the precision of the level 1 control to the level 2 control, the CV normalizes the variance to be independent of the mean. The analysis is more precise for the control with the lower CV.

12. A The Levey-Jennings plot is a graph of all QC results with concentration plotted on the *y*-axis and run number on the *x*-axis. The mean is at the center of the *y*-axis, and concentrations corresponding to −2s and +2s (or other specified control limits) are highlighted. Results are evaluated for multiple rule violations across both levels and runs. Corrective action for shifts and trends can be addressed before QC rules are broken.

13. B The Tonks-Youden plot is used for interlaboratory comparison of monthly means. The method mean for level 1 is at the center of the *y*-axis and the mean for level 2 is at the center of the *x*-axis. Lines are drawn from the means of both levels across the graph, dividing it into four equal quadrants. If a laboratory's monthly means both plot in the lower left or upper right quadrants, then SE exists in its method.

14. C CUSUM points are the algebraic sum of the difference between each QC result and the mean. The *y*-axis is the sum of differences, and the *x*-axis is the run number. The center of the *y*-axis is 0. Because QC results follow a random distribution, the points should distribute about the zero line. Results are out of control when the slope exceeds 45 degrees or a decision limit (e.g., ±2.7s) is exceeded.

15. All the following are requirements for QC material *except*:

A. Long-term stability
B. The matrix is similar to the specimens being tested
C. The concentration of analytes reflects the clinical range
D. Analyte concentration must be independent of the method of assay

Laboratory operations/Quality control/1

Answer to Question 15

15. D Ideal quality control materials are stable, made of the same components as the specimen, cover the dynamic linear range of the assay, and can be used for multiple analytes. The target mean for QC samples is determined from replicate assays by the user's method, not the "true" concentration of the analyte. Out-of-control results are linked to analytic performance rather than to the inherent accuracy of the method.

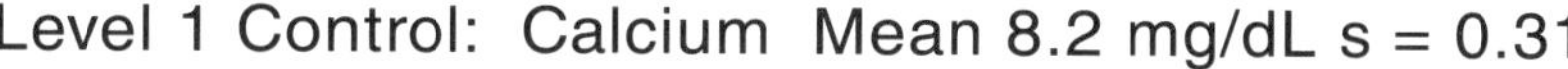

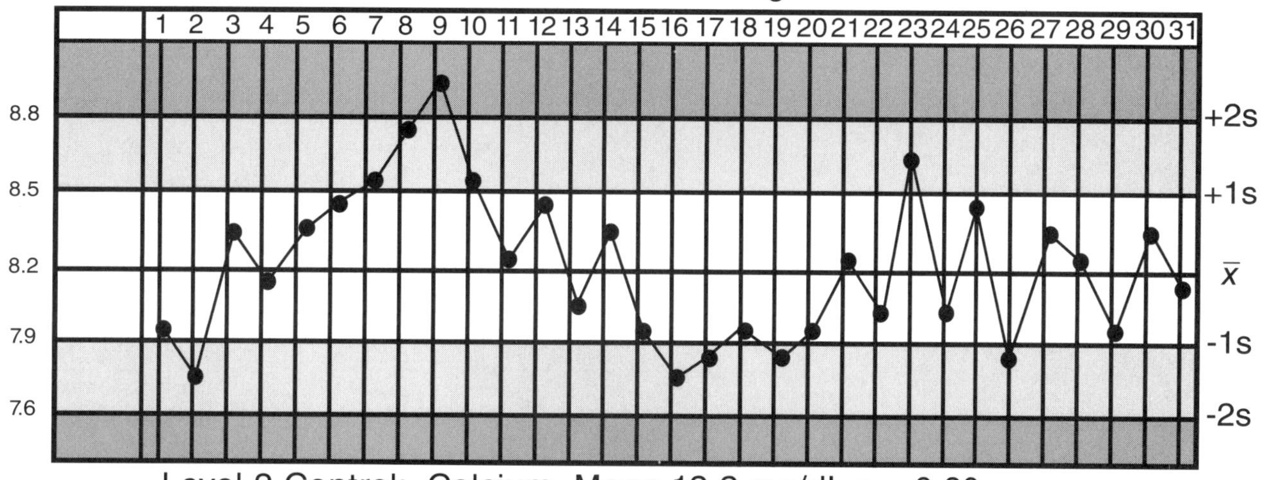

Level 2 Control: Calcium Mean 12.2 mg/dL s = 0.30

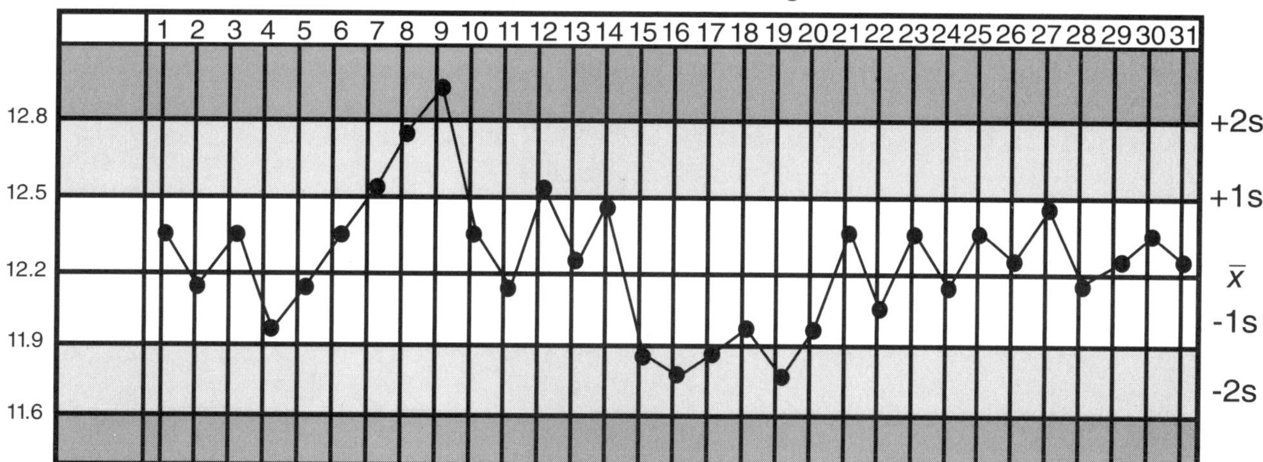

Questions 16–19 refer to the preceding Levey-Jennings chart.

16. Referring to the Levey-Jennings chart provided, identify the QC pattern that occurred during the first half of the month.
A. Shift
B. Trend
C. Random error
D. Kurtosis

Laboratory operations/Quality control/2

17. Referring to the Levey-Jennings chart provided, what is the first day in the month when the run should be rejected and patient results should be repeated using conventional QC limits and multirules?
A. Day 6
B. Day 7
C. Day 8
D. Day 9

Laboratory operations/Quality control/3

18. Referring to the Levey-Jennings chart provided, what analytical error is present beginning on day 15?
A. Shift
B. Trend
C. Random error
D. Kurtosis

Laboratory operations/Quality control/2

19. Referring to the Levey-Jennings chart provided, which of the following days would patient results be rejected using conventional QC limits and multirules?
A. Day 16
B. Day 17
C. Day 18
D. Day 19

Laboratory operations/Quality control/2

Answers to Questions 16–19 refer to the provided Levey-Jennings chart.

16. B A trend is characterized by six consecutive decreasing or increasing control results. The value for both controls becomes progressively higher from day 4 to day 9. Trends are caused by changes to the test system that increase over time, such as deterioration of reagents or calibrators, or progressive changes in temperature, evaporation, light exposure, and bacterial contamination. A trend is a type of SE because all results are affected. Conversely, RE affects some results (but not others) in an unpredictable manner. Control rules affected by RE are 1_{3s} and R_{4s}.

17. C Although the trend is apparent across QC levels by day 7, the patient results would not be rejected until day 8 when the 4_{1s} rule is broken. An advantage to plotting control data is that trends can be identified before results are out of control and patient data must be rejected. In this case, corrective steps should have been implemented by day 7 to avoid the delay and expense associated with having to repeat the analysis of patient samples. Because no action was taken on day 7 or 8, the 2_{2s} rule was broken on day 9.

18. A A shift is characterized by six consecutive points lying on the same side of the mean. This occurs from day 15 to day 20. Shifts are caused by a change in the assay conditions that affect the accuracy of all results, such as a change in the concentration of the calibrator; change in reagent; a new lot of reagent that differs in composition; or improper temperature setting, wavelength, or sample volume. The term *kurtosis* refers to the degree of flatness or sharpness in the peak of a set of values having a Gaussian distribution.

19. B The 4_{1s} rule is broken across both QC levels on day 17. This means that four consecutive controls are greater than ±1s from the mean. QC rules that are sensitive to SE are applied across both runs and levels to increase the probability of error detection. These are 2_{2s}, 4_{1s}, and $10\bar{x}$.

20. Given the following QC chart, identify the day in which a violation of the R_{4s} QC rule occurs:

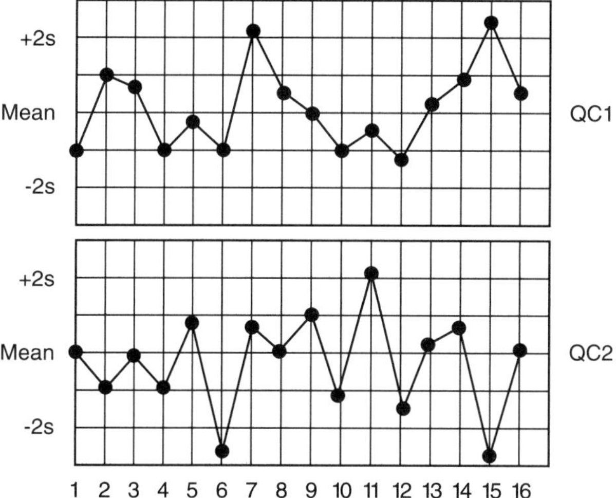

A. Day 3
B. Day 8
C. Day 10
D. Day 15

Laboratory operations/Quality control/2

21. What is the minimum requirement for performing QC for a nonwaived total protein assay?

A. One level assayed every 8 hours
B. Two levels assayed within 8 hours
C. Two levels assayed within 24 hours
D. Three levels assayed within 24 hours

Laboratory operations/Quality control/1

22. In which circumstances is a validation study (versus performing routine QC) required?

A. Instrument recalibration
B. Source lamp or ion selective electrode change
C. Change in reagent lot
D. Change in calibrator lot

Laboratory operations/Quality control/2

23. Which of the following statements *best* describes the QC requirements for clinical laboratories?

A. QC must be performed for all laboratory tests
B. QC for nonwaived tests must include at least one level of control every 24 hours
C. Equivalent quality control (eQC) is permitted for single-device and point-of-care tests
D. An individualized quality control plan (IQCP) can be used if approved by the lab's accrediting agency

Laboratory operations/Quality control/1

Answers to Questions 20–23

20. D An R_{4s} error is defined as the algebraic difference between two controls within the same run. In this Levey-Jennings plot, on day 15, level 1 is above the +2s limit (approximately +2.5s) and level 2 is below the −2s limit (approximately −2.5s). These controls are approximately 5s apart (+2.5s minus −2.5s = +5s).

21. C The minimum requirement by federal regulations (subpart K of the Clinical Laboratory Improvement Act, 1988 [CLIA 1988]) for frequency of QC for a nonwaived general chemistry analyte is two levels of control assayed every 24 hours, provided the manufacturer's QC requirements are no greater. Some laboratories prefer to assay two control levels every 8 hours to increase the opportunity for error detection. Two controls every 8 hours are required for blood gases, automated hematology, and point-of-care glucose testing to comply with College of American Pathology requirements. Three levels of control every 24 hours should be used for analytes that have significantly different CVs at low, normal, and high concentrations. These include blood gases, therapeutic drugs, and hormones.

22. C All of the listed conditions except a change in the reagent lot number can be validated by assaying two levels of control material after the procedure. A change in reagent lot number may alter the test system more dramatically, especially when the reagent was subjected to storage and shipping conditions that alter its performance. Therefore, both controls and patient samples should be analyzed and the results compared with the reagent in current use by utilizing criteria determined by the total allowable error for the analyte.

23. D QC is not required for diagnostic tests that are classified as waived tests under CLIA 1988 unless specified by the manufacturer or deemed accrediting agency. Subpart K specifies use of at least two levels of controls per 24 hours for all nonwaived tests (except for coagulation testing, which requires two levels every 8 hours, and blood gases, which requires three levels within 24 hours). eQC cannot be used to satisfy the requirements in subpart K as of January 1, 2016. An IQCP, if approved, permits laboratories to perform conventional QC with less frequency than required in subpart K.

24. What two parameters must be addressed in the risk assessment of an IQCP?

A. Risk of testing error and severity of harm when test failure occurs

B. Sigma level of the test and coefficient of variation index (CVI)

C. Bias and uncertainty of the test result

D. Analytical sensitivity and specificity

Laboratory operations/Quality control/1

25. Which *best* describes the appropriate way to use QC decision limits for a diagnostic laboratory test?

A. Always use the 2_{2s} rule with or without others to determine rejection

B. If QC is performed twice per day, use a combination of 2_{2s}, 1_{3s}, and 4_{1s}

C. If QC is performed more than twice per day, use only the 2_{2s} rule

D. Choose rules and number of controls based on the sigma performance of the test

Laboratory operations/Quality control/2

Answers to Questions 24–25

24. A IQCPs must determine the risk of testing error to include preanalytical, analytical, and postanalytical errors and risk of harm resulting from such errors. These are applied to a matrix that is used to determine whether the QC plan is at least equivalent to the CLIA standard. Generally, the laboratory must demonstrate that the frequency of device failure is unlikely and the severity of harm is mild when testing failure occurs.

25. D Tests that have extremely high reproducibility and low SE (bias) do not require as stringent QC limits as those that do not. Using the 4_{1s} and R_{4s} rules in such cases will result in rejecting tests that could have been reported because they fall within the CLIA range for allowable analytical error. In general, tests that perform above 5 sigma should not be rejected unless the 1_{3s} rule has been violated. In other words, results less than 3s from the mean are still within acceptable limits of error. For tests performing above 5 sigma, two controls measured every 1,000 samples and at least once per day are adequate for detection of clinically significant errors, but tests performing at 5 sigma or less require more frequent controls. For tests performing at 5 sigma, it is advisable to include the 2_{2s} and R_{4s} rules using two controls per run and at least once per day, and for tests performing at 4 sigma or below the 4_{1s} rule should be added using two controls per run and two runs per day. For tests performing below 4 sigma, use all of the conventional Westgard rules using four controls per run and two runs per day.

1.3

Laboratory Statistics

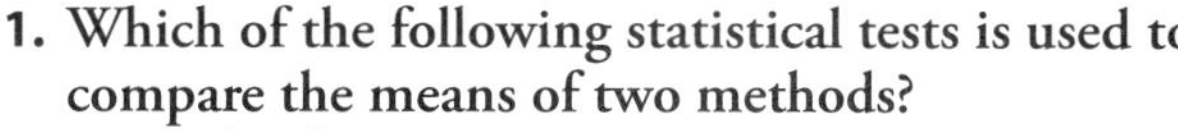

1. Which of the following statistical tests is used to compare the means of two methods?

A. Student's t test
B. F distribution
C. Correlation coefficient (r)
D. Linear regression analysis

Laboratory operations/Statistics/1

2. Two freezing point osmometers are compared by running 40 paired patient samples one time on each instrument, and the following results are obtained:

Instrument	Mean	Standard Deviation
Osmometer A	280 milliosmoles per kilogram(mOsm/kg)	3.1
Osmometer B	294 mOsm/kg	2.8

If the critical value for F = 2.8, then what conclusion can be drawn regarding the precision of the two instruments?

A. There is no statistically significant difference in precision
B. Osmometer A demonstrates better precision that is statistically significant
C. Osmometer B demonstrates better precision that is statistically significant
D. Precision cannot be evaluated statistically when single measurements are made on samples

Laboratory operations/Statistics/3

Answers to Questions 1–2

1. A Student's t test is the ratio of mean difference to the standard error of the mean difference (bias/RE) and tests for a significant difference in means. The F test is the ratio of variances and determines if one method is significantly less precise. The correlation coefficient is a measure of the association between two variables and should be high in any method comparison. An r value less than 0.90 in method comparisons usually occurs when the range of results is too narrow.

2. A The F test determines whether there is a statistically significant difference in the variance of the two sampling distributions. Assuming the samples are collected and stored in the same way and the analysis is done by a person who is familiar with the instruments, then differences in variance can be attributed to a difference in instrument precision. The F test is calculated by dividing the variance $(s_1)^2$ of the instrument having the higher standard deviation by the variance $(s_2)^2$ of the instrument having the smaller standard deviation.

$F = (s_1)^2 \div (s_2)^2 = (3.1)^2 \div (2.8)^2 = 9.61 \div 7.84 = 1.22$

If the value of F is smaller than the critical value at the 0.10 level of significance, then the hypothesis (there is no significant difference in the variance of the two instruments) is accepted. The 0.10 significance level is used for one-tailed statistical tests.

3. Two methods for total cholesterol are compared by running 40 paired patient samples in duplicate on each instrument. The following results are obtained:

Instrument	Mean	Standard Deviation
Method A (reference method)	235 mg/dL	3.8
Method B (candidate method)	246 mg/dL	3.4

Assuming the samples are collected and stored in the same way and the analysis is performed by a medical laboratory scientist (MLS) who is familiar with both methods, what is the bias in method B?

A. 0.4
B. 7.2
C. 10.6
D. 11.0

Laboratory operations/Statistics/2

4. When the magnitude of error increases with increasing sample concentration, it is called:

A. Constant error
B. Proportional error
C. Random error
D. Bias

Laboratory operations/Statistics/2

Answers to Questions 3–4

3. D Bias is defined as the difference between the means of the two methods and is calculated by using the formula: bias = $\bar{y} - \bar{x}$. The bias is an estimate of SE. The student's *t* test is used to determine if bias is statistically significant. The *t* statistic is the ratio of bias to the standard error of the mean difference. The greater the bias, the higher the *t* score.

4. B Proportional error (slope or percent error) results in greater absolute error (deviation from the target value) at higher sample concentration. Constant error refers to a difference between the target value and the result, which is independent of sample concentration. For example, if both level 1 and level 2 controls for laboratory A average 5 mg/dL below the cumulative mean reported by all other laboratories using the same method, then laboratory A has a constant error of −5 mg/dL for that method. Both proportional and constant error contribute to method bias.

5. Which explanation is the *best* interpretation of the following blood urea nitrogen (BUN) bias plot?

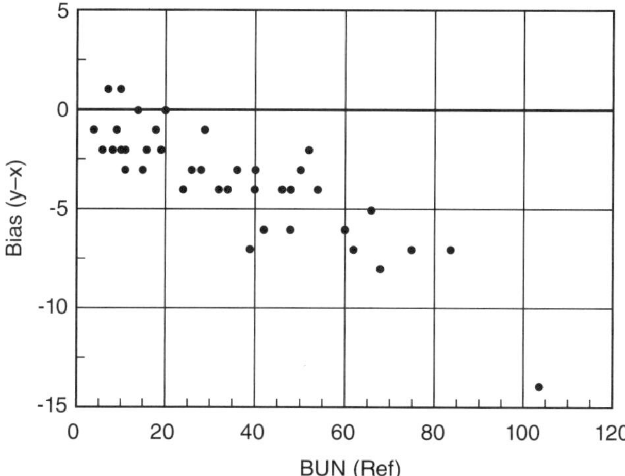

A. The new method consistently overestimates BUN by a constant concentration
B. The new method is greater than the reference method but not by a statistically significant margin
C. The new method is lower than the reference method by 5 mg/dL
D. The new method is lower than the reference and the magnitude is concentration dependent

Laboratory operations/Statistics/3

6. Serum samples collected from hospitalized patients over a 2-week period were split into two aliquots and analyzed for prostate-specific antigen (PSA) by using two methods. Each sample was assayed within 30 minutes of collection by a medical laboratory scientist familiar with both methods. The reference method was method *x* (upper reference limit = 4.0 μg/L). Linear regression analysis was performed by the least-squares method, and results are as follows:

Linear Regression	Correlation Coefficient (*r*)	Standard Error of Estimate ($s_{y/x}$)
$\hat{y} = 2.10 + 1.01x$	0.984	0.23

Which statement *best* characterizes the relationship between the methods?

A. There is a significant bias caused by constant error
B. There is a significant proportional error
C. There is no disagreement between the methods because the correlation coefficient approaches 1.0
D. There is no SE, but the RE of the new method is unacceptable

Laboratory operations/Statistics/3

Answers to Questions 5–6

5. D A bias (Bland-Altman) plot compares bias (candidate method–reference method) to the result of the reference method. Ideally, points should be scattered equally on both sides of the zero line. When the majority of points are below the zero line, the candidate method is negatively biased (lower than the reference). In this case, the difference between the methods increases in proportion to the BUN concentration. This type of scatter occurs when the slope of the linear regression line is low.

6. A The linear regression analysis is the most useful statistic to compare paired patient results because it estimates the magnitude of specific errors. The *y*-intercept of the regression line is a measure of constant error, and the slope is a measure of proportional error. Together, these represent the bias or SE of the new method. The range of the sample and RE. influence the correlation coefficient. Two methods that measure the same analyte will have a high correlation coefficient, provided the concentrations are measured over a wide range, and this statistic should not be used to judge the acceptability of the new method. The standard error of estimate is a measure of the closeness of data points to the regression line and is an expression of RE.

7. Which statement *best* summarizes the relationship between the new BUN method and reference method based on the following linear regression scatterplot?

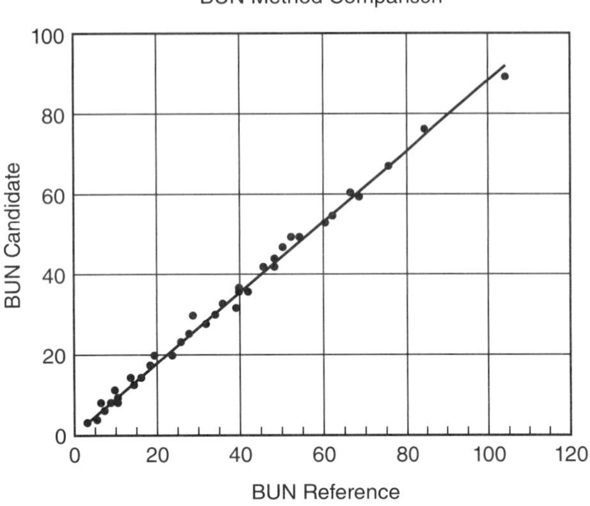

A. The methods agree very well but show a high standard error of estimate
B. There is little or no constant error, but some proportional error
C. There will be a significant degree of uncertainty in the regression equation
D. There is significant constant and proportional error but little RE

Laboratory operations/Statistics/3

8. A new method for BUN is evaluated by comparing the results of 40 paired patient samples to the urease–UV method. Normal and high controls were run on each shift for 5 days, five times per day. The results are as follows:

Linear Regression	Low Control	High Control
$\hat{y} = -0.3 + 0.90x$	$\bar{x} = 14.2$ mg/dL	$\bar{x} = 48.6$ mg/dL
	s = 1.24	s = 1.12

What is the total analytical error (TE) estimate for a sample having a concentration of 50 mg/dL?
A. –2.2 mg/dL
B. –2.8 mg/dL
C. –7.5 mg/dL
D. –10.0 mg/dL

Laboratory operations/Statistics/3

Answers to Questions 7–8

7. B The scatterplot shows that each sample produces a coordinate (*x* corresponds to the reference result and *y* to the candidate method result) that is remarkably close to the regression line. This means that the variance of regression is low and there is a high degree of certainty that the predicted value of *y* will be close to its measured value. Near zero concentration there is good agreement between methods; however, the higher the result, the greater is the difference between *x* and *y*. The regression equation for this scatterplot is $\hat{y} = -0.01 + 0.90x$, indicating a proportional error of –10%.

8. C Linear regression analysis gives an estimate of SE, which is equal to $(\hat{y} - xc)$, where *xc* is the expected concentration, and $\hat{y}$ is the value predicted by the linear regression equation.

$SE = [-0.3 + (0.9 \times 50\ mg/dL)] - 50.0\ mg/dL = 44.7 - 50.0 = -5.3\ mg/dL$

The standard deviation of the new method for the high control is used to estimate the RE because the mean of this control is nearer to the expected concentration of 50 mg/dL. RE is estimated by $\pm 1.96 \times s$.

$RE = 1.96 \times 1.12 = \pm 2.2\ mg/dL$

TE is equal to the sum of SE and RE.

$TE = SE + RE = -5.3\ mg/dL + (-2.2\ mg/dL) = -7.5\ mg/dL$

9. In addition to the number of true negatives (TNs), which of the following measurements is needed to calculate specificity?
A. True positives (TPs)
B. Prevalence
C. False negatives (FNs)
D. False positives (FPs)
Laboratory operations/Statistics/1

10. A new tumor marker for ovarian cancer is evaluated for sensitivity by testing serum samples from patients who have been diagnosed by staging biopsy specimens as having malignant or benign lesions. The following results were obtained:

Number of malignant patients who are positive for CA-125 = 21 out of 24
Number of benign patients who are negative for CA-125 = 61 out of 62

What is the sensitivity of the new CA-125 test?
A. 98.4%
B. 95.3%
C. 87.5%
D. 85.0%
Laboratory operations/Statistics/2

11. A new test for prostate cancer is found to have a sensitivity of 80.0% and a specificity of 84.0%. If the prevalence of prostate cancer is 4.0% in individuals older than 42 years, what is the predictive value of a positive test result (PVP) in this group?
A. 96.0%
B. 86.0%
C. 32.4%
D. 17.2%
Laboratory operations/Statistics/2

12. What measurement in addition to TNs and prevalence is required to calculate the predictive value of a negative test result (PVN)?
A. FNs
B. Variance
C. TPs
D. FPs
Laboratory operations/Statistics/2

Answers to Questions 9–12

9. D The clinical specificity of a laboratory test is defined as TNs divided by the sum of TNs and FPs.

$$\%\ Specificity = \frac{TN \times 100}{TN + FP}$$

Specificity is defined as the percentage of disease-free people who have a negative test result. The probability of FPs is calculated from the specificity as:

$$1 - \left(\frac{\%\ specificity}{100}\right)$$

10. C Sensitivity is defined as the percentage of persons with the disease who have a positive test result. It is calculated as TPs (the number of people with the disease who test positive) divided by the sum of TPs and FNs.

$$\%\ Sensitivity = \frac{TP \times 100}{TP + FN}$$

$$Sensitivity = (21 \times 100), (21 + 3) = 87.5\%$$

11. D The PVP is defined as the percentage of individuals with a positive test result who will have the disease or condition. It is dependent on the sensitivity of the test and the prevalence of the disease in the population tested. PVP is calculated by multiplying the TPs by 100 and then dividing by the sum of TPs and FPs.

$$\%\ PVP = \frac{TP \times 100}{(TP + FP)} \%\ PVP$$

where TP equals (sensitivity × prevalence) and FP equals (1 – specificity) × (1 – prevalence)

$$= \frac{0.80 \times 0.04 \times 100}{(0.80 \times 0.04) + [(1 - 0.84) \times (1 - 0.04)]}$$

$$= \frac{0.032 \times 100}{0.032 + (0.96 \times 0.16)}$$

$$= 17.2\%$$

12. A PVN is defined as the probability that a person with a negative test result is free of disease. A high PVN is a characteristic of a good screening test. The predictive value of a negative test is calculated by multiplying the TNs by 100 and then dividing by the sum of the TNs and FNs.

$$\%\ PVN = \frac{TN \times 100}{TN + FN}$$

13. A laboratory is establishing a reference range for a new analyte and wants the range to be determined by the regional population of adults aged 18 years or older. The analyte concentration is known to be independent of race and gender. Which is the most appropriate process to follow?

A. Determine the mean and standard deviation of the analyte from 40 healthy adults, and calculate the ±2s limit

B. Measure the analyte in 120 healthy adults, and calculate the central 95th percentile

C. Measure the analyte in 120 healthy adults, and use the lowest and highest values as the reference range limits

D. Measure the analyte in 60 healthy adults and 60 adults with conditions that affect the analyte concentration, and calculate the concentration of least overlap

Laboratory operations/Statistics/2

14. When comparing the laboratory's monthly mean to a peer group to determine if bias is present, what statistic is most appropriate?

A. F test

B. Linear regression analysis

C. Correlation coefficient

D. Standard deviation index (SDI)

Laboratory operations/Statistics/2

15. Which of the following methods is most useful to detect sample misidentification?

A. Cumulative summation

B. Critical limit

C. Delta limit

D. Significant change limit

Laboratory operations/Statistics/1

16. Which of the following total quality management (TQM) tools can be used to calculate the analytical error rate for an analyte in the clinical laboratory?

A. Lean production

B. Six sigma

C. International Standards Organization (ISO) 9000

D. Laboratory information system

Laboratory operations/Statistics/1

Answers to Questions 13–16

13. B Because the concentration of an analyte may not be normally distributed in a population, the reference range should not be determined from the standard deviation. It is more appropriate to determine the central 95th percentile (the range that encompasses 95% of the results). A minimum of 120 samples is required for statistical significance. Results are rank ordered from lowest to highest. The third result is the lowest value and the 118th is the highest value in the reference range. The laboratory can verify a pre-existing reference range (e.g., as determined by the manufacturer's study) by testing at least 20 healthy individuals. If no more than 10% fall outside the range, it can be considered valid for the patient population.

14. D The SDI equals the laboratory's mean minus the peer group's mean divided by the peer group's standard deviation. This normalizes the value and allows for performance comparisons for any analyte. It has a similar probability distribution to a *t* test and a value greater than 2.0 is considered significant.

15. C Cumulative summation is a statistical method used in quality assurance to detect a trend in QC results. Critical limits are used to define when medical intervention is likely needed to prevent injury or death. The significant change limit is the difference in test results that is medically significant, or that cannot be attributed to the sum of normal physiological and analytical variation. The delta limit (delta check) determines whether the difference between two measurements usually 24 to 48 hours apart exceeds the expected. Although this can result from an abrupt change in the patient's status, other causes are sample misidentification, contamination, and RE. Delta limits are expressed in percent and vary depending on analyte stability.

16. B All four of the answer choices are TQM tools used in the clinical laboratory to improve performance. Six sigma is a measurement of the frequency of product defects. In clinical laboratories, it refers to the frequency of an erroneous result. At the six-sigma level, the analytical process has such small variance that an error of six times the standard deviation would still be within acceptable limits for total allowable error. For example, a six-sigma process for an analyte produces a significant error in test result only 3.4 out of 1 million times the test is performed. Conversely, a method performing at the three-sigma level would give 66,807 errors per million.

17. The following plot represents a study of a screening test for malignant prostate cancer using plasma PSA (nanograms per milliliter [ng/mL]). The outcome measured was positive cytology results obtained through biopsy analysis. What concentration gives the highest sensitivity with the least number of unnecessary biopsy procedures?

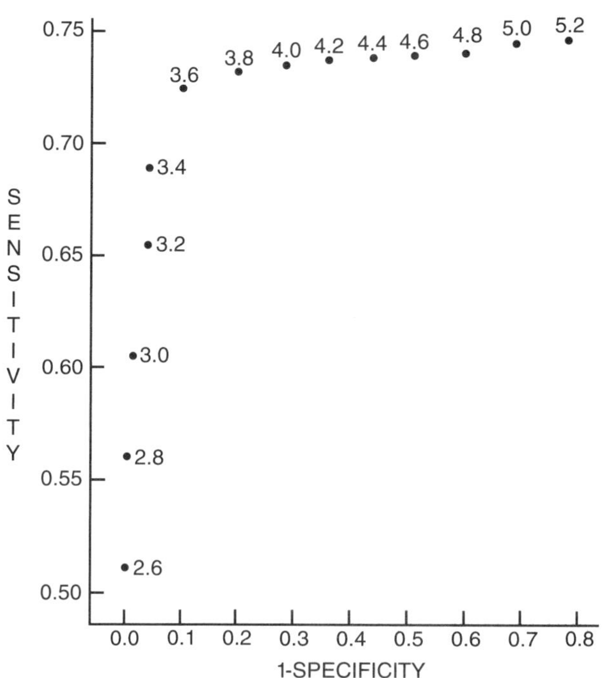

A. 2.6
B. 3.6
C. 3.8
D. 5.2

Laboratory operations/Statistics/3

18. A laboratory test for calcium has a bias of 0.5 mg/dL when compared with a peer group for proficiency testing. The CLIA total error allowable (TEa) for serum or plasma calcium is ±1.0 mg/dL. The laboratory's standard deviation for this test is 0.25 mg/dL. What is the laboratory's sigma?

A. 50
B. 2
C. 1
D. 0.25

Laboratory operations/Statistics/2

Answers to Questions 17–18

17. B A receiver operating characteristic (ROC) curve is used to identify the test result, giving the highest sensitivity with the least number of FPs. Sensitivity (TPs) is plotted against FPs. The number in the uppermost left corner represents the highest detection with the lowest number of FPs. In this case, a result of 3.6 ng/mL detects 72% of malignancies with one in 10 (10%) FPs.

18. B Sigma is calculated by subtracting bias from TEa (as defined by CLIA 1988) and dividing the difference (which signifies the RE that can be tolerated) by the laboratory's standard deviation. The result determines the probability (odds) of reporting a laboratory result that is beyond the CLIA error limit. A laboratory test functioning at two sigma is expected to produce 308,537 errors per million tests (called defects per million opportunities [DPMO]). In this example, almost one in three laboratory results would be above or below 1.0 mg/dL of the expected value. Conversely, a test performing at four sigma would produce 6,210 erroneous results per million, and one functioning at six sigma would have just 3.4 outside the CLIA limit for acceptable performance.

19. A new immunoassay for serum total cortisol is compared with a reference method, and the resultant data give a linear regression of $\hat{y}$ = 3.0 + 0.80x. The new method's standard deviation is 1.5 µg/dL. The CLIA TEa is ±25% at any concentration. Given a decision level of 20 µg/dL, what is the total error estimate, and would the new method be acceptable?

A. TEa = –1 µg/dL; acceptable
B. TEa = –3 µg/dL; acceptable
C. TEa = –4 µg/dL; acceptable
D. TEa = –5 µg/dL; unacceptable

Laboratory operations/Statistics/3

Answer to Question 19

19. C The regression equation is used to estimate the SE between the methods.

$\hat{y} = 3.0 + 0.8\,(20) = 19.0\ \mu g/dL$

$Bias = 19 - 20 = -1\ \mu g/dL$

On average, the new method measures 1 µg/dL lower than the reference method at a concentration of 20 µg/dL, but there is considerable uncertainty as to what the actual difference would be. Because the standard deviation of the new method is 1.5, the 95% confidence interval for this result by the new method is 19.0 ± 2(1.5) = 16.0 – 22.0 µg/dL. The total error estimate is bias + (–2s) or –1 + (–3) = –4 µg/dL. The CLIA TEa is ± 25% at any concentration. At 20 µg/dL, the TEa is 5 µg/dL. Therefore, the new method has an acceptable margin of error at this concentration based on the CLIA TEa limit for cortisol.

BIBLIOGRAPHY

1. Bishop ML, Fody EP, Van Siclen C, Mistler JM, Moy M. *Clinical Chemistry: Principles, Techniques, and Correlations.* 9th ed. Jones & Bartlet Learning; 2023.
2. Burtis CA, Bruns DE. *Tietz Fundamentals of Clinical Chemistry and Molecular Diagnostics.* 7th ed. Saunders; 2015.
3. Estridge BH, Reynolds AP. *Basic Clinical Laboratory Techniques.* 6th ed. Cengage Learning; 2012.
4. McPherson RA, Pinccus MR. *Henry's Clinical Diagnosis and Management by Laboratory Methods.* 23rd ed. Elsevier; 2017.
5. Westgard JO. *Basic QC Practices.* 4th ed. Westgard QC; 2016.

CHAPTER 2

Education and Management

2.1 *Education Theory and Practice*

2.2 *Management Theory and Practice*

2.3 *Laws and Regulations*

2.4 *Laboratory Economics*

2.5 *Laboratory Safety*

2.1
Education Theory and Practice

1. **A comparison of methods for the determination of alkaline phosphatase is categorized in which domain of educational objectives?**
   A. Affective
   B. Psychomotor
   C. Cognitive
   D. Behavioral

   Education and management/Education theory and practice/1

2. **Attitude, judgment, and interest refer to which domain of educational objectives?**
   A. Cognitive
   B. Affective
   C. Psychomotor
   D. Competency

   Education and management/Education theory and practice/1

3. **Criterion-referenced examinations are used to determine the:**
   A. Competency of a student according to a predetermined standard
   B. Validity of a test
   C. Status of one student compared to the whole group
   D. Accuracy of a test

   Education and management/Education theory and practice/1

4. **An instructor "curved" the final grades for a medical laboratory science blood bank examination. The highest grade was 85%, and the lowest grade was 60%. What type of exam evaluation is this?**
   A. Subjective
   B. Objective
   C. Norm referenced
   D. Criterion referenced

   Education and management/Education theory and practice/2

5. **A stated competency requirement for a medical laboratory science student is to perform calibration, plot data, and evaluate the acceptability of controls. This competency requirement encompasses which educational domains?**
   A. Cognitive, psychomotor, and affective
   B. Psychomotor and affective
   C. Affective and cognitive
   D. Cognitive and psychomotor

   Education and management/Education theory and practice/2

Answers to Questions 1–5

1. C The cognitive domain of educational objectives deals with application, analysis, synthesis, and evaluation of information or knowledge learned to be utilized in problem-solving.

2. B The affective domain of educational objectives includes those that emphasize values, attitudes, and interests that attach a value to an activity, situation, or phenomenon.

3. A A criterion-referenced test is used to determine the mastery of predetermined competencies, whereas a norm-referenced test evaluates students in comparison with the group. Criterion-referenced examinations use questions of known difficulty and can be calibrated against established criteria to evaluate the examinee's performance.

4. C This type of exam evaluation compares students with each other, rather than grading students on a set of standards or criteria that must be met.

5. D The student will perform the actual calibration (psychomotor skills), utilize the cognitive domain of analysis to plot the standards, construct a best-fit calibration line, determine the concentration of the controls, and evaluate the results as acceptable or repeat the calibration if an error is apparent.

6. A chemistry test result from a patient undergoing chemotherapy was within normal limits on Tuesday. The same test was reported to have an abnormal result on Monday ("flagged" high and approaching a critical value). The medical laboratory scientist (MLS) performing the test noted a delta-check error and remembered that both controls ran much higher on Monday, although they were within acceptable limits. The laboratory professional investigated the discrepancy before reporting the results. This is an example of which educational domain?

A. Cognitive
B. Affective
C. Psychomotor
D. Organizational

Education and management/Education theory and practice/2

7. In general, academic evaluation of students depends on the ability of the instructor to create a test that reflects the stated objectives of the course material as well as making the test:

A. Reliable and valid
B. Normally distributed and practical
C. Fair and short
D. Written and oral

Education and management/Education theory and practice/1

8. When dealing with the instruction of complex instrumentation, a demonstration by the instructor is necessary and should include the following:

A. Detailed diagrams of the electrical system
B. A blueprint of the optical system
C. A step-by-step narrative with comparisons to a manual method
D. A quiz as soon as the demonstration is complete

Education and management/Education theory and practice/2

9. An educational tool provided to students that includes a detailed real-world scenario in order to extrapolate data and solve complex issues is called:

A. Case study
B. Manual demonstration
C. Implementing new equipment
D. Histogram evaluation

Education and management/Education theory and practice/2

Answers to Questions 6–9

6. A The laboratory professional chose to investigate the situation to resolve a discrepancy. Comparing and evaluating the information refer to the cognitive domain. In doing so, a rule-based process, which includes evaluation of the specimen, instrument performance, potential sources of interference (e.g., the effects of drugs), and physiological variation, is followed before determining whether to report the result, repeat the test, or call for a new specimen.

7. A A test should be based on stated, measurable objectives and contain five attributes: reliability, validity, objectivity, fairness, and practicality.

8. C When demonstrating a complex instrument, the group of students assembled around the instrument should be kept small to permit clear visibility. A diagram with the major functioning parts should be provided, along with an assignment of a written summary or questions about the function, principle, testing performed, and reagents needed.

9. A The case study approach allows a student to engage in problem-solving and to utilize critical thinking skills based on a real, or potentially real, scenario. This allows for interaction and use of higher cognitive levels to determine the cause of the patient's illness and evaluate various laboratory test results.

10. An instructor in medical laboratory science is assigned to evaluate and expand the curriculum for entry level students. Which of the following subjects is most appropriate in the curriculum?

A. Cytology—cytogenetics
B. Histology—special stains
C. Computer (laboratory information systems [LIS])
D. Economics—budget analysis

Education and management/Education theory and practice/1

11. Your immediate supervisor requests that you back date and complete the quality control (QC) log for rapid plasma reagin (RPR) test controls that were supposed to have been performed the previous day. You did not work that day and suspect that the person who did work that day failed to enter the QC results. Such an ethical dilemma falls under which domain?

A. Cognitive
B. Psychomotor
C. Affective
D. None of these options

Education and management/Education theory and practice/2

Answers to Questions 10–11

10. C The ever-changing role of the laboratory professional in a clinical laboratory prompts the curriculum committee to reevaluate the courses required by the students on a yearly basis. The heart of the laboratory, the LIS, is one of the first important areas to which students are introduced when entering the professional clinical training portion of their degree.

11. C Ethical behavior in the laboratory falls under the affective domain of objectives. Laboratory workers should never enter results for a test that they did not perform. False documentation could lead to dismissal of the employee and loss of licensure for the laboratory.

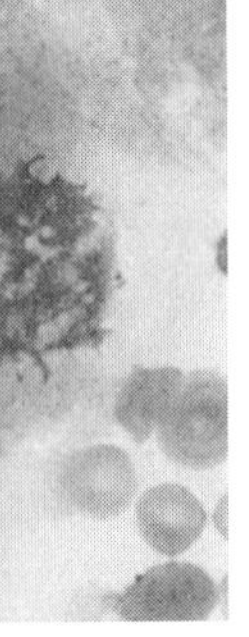

2.2
Management Theory and Practice

1. The McGregor X–Y theory advocates managing employees by stressing:
   A. Equal pay for equal work
   B. A pyramid of attainable goals for satisfaction at work
   C. Respect for the workers and acknowledgment of their ability to perform a task
   D. Collective bargaining

   Education and management/Management theory and practice/1

2. The Maslow theory of management is based on:
   A. The premise that all workers are unmotivated
   B. A pyramid of goals for the satisfaction of employee needs
   C. Use of detractors and perks to keep employees happy
   D. The professional development of the employee

   Education and management/Management theory and practice/1

3. The Herzberg theory relies on motivators that are part of the job design to instill employee satisfaction. These same motivators can become "dissatisfiers" if they are lacking. The Herzberg motivators are:
   A. Opportunity for achievement and advancement
   B. Performance evaluations every 24 months
   C. Continuing education sessions requiring supervisory approval
   D. Punitive actions taken when improvement diminishes

   Education and management/Management theory and practice/1

4. Management by objectives (MBO) is *least* effective for managing employees in which situation?
   A. Employees must be creative in their work
   B. The laboratory is converting to a new computer system
   C. The laboratory is undergoing a renovation
   D. Employees jointly agree to institutional goals

   Education and management/Management theory and practice/2

5. The four essential functions of a manager are:
   A. Staffing, decision making, cost analysis, evaluating
   B. Directing, leading, forecasting, and implementing
   C. Planning, organizing, directing, and controlling
   D. Innovating, designing, coordinating, and problem-solving

   Education and management/Management theory and practice/1

Answers to Questions 1–5

1. C The McGregor theory deals with participatory management in which the employee is considered a valuable asset.

2. B The Maslow theory of managing people deals with six levels. As the basic needs of an employee are met, the next highest need is substituted. The needs, in ascending order, are physiological, safety, security, social, esteem, and self-actualization. In expanded and updated versions of Maslow's theory, self-transcendence has been added beyond self-actualization. This level emphasizes the ability to focus beyond one's own needs to higher goals and purpose.

3. A According to Frederick Herzberg, achievement, opportunity for advancement, recognition, challenging work, responsibility, and a chance for advancement and personal growth are motivators and should be included as part of a job design.

4. A MBO stresses teamwork and shared goals and objectives but stifles creativity.

5. C Although managing may involve all the functions listed, the four core processes for all managers are planning, organizing, directing, and controlling. Planning includes formulating goals and objectives, organizing tasks, and establishing schedules. Organizing includes establishing effective communication, relationships, job descriptions, and training. Directing involves oversight of the various steps and stages of the plan, including coordination and leadership. Controlling involves evaluating resource utilization and outcomes, managing costs, and modifying the process to improve quality.

6. Unethical behavior by a laboratory supervisor that results in a compromise of employee safety should be:
- **A.** Reported to a lower authority
- **B.** Never confronted in fear of retaliation
- **C.** Reported to the Equal Employment Opportunity Commission
- **D.** Avoided and corrected the second time it happens

Education and management/Management theory and practice/2

7. When a new employee's performance is evaluated at the end of the probationary period, it should relate to:
- **A.** The individual's job description
- **B.** Verbal instructions
- **C.** Wage and salary policies
- **D.** Recruitment practices

Education and management/Management theory and practice/1

8. All the following are successful indicators of quality assurance (QA) and quality improvement (QI) programs in a clinical laboratory *except*:
- **A.** A "log" of incident report and solutions
- **B.** Emergency department and *STAT* turnaround times
- **C.** Positive patient identification wristbands for blood bank operations
- **D.** Employee recruitment practices

Education and management/Management theory and practice/2

9. Continuous quality improvement (CQI) is a team effort approach for clinical laboratories to:
- **A.** Identify potential problems and solutions
- **B.** Set annual laboratory financial benchmarks
- **C.** Create new Current Procedural Terminology codes
- **D.** Improve overall wages for laboratory employees

Education and management/Management theory and practice/2

10. Point-of-care testing (POCT) refers to:
- **A.** All testing performed on patients
- **B.** All laboratory testing performed in a central laboratory
- **C.** Any testing performed in the patient's location outside the laboratory
- **D.** Testing performed at a satellite laboratory

Education and management/Management theory and practice/2

Answers to Questions 6–10

6. C Direct confrontation is in order, followed by reporting the behavior to a higher authority at the clinical site. Major violations that are a threat to the safety of employees, patients, and the facility in general should be reported to the EEOC or the OSHA if the violations are not corrected in a timely fashion and if all avenues of action have been exhausted.

7. A The information used for the employee's performance review should reflect the job description used at the time of hire. An employee should receive a written job description that states the responsibilities and activities of the position. Job performance criteria and the rating system used should be clearly stated and available to the employee.

8. D These policies, along with laboratory performances on proficiency surveys, are a part of QA, QI, and total quality improvement (TQI). Although employee recruitment practices are very important, they are not considered part of the clinical laboratory QA or QI process.

9. A The CQI team identifies problems by collecting and analyzing data, and identifying solutions to correct any problems or discrepancies. By identifying potential problems and correcting existing problems, the laboratory demonstrates a commitment to high-quality patient care and outcomes.

10. C POCT refers to all tests performed outside the laboratory environment in the patient's specific location. This includes tests performed at the patient's bedside, in the emergency department, in the individual's home or long-term care facility, and tests performed in surgical and intensive care units.

11. Which of the following is addressed using the "six sigma" method?
- **A.** Human behavioral issues
- **B.** Items that need immediate attention
- **C.** Guaranteed customer satisfaction
- **D.** Improvement of performance and efficiency

Education and management/Management theory and practice/1

12. An LIS uses an algorithm based on the delta check process to identify erroneous results. Which process is a part of the LIS function?
- **A.** Inventory control management
- **B.** Real-time instrument interfacing
- **C.** Autoverification of test results
- **D.** Electronic crossmatching

Education and management/Management theory and practice/1

13. According to the Clinical Laboratory Improvement Act of 1988 (CLIA '88), when performing and documenting linearity, the following samples are required:
- **A.** A single calibrator and a zero-set point
- **B.** One normal level and one abnormal level
- **C.** Three levels of known concentration and a zero level
- **D.** A high control material and a low control material

Education and management/Management theory and practice/1

14. Which of the following would be *least* practical for POCT when rapid turnaround time (TAT) is required for immediate treatment?
- **A.** Cardiac markers
- **B.** Thyroid-stimulating hormone (TSH)
- **C.** Parathyroid hormone (PTH)
- **D.** Blood gases

Education and management/Management theory and practice/2

15. A shipment from a laboratory supply company arrived over the weekend. The shipment consisted of glass slides, latex gloves, and plastic test tubes—all nonperishable items. The shipment was left on the outside loading dock overnight. Are these supplies usable for patient care/testing?
- **A.** Yes, with no further QA testing required
- **B.** Yes, but only after quality analysis is performed to ensure that the items were not affected adversely
- **C.** No, the latex gloves might be contaminated, but the slides and test tubes may be used
- **D.** No, all supplies left outside for 24 hours unattended must be discarded

Education and management/Management theory and practice/3

Answers to Questions 11–15

11. D Six sigma management is a method for measuring the efficiency of a process, such as mass production, and it is applied in the clinical laboratory to reduce the frequency of test errors. The process consists of five steps: define, measure, analyze, improve, and control. The term *six sigma* denotes a process so precise that six times the standard deviation still results in a useful product (laboratory test result that is within acceptable limits for total allowable error). The error rate for a laboratory test performing at six sigma is only 3.4 per million test events.

12. C A laboratory information system (LIS) is used by laboratory professionals to perform many basic functions, such as test ordering and worklist generation, through real-time interfaces with laboratory instruments, QC and QA management, inventory control, and production of patient reports. In addition, they are capable of immediate decision making based on validated algorithms. This process, called autoverification, is used to determine whether a test result can be reported or whether another action is required.

13. C CLIA '88 guidelines require linearity testing by clinical laboratories on all nonwaived tests at least once before the test is performed on patient samples. The linearity test verifies the manufacturer's reportable range. In simplest terms, this consists of a reagent blank and three samples of known concentration that span the reportable range. A low, normal, and high control and reagent blank are adequate for this purpose.

14. B POCT is performed when the care of the patient is improved by obtaining the result immediately. Cardiac markers performed in the emergency department allow for urgent therapy for thromboembolism and other interventions. Blood gas analysis at the bedside permits immediate oxygen and ventilation adjustments and administration of medications to counteract acid–base imbalances. PTH assays performed in surgery allow the surgeon to determine whether a PTH-secreting mass has been successfully removed. While POCT is available for TSH, it is rarely used for emergency or urgent cases requiring immediate treatment.

15. B Laboratories must have written policies for determining whether laboratory reagents and supplies may be used. Nonperishable items should be inspected for contamination, damage, and manufacturing defects. Because items left in an uncontrolled environment may be exposed to adverse conditions, such as extreme temperatures, they should be inspected and tested to ensure that their performance is unaffected.

16. An immunology supervisor ordered several antinuclear antibody and influenza A kits. The outside packaging of both kits stated that the kits require a storage temperature of 2°C to 8°C. The kits were packed in dry ice but were unpacked at 7:00 p.m. and left in the mailroom at room temperature for approximately 1 hour. What follow-up action is required?

A. The kits can be placed into inventory
B. The kits must be tested using quality controls before use and used only if QC performance is acceptable
C. The kits should not be used for clinical testing
D. The decision to use or discard the kits depends on the manufacturer's documentation for stability and the laboratory's lot-to-lot analysis

Education and management/Management theory and practice/3

17. A patient refuses to have blood drawn for a routine laboratory test request made by a primary care provider. What is the *most* appropriate course of action?

A. Perform the venipuncture against the patient's will
B. Do not attempt the venipuncture, and file an incident report with the laboratory manager
C. Request that the patient be sedated, and then collect the sample
D. Request assistance from the legal department

Education and management/Management theory and practice/2

18. Which of the following accurately describes the steps involved in the LEAN process?

A. Lower cost, efficient flow, added value, and net result
B. Customer value, value stream map, flow, pull, and improved outcome
C. Satisfaction, cost savings, and turnaround time
D. Efficiency study, modeling, construct, and step-by-step process

Education and management/Management theory and practice/2

Answers to Questions 16–18

16. D All laboratory kits and reagents must be stored according to the manufacturer's instructions. The manufacturer should be consulted to determine whether storage time and temperature limits have been established for the kits. If these have not been exceeded, and the lot-to-lot analysis confirms that they are unaffected, then the kits may be used.

17. B Patients have the right to refuse treatment, even if they signed a document upon admission giving consent for treatment. In this situation, the supervisor should be notified, the incident documented, and the provider notified. The issue of informed consent is a legal one, and the laboratory personnel should act in accordance with the laws governing their jurisdiction. For example, some courts will not admit results of blood tests into evidence if the subject had not been formally arrested and the sample was collected against the subject's will.

18. B LEAN is a method used to improve customer satisfaction. It is used often in clinical laboratories to improve a process, such as ensuring faster test turnaround time. LEAN is not an acronym; it refers to streamlining a process so that there is no waste. The five steps in the LEAN method are value, value stream map, flow, pull, and improvement.

19. A laboratory wishes to evaluate its specimen-processing operations to improve test turnaround time for cardiac markers using the LEAN process. To accomplish this, the laboratory manager measures the specimen collection and transport time to the laboratory, along with when the sample arrived in the laboratory, evident by recording in the LIS and instrument data link, centrifuged, and placed on the automated track. This process is called:

A. Establishing pull
B. Creating a flow diagram
C. Mapping the value stream
D. Process analysis

Education and management/Management theory and practice/2

20. A breach of confidentiality involving a patient's chemistry test result occurred when it was willfully given to another employee who was closely acquainted with the patient but was not a family member. What is the laboratory supervisor's *most* appropriate course of action?

A. Terminate both employees
B. Let it go and do nothing
C. Reprimand both employees, note the incident in their files, and require confidentiality retraining
D. Call for a meeting of all laboratory employees to discuss the incident and initiate retraining for all

Education and management/Management theory and practice/3

Answers to Questions 19–20

19. C A value stream map is a diagram of all steps involved in a process. The map is used to identify areas of waste where efficiency can be improved. Flow is the refinement of the value stream, eliminating waste and improving efficiency. Pull is the process of merging the steps into the next part of the process so that it works seamlessly, and problems can be easily identified and corrected.

20. C The supervisor must enforce the rules and regulations of the laboratory. The ethical position taken by the supervisor—reprimanding the involved employees and then requiring further training of those individuals—is also part of weighing the consequences of the action and is meant to prevent any future breaches of confidentiality by other employees.

2.3
Laws and Regulations

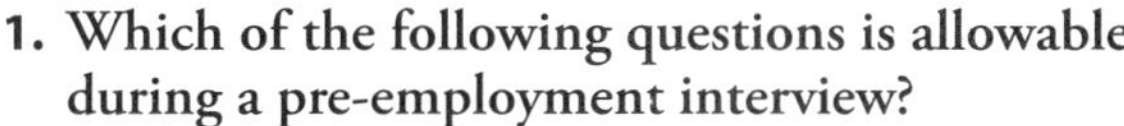

1. **Which of the following questions is allowable during a pre-employment interview?**
   A. How many times have you been pregnant?
   B. Have you been convicted of any felonies?
   C. Does your husband belong to any religious societies?
   D. Are you planning to use the hospital day-care center?

   Education and management/Laws and regulations/2

2. **A chemistry profile that includes electrolytes, glucose, blood urea nitrogen (BUN), and creatinine is ordered on an 80-year-old patient with vomiting and dizziness. How should the laboratory submit the charge for these tests for reimbursement by Medicare?**
   A. Submit as one test
   B. Submit each test separately
   C. Submit Medicare-approved tests only
   D. Submit as four individual tests

   Education and management/Laws and regulations/2

3. **According to CLIA '88, control of laboratory test reliability is accomplished by all the following requirements *except*:**
   A. Documentation of quality control results and corrective actions
   B. Participation in proficiency testing for all nonwaived tests
   C. Professional certification of all testing personnel
   D. Demonstration that all quantitative tests meet manufacturer's performance specifications

   Education and management/Laws and regulations/2

4. **CLIA '88 specifies that the minimum requirements for proficiency testing (PT) of analytes (excluding cytology) are:**
   A. One challenge per analyte and one testing event per year
   B. Ten challenges per analyte and five testing events per year
   C. Five challenges per analyte and at least three testing events per year
   D. Twelve challenges per analyte and one testing event per month

   Education and management/Laws and regulations/1

Answers to Questions 1–4

1. B Title VII of the Civil Rights Act of 1964 states that questions are permissible during interviews if they are related to legitimate occupational qualifications; however, the Equal Employment Opportunity Commission (EEOC) discourages doing so to prevent discriminatory practices. Some states and localities may have stricter laws regarding when and how you may inquire about criminal history of a potential employee.

2. A A chemistry profile that includes electrolytes, glucose, BUN, and creatinine is considered a billable procedure and has a single CPT code (currently this panel is called the Basic Metabolic Panel and is coded as CPT 80048). Splitting a profile into many individual tests for billing purposes may be prohibited by law. For example, a complete blood count (CBC) cannot be split into five parts, with each component being charged separately.

3. C CLIA '88 requires all clinical laboratories to be certified, but the requirements differ for each of the three certification levels—waivered, moderate, or high complexity. For example, quality control must be practiced by all laboratories, but standards for testing personnel differ for all three levels and do not specify certification, only educational levels.

4. C Analytes for which proficiency testing is required are identified in Section 493 Subpart I of the CLIA rules. A minimum number of five challenges for each analyte and at least three testing events per year are required. The testing events are evenly spaced throughout the year. Unsatisfactory performance for the same analyte for two out of two events or two out of the three most recent events constitutes unsuccessful participation and may result in punitive action.

5. According to CLIA '88, satisfactory performance for ABO, Rh, and compatibility tests requires a score of:
A. 100%
B. 90%
C. 80%
D. 75%
Education and management/Laws and regulations/1

6. To comply with CLIA '88, calibration materials must:
A. Be purchased by an authorized agency, such as the College of Pathology
B. Have concentration values that cover the laboratory's reportable range
C. Be traceable to the National Calibration Board
D. Be identical in concentration to those sold by the reagent manufacturer
Education and management/Laws and regulations/1

7. According to CLIA '88, calibration materials should be appropriate for the methodology and be:
A. Of bovine origin
B. Three times the normal range for the specific analyte
C. Traceable to a reference method and reference material of known value
D. Twice the laboratory's reference range for the analyte
Education and management/Laws and regulations/1

8. Under CLIA '88, testing personnel with an associate degree and appropriate training in the clinical laboratory are authorized to perform:
A. Waived tests only
B. Tests that are qualitative or waived and some moderate-complexity tests
C. Waived and moderate-complexity tests
D. Waived, moderate-complexity, and high-complexity tests
Education and management/Laws and regulations/1

9. Sexual harassment is a form of discrimination and therefore is prohibited by the:
A. Occupational Safety and Health Administration (OSHA)
B. Civil Rights Act of 1964 (Title VII)
C. Right to Privacy Act of 1974
D. U.S. Department of Health and Human Services (USDHHS)
Education and management/Laws and regulations/1

10. Records of a patient's laboratory test results may not be released without consent to anyone outside the clinical laboratory *except* to the:
A. American Red Cross
B. U.S. Department of Health and Human Services
C. Insurance carrier
D. Provider who ordered the tests
Education and management/Laws and regulations/2

Answers to Questions 5–10

5. A Unsatisfactory performance occurs when any challenge for ABO, Rh, or compatibility testing is in error. For all other tests, a score below 80% is defined as unsatisfactory performance. Unsatisfactory performance for the same analyte for two out of two events or two out of the three most recent events constitutes unsuccessful participation.

6. B According to CLIA '88, the minimum requirement for calibration is every 6 months or more frequently if specified by the manufacturer. The calibrators must cover the reportable range of the method. A minimum of two levels of calibrant must be used (more if specified by the manufacturer).

7. C Calibrators must have an assigned concentration determined by assay using a reference method. The reference method should be calibrated using standards that are traceable to National Bureau of Standards material or acceptable primary standards.

8. D Testing personnel with an associate degree and approved laboratory training may perform high-complexity tests as well as waived and moderate-complexity tests. However, the laboratory must be certified at all three levels.

9. B The Civil Rights Act of 1964, by federal law, prohibits discrimination in employment based on race, color, religion, or gender. The law established the Equal Employment Opportunity Commission (EEOC) to hear complaints of discrimination by employees and initiate legal action as appropriate.

10. D The Privacy Act of 1974 prohibits the release of medical records without the patient's consent, except to the patient's attending physician, attorney, or next of kin (if the patient is deceased), unless solicited by a valid subpoena.

11. The most common deficiency cited during an onsite laboratory inspection by the College of American Pathologists (CAP) and The Joint Commission is:

A. Improper documentation
B. Insufficient workspace area
C. Improper reagent storage
D. Improper instrument calibration frequency

Education and management/Laws and regulations/2

12. Which of the following circumstances is considered a form of sexual harassment?

A. Unwelcome sexual advances by a supervisor
B. Requests for favors of a sexual nature from a fellow laboratory employee
C. Physical conduct of a sexual nature from an employee working in another department
D. All circumstances listed are considered sexual harassment

Education and management/Laws and regulations/2

13. Which regulatory agency mandates the following requirements for protection of employees of clinical laboratories?
Provide personal protective equipment (PPE)
Require hepatitis B vaccinations at no cost
Require specific biohazard materials labelling
Provide training and updating yearly of safety standards

A. U.S. Food and Drug Administration (FDA)
B. Occupational Safety and Health Administration (OSHA)
C. American Association of Blood Banks (AABB)
D. American Society of Clinical Pathologists (ASCP)

Education and management/Laws and regulations/1

14. The CLIA '88 was enacted to regulate the following:

A. All clinical laboratories in the United States
B. Independent laboratories not regulated by the OSHA
C. Environmental Protection Agency laboratories
D. Industrial laboratories

Education and management/Laws and regulations/1

15. Records of a patient's laboratory test results may be released *without the prior consent* of the patient to all the following *except*:

A. An insurance carrier
B. Primary provider on call
C. Nursing staff
D. An employer

Education and management/Laws and regulations/2

Answers to Questions 11–15

11. A Improper documentation accounts for most laboratory deficiencies, specifically, the records of competency and assessment for laboratory personnel performing nonwaived testing.

12. D Sexual harassment is a form of discrimination, and it is prohibited by the Civil Rights Act of 1964 (Title VII). The suggestion that a sexual favor must be performed to avoid punitive action or receive a favorable performance evaluation constitutes sexual harassment. Additionally, offensive language and behavior with sexual connotations are forms of sexual harassment, regardless of the department in which the offending employee works.

13. B The U.S. Department of Labor, through the OSHA, mandates a workplace that is safe and healthy. Other agencies that inspect clinical laboratories (CLIA '88, College of American Pathologists, The Joint Commission, etc.) also require safety guidelines for the health care workers in the clinical laboratory.

14. A The regulations for clinical laboratories (CLIA '88) were finally published in 1992 in the *Federal Register*. The federal mandate was designed to regulate a specific standard for each laboratory test, as well as categorize the laboratories according to the level of testing and the laboratory personnel.

15. D The Health Insurance Portability and Accountability Act of 1996 (HIPAA) provides for increased access to health care by making it easier for providers to send medical information to insurance companies electronically. The law requires health care providers to safeguard the confidentiality of patient medical information and to provide patients with a compliance statement that defines who is entitled to receive their health information. The provider ordering the tests and the health care workers directly involved in patient care are allowed to see laboratory results. Laboratory results may also be released to the patient's insurance provider, medical review officers, and public health officials. They may also be released to the patient's family, provided the patient is notified of this policy beforehand and is given the right to agree or disagree.

16. Which of the following is *not* an appropriate guideline for phlebotomists to follow to prevent a malpractice lawsuit?
A. Use one form of patient identification, such as the last name
B. Always keep patient confidentiality
C. Always use aseptic venipuncture technique
D. Label specimens only after the blood has been drawn

Education and management/Laws and regulations/2

17. According to CLIA '88, testing personnel performing high-complexity laboratory tests must have at least a:
A. Bachelor of Arts degree
B. Bachelor of Science degree in medical laboratory science
C. Associate degree in medical laboratory science (medical laboratory technician [MLT])
D. High school diploma

Education and management/Laws and regulations/2

18. During an interview, an employer may request the following from a prospective new employee:
A. Marital status
B. Age of children
C. Arrest record for driving under the influence of alcohol
D. Professional certification

Education and management/Laws and regulations/2

19. Safety data sheets (SDSs) for hazardous materials must be reviewed by personnel per OSHA regulations:
A. Weekly
B. Monthly
C. Every 6 months
D. Yearly

Education and management/Laws and regulations/1

20. What documents are needed to meet the ISO-9000 standards for laboratory certification?
A. Quality manual, document control, internal audits, and corrective and preventive actions
B. Work performance evaluation, maintenance, and budgeting
C. Inventory, quality control, and customer satisfaction
D. Risk prevention, quality control, and personnel

Education and management/Laws and regulations/2

Answers to Questions 16–20

16. A Outpatient identification through two means (name and date of birth) is a standard procedure to avoid drawing the wrong patient. Other malpractice prevention measures include treating people equally, securing informed consent before testing, and listening to patients' concerns.

17. C CLIA '88 requires personnel performing high-complexity tests to have earned at least an associate degree in medical laboratory science or attained a level of college education and clinical laboratory training equivalent to an associate degree in medical laboratory science.

18. D All of the options are in violation of Title VII of the Civil Rights Act of 1964, except the request for certification. The certification is usually a requirement for job performance and is listed in the job description.

19. D OSHA requires safety training and the review of safety documents, including SDSs, on a yearly basis. The laboratory must maintain an SDS inventory for all hazardous materials it uses. The inventory must be readily available to all employees who may have contact with or handle the materials.

20. A ISO refers to the International Organization for Standardization. ISO-9000 is a set of three standards—ISO-9000, -9001, and -9004 (ISO-9003 is no longer used)—for quality management that can be applied to any business or organization, such as a clinical laboratory. When an organization demonstrates compliance with ISO-9000 standards, it is said to be certified. ISO certification tells an organization's customers that it adheres to quality improvement standards and guidelines that improve performance and ensure the highest quality possible.

21. In the field of clinical laboratory testing and *in vitro* diagnostic test systems, ISO TC 212 is the document used for standardization and guidance in all the following areas *except*:
- **A.** Quality management and quality assurance
- **B.** Scheduling, yearly evaluations, and workloads
- **C.** Pre- and postanalytical procedures
- **D.** Laboratory safety and reference systems

Education and management/Laws and regulations/1

22. Which of the following organizations is responsible for promulgating hospital-wide compliance standards?
- **A.** CAP (College of American Pathologists)
- **B.** COLA (Commission on Office Laboratory Accreditation)
- **C.** TJC (The Joint Commission)
- **D.** CLIAC (Clinical Laboratory Improvement Advisory Committee)

Education and management/Laws and regulations/1

23. According to CLIA regulations, which credentials would *not* meet the qualifications to be a technical consultant for a moderately complex laboratory?
- **A.** Board-certified podiatrist with at least 1 year of training in the respective laboratory specialty in a nonwaived laboratory
- **B.** Bachelor of Science degree in chemistry, physical science, or biology and 2 years of training in the respective laboratory specialty in a nonwaived laboratory
- **C.** Master's degree in chemistry, biology, or physics and 1 year of training in the respective laboratory specialty in a nonwaived laboratory
- **D.** Doctorate in chemistry and 6 months' experience in the respective laboratory specialty in a nonwaived laboratory

Education and management/Laws and regulations/2

24. According to CLIA regulations, which person qualifies as a clinical laboratory consultant?
- **A.** CLIA qualified laboratory director
- **B.** Medical laboratory scientist with baccalaureate degree and 1 year of laboratory training or experience
- **C.** Medical laboratory technician with an associate degree and 2 years of laboratory training or experience
- **D.** All the above

Education and management/Laws and regulations/2

Answers to Questions 21–24

21. B TC 212 is an ISO standard written for clinical laboratory testing and manufacturing of *in vitro* diagnostic products. The standards deal with the analytical test process, pre- and postanalytical processes, laboratory safety, and QA, including personnel qualifications and accreditation. The standards committee for ISO TC 212 in the United States works under the auspices of the American National Standards Institute (ANSI) and has designated the Clinical and Laboratory Standards Institute (CLSI) to oversee the standards committee.

22. C TJC is an agency that accredits and inspects all departments of hospitals, as well as laboratories. The other organizations are responsible for accreditation or, in the case of CLIAC certification, for only laboratory testing sites.

23. D A technical consultant, according to definition by the CLIA, may be a licensed and board certified doctor of medicine, osteopathy, or podiatry with at least 1 year of training or experience in the laboratory specialty for which they consult. One year of laboratory training or experience is needed for someone with an earned doctor of clinical laboratory science (DCLS) or master's degree in biology, chemistry, or medical laboratory science (MLS). A person with a baccalaureate degree in biology, chemistry, or MLS must have 2 years of training or experience, while a person with an associate degree in medical laboratory technology (MLT), MLS, or clinical laboratory science (CLS) must have 4 years of training or experience.

24. A A clinical consultant, according to the definition by the CLIA, may be a laboratory director approved by CLIA or a licensed doctor of medicine, osteopathy, or podiatry. Individuals holding a doctoral degree in a chemical, biological, or clinical or medical laboratory science or medical technology that meet specific educational requirements and have 2 years of laboratory training or experience, and 2 years of laboratory experience directing or supervising high-complexity testing may also serve as a clinical consultant. These individuals must also obtain 20 continuing education (CE) hours in laboratory practice that cover the director responsibilities as defined by CLIA.

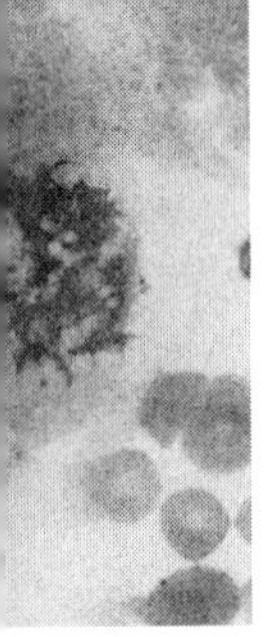

2.4

Laboratory Economics

1. **Direct laboratory costs for a diagnostic test include which of the following?**
   A. Equipment maintenance
   B. Insurance
   C. Depreciation
   D. Overtime pay
   Education and management/Laboratory economics/1

2. **Which of the following accounts for the largest portion of the direct cost of a diagnostic laboratory test?**
   A. Reagents
   B. General supplies
   C. Labor
   D. Instrument depreciation
   Education and management/Laboratory economics/1

3. **Using the surcharge/cost-plus method for determining diagnostic test charges, determine the charge for an ova and parasite examination on fecal specimens, given the following information:**

   Collection, handling, transport, clerical, and reporting = $2.00
   Reference laboratory charge = $20.00
   Laboratory "markup" = 100%

   A. $22.00
   B. $32.00
   C. $42.00
   D. $122.00
   Education and management/Laboratory economics/2

4. **In deciding whether to adopt a new test on the laboratory's automated chemistry analyzer, which parameters are needed to determine the number of tests required to break even?**
   A. Test turnaround time
   B. Cost of labor per hour
   C. Number of other tests performed per month
   D. Total fixed laboratory costs
   Education and management/Laboratory economics/2

5. **Which statement *best* represents the relationship between test volume and revenue or costs for batch-run tests?**
   A. As volume increases, the fixed cost per test also increases
   B. As volume increases, the revenue also increases
   C. Revenue is approximately equal for both high- and low-volume tests
   D. 90% of the revenue is generated by 5% of the tests offered
   Education and management/Laboratory economics/2

Answers to Questions 1–5

1. D All costs that are specifically linked to a test (e.g., personnel, overtime, chemicals, and supplies) are direct costs.

2. C Labor accounts for 60% to 70% of the direct cost per test in most laboratories. The cost of labor, reagents, and supplies are direct costs, but instrument depreciation is not.

3. C The "markup" factor is used to establish part of the cost of a test to obtain the desired profit margin. Tests sent to reference laboratories or done in-house have some additional costs, and this is referred to as the surcharge/cost-plus method of determining test charges.

4. D The formula for calculating the break-even point in test volume is:

No. of tests = total fixed costs ÷ (average reimbursement – variable cost per test)

The total fixed costs are the expenses that are not expected to change as the workload increases (e.g., cost of the instrument). The variable cost per test includes any costs that increase as the workload increases (e.g., cost of reagents). The average reimbursement represents the expected revenue generated per billable test result.

5. B As volume increases, costs should decrease, and revenues should increase. The large, fixed costs, such as instrumentation, labor, and management, do not change with the size of the batch. As volume increases, reagent and consumable costs per test often become lower, thus reducing the variable cost per test. In most laboratories, about 80% of the revenue is generated by laboratory tests that make up the top 20% of the test volume.

6. A hospital submits a bill for $200 to the patient's insurance company for the cost of outpatient laboratory tests. The laboratory services rendered by the hospital are paid according to an agreed fee schedule. The specific laboratory procedures are billed according to which system of coding?
A. Diagnosis-Related Group (DRG)
B. Current Procedural Terminology (CPT)
C. Medicare
D. Medicaid
Education and management/Laboratory economics/1

7. A hospital has a contract with a major medical insurer that reimburses the laboratory at a rate of $1 per insured life per year. This type of reimbursement is called:
A. A prospective payment system
B. A preferred provider discount
C. Capitation
D. Diagnosis-related group
Education and management/Laboratory economics/1

8. According to federal and state regulations, a hospital's capital budget should include which of the following before projects are submitted for approval?
A. A timetable of completion
B. A cost analysis
C. Salaries and wages for new employees
D. A certificate of need
Education and management/Laboratory economics/1

9. A rural hospital laboratory employs 8.25 full-time equivalents (FTEs). To budget for next year's salaries for the employees, the laboratory manager needs to submit what figures for the laboratory's projected annual budget?
A. Total (paid) hours
B. Productive (worked) hours
C. Total hours of full-time employees
D. Total hours of part-time employees
Education and management/Laboratory economics/1

10. A new LIS will be evaluated by the laboratory staff. All the following points should be considered in the evaluation *except*:
A. Cost of updating software
B. Interface ability with existing laboratory instruments
C. Tracking of non-crossmatched blood units in the blood bank
D. Knowledge of technology of the laboratory staff
Education and management/Laboratory economics/2

11. The following are considered indirect costs when calculating costs for laboratory tests *except*:
A. Public relations
B. Secretarial staff
C. Insurance
D. Specimen collection process
Education and management/Laboratory economics/2

Answers to Questions 6–11

6. B The CPT code refers to Current Procedural Terminology. Codes are assigned to all medical procedures, which are grouped according to common disease characteristics. The insurance company or payer (e.g., Medicare) usually has agreed to a reimbursement amount per test or procedure. The American Medical Association issues the publication titled *Current Procedural Terminology*, which is updated yearly.

7. C Capitation plans provide the laboratory with a fixed (known) revenue based on a negotiated per-capita fee for the members of the group. To achieve a profit, the laboratory must manage its resources to provide covered laboratory tests to the group at a cost that does not equal or exceed its reimbursement.

8. D A certificate of need (CON) is an authorization to proceed with a needed project, such as a new obstetrics department or new wing to the laboratory. While the federal government removed this mandate in 1986, 35 states maintain a CON program or variation of one. The capital limit can vary widely based on which state program is applicable.

9. A The total (paid) hours are the total number of hours for which employees are paid. This includes vacation time, sick time, and the actual time spent working in the laboratory. However, "productive (worked) hours" refers only to the actual hours worked, including overtime. A budget must include the total (paid) hours to give a clear picture of what is needed for the next year of wages and salaries.

10. D Each laboratory will have specific needs to determine the appropriate LIS. However, storage capacity, reliability, security, upgrade costs, instrument interface availability, inventory management, and quality control functions are common parameters that must be considered. Technology knowledge of the laboratory staff is irrelevant. The laboratory is responsible for implementation and proper training of all staff.

11. D Indirect costs refer to other costs not associated with the actual testing (reagents, testing personnel time, specimen collection, etc.).

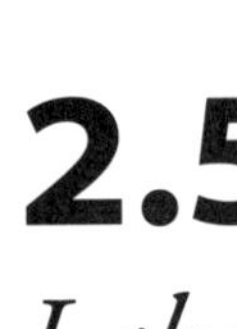

2.5
Laboratory Safety

1. **Which order of events should be followed at the conclusion of a laboratory worker's shift to prevent the spread of bloodborne pathogens?**
   A. Remove gloves, disinfect area, wash hands, and remove laboratory coat
   B. Disinfect area, remove gloves, remove laboratory coat, and wash hands
   C. Disinfect area, remove gloves, wash hands, and remove laboratory coat
   D. Remove gloves, wash hands, remove laboratory coat, and disinfect area
   Education and management/Laboratory safety/2

2. **The safety data sheets (SDSs) for hazardous chemicals address which of the following conditions?**
   A. Physical characteristics of the chemical
   B. Safe handling and storage of the chemical
   C. Specific health hazards associated with the chemical
   D. All the items are addressed by an SDS
   Education and management/Laboratory safety/1

3. **A medical laboratory science student accidentally splashed a few drops of an extraction reagent from an enzyme immunoassay (EIA) kit for group A *Streptococcus* into their right eye and felt an immediate burning sensation. What should the student do first?**
   A. Locate the SDS for the EIA test kit
   B. Go directly to the emergency department for treatment
   C. Go to the eyewash station and rinse the eye thoroughly with water
   D. Report directly to their immediate supervisor
   Education and management/Laboratory safety/2

4. ***Bacillus anthracis* is recovered from a patient sample in the clinical microbiology laboratory. Such an organism would fall under which Centers for Disease Control and Prevention (CDC) category of biological agent?**
   A. Category A
   B. Category B
   C. Category C
   D. Category D
   Education and management/Laboratory safety/1

Answers to Questions 1–4

1. B According to the OSHA Bloodborne Pathogens Rule of 1992, gloves then laboratory coats are to be removed after disinfection of the work area. Hands are washed last.

2. D SDSs describe the chemical and physical characteristics, safe handling and storage, and potential health hazards of reagents used in the laboratory. These documents must be easily accessible to all employees. They should be reviewed at least once per year during safety in-service training.

3. C OSHA regulations require that new employees and students be informed of all occupational hazards at the laboratory, that the laboratory testing personnel be provided with PPE and receive training in procedures to be followed when exposed to hazardous materials. When a chemical compound comes into contact with the skin or eyes, the first course of action is to dilute the chemical by flooding it with a large volume of water. If further treatment is necessary, obtain the SDS and seek appropriate medical advice. All issues involving chemical or biological exposure should be reported to the relevant individuals. This process will be documented in the laboratory's chemical hygiene plan.

4. A The CDC groups biological agents that may be used to carry out terrorist threats into three categories: A, B, or C. Category A agents are those that would cause the most harm because of their highly infectious nature, mode of transmission, and high mortality risk. This group includes *Bacillus anthracis, Clostridium botulinum, Francisella tularensis, Yersinia pestis,* smallpox virus, and viruses that cause hemorrhagic fever, such as Ebola and Marburg viruses. Category B includes bacteria and viruses that pose a lesser threat, such as the organisms that produce ricin, gangrene, and Q fever. Category C includes emergent infectious agents.

BIBLIOGRAPHY

1. Clinical Laboratory Improvement Amendments of 1988 (CLIA) Proficiency Testing Regulations Related to Analytes and Acceptable Performance. 42 CFR Pt 493. 57 *Fed Regist.* 7002 (February 28, 2024).
2. Harmening, DM. *Laboratory Management, Principles and Processes.* 4th ed. D.H. Publishing & Consulting; 2020.
3. Isabel JM, Ellinger PJ, Griffin DM. *Laboratory Operations and Management: Foundations of Practice.* F.A. Davis Company; 2024.
4. Pozgar GD, Santucci NM, Pinella JW. *Legal and Ethical Issues for Health Professionals.* 2nd ed. Jones and Bartlett; 2005.
5. Varnadoe LA. *Medical Laboratory Management and Supervision.* 2nd ed. PriorityEd; 2008.

CHAPTER 3

Immunology

3.1 *Basic Principles of Immunology*

3.2 *Immunologic Techniques*

3.3 *Infectious Disease Methods*

3.4 *Autoimmune Disorders*

3.5 *Hypersensitivity*

3.6 *Immunodeficiency, Immunoglobulins, Complement, and Cellular Testing*

3.7 *Tumors, Transplantation, and Genetics*

3.1
Basic Principles of Immunology

1. From the following, identify a specific component of the adaptive immune system that is formed in response to antigenic stimulation:
A. Lysozyme
B. Complement
C. Commensal organisms
D. Immunoglobulin (Ig)
Immunology/Basic principles/1

2. Which two organs are considered the primary lymphoid organs in which immunocompetent cells originate and mature?
A. Thyroid and Peyer patches
B. Thymus and bone marrow
C. Spleen and mucosal-associated lymphoid tissue (MALT)
D. Lymph nodes and thoracic duct
Immunology/Basic principles/1

3. What type of B cells are formed after antigen stimulation?
A. Plasma cells and memory B cells
B. Mature B cells
C. Antigen-dependent B cells
D. Receptor-activated B cells
Immunology/Basic principles/1

4. T cells travel from bone marrow to the thymus for maturation. What is the correct order of the maturation sequence for T cells in the thymus?
A. Bone marrow to the cortex; after thymic education, released back to peripheral circulation
B. Maturation and selection occur in the cortex; migration to the medulla; release of mature T cells to secondary lymphoid organs
C. Storage in either the cortex or medulla; release of T cells into the peripheral circulation
D. Activation and selection occur in the medulla; mature T cells are stored in the cortex until activated by antigen
Immunology/Basic principles/1

5. Which cluster of differentiation (CD) marker is the most specific identifying marker for mature T cells?
A. CD1
B. CD2
C. CD3
D. CD4 or CD8
Immunology/Basic principles/1

Answers to Questions 1–5

1. D Ig (immunoglobulin or antibody) is a specific molecule produced by the adaptive immune system in response to the exposure to a specific antigen.

2. B Immunocompetent cells either originate or mature in the bone marrow and the thymus. These tissues are considered primary lymphoid organs. Some immunocompetent cells mature or reside in bone marrow (the source of all hematopoietic cells) until transported to the thymus, spleen, or Peyer patches, where they process antigen or manufacture antibody. T lymphocytes, after originating in bone marrow, travel to the thymus to mature and differentiate.

3. A Mature B cells exhibit surface Ig that cross-links with a foreign antigen activating the B cell and leading to capping and internalization of antigen. An activated B cell is termed a plasma cell that produces and secretes Igs. Some B cells will also become memory cells that reside in lymphoid organs until a second exposure to the foreign antigen occurs.

4. B Immature T cells travel from bone marrow to the thymus to mature into functional T cells. Once in the thymus, T cells undergo a selection and maturation sequence that begins in the cortex and moves to the medulla of the thymus. Thymic factors, such as thymosin and thymopoietin, and cells within the thymus, such as macrophages and dendritic cells, assist in this sequence. After completion of the maturation cycle, T cells are released to secondary lymphoid organs to await antigen recognition and activation.

5. C The CD3 marker appears during the early stages of T-cell development and can be used to differentiate T cells from other lymphocytes.

6. Which markers are found on mature, peripheral helper T cells?
A. CD1, CD2, CD4
B. CD2, CD3, CD8
C. CD1, CD3, CD4
D. CD2, CD3, CD4
Immunology/Basic principles/1

7. Which T cells express the CD8 marker and act specifically to kill tumors or virally infected cells?
A. Helper T cells
B. Suppressor T cells
C. Cytotoxic T cells (T_C cells)
D. Regulator T cells
Immunology/Basic principles/1

8. How are T_C cells and natural killer (NK) cells similar?
A. Require antibody to be present
B. Effective against virally infected cells
C. Recognize antigen in association with HLA class II markers
D. Do not bind to infected cells
Immunology/Basic principles/1

9. What is the name of the process by which phagocytic cells are attracted to a substance, such as a bacterial peptide?
A. Diapedesis
B. Degranulation
C. Chemotaxis
D. Phagotaxis
Immunology/Basic principles/1

10. All the following are immunologic functions of complement *except*:
A. Induction of an antiviral state
B. Opsonization
C. Chemotaxis
D. Anaphylatoxin formation
Immunology/Basic principles/1

11. Which complement component is found in both the classic and alternate pathways?
A. C1
B. C4
C. Factor D
D. C3
Immunology/Basic principles/1

12. Which Ig(s) can activate the classic complement pathway?
A. IgA and IgD
B. IgM only
C. IgG and IgM
D. IgG only
Immunology/Basic principles/1

13. How is complement activity inactivated *in vitro*?
A. Heating serum at 56°C for 30 minutes
B. Keeping serum at room temperature of 22°C for 1 hour
C. Heating serum at 37°C for 45 minutes
D. Freezing serum at 0°C for 24 hours
Immunology/Basic principles/1

Answers to Questions 6–13

6. D Mature, peripheral helper T cells have the CD2, CD3 (mature T cell), and CD4 (helper) markers.

7. C T_C cells recognize antigen in association with major histocompatibility complex (MHC) class I complexes and act against target cells that express foreign antigens on their surface. These include viral antigens and the human leukocyte antigens (HLAs) that are the target of graft rejection.

8. B Both T_C and NK cells are effective against virally infected cells, and neither requires an antibody to bind to infected cells. NK cells do not exhibit MHC class restriction, whereas activation of T_C cells requires the presence of MHC class I molecules in association with the viral antigen.

9. C Chemotaxis is the process by which phagocytic cells are attracted toward an area where they detect a disturbance in the normal functions of body tissues. Products from bacteria and viruses, complement components, coagulation proteins, and cytokines from other immune cells all act as chemotactic factors.

10. A Complement molecules are serum proteins that function in opsonization, chemotaxis, and anaphylatoxin formation but do not induce an antiviral state in target cells. This function is performed by interferons.

11. D C3 is found in both the classic and alternate pathways of the complement system. In the classic pathway, C3b forms a complex on the cell with C4b2a that enzymatically cleaves C5. In the alternate pathway, C3b binds to an activator on the cell surface and forms a complex with factor B called C3bBb, which, like C4b2a3b, cleaves C5 into C5a and C5b.

12. C Both IgG and IgM can activate the classic complement pathway. IgM is, however, a more potent complement activator.

13. A Complement activity in serum, *in vitro*, is inactivated by heating at 56°C for 30 minutes. In test procedures where complement may interfere with the test system, it may be necessary to inactivate complement to prevent interference with the testing process.

14. What is the purpose of C3a, C4a, and C5a, the cleavage products of the complement cascade?
A. To bind with specific membrane receptors of lymphocytes and stimulate release of cytotoxic substances
B. To increase vascular permeability, contraction of smooth muscle, and release of histamine from basophils
C. To bind with membrane receptors of macrophages to facilitate phagocytosis and the removal of debris and foreign substances
D. To regulate and degrade membrane cofactor protein after activation by C3 convertase
Immunology/Basic principles/1

15. Which region of the Ig molecule binds antigen?
A. Fragment antigen binding (Fab)
B. Fragment crystallizable (Fc)
C. Constant light (C_L)
D. Constant heavy (C_H)
Immunology/Basic principles/1

16. Which region determines whether an Ig molecule binds to complement?
A. Variable heavy (V_H)
B. Constant heavy (C_H)
C. Variable light (V_L)
D. Constant light (C_L)
Immunology/Basic principles/1

17. Which Ig class(es) contains a J chain?
A. IgM
B. IgE and IgD
C. IgM and surface IgA (sIgA)
D. IgG3 and IgA
Immunology/Basic principles/1

18. Which Ig is produced first during the primary immune response to an antigen?
A. IgG
B. IgM
C. IgA
D. IgE
Immunology/Basic principles/1

19. During a secondary immune response, which immunoglobulin is produced in the highest quantity or titer?
A. IgG
B. IgM
C. IgA
D. IgE
Immunology/Basic principles/1

20. Which Ig can cross the placenta?
A. IgG
B. IgM
C. IgA
D. IgE
Immunology/Basic principles/1

Answers to Questions 14–20

14. B C3a, C4a, and C5a are cleavage products of the complement cascade that participate in various biological functions, such as vasodilation and smooth muscle contraction. These small peptides act as anaphylatoxins, for example, effector molecules that participate in the inflammatory response to assist in the destruction and clearance of foreign antigens.

15. A Fab is the region of the Ig molecule that binds antigen. Two Fab fragments are formed from hydrolysis of the Ig molecule by papain. Each consists of a light chain and the V_H and C_{H1} regions of the heavy chain. The variable regions of the light and heavy chains interact, forming a specific antigen-combining site.

16. B The composition and structure of the constant region of the heavy chain determine whether that Ig will bind complement.

17. C Both IgM and surface IgA (sIgA) contain a J chain joining individual molecules together; the J chain in IgM joins five molecules, and the J chain in sIgA joins two molecules.

18. B The first antibody produced during the primary immune response to an antigen is IgM.

19. A A high titer of IgG characterizes the secondary immune response. This is a result of memory B cells that are preprogrammed to respond to a specific antigen. This eliminates some of the initial activation of naïve B cells as the sole immune response to a foreign antigen.

20. A IgG is the only Ig class that can cross the placenta. All subclasses of IgG can cross the placenta, but IgG2 crosses more slowly. This process requires recognition of the Fc region of the IgG by placental cells. These cells take up the IgG from maternal blood and secrete it into fetal blood, providing humoral immunity to the neonate for the first few months after delivery.

21. Which Ig cross-links mast cells activating the release of histamine?

A. IgG
B. IgM
C. IgA
D. IgE

Immunology/Basic principles/1

22. All the following are functions of Igs *except*:

A. Neutralizing toxic substances
B. Facilitating phagocytosis through opsonization
C. Interacting with T_C cells to lyse viruses
D. Combining with complement to destroy cellular antigens

Immunology/Basic principles/1

23. Which of the following cell surface molecules is classified as an MHC class II antigen?

A. HLA-A
B. HLA-B
C. HLA-C
D. HLA-DR

Immunology/Basic principles/1

24. Which MHC class molecule is necessary for antigen recognition by CD4-positive T cells?

A. Class I
B. Class II
C. Class III
D. No MHC molecule is necessary for antigen recognition

Immunology/Basic principles/1

25. Which of the following are products of HLA class III genes?

A. T-cell immune receptors
B. HLA-D antigens on immune cells
C. Complement proteins C2, C4, and factor B
D. Ig V_L regions

Immunology/Basic principles/1

26. What molecule on the surface of most T cells recognize antigens?

A. IgT, a four-chain molecule that includes the tau heavy chain
B. MHC protein, a two-chain molecule encoded by the HLA region
C. CD3, consisting of six different chains
D. T-cell receptor (TcR), consisting of two chains: α-chain and β-chain

Immunology/Basic principles/1

Answers to Questions 21–26

21. D IgE is the Ig that cross-links with basophils and mast cells. IgE stimulates the release of histamine and mediates an allergic immune response.

22. C T_C cells lyse virally infected cells directly, without requirement for a specific antibody. The T_C cell is activated by a viral antigen that is associated with MHC class I molecules on the surface of the infected cell. The activated T_C cell secretes several toxins, such as tumor necrosis factor, which destroy the infected cell and virions.

23. D The MHC region is located on the short arm of chromosome 6 and codes for antigens expressed on the surface of leukocytes and tissues. The MHC genes control immune recognition; their products include the antigens that determine transplant rejection.

24. B Helper T lymphocytes (CD4-positive T cells) recognize antigens only in the context of a class II molecule. Because class II antigens are expressed on macrophages, monocytes, and B cells, the helper T-cell response is mediated by interaction with processed antigen on the surface of the cells.

25. C Complement components C2 and C4 of the classic pathway and factor B of the alternate pathway are class III molecules. HLA-A, HLA-B, and HLA-C antigens are classified as class I antigens, and HLA-D, HLA-DR, HLA-DQ, and HLA-DP antigens are classified as class II antigens.

26. D T cells have a membrane-bound receptor (TcR) that is antigen specific. This two-chain molecule consists of a single α-chain, like an Ig light chain, and a single β-chain, like an Ig heavy chain. Some T cells may express a γ-δ receptor instead of the α-β molecule. There is no τ heavy chain. MHC and CD3 molecules are present on T cells, but they are not the molecules that influence antigen specificity to the cell.

27. TcR is similar to Ig molecules in that it:
- **A.** Remains bound to the cell surface and is never secreted
- **B.** Contains V and C regions on each of its chains
- **C.** Binds complement
- **D.** Can cross the placenta and provide protection to a fetus

Immunology/Basic principles/1

28. Toll-like receptors (TLRs) are found on which cells?
- **A.** T cells
- **B.** Dendritic cells
- **C.** B cells
- **D.** Large granular lymphocytes

Immunology/Basic principles/1

29. Macrophages produce the following proteins during antigen processing?
- **A.** IL-1 and IL-6
- **B.** γ-Interferon
- **C.** IL-4, IL-5, and IL-10
- **D.** Complement components C1 and C3

Immunology/Basic principles/1

30. A superantigen, such as toxic shock syndrome toxin-1 (TSST-1), bypasses the normal antigen-processing stage by binding to and cross-linking:
- **A.** A portion of an Ig molecule and complement component C1
- **B.** TLRs and an MHC class 1 molecule
- **C.** A portion of an Ig and a portion of a TcR
- **D.** A portion of a TcR and an MHC class II molecule

Immunology/Basic principles/1

31. T-regulator cells, responsible for controlling autoimmune antibody production, express which of the following phenotypes?
- **A.** CD3, CD4, CD8
- **B.** CD3, CD8, CD25
- **C.** CD3, CD4, CD25
- **D.** CD8, CD25, CD56

Immunology/Basic principles/1

32. The interaction between individual antigen and antibody molecules depends on several types of bonds, such as ionic bonds, hydrogen bonds, hydrophobic bonds, and van der Waals forces. What term describes the strength of this interaction?
- **A.** Avidity
- **B.** Affinity
- **C.** Reactivity
- **D.** Valency

Immunology/Basic principles/2

Answers to Questions 27–32

27. B The antigen-binding regions of both the α- and β-chains of the TcR are encoded by V genes that undergo rearrangement like that observed in Ig genes. The α-chain gene consists of V and J segments, like an Ig light chain. The β-chain consists of V, D, and J segments, like an Ig heavy chain. The α- and β-chains each have a single C-region gene encoding the constant region of the molecule. Although answer A is true for TcRs, it is not true for immunoglobulins that can be cell bound or secreted. Answers C and D are true for certain Ig heavy-chain isotypes but are not true for the TcR.

28. B TLRs are the primary antigen recognition proteins of the innate immune system. They are located on antigen-presenting cells, such as dendritic cells and macrophages. TLRs recognize structural motifs common to infecting organisms. TLR4, for example, recognizes bacterial lipopolysaccharide (LPS).

29. A Interleukin 1 (IL-1) and IL-6 are proinflammatory cytokines produced by macrophages. In addition to their inflammatory properties, the interleukins activate T-helper cells during antigen presentation. γ-Interferon, IL-4, IL-5, and IL-10 are all produced by T cells. Complement components are produced by a variety of cells but are not part of the macrophage antigen-presentation process.

30. D A superantigen binds to the V β-portion of the TcR and an MHC class II molecule. This binding can activate T cells without the involvement of an antigen-presenting cell. The simultaneous activation of many T cells causes a rapid cytokine release, resulting in the vascular collapse and pathology of toxic shock syndrome.

31. C T-regulator cells are believed to be the primary immune suppressor cells and express CD3, CD4, and CD25. CD25 is the IL-2 receptor. CD25 may be expressed by activated T cells but is constitutively expressed by the T-regulator cells. CD25 expression on T-regulator cells occurs in the thymus and is regulated by the FOXP3 protein.

32. B Affinity refers to the strength of a single antibody–antigen interaction. Avidity is the strength of interactions between many different antibodies against a particular antigen (i.e., the sum of many affinities).

33. Inflammation involves a variety of biochemical and cellular mediators. Which of the following may be increased within 72 hours after an initial infection?

A. Neutrophils, macrophages, antibody, complement, α_1-antitrypsin
B. Macrophages, T cells, antibody, haptoglobin, fibrinogen
C. Neutrophils, macrophages, complement, fibrinogen, C-reactive protein
D. Macrophages, T cells, B cells, ceruloplasmin, complement

Immunology/Basic principles/2

Answer to Question 33

33. C The correct list, in which *all* mediators are involved in an inflammatory response within 72 hours after the initial infection, is neutrophils, macrophages, complement, fibrinogen, and C-reactive protein. Phagocytic cells, acute phase reactants, and fibrinolytic factors enter the site of inflammation. Antibody and lymphocytes do not enter until later.

3.2

Immunologic Techniques

1. A laboratory is evaluating an enzyme-linked immunosorbent assay (ELISA) for detecting an antibody to cyclic citrullinated peptide (CCP), which is a marker for rheumatoid arthritis (RA). The laboratory includes serum from healthy volunteers and from patients with other connective tissue diseases in the evaluation. These specimens determine which factor of the assay?

A. Sensitivity
B. Precision
C. Bias
D. Specificity

Immunology/Techniques/2

2. The detection of precipitation reactions depends on the presence of optimal proportions of antigen and antibody. A patient's sample contains a large amount of antibody, but the reaction in a test system containing antigen is negative. What is the explanation for this phenomenon?

A. Performance error
B. Low specificity
C. A shift in the zone of equivalence
D. Prozone

Immunology/Techniques/3

3. The positive and negative control values for an ELISA are below the acceptable ranges. What is the most likely cause?

A. Decay of the positive and negative controls
B. Incomplete washing following specimen addition
C. Overly long incubation times
D. Decay of the antibody–enzyme conjugate

Immunology/Techniques/3

4. Which of the responses is the correct interpretation of an Ouchterlony plate that demonstrates crossed lines between wells 1 and 2 (antigen is placed in the center well and antisera in wells 1 and 2)?

A. No reaction between wells 1 and 2
B. Partial identity between wells 1 and 2
C. Nonidentity between wells 1 and 2
D. Identity between wells 1 and 2

Immunology/Techniques/2

Answers to Questions 1–4

1. D Specificity is defined as a negative result in the absence of the disease. The non-RA specimens would be expected to test negative if the assay has high specificity. Precision is the ability of the assay to repeatedly yield the same results on a single specimen. Both bias and sensitivity calculations would include specimens from RA persons. Although those specimens would be included in the evaluation, they are not listed in the question.

2. D Although performance errors and low specificity should be considered, if a test system fails to yield the expected reaction, excessive antibody preventing a precipitation reaction is usually the cause. Prozone occurs when antibody molecules saturate the antigen sites, preventing cross-linking of the antigen–antibody complexes by other antibody molecules. Because antigen and antibody do not react at equivalence, a visible product is not formed, leading to a false-negative result.

3. D The antibody–enzyme conjugate is very sensitive to storage conditions and is easy to dissociate. Control specimens are unlikely to decay, and the other options would lead to higher values.

4. C Crossed lines indicate nonidentity of the antibodies in wells 1 and 2. The antibody from well 1 recognizes a different antigenic determinant than the antibody from well 2; there is no cross-linking between the two antibodies and antigen complex.

5. A weightlifter taking many supplements is tested monthly for thyroid-stimulating hormone (TSH) in a direct capture assay, which uses a streptavidin–biotin indicator system. The individual has had normal TSH levels for the past 3 months on specimens collected in the late evening. This month the patient has a blood sample drawn right after breakfast. The TSH level is three times the patient's previous level. What is the most likely cause for the difference in TSH levels?

A. Diurnal variation in TSH levels
B. Exogenous biotin in the patient's system from a supplement taken that morning
C. Reduced thyroid function caused by an unidentified pathology
D. Pipetting error

Immunology/Techniques/3

6. What makes up the indicator system in an indirect ELISA for detecting antibody?

A. Enzyme-conjugated antibody + chromogenic substrate
B. Enzyme-conjugated antigen + chromogenic substrate
C. Enzyme + antigen
D. Substrate + antigen

Immunology/Techniques/1

7. What outcome results from improper washing of a tube or well after adding the enzyme–antibody conjugate in an ELISA system?

A. Result will be falsely decreased
B. Result will be falsely increased
C. Result will be unaffected
D. Result is impossible to determine

Immunology/Techniques/3

8. What would happen if the color reaction phase were prolonged in one tube or well of an ELISA test?

A. Result will be falsely decreased
B. Result will be falsely increased
C. Result will be unaffected
D. Impossible to determine

Immunology/Techniques/3

9. The absorbance of a sample measured by ELISA is greater than the highest standard. What corrective action should be taken?

A. Extrapolate an estimated value from the highest reading
B. Repeat the test using a standard of higher concentration
C. Repeat the assay using one half the volume of the sample
D. Dilute the test sample

Immunology/Techniques/3

Answers to Questions 5–9

5. B High levels of exogenous biotin may be present in blood up to 10 to 15 hours after ingestion and will usually cause falsely elevated values in avidin–biotin direct ELISA assays and competitive immunoassays but lower values in sandwich (immunometric) assays. Monthly variation in TSH should not approach the level seen in this situation.

6. A ELISA measures antibody by using immobilized reagent antigen. The antigen is fixed to the walls of a tube or bottom of a microtiter well. Serum is added (and incubated) and the antibody binds, if present. After washing, the antigen–antibody complexes are detected by adding an enzyme-labeled anti-immunoglobulin (anti-Ig). The unbound enzyme label is removed by washing, and the bound enzyme label is detected by adding chromogenic substrate. The enzyme catalyzes the conversion of substrate to a colored product.

7. B If unbound enzyme-conjugated anti-Ig is not washed away, it will catalyze the conversion of the substrate to a colored product, yielding a falsely elevated result.

8. B If the color reaction is not stopped within the time limits specified by the procedure, the enzyme will continue to act on the substrate, producing a falsely elevated test result.

9. D Usually, when a test sample reads at a value above the highest standard in an ELISA, the sample is diluted, and the ELISA is repeated. In those instances where no additional clinical value can be obtained by dilution, the result may be reported as greater than the highest standard (citing the upper reportable limit of the assay).

10. A patient was suspected of having a lymphoproliferative disorder. After several laboratory tests were completed, the patient was found to have an IgMκ paraprotein. In what sequence should the laboratory tests leading to this diagnosis have been performed?

A. Serum protein electrophoresis (SPE) followed by immunofixation electrophoresis (IFE)
B. Ig levels, followed by SPE
C. Total lymphocyte count, followed by Ig levels
D. Ig levels, followed by urine protein electrophoresis

Immunology/Techniques/3

11. An IFE performed on a serum sample showed a narrow dark band in the lanes containing anti-γ and anti-λ. How should this result be interpreted?

A. Abnormally decreased IgG concentration
B. Abnormal test result demonstrating monoclonal IgGλ
C. Normal test result
D. Impossible to determine without densitometric quantitation

Immunology/Techniques/2

12. Which type of nephelometry is used to measure immune complex formation almost immediately after reagent has been added?

A. Rate
B. Endpoint
C. Continuous
D. One-dimensional

Immunology/Techniques/2

13. An antinuclear antibody (ANA) test was performed by using immunofluorescence microscopy assay (IFA), and a clinically significant pattern and titer were reported. Positive and negative controls performed as expected. However, the clinical evaluation of the patient was not consistent with the reported pattern. What is the most likely explanation for this situation?

A. The clinical condition of the patient changed since the sample was tested
B. The pattern of fluorescence was misinterpreted
C. The control results were misinterpreted
D. The wrong cell line was used for the test

Immunology/Techniques/3

Answers to Questions 10–13

10. A SPE should be performed initially to detect the presence of an abnormal Ig that demonstrates restricted electrophoretic mobility. A patient producing only monoclonal light chains may not show an abnormal serum finding because the light chains may be excreted in urine. A positive finding for either serum or urine should be followed by IFE on the positive specimen. This is required to confirm the presence of monoclonal Ig and to identify the heavy and light chain types. In lymphoproliferative disorders, flow cytometry and cellular characterization are often performed.

11. B A *narrow* dark band formed in both the lane containing anti-γ and anti-λ indicates the presence of a monoclonal IgGλ. A diffuse dark band would indicate a polyclonal increase in IgG that often accompanies chronic inflammatory disorders, such as systemic lupus erythematosus (SLE).

12. A Rate nephelometry is used to measure the formation of small immune complexes as they are formed under conditions of antibody excess. The rate of increase in the photodetector output is measured within seconds or minutes, and the rate increases with increasing antigen concentration. Antigen concentration is determined by comparing the rate for the sample with that for standards by using an algorithm that compensates for nonlinearity. In endpoint nephelometry, reactions are read after equivalence. Immune complexes are of maximal size but may tend to settle out of solution, thereby decreasing the amount of scatter.

13. B In an IFA for antinuclear antibodies, the fluorescence pattern must be correlated correctly with the specificity of the antibodies. Both pathological and nonpathological antibodies can occur, and antibodies may be detected at a significant titer in a patient whose disease is inactive. Failure to correctly identify subcellular structures may result in misinterpretation of the antibody specificity or a false-positive result caused by nonspecific fluorescence.

14. What corrective action should be taken when a specific pattern cannot be identified in a specimen with a positive ANA IFA?

A. Repeat the test using a larger volume of sample
B. Call the physician
C. Have another medical laboratory scientist read the slide
D. Dilute the sample and retest

Immunology/Techniques/3

15. Which statement *best* describes passive agglutination reactions used for serodiagnosis?

A. Such agglutination reactions are more rapid because they are a single-step process
B. Reactions require the addition of a second antibody
C. Passive agglutination reactions require biphasic incubation
D. Carrier particles for antigen, such as latex particles, are used

Immunology/Techniques/2

16. What has happened in a titer if tube Nos. 5 to 7 demonstrate a stronger reaction than tube Nos. 1 to 4?

A. Prozone reaction
B. Postzone reaction
C. Equivalence reaction
D. Poor technique

Immunology/Techniques/3

17. What is the titer in tube No. 8 if tube No. 1 is undiluted and dilutions are doubled?

A. 64
B. 128
C. 256
D. 512

Immunology/Techniques/2

18. The directions for a slide agglutination test are as follows: After mixing the patient's serum and antigen-coated latex particles, the slide must be rotated for 2 minutes. What would happen if the slide is rotated for 10 minutes?

A. Possible false-positive result
B. Possible false-negative result
C. No effect
D. Depends on the amount of antibody present in the sample

Immunology/Techniques/3

19. Which outcome indicates a negative result in a complement fixation test?

A. Hemagglutination
B. Absence of hemagglutination
C. Hemolysis
D. Absence of hemolysis

Immunology/Techniques/1

Answers to Questions 14–19

14. D An unexpected pattern may indicate the presence of more than one antibody. Diluting the sample may improve visualization of the antibody specificities if each antibody is present in a different concentration and evident in different titers. If the pattern is still atypical, a new sample should be collected and the test repeated, or the specimen should be tested by an alternative method, such as ELISA or multiplex.

15. D Most agglutination tests used in serology employ passive or indirect agglutination, in which carrier particles are coated with the antigen. The carrier molecule is of sufficient size so that the reaction of the antigen with antibody results in the formation of a complex that is easily visible.

16. A In tubes Nos. 1 to 4, insufficient antigen is present to give a visible reaction because excess antibody has saturated all available antigen sites. After dilution of antibody, tubes Nos. 1 to 4 have the equivalent concentrations of antigen and antibody to allow formation of visible complexes.

17. B The antibody titer is reciprocal of the highest dilution of serum giving a positive reaction. For doubling dilutions, each tube has one half the amount of serum as the previous tube. Because the first tube was undiluted, the dilution in tube No. 8 is $(1/2)^7$ and the titer equals 2^7 or 128.

18. A Failure to follow directions, as in this case where the reaction was allowed to proceed beyond the recommended time, may result in a false-positive reading. Drying causes the clumping of latex particles in the absence of an actual positive reaction.

19. C In complement fixation, hemolysis indicates a negative test result. The absence of hemolysis indicates that complement was fixed in an antigen–antibody reaction and, therefore, the specific complement binding antibody was present in the patient's serum. Consequently, it was not available to react in the indicator system.

20. What effect does selecting the wrong gate have on the results when cells are counted by flow cytometry?
A. No effect
B. Failure to count the desired cell population
C. Falsely elevated results
D. Impossible to determine
Immunology/Techniques/3

21. Which statement *best* describes immunophenotyping?
A. Lineage determination by detecting antigens on the surface of the gated cells by using fluorescent antibodies
B. Identification of cell maturity by using antibodies to detect antigens within the nucleus
C. Identification and sorting of cells by front and side scatter of light from a laser
D. Analysis of cells collected by flow cytometry by using traditional agglutination reactions
Immunology/Techniques/2

22. A flow cytometry scattergram of a bone marrow sample identified a dense population of cells located in between normal lymphoid and normal myeloid cells. What is the most likely explanation?
A. The sample was improperly collected
B. An abnormal cell population is present
C. The laser optics are out of alignment
D. The cells are most likely not leukocytes
Immunology/Techniques/3

23. Which of the following serial dilutions contains an incorrect factor?
A. 1:4, 1:8, 1:16
B. 1:1, 1:2, 1:4
C. 1:5, 1:15, 1:45
D. 1:2, 1:6, 1:12
Immunology/Techniques/3

Answers to Questions 20–23

20. B Gating is the step performed to select the correct cells to be counted. Failure to properly perform this procedure will result in problems in isolating and counting the desired cells. It is impossible to determine whether the result would be falsely elevated or falsely lowered by problems with gating.

21. A *Immunophenotyping* refers to classification of cells (lineage and maturity assignment) with use of a panel of fluorescent-labeled antibodies directed against specific surface antigens on the cells. Antibodies are named according to the CD number. Monoclonal antibodies having a common CD number do not necessarily bind to the same epitope but recognize the same antigen on the cell surface. Reactivity of the selected cells with a panel of antibodies differentiates lymphoid cells from myeloid cells and identifies the stage of cell maturation.

22. B Lymphoid cells and myeloid cells display in predictable regions of the scatterplot because of their characteristic size and density. Lymphoid cells cause less forward scatter and side scatter from the laser compared with myeloid cells. A dense zone of cells in between those regions is caused by the presence of many abnormal cells, usually blasts. The lineage of the cells can be determined by immunophenotyping with a panel of fluorescent-labeled antibodies.

23. D All the dilutions are multiplied by the same factor in a progression except the last one: 1:2 to 1:6 is ×3, whereas 1:6 to 1:12 is ×2. Threefold dilutions of a 1:2 dilution would result in a 1:6 followed by a 1:18.

24. On January 4, an SPE on a specimen obtained at the hospital in North Dakota from a 58-year-old patient shows a band at the β–γ junction. The specimen was also positive for RF. The laboratorian recommends that an immunofixation test be performed to determine whether the band represents a monoclonal Ig. Another specimen is obtained 2 weeks later by the provider in the clinic 30 miles away, and whole blood is submitted to the laboratory for IFE. The courier placed the whole blood specimen in an ice chest for transport. In this specimen, no β–γ band is seen in the serum protein lane, and the IgM lane is very faint. The RF on this specimen was negative. What is the explanation for the results?

A. Nothing went wrong in the laboratory; the patient had an infection 2 weeks ago and it is no longer present

B. Something went wrong in the laboratory—one of the specimens was likely mislabeled, requiring a new specimen, and retest the new specimen

C. The laboratory needs to run a second specimen after 2-mercaptoethanol treatment, which will eliminate IgM aggregates and allow for more sensitive monoclonal IgM detection

D. The sample requires a redraw from the patient, and this time, separate the serum from the clot in the provider's office before placing the specimen on ice and sending it to the laboratory by courier

Immunology/Techniques/3

25. The laboratorian is evaluating an ELISA assay as a replacement for the IFA ANA test. The laboratorian tests 50 specimens in duplicate on each assay. The ELISA assay uses a human epithelial type 2 (HEp-2) extract as an antigen source. The correlation between the ELISA and IFA tests is only 60% (30 of 50 specimens agree). Which of the following is the next *best* course of action?

A. Test another 50 specimens

B. Perform a competency check on the medical laboratory scientists who performed the tests

C. Order a new lot of both kits and then retest the new lots

D. Refer the discrepant specimens for testing by another method

Immunology/Techniques/3

Answers to Questions 24–25

24. D The most likely cause of the discrepant results is the presence of a type II cryoglobulin. This is a monoclonal RF. The protein likely precipitated during the courier ride and was, thus, in the clot when the laboratory separated the serum.

25. D In this situation, the laboratorian has already tested the specimens in duplicate. Testing an additional 50 specimens will not change the fact that there are 20 discrepant specimens. The best course of action is to determine what antibodies are present in these specimens. Then, determine whether ELISA or IFA is a better procedure for detecting the most clinically relevant antibodies. The laboratory professional could perform clinical chart reviews as an alternative but obtaining that data would be difficult and much of it may be subjective.

3.3
Infectious Disease Methods

1. Which serum antibody response usually characterizes the primary (early) stage of syphilis?
A. Antibodies against syphilis are undetectable
B. Detected 1 to 3 weeks after appearance of the primary chancre
C. Detected in 50% of cases before the primary chancre disappears
D. Detected within 2 weeks after infection
Immunology/Infectious disease methods/Syphilis/1

2. What substance is detected in the sample by the rapid plasma reagin (RPR) and Venereal Disease Research Laboratory (VDRL) tests for syphilis?
A. Cardiolipin
B. Anticardiolipin antibody (ACA)
C. Anti–*Treponema pallidum* antibody
D. *T. pallidum*
Immunology/Infectious disease methods/Syphilis/1

3. What type of antigen is used in the RPR test?
A. Live treponemal organisms
B. Killed suspension of treponemal organisms
C. Cardiolipin
D. Tanned sheep cells
Immunology/Infectious disease methods/Syphilis/1

4. Which of the following is the most sensitive test to detect congenital syphilis?
A. VDRL
B. RPR
C. *T. pallidum* particle agglutination (TP-PA)
D. Polymerase chain reaction (PCR)
Immunology/Infectious disease methods/Syphilis/1

5. A biological false-positive reaction is *least* likely with which test for syphilis?
A. VDRL
B. TP-PA
C. RPR
D. All are equally likely to yield a false-positive result
Immunology/Infectious disease methods/Syphilis/2

6. A 12-year-old patient has symptoms of fatigue and localized lymphadenopathy. Laboratory tests reveal peripheral blood lymphocytosis, positive RPR, and positive spot test for infectious mononucleosis (IM). What test should be performed next?
A. HIV screen
B. VDRL
C. Epstein-Barr virus (EBV)–specific antigen test
D. TP-PA test
Immunology/Infectious disease methods/3

Answers to Questions 1–6

1. B During the primary stage of syphilis, about 90% of patients develop antibodies between 1 and 3 weeks after the appearance of the primary chancre.

2. B *Reagin* is a nontreponemal antibody that appears in the serum of individuals with syphilis and is detected by the RPR and VDRL assays. Reagin reacts with cardiolipin, a lipid-rich extract of beef heart and other animal tissues.

3. C Cardiolipin is extracted from animal tissues, such as beef hearts, and attached to carbon particles. In the presence of reagin, the particles will agglutinate.

4. D PCR will amplify a very small amount of DNA from *T. pallidum* and allow for the detection of the organism in the infant. Antibody tests, such as VDRL and RPR, may detect maternal antibody only and do not indicate whether the infant has been infected.

5. B The TP-PA test is more specific for *T. pallidum* compared with nontreponemal tests, such as the VDRL and RPR tests, and would be the least likely to yield a biological false-positive result. Nontreponemal tests have a biologically false-positive rate of 1% to 10%, depending on the patient population tested. False-positive findings are caused commonly by infectious mononucleosis (IM), SLE, viral hepatitis, and human immunodeficiency virus (HIV) infection.

6. D The patient's symptoms are nonspecific and could be attributed to many potential causes. However, the patient's age, lymphocytosis, and serological results point to IM. The rapid spot test for antibodies seen in IM is highly specific. The EBV-specific antigen test is more sensitive but is unnecessary when the spot test is positive.

7. Which test is most likely to be positive in the tertiary stage of syphilis?

A. Treponemal-specific antibody
B. RPR
C. VDRL
D. Reagin screen test (RST)

Immunology/Infectious disease methods/Syphilis/3

8. What is the most likely interpretation of the following syphilis serological results?

RPR: reactive; TP-PA: nonreactive

A. Neurosyphilis
B. Secondary syphilis
C. Syphilis that has been successfully treated
D. Biological false positive

Immunology/Infectious disease methods/Syphilis/2

9. Which specimen is recommended to evaluate latent or tertiary syphilis?

A. Serum sample
B. Chancre fluid
C. Cerebrospinal fluid (CSF)
D. Joint fluid

Immunology/Infectious disease methods/Syphilis/1

10. Interpret the following quantitative RPR test results.

RPR titer: weakly reactive—1:4; reactive—1:8 to 1:64

A. Excess antibody, prozone effect
B. Excess antigen, postzone effect
C. Equivalence of antigen and antibody
D. Impossible to interpret; testing error

Immunology/Infectious disease methods/Syphilis/3

11. Tests to identify infection with HIV fall into which three general types of tests?

A. Tissue culture, antigen, and antibody tests
B. Tests for antigens, antibodies, and nucleic acid
C. DNA probe, DNA amplification, and Western blot tests
D. ELISA, Western blot, and Southern blot tests

Immunology/Infectious disease methods/HIV/1

12. Which tests are considered screening tests for HIV?

A. ELISA, chemiluminescent, and rapid antibody tests
B. IFA, Western blot, radioimmunoprecipitation assay
C. Culture, antigen capture assay, DNA amplification
D. Reverse transcriptase and messenger RNA (mRNA) assay

Immunology/Infectious disease methods/HIV/1

13. Which tests are the recommended confirmatory tests for HIV?

A. ELISA and rapid antibody tests
B. HIV-1,2 antibody differentiation assays and qualitative PCR test
C. Culture, antigen capture assay, quantitative PCR
D. Reverse transcriptase and mRNA assay

Immunology/Infectious disease methods/HIV/1

Answers to Questions 7–13

7. A A treponemal-specific antibody test is more likely to be positive compared with a nontreponemal test in the tertiary stage of syphilis. In some cases, systemic lesions have subsided by the tertiary stage, and the nontreponemal tests become seronegative. Although the treponemal-specific antibody test is the most sensitive test for tertiary syphilis, it will be positive in both treated and untreated cases.

8. D A positive reaction with nontreponemal antigen and a negative reaction with a treponemal antigen is most likely caused by a biological false-positive non-treponemal test result.

9. C Latent syphilis usually begins after the second year of untreated infection. In some cases, the serological tests become negative. However, if neurosyphilis is present, CSF serology will be positive, and the CSF will display increased protein and pleocytosis characteristic of central nervous system infection.

10. A This patient may be in the secondary stage of syphilis and is producing large amounts of antibody to *T. pallidum* sufficient to cause a prozone reaction because of antibody excess in the test. The test became strongly reactive only after the antibody was diluted.

11. B The three types of screening tests for HIV include antibody tests, antigen–antibody combination tests, and nucleic acid methods.

12. A The fourth- and fifth-generation HIV assays detect both antibody and the p24 antigen. These assays are available in ELISA, automated chemiluminescent systems, multiplex systems, and in a rapid card format.

13. B The current HIV testing algorithm begins with a screening assay, followed by an HIV-1,2 antibody differentiation assay (HIV-1,2 supplemental assay); if those results are discordant, an HIV qualitative PCR assay is performed. Western blot is no longer included in this algorithm.

14. How do fourth- and fifth-generation HIV tests reduce the time from infection to the test becoming positive?

A. They are PCR tests detecting viral RNA
B. They detect p24 antigen in addition to HIV antibody
C. They detect proviral DNA
D. They detect antibodies to more antigens than earlier generations of HIV tests

Immunology/Infectious disease methods/HIV/2

15. A female who has had five pregnancies subsequently tests positive for HIV on a fourth-generation assay and is negative on an HIV-1,2 differentiation assay and a follow-up molecular assay. The initial reactivity may be caused by:

A. Possible cross reaction with herpes or EBV antibodies
B. Interference from medication
C. Cross-reacting antibodies elicited during pregnancy
D. Possible technical error; a repeat specimen should be requested

Immunology/Infectious disease methods/HIV/3

16. Interpret the following results for HIV testing:

Fourth-generation ELISA: positive; repeat ELISA: positive; HIV 1,2 antibody differentiation assay: negative; qualitative HIV RNA rtPCR assay: positive

A. False-positive fourth-generation assay
B. False-negative antibody differentiation assay
C. Indeterminate; further testing indicated
D. HIV p24 antigen detected on fourth-generation ELISA

Immunology/Infectious disease methods/HIV/3

17. What is the most likely explanation when antibody tests for HIV are negative, but the PCR test is positive?

A. Probably not HIV infection
B. Patient is in the "window phase" before antibody production
C. Tests were performed incorrectly
D. Clinical signs may be misinterpreted

Immunology/Infectious disease methods/HIV/3

18. What criteria constitute the classification system for HIV infection?

A. CD4-positive T-cell count and clinical symptoms
B. Clinical symptoms, condition, duration, and strength of reactivity on a fourth-generation HIV test
C. Presence or absence of lymphadenopathy
D. Strong fourth-generation HIV test reactivity and CD8-positive T-cell count

Immunology/Infectious disease methods/HIV/2

Answers to Questions 14–18

14. B Including the p24 antigen in the fourth- and fifth-generation tests allows for the detection of HIV infection approximately 1 week earlier compared with the third-generation antibody-only assays and up to 3 weeks earlier compared with Western blot. Western blot is no longer a recommended test in the diagnostic algorithm.

15. C Pregnancy is a common cause of false-positive HIV screening results.

16. D The fourth-generation HIV assay detects antibody and the p24 antigen but does not differentiate between those results. In this case, the antibody-confirming test is negative, suggesting the initial reactive fourth-generation test result is either a false positive or is caused by the presence of p24 in the specimen. The positive molecular assay confirms the presence of the virus in the specimen. This usually occurs in early infection, prior to antibody being produced.

17. B In early seroconversion, patients may not be making antibodies in sufficient amounts to be detected by antibody tests. The period between infection with HIV and the appearance of detectable antibodies is called the *window phase*. This period has been reduced to a few weeks by antibody and antigen-detecting fourth- and fifth-generation assays and an algorithm that includes PCR testing.

18. A The classification (not diagnostic) system for HIV infection is based on a combination of CD4-positive T-cell count (helper T cells) and various categories of clinical symptoms. Classification is important in determining treatment options and the progression of the disease.

19. What is the main difficulty associated with the development of an HIV vaccine?
A. The virus has been difficult to culture; antigen extraction and concentration are extremely laborious
B. Human trials cannot be performed
C. Different strains of the virus are genetically diverse
D. Anti-idiotype antibodies cannot be developed
Immunology/Infectious disease methods/HIV/2

20. Which CD4:CD8 ratio is most likely in a patient with acquired immunodeficiency syndrome (AIDS)?
A. 2:1
B. 3:1
C. 2:3
D. 1:3
Immunology/Infectious disease methods/HIV/2

21. What is the advantage of fourth-generation rapid HIV tests over earlier rapid HIV tests?
A. They use recombinant antigens
B. They detect multiple strains of HIV
C. They detect p24 antigen
D. They are quantitative
Immunology/Infectious disease methods/HIV/2

22. Which method is used to diagnose an HIV infection in infants who are born to HIV-positive mothers?
A. ELISA
B. Western blot test
C. PCR test
D. Viral culture
Immunology/Infectious disease methods/HIV/2

23. What is the most likely cause when a fourth-generation HIV assay is positive for all controls and samples?
A. Improper pipetting
B. Improper washing
C. Improper addition of sample
D. Improper reading
Immunology/Infectious disease methods/HIV/3

24. All the following results indicate a diagnosis of acute viral hepatitis, *except*:
A. Abnormal test results for liver enzymes
B. Clinical signs and symptoms
C. Positive results for hepatitis markers
D. Total anti-HAV (IgM and IgG)
Immunology/Infectious disease methods/Hepatitis/2

Answers to Questions 19–24

19. C Vaccine development has been difficult primarily because of the genetic diversity among different strains of the virus, and new strains are constantly emerging. HIV-1 can be divided into two main subtypes designated M (for main) and O (for outlier). The M group is further divided into nine subgroups, designated A through K (there is no E or I subgroup), based on differences in the nucleotide sequence of the *gag* gene. Two remaining subtypes are designated N (non-M and non-O) and P (a subtype related to SIVgor). In addition, different subtypes can combine to form new recombinant viruses. A vaccine that is effective for all the subgroups and circulating recombinant forms is yet to be developed.

20. D An inverted CD4:CD8 ratio (less than 1.0) is a common finding in a patient with AIDS. The Centers for Disease Control and Prevention (CDC) requires a CD4-positive (helper T) cell count of less than 200/μL or 14% in the absence of an AIDS-defining illness in the case surveillance definition of AIDS.

21. C Both third-generation and fourth-generation rapid tests for HIV use recombinant and synthetic HIV antigens conjugated to a solid phase. The multivalent nature of these tests allows for detection of less common subgroups of HIV-1 and simultaneous detection of both HIV-1 and HIV-2. However, the fourth-generation assays also use solid-phase antibodies to p24 antigen to detect its presence. Because p24 antigen appears before antibodies to HIV, fourth-generation tests can detect infection 4 to 7 days earlier compared with tests based on antibody detection alone.

22. C Fourth- and fifth-generation ELISA and chemiluminescent assays reflect the presence of maternal antibody. The PCR test uses small amounts of blood and does not rely on the antibody response. PCR amplifies small amounts of viral nucleic acid and can detect less than 20 copies of viral RNA per milliliter of plasma. These qualities make PCR ideal for the testing of infants. Nucleic acid methods for HIV RNA include both qualitative (for diagnosis) and quantitative (for monitoring) reverse-transcriptase real-time PCR (RT-PCR) assays.

23. B Improper washing may not remove unbound, enzyme-conjugated anti-human Ig, and every sample may appear positive.

24. D To diagnose a case of hepatitis, the physician must consider clinical signs as well as the results of laboratory tests that measure liver enzymes and hepatitis markers. However, a combined test for hepatitis A IgM and IgG is not useful to diagnose acute hepatitis. A test for IgM antibodies to hepatitis A virus (anti-HAV) is recommended in symptomatic patients.

25. Which of the following statements regarding infection with hepatitis D virus (HDV) is true?
A. Occurs in patients with HIV infection
B. Does not progress to chronic hepatitis
C. Occurs in patients with hepatitis B virus (HBV) infection
D. Is not spread through blood or sexual contact
Immunology/Infectious disease methods/Hepatitis/1

26. All the following hepatitis viruses are spread through blood or blood products *except*:
A. Hepatitis A virus (HAV)
B. HBV
C. Hepatitis C virus (HCV)
D. HDV
Immunology/Infectious disease methods/Hepatitis/1

27. Which hepatitis B marker is the *best* indicator of early acute infection?
A. Hepatitis B surface antigen (HBsAg)
B. Hepatitis B e-antigen (HBeAg)
C. Hepatitis B core antibody (anti-HBc)
D. Hepatitis B surface antibody (anti-HBs)
Immunology/Infectious disease methods/Hepatitis/2

28. Which is the first antibody detected in serum after infection with HBV?
A. Anti-HBs
B. Anti-HBc IgM
C. Anti-HBe
D. All are detectable at the same time
Immunology/Infectious disease methods/Hepatitis/2

29. Which antibody persists in low-level carriers of HBV?
A. IgM anti-HBc
B. IgG anti-HBc
C. IgM anti-HBe
D. IgG anti-HBs
Immunology/Infectious disease methods/Hepatitis/2

30. What is the most likely explanation when a patient has clinical signs of viral hepatitis but tests negative for HAV IgM, HBsAg, and HCV antibody?
A. Tests were performed improperly
B. The patient does not have hepatitis
C. The patient may be in the "core window"
D. Clinical evaluation was performed improperly
Immunology/Infectious disease methods/Hepatitis/3

31. Which hepatitis B markers should be performed on blood products?
A. HBsAg and anti-HBc
B. Anti-HBs and anti-HBc
C. HBeAg and HBcAg
D. Anti-HBs and HBeAg
Immunology/Infectious disease methods/Hepatitis/1

Answers to Questions 25–31

25. C HDV is an RNA virus that requires the surface antigen or envelope of the HBV for entry into the hepatocyte. Consequently, HDV can infect only patients who are coinfected with hepatitis B.

26. A HAV is spread through the fecal–oral route and is the cause of infectious hepatitis. HAV has a shorter incubation period (2–7 weeks) than HBV (1–6 months). Epidemics of HAV can occur, especially when food and water become contaminated with raw sewage.

27. A HBsAg is the first marker to appear in HBV infection. It is usually detected within 4 weeks of exposure (prior to the rise in transaminases) and persists for about 3 months after serum enzyme levels return to normal.

28. B Antibody to the hepatitis B core antigen (anti-HBc) is the first detectable hepatitis B antibody. It persists in serum for years after infection and is found in the serum of asymptomatic carriers of HBV. Because levels of total anti-HBc are high after recovery, IgM anti-HBc is a more useful marker for acute infection. Both anti-HBc and anti-HBs can persist for life, but only anti-HBs is considered protective.

29. B IgG anti-HBc can be detected in carriers who are HBsAg and anti-HBs negative. These individuals are hepatitis B DNA positive also and, thus, are presumed infective, even though the level of HBsAg is too low to detect. No specific B core IgG test is available, however. This patient would be positive in the anti-B core total antibody assay and negative in the anti-HB core IgM test.

30. C The patient may be in the "core window," the period of HBV infection when both the surface antigen and surface antibody are undetectable. The IgM anti-HBc and the anti-HBc total antibody assays, along with the hepatitis B DNA PCR assay, would be the only detectable markers in the serum of a patient in the core window phase of HBV infection.

31. A Blood products that consist of different components derived from whole blood are tested for HBsAg, an early indicator of infection, and anti-HBc, a marker that may persist for life. Following recovery from HBV infection, some patients demonstrate negative serology for HBsAg and anti-HBs but are positive for anti-HBc. Such patients are considered infective.

32. Which hepatitis antibody confers immunity against reinfection with HBV?
A. Anti-HBc IgM
B. Anti-HBc IgG
C. Anti-HBe
D. Anti-HBs

Immunology/Infectious disease methods/Hepatitis/1

33. Which test, other than serological markers, is most consistently elevated in viral hepatitis?
A. Antinuclear antibodies
B. Alanine aminotransferase (ALT)
C. Absolute lymphocyte count
D. Lactate dehydrogenase

Immunology/Infectious disease methods/Hepatitis/2

34. If only anti-HBs is positive, which of the following can be ruled out?
A. HBV vaccination
B. Distant past infection with HBV
C. Hepatitis B immune globulin (HBIG) injection
D. Chronic HBV infection

Immunology/Infectious disease methods/Hepatitis/2

35. Interpret the following results for EBV infection: IgG and IgM antibodies to viral capsid antigen (VCA) are positive.
A. Infection in the past
B. Infection with a mutual enhancer virus, such as HIV
C. Current infection
D. Impossible to interpret; need more information

Immunology/Infectious disease methods/EBV/3

36. Rapid mono tests use latex particles coated with which of the following?
A. Guinea pig antigen
B. Beef proteins
C. Horse proteins
D. Sheep proteins

Immunology/Infectious disease methods/EBV/1

37. Blood products are tested for which virus before being transfused to newborns?
A. EBV
B. Human T-lymphotropic virus II (HTLV-II)
C. Cytomegalovirus (CMV)
D. HDV

Immunology/Infectious disease methods/1

38. What is the endpoint for the antistreptolysin O (ASO) latex agglutination assay?
A. Highest serum dilution that shows no agglutination
B. Highest serum dilution that shows agglutination
C. Lowest serum dilution that shows agglutination
D. Lowest serum dilution that shows no agglutination

Immunology/Infectious disease methods/Streptococcus/2

Answers to Questions 32–38

32. D Anti-HBs appears later in infection compared with anti-HBc and is used as a marker for immunity after infection or vaccination, rather than for diagnosis of current infection.

33. B Alanine transaminase (ALT) is a liver enzyme and may be increased in hepatic disease. Highest levels occur in acute viral hepatitis, reaching 20 to 50 times the upper limit of normal.

34. D Individuals with chronic HBV infection show a positive test result for anti-HBc (IgG or total) and HBsAg but not anti-HBs. Patients with active chronic hepatitis have not become immune to the virus.

35. C IgM and IgG antibodies to VCA are found in a current infection with EBV. The IgG antibody may persist for life, but the IgM anti-VCA disappears within 4 months after the infection resolves.

36. B Rapid mono tests detect a heterophile antibody directed against beef proteins. Although these antibodies may also react with horse or sheep red blood cells (RBCs), those proteins are not used in these tests.

37. C CMV can be life threatening if transmitted to a newborn through a blood product. HTLV-II is a rare virus, which, like HIV, is a T-cell tropic RNA retrovirus. The virus has been associated with hairy cell leukemia, but this is not a consistent finding.

38. B The latex test for ASO includes latex particles coated with streptolysin O. Serial dilutions are prepared and the highest dilution showing agglutination is the endpoint.

39. A patient with clinical signs of streptococcal pharyngitis tested negative with the streptozyme test. What is the correct follow-up serological test for this patient?

A. Either ASO or anti-deoxyribonuclease B (anti-DNase B) test
B. Another streptozyme test using diluted serum
C. Antihyaluronidase test
D. Wait for 3 to 5 days and repeat the streptozyme test

Immunology/Infectious disease methods/Streptococcus/3

40. Rapid assays for influenza that utilize specimens obtained from nasopharyngeal swabs detect:

A. IgM anti-influenza
B. IgA anti-influenza
C. IgA–influenza antigen immune complexes
D. Influenza nucleoprotein antigens

Immunology/Infectious disease methods/Influenza/2

41. How can interfering cold agglutinins be removed from a test sample?

A. Centrifuge the serum and remove the top layer
B. Incubate the clot at 1°C to 4°C for several hours and then remove the serum
C. Incubate the serum at 56°C in a water bath for 30 minutes
D. Use an anticoagulated sample

Immunology/Infectious disease methods/Cold agglutinins/2

42. All tubes (dilutions) except the negative control are positive for cold agglutinins. This indicates:

A. Contaminated RBCs
B. A rare antibody against RBC antigens
C. The sample was stored at 4°C prior to separating serum and cells
D. Further serial dilution is necessary

Immunology/Infectious disease methods/Cold agglutinins/3

43. All positive cold agglutinin tubes remain positive after 37°C incubation except the positive control. What is the most likely explanation for this result?

A. High-titer cold agglutinins
B. Contamination of the test system
C. Antibody other than cold agglutinins
D. Faulty water bath

Immunology/Infectious disease methods/Cold agglutinins/3

44. Which increase in antibody titer (dilution) *best* indicates an acute infection?

A. From 1:2 to 1:8
B. From 1:4 to 1:16
C. From 1:16 to 1:256
D. From 1:64 to 1:128

Immunology/Infectious disease methods/2

Answers to Questions 39–44

39. A The streptozyme test is used for screening and contains several of the antigens associated with streptococcal products. Because some patients produce an antibody response to a limited number of streptococcal products, no single test is sufficiently sensitive to rule out infection. Clinical sensitivity is increased by performing additional tests when initial results are negative. The streptozyme test generally yields more false-positive and false-negative results compared with the ASO and anti-DNase B tests. A positive result occurs in a smaller number of patients with recent streptococcal infections in the antihyaluronidase test compared with the ASO and anti-DNase B tests.

40. D The rapid influenza assays are antigen detection methods. The tests contain the nucleoprotein antigens for influenza A and B. They are designed to detect early infections, before antibody is produced.

41. B Cold agglutinins will attach to autologous RBCs if incubated at 1°C to 4°C. The absorbed serum will be free of cold agglutinins.

42. D Cold agglutinins may be measured in patients who have cold agglutinin disease, that is, cold autoimmune hemolytic anemia. In such cases, titers can be as high as 10^6. If all tubes (dilutions) for cold agglutinins are positive, except the negative control, then a high titer of cold agglutinins is present in the sample. Further serial dilutions should be performed.

43. C Cold agglutinins do not remain reactive above 30°C, and agglutination must disperse after incubation at 37°C. The most likely explanation when agglutination remains after 37°C incubation is that a warm alloantibody or autoantibody is present.

44. C A fourfold (two-tube) or greater increase in antibody titer is usually indicative of an acute infection. Although answers A and B show a fourfold rise in titer, answer C shows a 16-fold rise in titer and is the most definitive. In most serological tests, a single high titer is insufficient evidence of acute infection unless specific IgM antibodies are measured because age, individual variation, immunologic status, and history of previous exposure (or vaccination) cause a wide variation in normal serum antibody titers.

45. Which of the following positive antibody tests may be an indication of recent vaccination or early primary infection for rubella in a patient with no clinical symptoms?
A. Only IgG antibodies positive
B. Only IgM antibodies positive
C. Both IgG and IgM antibodies positive
D. Fourfold rise in titer for IgG antibodies

Immunology/Infectious disease methods/Rubella/2

46. Why is laboratory diagnosis difficult in cases of Lyme disease?
A. Clinical response may not be apparent upon initial infection; IgM antibody may not be detected until 3 to 6 weeks after the infection
B. Laboratory tests may be designed to detect whole *Borrelia burgdorferi*, not flagellar antigen found early in infection
C. Most laboratory tests are technically demanding and lack specificity
D. Antibodies formed initially to *B. burgdorferi* may cross-react in antigen tests for autoimmune diseases

Immunology/Infectious disease methods/Borrelia burgdorferi/2

47. Serological tests for which disease may give a false-positive result if the patient has Lyme disease?
A. HIV
B. Syphilis
C. EBV
D. Hepatitis C

Immunology/Infectious disease methods/2

48. In monitoring a patient with HIV infection, which parameter may be expected to be the most sensitive indicator of the effectiveness of antiretroviral treatment?
A. HIV antibody titer
B. CD4:CD8 ratio
C. HIV viral load
D. Absolute total T-cell count

Immunology/Infectious disease methods/HIV/2

49. A renal transplant recipient is found to have a rising creatinine level and reduced urine output. The physician orders a "urine PCR" assay. What infectious disease is the potential etiological agent responsible for this reaction?
A. HCV
B. *Legionella pneumophila*
C. EBV
D. BK virus

Immunology/Infectious disease methods/2

50. A newborn is to be tested for vertically transmitted HIV infection. Which of the following tests is most useful?
A. HIV PCR
B. CD4 count
C. Rapid HIV antibody test
D. HIV IgM antibody test

Immunology/Infectious disease methods/HIV/2

Answers to Questions 45–50

45. B If only IgM antibodies are positive, this result indicates recent vaccination or early primary infection.

46. A Lyme disease is caused by *B. burgdorferi*, a spirochete, and typical clinical symptoms, such as rash or erythema chronicum migrans, may be absent in some infected individuals. Additionally, IgM antibody is not detectable by laboratory tests until 3 to 6 weeks after a tick bite, and IgG antibody develops later.

47. B Lyme disease is caused by a spirochete, and positive results may occur with some specific treponemal antibody tests for syphilis.

48. C The HIV viral load will rise or fall in response to treatment more quickly compared with any of the other listed parameters. The absolute CD4 count is also an indicator of treatment effectiveness and is used in resource-poor areas that might not have facilities for molecular testing. Note, however, that the absolute CD4 count is not one of the choices.

49. D BK virus is a polyomavirus that can cause renal and urinary tract infections. The virus is an opportunistic pathogen and has become a well-recognized cause of poor renal function in kidney transplant recipients.

50. A Neonatal HIV diagnosis is performed by screening for the presence of the virus nucleic acid. The current antibody tests are either an IgG-specific assay or an IgG/IgM combination assay. Thus, an infant whose mother is HIV positive will also be positive in the HIV antibody assay. Although the CD4 count may be a useful assay to determine disease activity, there are many causes of reduced CD4 numbers, so this assay should not be used to diagnose HIV infection.

51. Which of the following fungal organisms is *best* diagnosed by an antigen detection test as opposed to an antibody detection assay?
A. *Histoplasma*
B. *Cryptococcus*
C. *Candida*
D. *Aspergillus*

Immunology/Infectious disease methods/Mycology/2

52. The cytology laboratory refers a Papanicolaou smear specimen to the laboratory for an assay designed to detect the presence of a virus associated with cervical cancer. What test should be performed?
A. An ELISA for anti-human simplex virus 2 (anti-HSV-2) antibodies
B. A molecular assay for HSV-2
C. An ELISA for human papillomavirus (HPV) antibodies
D. A molecular assay for HPV

Immunology/Infectious disease methods/2

53. An immunosuppressed patient has unexplained anemia. The provider suspects a parvovirus B19 infection. The parvovirus IgM test result is negative. The next course of action is:
A. The patient does not have parvovirus
B. A convalescent specimen is recommended in 4 weeks to determine if a fourfold rise in titer has occurred
C. A parvovirus PCR is recommended
D. A recent transfusion for the patient's anemia may have resulted in a false-negative result and the patient should be retested in 4 weeks

Immunology/Infectious disease methods/Parvovirus/2

54. A patient was tested for syphilis by the RPR method and was reactive. A TP-PA test was performed, and the result was negative. Subsequent testing showed the patient to have a high titer of anticardiolipin antibodies (ACAs) by the ELISA method. Which routine laboratory test is most likely to be abnormal for this patient?
A. Activated partial thromboplastin time (aPTT)
B. Anti–smooth muscle antibodies
C. Aspartate aminotransferase (AST)
D. C3 assay by immunonephelometry

Immunology/Infectious disease methods/Syphilis/3

Answers to Questions 51–54

51. B The *Cryptococcus* antibody response is not a reliable indicator of a current infection; thus, an antigen assay is normally used to monitor the disease. The antigen assay may be used for serum or CSF and will decline in response to treatment much faster than a traditional antibody test. A urinary antigen test is available for histoplasmosis, and a serum galactomannan assay is available for *Aspergillus*. The two assays perform better than antibody detection. No antigen test is available for *Candida*, and thus, antibody detection is the best serological procedure for this organism.

52. D Cervical cell atypia and cervical cancer are associated with specific high-risk serotypes of HPV infections. Although HPV antibody assays are available, they are not serotype specific, nor do they relate to disease activity. Thus, molecular probe assays are the tests of choice to detect high-risk HPV infection. Although HSV-2 is associated with genital herpesvirus, that virus has not been shown to cause cervical cancer.

53. C A negative IgM assay rarely rules out an infection. Although a convalescent specimen may be useful in many cases, in an immunosuppressed patient the convalescent specimen may remain negative in the presence of an infection. Thus, a parvovirus PCR test is the preferred choice in this case. A false-negative result could be caused by multiple whole blood or plasma transfusions, but retesting for an antibody a month later would not be beneficial to the patient.

54. A Approximately 50% to 70% of patients with ACAs also have the lupus anticoagulant (LAC) in their serum. LAC is an Ig that interferes with the in vitro coagulation tests: prothrombin time (PT), aPTT, and dilute Russell viper venom (DRVV) time. The tests require phospholipid for the activation of factor X. About 30% of patients with antibodies to cardiolipin or phospholipids have a biologically false-positive RPR result. Anti–smooth muscle antibodies are commonly associated with chronic active hepatitis, and increased AST with necrotic liver diseases. Although ACA and LAC may be associated with SLE, many patients with these antibodies do not have SLE and would have a normal C3 level.

55. A 54-year-old individual was admitted to the hospital after having a seizure. Many laboratory tests were performed, including an RPR, but none of the results were positive. The provider suspects a case of late (tertiary) syphilis. Which test should be performed next?

A. Repeat RPR, followed by VDRL
B. Treponemal test, such as TP-PA on serum
C. VDRL on CSF
D. No laboratory test is positive for late (tertiary) syphilis

Immunology/Infectious disease methods/Syphilis/3

56. A patient presented at the clinic complaining of a rash, severe headaches, stiff neck, and sleep problems. Laboratory tests of significance include an elevated sedimentation rate (ESR) and slightly increased liver enzymes. Further questioning of the patient revealed that they had returned from a hunting trip in upstate New York 4 weeks ago. The provider ordered a serological test for Lyme disease, and the assay was negative. What is the most likely explanation for these results?

A. The antibody response is not sufficient to be detected at this stage
B. The clinical symptoms and laboratory results are not characteristic of Lyme disease
C. The patient is likely to have early-stage HBV infection
D. Laboratory error has caused a false-negative result

Immunology/Infectious disease methods/3

57. A 19-year-old presented at the clinic complaining of a sore throat and fatigue. Upon physical examination, lymphadenopathy was noted. Reactive lymphocytes were noted on the differential, but a rapid test for antibodies to IM was negative. Liver enzymes were only slightly elevated. What test(s) should be ordered next?

A. Hepatitis testing
B. EBV serological panel
C. HIV confirmatory testing
D. Bone marrow biopsy

Immunology/Infectious disease methods/3

58. A patient received 2 units of RBCs following surgery. Two weeks after the surgery, the patient was seen by a provider and was found to have mild jaundice and slightly elevated liver enzymes. Hepatitis testing, however, was negative. What follow-up is recommended?

A. Nothing until more severe or definitive clinical signs develop
B. Repeat hepatitis testing immediately
C. Repeat hepatitis testing in a few weeks
D. Check blood bank donor records and contact donor(s) of transfused units

Immunology/Infectious disease methods/Hepatitis/3

Answers to Questions 55–58

55. B Serum antibody tests, such as RPR and VDRL, are often negative in cases of late syphilis. However, treponemal tests remain positive in greater than 95% of cases. The VDRL test on CSF is the most specific test for diagnosis of neurosyphilis because treponemal test results remain positive after treatment. It should be used as the confirmatory test when the serum treponemal test result is positive. However, the CSF VDRL is limited in sensitivity and would not be positive if the serum treponemal-specific antibody test was negative.

56. A The antibody response to *B. burgdorferi* may not develop until several weeks after initial infection. The antibody test should be repeated 2 to 4 weeks later. To confirm a positive EIA, samples that initially test positive or equivocal (indeterminate) should be retested using a second enzyme immunoassay or immunoblot method. Regardless of the laboratory results, if the provider suspects Lyme disease, treatment should begin immediately.

57. B An EBV serological panel would give a more accurate assessment than a rapid slide IM test. The time of appearance of the various antibodies to the viral antigens differs according to the clinical course of the infection.

58. C The level of HBsAg may not have reached detectable levels, and antibodies to HBc and HCV would not have yet developed. Waiting 1 or 2 weeks and repeating the tests may reveal evidence of hepatitis virus infection.

59. A hospital employee received the final dose of the hepatitis B vaccine 3 weeks ago. The employee wants to donate blood. Which of the following results are expected from the hepatitis screen, and will the employee be allowed to donate blood?

A. HBsAg, positive; anti-HBc, negative—they may donate
B. HBsAg, negative; anti-HBc, positive—they may not donate
C. HBsAg, positive; anti-HBc, positive—they may not donate
D. HBsAg, negative; anti-HBc, negative—they may donate

Immunology/Infectious disease methods/Hepatitis/3

60. A pregnant female presented with a maculopapular rash on the face and neck with a temperature was 37.7°C. Rubella tests for both IgG and IgM antibody were positive. What positive test(s) would reveal a diagnosis of congenital rubella syndrome in the baby after birth?

A. Positive rubella tests for both IgG and IgM antibody
B. Positive rubella test for IgM
C. Positive rubella test for IgG
D. No positive test is revealed in congenital rubella syndrome

Immunology/Infectious disease methods/Rubella/3

61. A patient with rheumatoid arthritis (RA) has acute pneumonia but a negative result on throat culture. The provider suspects an infection with *Mycoplasma pneumoniae* and requests an IgM-specific antibody test. The test is performed directly on serial dilutions of serum less than 4 hours old. The result is positive, giving a titer of 1:32. However, the test is repeated 3 weeks later, and the titer remains at 1:32. What test should be performed to determine if the patient is truly infected with *M. pneumoniae*?

A. IgG anti-*M. pneumoniae*
B. Cold agglutinins
C. *M. pneumoniae* PCR or another molecular assay
D. Respiratory culture

Immunology/Infectious disease methods/3

62. An initial and repeat fourth-generation HIV screening test are both positive. The antibody differentiation assay is negative, as is the qualitative RNA PCR test. The patient shows no clinical signs of HIV infection, and the patient's CD4 T-cell count is normal. Based on these results, which conclusion is correct?

A. Patient is diagnosed as HIV-1 positive
B. Patient is diagnosed as HIV-2 positive
C. Results are inconclusive
D. Patient is diagnosed as HIV-1 negative

Immunology/Infectious disease methods/HIV/3

Answers to Questions 59–62

59. D The employee may donate if they are symptom free. The response to hepatitis B vaccine would include a positive result for anti-HBs, a test not normally a part of routine donor testing. The employee will be negative for HBsAg and anti-HBc; however, transient antigen positivity (less than 2 weeks) may be seen following vaccination.

60. B A finding of IgG is not definitive for congenital rubella syndrome because IgG crosses the placenta from the mother; however, demonstration of IgM, even in a single neonatal sample, is diagnostic.

61. C The IgM-specific antibody test for *M. pneumoniae* detects antibodies to mycoplasmal membrane antigens and, unlike cold agglutinins, is specific for *M. pneumoniae*. A positive result (titer of 1:32 or higher) occurs during the acute phase in about 87% of *M. pneumoniae* infections and does not need to be confirmed by assay of convalescent serum. However, *Mycoplasma* IgM may last a year or more; thus, its presence does not always indicate a current infection. PCR performed on a respiratory specimen is the definitive test and should be performed if there is a question about an IgM result.

62. D The fourth-generation algorithm detects infection approximately 2 weeks after exposure. This patient has negative follow-up test results for both antibody and nucleic acid, the patient would be considered HIV negative. The lack of symptoms would not be consistent with a very recent infection; the patient would likely have an acute retroviral syndrome. However, a repeat test may be performed if clinical suspicion remains high.

63. A female who has been pregnant for 12 weeks is tested for toxoplasmosis. The patient's IgM ELISA titer is 2.6 (reference range less than 1.6), and IgG ELISA value is 66 (reference range less than 8). The provider asks the laboratorian if these results indicated an infection during the past 12 weeks. Which of the following tests are recommended to determine whether the patient was infected during pregnancy?

A. Toxoplasmosis PCR on amniotic fluid
B. Toxoplasmosis IgM on amniotic fluid
C. Toxoplasmosis IgG avidity
D. Amniotic fluid culture

Immunology/Infectious disease methods/Toxoplasmosis/3

64. A patient undergoing dialysis is positive for both HBsAg and anti-HBs. The provider suspects a laboratory error. Is the provider's interpretation correct?

A. Yes; the patient should not test positive for both HBsAg and anti-HBs
B. No; incomplete dialysis of a patient in the core window phase of HBV infection will yield this result
C. No; it is likely the patient has recently received a hepatitis B booster vaccination within the past week, and this could have caused these results
D. Perhaps a new specimen should be submitted to clear up the confusion

Immunology/Infectious disease methods/Hepatitis/3

Answers to Questions 63–64

63. C Although IgM is positive, in toxoplasmosis specific IgM may remain detectable for a year or more following infection. IgG avidity, or the strength of binding of a serum to the antigen of interest, is a useful method to determine whether an infection is recent or in the distant past. IgG avidity will increase with time following an infection. Amniotic fluid testing is not useful for determining when the mother might have been infected.

64. C HBsAg will remain detectable at low levels following a vaccination for up to 1 to 2 weeks. Thus, patients who have received a second injection of hepatitis B vaccine may have anti-HBs and detectable antigen for a brief period. This has been reported more frequently in patients undergoing dialysis and in pediatric populations.

3.4

Autoimmune Disorders

1. What is the general definition for autoimmunity?
A. Increase of tolerance to self-antigens
B. Loss of tolerance to self-antigens
C. Increase in clonal deletion of mutant cells
D. Manifestation of immunosuppression

Immunology/Autoimmune disorders/1

2. An ANA test is performed on a specimen from a 55-year-old patient who has unexplained joint pain. The IFA result shows a titer of 40 and a homogeneous pattern. The appropriate follow-up for this patient is:
A. Anti-DNA assay
B. Extractable nuclear antigen (ENA) testing
C. Retest ANA in 3 to 6 months
D. CH_{50} complement assay

Immunology/Autoimmune disorders/2

3. Which disease is likely to show a rim (peripheral) pattern in an immunofluorescence (IF) microscopy test for ANA?
A. Mixed connective tissue disease (MCTD)
B. **Rheumatoid arthritis** (RA)
C. **Systemic lupus erythematosus** (SLE)
D. Scleroderma

Immunology/Autoimmune disorders/2

4. A patient's specimen is strongly positive in an ANA ELISA. Which of the following would *not* be an appropriate follow-up to this result?
A. IFA on human epithelial type 2 (HEp-2) cells
B. Specific ENA ELISA tests
C. Specific anti-DNA ELISA
D. Rheumatoid factor (RF) assay

Immunology/Autoimmune disorders/2

5. What type of antibodies are represented by the homogeneous pattern in the IFA for ANAs?
A. Antihistone antibodies
B. Anticentromere antibodies
C. Anti-ENA (anti-Smith [anti-Sm] and anti-ribonucleoprotein [anti-RNP]) antibodies
D. Anti-RNA antibodies

Immunology/Autoimmune disorders/1

6. What disease is indicated by a high titer of anti-Sm antibody?
A. **Mixed connective tissue disease** (MCTD)
B. **Rheumatoid arthritis** (RA)
C. **Systemic lupus erythematosus** (SLE)
D. Scleroderma

Immunology/Autoimmune disorders/2

Answers to Questions 1–6

1. B Autoimmunity is a loss of tolerance to self-antigens and the subsequent formation of autoantibodies.

2. C Approximately 25% of females in this age range may have low titer–positive ANA assays with no demonstrable connective tissue disease. A patient with anti-DNA–positive SLE would be expected to have a much higher titer (greater than 160) in an IFA. A similar titer would be expected for an ENA-positive specimen, although the pattern would be speckled. Complement testing would not be indicated with this low titer in a 55-year-old female.

3. C The rim or peripheral pattern seen in indirect immunofluorescence techniques is commonly found in cases of active SLE. The responsible autoantibody is highly correlated to anti–double-stranded DNA (anti-dsDNA).

4. D The ANA ELISA is a screening assay. A positive result may be followed up by more specific antibody ELISA tests or an ANA IFA to determine the pattern and titer. The ANA ELISA does not screen for RF.

5. A Antihistone antibodies (and anti-DNA antibodies) cause the solid or homogeneous pattern, which is commonly found in patients with SLE, RA, MCTD, and Sjögren syndrome. Antibodies to the centromere of chromosomes is a marker for the CREST (calcinosis, Raynaud phenomenon, esophageal dysfunction, sclerodactyly, and telangiectasia) form of systemic sclerosis.

6. C High-titer anti-Sm is indicative of SLE. Anti-Sm is an antibody against saline ENAs and causes a speckled pattern of immunofluorescence.

7. Which disease is *least* likely when a nucleolar pattern occurs in an IFA for ANAs?
A. Mixed connective tissue disease (MCTD)
B. Sjögren syndrome
C. Systemic lupus erythematosus (SLE)
D. Scleroderma

Immunology/Autoimmune disorders/2

8. What antibodies are represented by the nucleolar pattern in the IFA for ANAs?
A. Antihistone antibodies
B. Anti-dsDNA antibodies
C. Anti-ENA (anti-Sm and anti-RNP) antibodies
D. Anti-RNA antibodies

Immunology/Autoimmune disorders/1

9. Which test would *best* distinguish between SLE and MCTD?
A. Multiplex or ELISA test for anti-Sm and anti-RNP antibodies
B. IFA using *Crithidia* as substrate
C. Slide agglutination testing
D. Laboratory tests cannot distinguish between these disorders

Immunology/Autoimmune disorders/3

10. An ANA test on HEp-2 cells shows nucleolar staining in interphase cells and dense chromatin staining in mitotic cells. The most likely cause of this staining pattern is:
A. Antifibrillarin antibody
B. Anti–ribosomal P antibody
C. A serum with nucleolar and homogeneous patterns
D. Technical artifact

Immunology/Autoimmune disorders/2

11. Which immunofluorescence pattern indicates the need for ENA testing by multiplex, line blots, or ELISA assays?
A. Homogeneous or solid
B. Peripheral or rim
C. Speckled
D. Nucleolar

Immunology/Autoimmune disorders/3

12. Which of the following is used in rapid slide tests for detection of RFs?
A. Whole IgM molecules
B. Fc portion of the IgG molecule
C. Fab portion of the IgG molecule
D. Fc portion of the IgM molecule

Immunology/Autoimmune disorders/Rheumatoid factor/2

Answers to Questions 7–12

7. A All the diseases except MCTD may cause a nucleolar pattern of immunofluorescence. Nucleolar fluorescence is caused by anti-RNA antibodies and is seen in about 50% of patients with scleroderma.

8. D Anti-RNA antibodies are represented by the nucleolar pattern. This pattern may be seen in most systemic autoimmune diseases and is especially common in patients with scleroderma. Anti-RNA and anti-Sm are not usually found in patients with MCTD. This is a syndrome involving aspects of SLE, RA, scleroderma, and polymyositis. The immunofluorescence pattern most often seen in MCTD is the speckled pattern caused by anti-RNP.

9. A Line blots, multiplex, and ELISA assays, using purified or recombinant antigens, are available for differentiating anti-RNP from anti-Sm antibodies. Anti-Sm with or without anti-RNP is found in approximately one third of patients with SLE. Anti-RNP in the absence of anti-Sm is found in over 95% of patients with MCTD (mixed connective tissue disease).

10. A Antifibrillarin antibody has this appearance. Ribosomal P antibody has nucleolar staining and a background homogeneous and cytoplasmic stain. A combination nucleolar/homogeneous specimen will also show homogeneous staining in the interphase cells. This pattern is not seen in typical technical artifacts.

11. C A speckled pattern is often caused by the presence of antibodies against the ENAs, such as Sm, RNP, SSA, and SSB. Homogeneous and rim patterns suggest antibodies to dsDNA. The homogeneous pattern may also be seen with antibodies to deoxyribonuclear protein, which is not an ENA. Nucleolar patterns often indicate antibodies to RNA or fibrillarin.

12. B RFs react with the Fc portion of the IgG molecule and are usually IgM. This is the basis of rapid agglutination tests for RA. Particles of latex or cells are coated with IgG. Addition of serum containing RF results in visible agglutination.

13. Which of the following methods is least likely to give a definitive result for the diagnosis of RA?
A. Nephelometric measurement of anti-IgG
B. Agglutination testing for RF
C. Anti-CCP
D. IFA for ANAs

Immunology/Autoimmune disorders/Rheumatoid arthritis/2

14. Which disease might be indicated by antibodies to smooth muscle?
A. Atrophic gastritis
B. Autoimmune hepatitis
C. Myasthenia gravis
D. Sjögren syndrome

Immunology/Autoimmune disorders/1

15. Antibodies to thyroid peroxidase may appear in which of the following diseases?
A. Graves disease and Hashimoto thyroiditis
B. Myasthenia gravis
C. Granulomatous thyroid disease
D. Addison disease

Immunology/Autoimmune disorders/1

16. What is the main use of laboratory tests to detect antibodies to islet cells and insulin in cases of insulin-dependent diabetes mellitus (IDDM)?
A. To regulate levels of injected insulin
B. To diagnose IDDM
C. To rule out the presence of other autoimmune diseases
D. To screen susceptible individuals prior to destruction of β-cells

Immunology/Autoimmune disorders/Diabetes/2

17. A patient presents clinical symptoms of celiac disease. Tests for anti-tissue transglutaminase and antigliadin antibodies are negative. Which of the following tests should be ordered?
A. IgG level
B. HLA-DQ2 and -DQ8 typing
C. HLA-DR3 and -DR7 typing
D. IgM level

Immunology/Autoimmune disorders/Celiac disease/2

Answers to Questions 13–17

13. D Patients with RA often show a homogeneous pattern of fluorescence in tests for ANAs. However, this pattern is seen in a wide range of systemic autoimmune diseases and in many normal persons at a titer below 10. The first two methods listed may be used to identify anti-IgG, which is one laboratory criterion used to establish a diagnosis of RA. Anti-CCP is an additional laboratory criterion used in the RA diagnostic algorithm.

14. B Antibodies to smooth muscle are found in the serum of up to 70% of patients with active chronic hepatitis and up to 50% of patients with primary biliary cirrhosis.

15. A Antibodies to thyroid peroxidase may be detected in both Graves disease (hyperthyroidism) and Hashimoto thyroiditis (hypothyroidism). If a positive result is found to thyroid peroxidase, thyroxine levels and clinical presentation can be used to distinguish between the two diseases.

16. D Fasting hyperglycemia and hemoglobin A1c levels are the primary findings used to diagnose IDDM. For individuals with an inherited susceptibility to the development of IDDM, laboratory tests for the detection of antibodies to islet cells and insulin may help to initiate early treatment before complete destruction of β-cells.

17. B Although antibodies to tissue transglutaminase and gliadin are often found in celiac disease, their combined sensitivity is less than 100%. Celiac disease is almost exclusively associated with the presence of HLA-DQ2 and/or HLA-DQ8. These HLA genes are not diagnostic of celiac disease but provide a testing alternative in antibody-negative individuals who meet the clinical diagnostic criteria for celiac disease.

18. A specimen appears to have a perinuclear staining pattern in an antineutrophil cytoplasmic antibody (ANCA) immunofluorescent assay using ethanol-fixed neutrophils, suggesting the possibility of a perinuclear ANCA (pANCA). On which of the following substrates would this specimen display cytoplasmic speckling?

A. Formalin-fixed neutrophils
B. Unfixed neutrophils
C. HEp-2 cells
D. Rabbit kidney tissue

Immunology/Autoimmune disorders/3

19. A patient with symptoms associated with SLE and scleroderma was evaluated by immunofluorescence microscopy for ANAs by using the HEp-2 cell line as substrate. The cell line displayed a mixed pattern of fluorescence that could not be separated by serial dilutions of the serum. Which procedure would be most helpful in determining the antibody profile of this patient?

A. Use of a different tissue substrate
B. Absorption of the serum using the appropriate tissue extract
C. Requesting a new specimen
D. ELISA tests for specific antibodies

Immunology/Autoimmune disorders/3

20. A patient with joint swelling and pain tested negative for serum RF by both latex agglutination and ELISA methods. What additional test would help establish a diagnosis of RA in this patient?

A. Anti-CCP
B. ANA testing
C. Flow cytometry
D. Complement levels

Immunology/Autoimmune disorders/Rheumatoid arthritis/3

Answers to Questions 18–20

18. A Antibodies to neutrophil cytoplasmic antigen demonstrating a perinuclear pattern of fluorescence indicate a diagnosis of vasculitis. However, atypical ANCAs and ANAs also demonstrate a perinuclear staining pattern on ethanol-fixed neutrophils. To differentiate these from pANCA, specimens appearing as pANCAs on ethanol-fixed cells are tested on formalin-fixed neutrophils. The myeloperoxidase-containing granules that coalesce around the nuclear membrane during ethanol fixation will remain in the cytoplasm during formalin fixation. Thus, pANCAs will have a cytoplasmic (cANCA) pattern on a formalin-fixed slide, but ANAs will retain a perinuclear pattern, and the fluorescence will be diminished.

19. D Many patients with multiorgan autoimmune disease display symptoms that overlap two or more diseases and have complex mixtures of serum autoantibodies. The HEp-2 substrate is the most sensitive cell line for immunofluorescent microscopy because it contains cells in various mitotic stages, which expose the serum to more antigens. Use of a nonhuman substrate, such as *Crithidia*, may help identify dsDNA antibodies but would not aid in differentiating all the antibodies in a complex mixture. The best methods are ELISA, line blots, and multiplex tests because they are more specific than immunofluorescence microscopy for identifying antibodies to specific antigens. These assays are often used to measure antibodies to ENAs, which may be partially or completely lost during fixation of cells used for immunofluorescent microscopy. These antibodies cause a speckled pattern and are seen in a wide range of autoimmune diseases. Identification of the anti-ENA specificities is helpful in differentiating these diseases.

20. A Antibodies to CCP are often found in RF-negative patients with RA. The absence of RFs from serum does not rule out a diagnosis of RA, and more than half the patients who are diagnosed with RA present initially with a negative serum RF result. Both RF and anti-CCP are criteria assays for diagnosing RA, and at least one of them must be positive for a confirmed diagnosis.

3.5 Hypersensitivity

1. Which of the following is a description of a type I hypersensitivity reaction?

A. Ragweed antigen cross-links with IgE on the surface of mast cells, causing release of preformed mediators and resulting in symptoms of an allergic reaction

B. Anti-Fy[a] from a pregnant female crosses the placenta and attaches to the Fy[a] antigen-positive RBCs of the fetus, destroying the RBCs

C. Immune complex deposition occurs on the glomerular basement membrane of the kidney, leading to renal failure

D. Exposure to poison ivy causes sensitized T cells to release lymphokines that cause a localized inflammatory reaction

Immunology/Hypersensitivity/2

2. Why is skin testing the most widely used method to test for a type I hypersensitivity reaction?

A. It causes less trauma and is more cost effective than other methods

B. It has greater sensitivity than *in vitro* measurements

C. It is more likely to be positive for IgE-specific allergens compared with other methods

D. It may be used to predict the development of further allergen sensitivity

Immunology/Hypersensitivity/1

3. Which *in vitro* test measures IgE levels against a specific allergen?

A. Histamine release assay

B. Radioimmunosorbent test (RIST)

C. Fluorescent allergosorbent test (FAST)

D. Precipitin radioimmunosorbent test (PRIST)

Immunology/Hypersensitivity/1

4. A patient who is blood group O is accidentally transfused with group A blood and develops a reaction during the transfusion. What antibody is involved in this type II reaction?

A. IgM

B. IgE

C. IgG and IgE

D. IgG

Immunology/Hypersensitivity/1

5. Which test would measure the coating of RBCs by antibody as occurs in hemolytic transfusion reactions?

A. Indirect antiglobulin test (IAT)

B. Direct antiglobulin test (DAT)

C. ELISA

D. Hemagglutination

Immunology/Hypersensitivity/1

Answers to Questions 1–5

1. A Type I immediate hypersensitivity (anaphylactic) responses are characterized by IgE molecules binding to mast cells via the Fc receptor. Cross-linking of surface IgE caused by binding of allergens causes the mast cell to degranulate, releasing histamine and other chemical mediators of allergy.

2. B Skin testing is considered much more sensitive than *in vitro* tests that measure either total or antigen-specific IgE.

3. C FAST is a fluorescent assay that measures specific IgE; RIST and PRIST tests are radioimmunoassays that measure total IgE. The FAST procedure and a chemiluminescent assay have replaced the radioallergosorbent test (RAST) for measuring allergen-specific IgE. The histamine release assay is a more general assay.

4. A IgG and IgM are the antibodies involved in a type II cytotoxic reaction. Naturally occurring anti-A in the form of IgM is present in the blood of a group O individual and would cause an immediate transfusion reaction. Cell destruction occurs when antibodies bind to cells, causing destruction via complement activation, thereby triggering intravascular hemolysis.

5. B The DAT measures antibody that has already coated RBCs *in vivo*. DAT and direct IFAs use anti-Ig to detect antibody-sensitized cells.

6. Which test detects antibodies that have attached to tissues, resulting in a type II cytotoxic reaction?
A. Indirect immunofluorescence
B. Direct immunofluorescence (D-IFA)
C. Immunofixation electrophoresis (IFE)
D. Hemagglutination
Immunology/Hypersensitivity/1

7. Which of the following conditions will most likely result in a false-negative DAT?
A. Insufficient washing of RBCs
B. Use of heavy chain–specific polyclonal anti-human Ig
C. Use of excessive centrifugal force
D. Use of a sample obtained by finger puncture
Immunology/Hypersensitivity/3

8. Which of the following tests will detect circulating immune complexes in the serum of some patients with systemic autoimmune diseases, such as RA?
A. Direct IFA
B. Enzyme immunoassay (EIA)
C. Assay of cryoglobulins
D. IAT
Immunology/Hypersensitivity/2

9. What immune elements are involved in a positive skin test for tuberculosis?
A. IgE antibodies
B. T cells and macrophages
C. NK cells and IgG antibody
D. B cells and IgM antibody
Immunology/Hypersensitivity/1

10. A patient receives a transfusion of packed RBCs and fresh frozen plasma (FFP) and develops an anaphylactic, nonhemolytic reaction. The patient reports receiving a transfusion 20 years earlier and had no reaction to the transfusion. The patient did indicate feeling "poorly" a few weeks later. Which of the following transfused substances most likely elicited the reaction?
A. IgA
B. Group A antigen
C. Rho (D) antigen
D. An antigen belonging to the Duffy system
Immunology/Hypersensitivity/3

11. A patient deficient in the C3 complement component would be expected to mount a normal:
A. Type I and IV hypersensitivity response
B. Type II and IV hypersensitivity response
C. Type I and III hypersensitivity response
D. Type II and III hypersensitivity response
Immunology/Hypersensitivity/2

Answers to Questions 6–11

6. B The direct immunofluorescence (D-IFA) detects the presence of antibody that may cause a type II cytotoxic reaction. For example, renal biopsies from patients with Goodpasture syndrome exhibit a smooth pattern of fluorescence along the basement membrane after reaction with fluorescein isothiocyanate (FITC)–conjugated anti-Ig. The reaction detects antibodies against the basement membrane of the glomeruli.

7. A Insufficient washing can cause incomplete removal of excess or unbound Ig and other proteins, which may neutralize the antiglobulin reagent.

8. C Most autoimmune diseases involve the formation of antigen–antibody complexes that deposit in tissues, causing local inflammation and necrosis induced by complement activation, phagocytosis, white blood cell (WBC) infiltration, and lysosomal damage. Some patients make monoclonal or polyclonal antibodies with RF activity that bind to serum Igs, forming aggregates that are insoluble at 4°C. These circulating immune complexes are detected by allowing a blood sample to clot at 37°C, transferring the serum to a sedimentation rate tube, and then incubating the serum at 4°C for 3 days.

9. B T cells and macrophages are the immune elements primarily responsible for the clinical manifestations of a positive tuberculosis test. Reactions usually take 48 to 72 hours to reach peak development and are characteristic of localized type IV cell-mediated hypersensitivity. The skin reaction is characterized by a lesion containing a mononuclear cell infiltrate.

10. A The fact that this is a nonhemolytic reaction suggests that a non-RBC antigen may be involved. Selective IgA deficiency occurs in approximately one in 700 individuals and is often asymptomatic. Individuals deficient in IgA may make an antibody against the α-heavy chain if they are exposed to IgA via a transfusion. This antibody may lead to a serum sickness reaction if the IgA is still present after antibody formation. This could explain the patient feeling "poorly" after the initial transfusion. A subsequent transfusion may lead to an Arthus reaction if IgG anti-IgA is present or an anaphylactic reaction if IgE anti-IgA is present.

11. A Complement is involved in types II and III hypersensitivity; thus, an individual deficient in C3 will be deficient in those responses. The complement deficiency should have no effect on IgE (type I) or cell-mediated (type IV) hypersensitivities.

3.6

Immunodeficiency, Immunoglobulins, Complement, and Cellular Testing

1. Which of the following symptoms in a young child may indicate an immunodeficiency syndrome?
A. Anaphylactic reactions
B. Severe rashes and myalgia
C. Recurrent bacterial, fungal, and viral infections
D. Weight loss, rapid heartbeat, breathlessness
Immunology/Immunodeficiency/1

2. What screening test should be performed first in a young patient suspected of having an immune dysfunction disorder?
A. Complete blood count (CBC) and WBC differential
B. Chemotaxis assay
C. Complement levels
D. Bone marrow biopsy
Immunology/Immunodeficiency/2

3. Which test should be performed when a patient has a reaction to transfused plasma products?
A. Ig levels
B. T-cell count
C. Hemoglobin levels
D. RBC enzymes
Immunology/Immunodeficiency/2

4. What is the "M" component in monoclonal gammopathies?
A. IgM produced in excess
B. Heavy chain produced in excess
C. Malignant proliferation of B cells
D. Monoclonal antibody or cell line
Immunology/Immunoglobulins/1

5. A child suspected of having an inherited humoral immunodeficiency disease is given diphtheria/tetanus vaccine. Two weeks after the immunization, the patient's level of antibody to the specific antigens is measured. Which result is expected for this patient if there is a humoral deficiency?
A. Increased levels of specific antibody
B. No change in the level of specific antibody
C. An increase in IgG-specific antibody but not IgM-specific antibody
D. Increased levels of nonspecific antibody
Immunology/Immunodeficiency/3

Answers to Questions 1–5

1. C An immunodeficiency syndrome should be considered in a young child who has a history of recurrent bacterial, fungal, and viral infections manifested after the disappearance of maternal IgG. Immunodeficiency disorders may involve deficiencies in production and/or function of lymphocytes and phagocytic cells or a deficiency in production of a complement factor. The choice of laboratory tests is based on the patient's clinical presentation, age, and history.

2. A The first screening tests performed in the initial evaluation of a young patient who is suspected of having an immune dysfunction are the CBC and differential. WBCs that are decreased in number or abnormal in appearance may indicate further testing.

3. A A reaction to plasma products may be found in an IgA-deficient person who has formed anti-IgA antibodies. Ig levels would aid in this determination. Selective IgA deficiency is the most common immunodeficiency disease and is characterized by serum IgA levels below 5 mg/dL. IgA is usually absent from secretions, but the B-cell count is usually normal.

4. D The "M" component refers to any monoclonal protein or cell line produced in a monoclonal gammopathy, such as multiple myeloma.

5. B In a patient with immunodeficiency, the expected levels of specific antibody to the antigens in the vaccine would be decreased or not present. This response provides evidence of deficient antibody production.

6. Which disease may be expected to show an IgM spike on an electrophoretic pattern?
A. Hypogammaglobulinemia
B. Multicystic kidney disease
C. Waldenström macroglobulinemia
D. Wiskott-Aldrich syndrome
Immunology/Immunoglobulins/2

7. In testing for DiGeorge syndrome, what type of laboratory analysis would be most helpful in determining the number of mature T cells?
A. CBC
B. Dihydrorhodamine reduction (DHR) test
C. T-cell mitogen assays
D. Flow cytometry
Immunology/Cellular testing/2

8. Interpret the following description of an IFE assay of urine: Dense wide bands in both the κ- and λ-chain lanes. No bands present in the heavy-chain lanes.
A. Normal
B. Light-chain disease
C. Increased polyclonal Fab fragments
D. Multiple myeloma
Immunology/Immunoglobulins/2

9. Free monoclonal light chains are often present in the serum of patients with multiple myeloma and may be useful for disease monitoring. Which of the following assays would be recommended to detect the presence of free light chains in serum?
A. SPE
B. Urine immunofixation
C. Nephelometry
D. ELISA
Immunology/Immunoglobulins/2

10. What is measured in the CH_{50} assay?
A. RBC quantity needed to agglutinate 50% of antibody
B. Complement needed to lyse 50% of RBCs
C. Complement needed to lyse 50% of antibody-sensitized RBCs
D. Antibody and complement needed to sensitize 50% of RBCs
Immunology/Complement/1

11. What type of disorders would show a decrease in C3, C4, and CH_{50}?
A. Autoimmune disorders, such as SLE and RA
B. Immunodeficiency disorders, such as common variable immunodeficiency
C. Tumors
D. Bacterial, viral, fungal, or parasitic infections
Immunology/Complement/2

Answers to Questions 6–11

6. C Waldenström macroglobulinemia is a malignancy of plasmacytoid lymphocytes involving both bone marrow and lymph nodes. The malignant cells secrete monoclonal IgM and are in transition from B cells to plasma cells. In contrast to multiple myeloma, osteolytic bone lesions are not found.

7. D DiGeorge syndrome is caused by a developmental failure or hypoplasia of the thymus and results in deficiency of T lymphocytes and cell-mediated immune function. The T-cell count is low, but the level of immunoglobulins is usually normal. Flow cytometry is most helpful in determining numbers and subpopulations of T cells.

8. C Heavy wide bands seen with both anti-κ and anti-λ antisera indicate excessive polyclonal light-chain excretion. Light-chain disease would show a heavy restricted band for one of the light-chain reactions, but not both. The finding of excess λ- and κ-chains indicates a polyclonal gammopathy with increased Ig turnover and excretion of the light chains as Fab fragments.

9. C Free light chains in serum are a sensitive indicator of monoclonal gammopathy. They are often not present in sufficient quantity to show a band on a protein electrophoresis gel. Detecting light chains in urine is not an indicator of what the serum levels may be. Serum Ig heavy and light chains are commonly measured by using rate or endpoint nephelometry. ELISA assays are most often used to measure specific antibody levels, not to quantitate Ig heavy- or light-chain isotypes.

10. C CH_{50} is the amount of complement needed to lyse 50% of standardized antibody-sensitized sheep RBCs. It is expressed as the reciprocal of the serum dilution resulting in 50% hemolysis. Low levels are associated with deficiency of some complement components and active systemic autoimmune diseases in which complement is being consumed.

11. A The pattern of decreased C3, C4, and CH_{50} indicates classic pathway activation. This results in consumption of complement and is associated with SLE, serum sickness, subacute bacterial endocarditis, and other immune complex diseases. The inflammatory response seen in malignancy and acute infections gives rise to an increase in complement components. Immunodeficiency caused by an inherited deficiency in complement constitutes only about 1% of immunodeficiency diseases. Such disorders reduce the CH_{50} but involve a deficient serum level of only one complement factor.

12. All the following tests measure phagocyte function *except*:
A. Leukocyte adhesion molecule analysis
B. DHR (dihydrorhodamine) assay
C. Nitro blue tetrazolium (NBT) test
D. IL-2 assay

Immunology/Cellular testing/1

13. An 18-month-old child has recurrent sinopulmonary infections and septicemia. Bruton thymidine kinase deficiency is suspected. Which test result would be markedly decreased?
A. Serum IgG, IgA, and IgM
B. Total T-cell count
C. Both B- and T-cell counts
D. Lymphocyte proliferation with phytohemagglutinin (PHA) stimulation

Immunology/Immunodeficiency/3

14. A patient received 5 units of FFP and developed a severe anaphylactic reaction. The patient has a history of respiratory and gastrointestinal infections. Post-transfusion studies showed all 5 units to be ABO compatible. What immunologic test would help to determine the cause of this transfusion reaction?
A. Complement levels, particularly C3 and C4
B. Flow cytometry for T-cell counts
C. Measurement of immunoglobulins
D. NBT test for phagocytic function

Immunology/Immunodeficiency/3

15. IFE revealed excessive amounts of polyclonal IgM and low concentrations of IgG and IgA. What is the most likely explanation of these findings and the recommended follow-up or result?
A. Proper amounts of antisera were not added; repeat both tests
B. Test specimen was not added properly; repeat both procedures
C. Patient has common variable immunodeficiency; perform B-cell count
D. Patient has immunodeficiency with hyper-IgM; perform CD40 ligand (CD154) analysis

Immunology/Immunodeficiency/3

16. Would an hCG test using a monoclonal antibody against the β-subunit of hCG likely be affected by an increased level of follicle-stimulating hormone (FSH)?
A. Yes, the β-subunit of FSH is identical to that of hCG
B. No, the test would be specific for the β-subunit of hCG
C. Yes, a cross reaction would occur because of structural similarities
D. No, the structure of FSH and hCG are not at all similar

Immunology/Immunoglobulins/3

Answers to Questions 12–16

12. D The DHR assay and the older NBT tests are used to diagnose chronic granulomatous disease, an inherited disorder in which phagocytic cells fail to kill microorganisms because of a defect in peroxide production (respiratory burst). Leukocyte adhesion deficiency is associated with a defect in the production of integrin molecules on the surface of WBCs and their granules. IL-2 is a cytokine produced by activated T-helper and B cells. It causes B-cell proliferation and increased production of antibody, interferon, and other cytokines. IL-2 can be measured by EIA and is used to detect transplant rejection, which is associated with an increase in the serum and urine levels.

13. A The patient with Bruton thymidine kinase deficiency presents with clinical symptoms related to recurrent infections, demonstrated in the laboratory by decreased or absent Igs. Peripheral blood B cells are absent or markedly reduced, but T cells are normal in number and function. Because PHA a T-cell mitogen, the lymphocyte proliferation test using PHA would be normal for this patient.

14. C The patient had an anaphylactic reaction to a plasma product. This, combined with the history of respiratory and gastrointestinal infections, suggests a selective IgA deficiency. Measurement of immunoglobulins would be helpful in this case. A low serum IgA and normal IgG substantiate the diagnosis of selective IgA deficiency. Such patients frequently produce anti-IgA, which is often responsible for a severe transfusion reaction when ABO-compatible plasma is administered.

15. D Low plasma concentrations of IgG and IgA and an abundance of IgM is consistent with the CD40 ligand deficiency. Most cases are X-linked and result from a mutation of the gene *TNFSF5*, which encodes a receptor needed for switching Ig production. Patients with common variable immunodeficiency have low serum IgG, IgA, and IgM.

16. B Luteinizing hormone, FSH, and hCG share a common α-subunit but have different β-subunits. A test for hCG using a monoclonal antibody would be specific for hCG, provided that the antibody was directed against an antigenic determinant on the carboxy terminal end of the β-subunit.

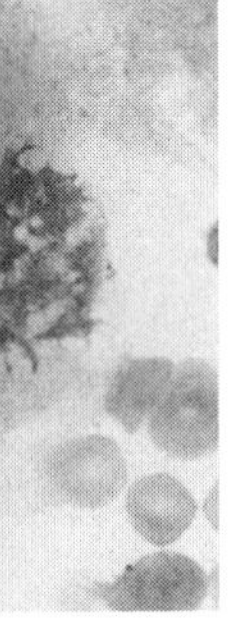

3.7

Tumors, Transplantation, and Genetics

1. A patient had surgery for colorectal cancer, after which they received chemotherapy for 6 months. The test for carcinoembryonic antigen (CEA) was normal at this time. One year later, the bimonthly level of CEA was elevated (above 10 ng/mL). An examination and biopsy revealed the recurrence of a small tumor. What was the value of the results provided by the CEA test in this clinical situation?

A. Diagnostic information
B. Information for further treatment
C. Information on the immunologic response of the patient
D. No useful clinical information in this case

Immunology/Tumors/3

2. A cancerantigen 125 assay (CA-125) was performed on a female with ovarian cancer. After treatment, the levels fell significantly. An examination performed later revealed recurrence of the tumor, but the CA-125 levels remained low. What is the explanation for these results?

A. Test error
B. CA-125 was the wrong laboratory test; α-fetoprotein (AFP) is a better test to monitor ovarian cancer
C. CA-125 may not be sensitive enough when used alone to monitor tumor development
D. CA-125 is not specific enough to detect only one type of tumor

Immunology/Tumors/3

3. What is the correct procedure upon receiving a test request for human chorionic gonadotropin (hCG) on the serum of a 60-year-old male?

A. Return the request; hCG is not performed on men
B. Perform a qualitative hCG test to see if hCG is present
C. Perform the test; hCG may be increased in testicular tumors
D. Perform the test but use different standards and controls

Immunology/Tumors/3

Answers to Questions 1–3

1. B CEA is a glycoprotein that is elevated in about 60% of patients with colorectal cancer and one third or more patients with pulmonary, gastric, and pancreatic cancers. CEA may be positive in smokers and in patients with cirrhosis, Crohn disease, and other nonmalignant conditions. Because sensitivity for malignant disease is low, CEA is not recommended for use as a diagnostic test. However, an elevated CEA level after treatment is evidence of tumor recurrence and the need for second-look surgery.

2. C CA-125 is a tumor-associated glycoprotein antigen that is elevated in 70% to 80% of patients with ovarian cancer and about 20% of patients with pancreatic cancer. Although an increase in CA-125 may indicate recurrent or progressive disease, low levels do not necessarily indicate the absence of tumor growth.

3. C hCG is normally tested for in pregnancy; it is increased in approximately 60% of patients with testicular tumors and a lower percentage of those with ovarian, gastrointestinal, breast, and pulmonary tumors. Malignant cells secreting hCG may produce only the β-subunit; therefore, qualitative and quantitative tests that detect both intact hCG and free β-subunits provide better sensitivity than either test alone.

4. Which of the following substances, sometimes used as a tumor marker, is increased two- or threefold in a normal pregnancy?
A. Alkaline phosphatase (ALP)
B. Calcitonin
C. Adrenocortocotropic hormone (ACTH)
D. Neuron-specific enolase
Immunology/Tumors/2

5. What is an advantage of performing a prostate-specific antigen (PSA) test for prostate cancer?
A. PSA is stable in serum and not affected by digital rectal examination
B. PSA is increased only in prostatic malignancy
C. A normal serum level rules out malignant prostatic disease
D. The percentage of free PSA is elevated in persons with malignant disease
Immunology/Tumors/2

6. Which method is the most sensitive for quantitation of alpha-fetoprotein (AFP)?
A. Double immunodiffusion
B. Electrophoresis
C. Enzyme immunoassay
D. Particle agglutination
Immunology/Tumors/1

7. How is human leukocyte antigen (HLA) typing used in the investigation of genetic diseases?
A. For prediction of the severity of the disease
B. For genetic linkage studies
C. For direct diagnosis of disease
D. It is not useful in this situation
Immunology/Genetics/1

Answers to Questions 4–7

4. A Isoenzymes of ALP are sometimes used as tumor markers, but they have a low specificity because they are also increased in nonmalignant diseases. These include placental-like (heat-stable) ALP isoenzymes, which are found (infrequently) in some malignancies, such as cancer of the lung; bone-derived ALP, which is a marker for metastatic bone cancer; and the fast-migrating liver isoenzyme, which is a marker for metastatic liver cancer. ACTH is secreted as an ectopic hormone in some patients with cancer of the lung. Calcitonin is a hormone produced by the medulla of the thyroid and is increased in the serum of patients with medullary thyroid carcinoma. Neuron-specific enolase is an enzyme that is used as a tumor marker primarily for neuroblastoma.

5. A PSA is a glycoprotein with protease activity that is specific for the prostate gland. High levels may be caused by prostate malignancy, benign prostatic hypertrophy, or prostatitis, but PSA is not increased by physical examination of the prostate. PSA has a sensitivity of 80% and a specificity of about 75% for prostate cancer. The sensitivity is sufficiently high to warrant its use in screening tests, but its sensitivity for stage A cancer is below 60%. Most of the serum PSA is bound to protease inhibitors, such as α_1-antitrypsin and α_1-antichymotrypsin. Patients with borderline PSA levels (4–10 ng/mL) and a low percentage of free PSA are more likely to have cancer of the prostate compared with patients with a normal percentage of free PSA.

6. C AFP is a glycoprotein that is produced in about 80% to 90% of patients with hepatoma and in a lower percentage of patients with other tumors, including retinoblastoma, breast cancer, uterine cancer, and pancreatic cancer. The upper reference limit for serum is only 10 ng/mL, which requires a sensitive method of assay, such as EIA. The high analytical sensitivity of chemiluminescent immunoassays permits detection of reduced AFP levels in maternal serum associated with Down syndrome, as well as elevated levels associated with spina bifida.

7. B HLA typing is useful in predicting some genetic diseases and for genetic counseling because certain HLA types show strong linkage to some diseases. HLA typing is not specifically used to diagnose a disease or assess its severity. In linkage studies, a disease gene can be predicted because it is located next to the locus of a normal gene with which it segregates. For example, the relative risk of developing ankylosing spondylitis is 87% in individuals who are positive for HLA-B27. Analysis of family pedigrees for the linkage marker and disease can be used to determine the probability that a family member will inherit the disease gene.

8. Select the *best* donor for a male, blood type AB, in need of kidney transplantation.

A. His brother, type AB, HLA matched for class II antigens
B. His mother, type B, HLA matched for class I antigens
C. His cousin, type O, HLA matched for major class II antigens
D. Deceased donor, type O, HLA matched for some class I and II antigens

Immunology/Transplantation/Genetics/3

9. Interpret the following microcytotoxicity target cell results:

A9 and B12 cells = damaged; A1 and Aw19 cells = intact

A. Positive for A1 and Aw19; negative for A9 and B12
B. Negative for A1 and Aw19; positive for A9 and B12
C. Error in test system; retest
D. Impossible to determine

Immunology/Transplantation/3

10. Which method, classically used for HLA-D typing, is often used to determine the compatibility between a living organ donor and a recipient?

A. Flow cytometry
B. Mixed lymphocyte culture (MLC)
C. Primed lymphocyte test
D. Restriction fragment length polymorphism (RFLP)

Immunology/Transplantation/2

11. Cells type negative for all HLA antigens in a complement-dependent cytotoxicity assay. What is the most likely cause?

A. Too much supravital dye was added
B. Rabbit complement is inactivated
C. All leukocytes are dead
D. Antisera is too concentrated

Immunology/Transplantation/3

12. What method may be used for tissue typing instead of serological HLA typing?

A. PCR
B. Southern blotting
C. RFLP
D. All of these options

Immunology/Transplantation/1

Answers to Questions 8–12

8. A A twin or sibling donor of the same blood type and HLA matched for class II antigens is the best donor in this situation. Class II antigens (HLA-D, -DR, -DQ, and -DP) determine the ability of the transplant recipient to recognize the graft. The HLA genes are located close together on chromosome 6, and crossover between HLA genes is rare. Siblings with closely matched class II antigens most likely inherited the same class I genes. The probability of siblings inheriting the same HLA haplotypes from both parents is 1:4.

9. B The microcytotoxicity test is based on the reaction of specific antisera and HLA antigens on test cells. Cells damaged by the binding of antibody and complement are detected with supravital dye, such as eosin.

10. B Flow cytometry can be used in transplantation to type serologically defined HLA antigens. The one-way mixed lymphocyte reaction is used to identify HLA-D antigens on the donor's lymphocytes and is used for crossmatching living donors with transplant recipients. The assay is time consuming and would not be used as part of the laboratory testing process for a transplant from a deceased donor. HLA-D incompatibility is associated with the recognition phase of allograft rejection. The primed lymphocyte test is used to identify HLA-DP antigens.

11. B Inactive rabbit complement may not become fixed to antibodies that have bound test leukocytes; therefore, no lysis of cells will occur. When the supravital dye is added, all cells will appear negative (exclude the dye) for all HLAs.

12. D PCR, Southern blotting, next-generation sequencing, and testing for RFLPs may all be used to identify HLA genes. Many laboratories use PCR technology for the routine determination of HLA type.

13. A patient had a PSA level of 60 ng/mL the day before surgery to remove a localized prostate tumor. One week after surgery, serum PSA was determined to be 8 ng/mL by the same method. What is the most likely cause of these results?
- **A.** Incomplete removal of the malignancy
- **B.** Cross reactivity of the antibody with another tumor antigen
- **C.** Testing too soon after surgery
- **D.** Hook effect with the PSA assay

Immunology/Tumors/3

14. What is the main advantage of the recovery and reinfusion of autologous stem cells?
- **A.** It slows the rate of rejection of transplanted cells
- **B.** It prevents graft-versus-host disease
- **C.** No HLA testing is required
- **D.** Engraftment occurs in a more efficient sequence

Immunology/Transplantation/2

15. A transplant recipient began to show signs of rejection 8 days after transplantation, and the organ was removed. What immune elements might be found in the rejected organ?
- **A.** Antibody and complement
- **B.** Primarily antibody
- **C.** Macrophages
- **D.** T cells

Immunology/Transplantation/3

16. A patient with ovarian cancer who has been treated with chemotherapy is being monitored for recurrence by using serum CA-125, CA-50, and CA 15–3. Six months after treatment the CA 15–3 is elevated, but the CA-125 and CA-50 remain low. What is the most likely explanation of these findings?
- **A.** Ovarian malignancy has recurred
- **B.** CA 15–3 is specific for breast cancer and indicates metastatic breast cancer
- **C.** Testing error occurred in the measurement of CA 15–3 caused by poor analytical specificity
- **D.** The CA 15–3 elevation is spurious and probably benign

Immunology/Tumors/3

Answers to Questions 13–16

13. C When monitoring the level of a tumor marker for treatment efficacy or recurrence, the half-life of the protein must be considered when determining the testing interval. PSA has a half-life of almost 4 days and would not reach normal levels after surgery for approximately 3 to 4 weeks. The hook effect is the result of very high antigen levels giving a lower-than-expected result in a double antibody sandwich assay when both antibodies and sample are added at the same time.

14. B The main advantage to the patient from the reinfusion of autologous stem cells is that the procedure prevents graft-versus-host disease, especially in the immunocompromised patient. Although HLA testing is not required, this is not the primary advantage for patient care.

15. D Acute rejection occurs within 3 weeks of transplantation. The immune component most likely to be involved in acute rejection is the T cell in a type IV, delayed hypersensitivity (cell-mediated) reaction. Preformed antibody, and possibly complement, is usually involved in hyperacute (immediate) rejection and chronic rejection.

16. A Although CA-125 is the commonly used tumor marker for ovarian cancer, not all ovarian tumors produce CA-125. Greatest sensitivity in monitoring for recurrence is achieved when several markers known to be increased in the malignant tissue type are measured simultaneously and when the markers are elevated (by malignancy) prior to treatment. In addition to limited sensitivity, no single tumor marker is entirely specific. Carbohydrate and other oncofetal antigens are produced by several malignant and benign conditions. Although testing errors may occur in any situation, measurements of carbohydrate antigens use purified monoclonal antibodies with very low cross reactivities.

BIBLIOGRAPHY

1. Abbas AK, Lichtman AH, Pillai S. *Cellular and Molecular Immunology.* 10th ed. Elsevier; 2022.
2. Stevens CD, Miller LE. *Clinical Immunology and Serology: A Laboratory Perspective.* 5th ed. F.A. Davis Company; 2021.
3. Tille PM. *Bailey and Scott's Diagnostic Microbiology.* 16th ed. Elsevier; 2026.

CHAPTER 4

Molecular Diagnostics

4.1 *Nucleic Acid Chemistry*

4.2 *Basic Concepts*

4.3 *Biochemical Reagents*

4.4 *Genetics*

4.5 *Molecular Techniques*

4.6 *Molecular Laboratory Practices*

4.1
Nucleic Acid Chemistry

1. **The difference between the sugar in deoxyribonucleic acid and ribonucleic acid is:**
   - A. Deoxyribose is significantly less stable than ribose in nucleic acid structures
   - B. Deoxyribose lacks one oxygen atom on the 2′ carbon
   - C. Deoxyribose is responsible for carrying oxygen
   - D. Ribose is a six-carbon sugar

   Molecular/Nucleic acid chemistry/1

2. **A molecule that is formed between a phosphorylated ribose sugar and a nitrogenous base is a:**
   - A. Deoxyribose
   - B. DNA polymerase
   - C. Nucleotide
   - D. Nucleon

   Molecular/Nucleic acid chemistry/1

3. **Nucleic acids are composed of a sugar phosphate backbone and nitrogenous bases that include:**
   - A. Adenine, celluline, guanine, and thymine
   - B. Alanine, celluline, guanine, uracil, and thymine
   - C. Adenine, cytosine, guanine, uracil, and thymine
   - D. Adenine, cytosine, guanine, and thymine

   Molecular/Nucleic acid chemistry/1

4. **The secondary structure or double helix of a DNA molecule is stabilized by:**
   - A. Hydrogen bonding between nitrogenous bases, and the hydrophobicity of the internal molecules and hydrophilic molecules on the outside of the helix
   - B. The secondary structure or double helix is stabilized solely by ionic or van der Waals forces
   - C. Covalent bonds stabilize the interactions between the adenine and guanine bases resulting in double-stranded formation
   - D. DNA is highly ionic and dissolves readily in aqueous fluid, becoming unstable

   Molecular/Nucleic acid chemistry/2

Answers to Questions 1–4

1. B The major difference in deoxyribose and ribose is the absence of an oxygen atom on the number 2 carbon of the ribose molecule. Ribose is a pentose, or 5-carbon sugar.

2. C The assembly of a nucleic acid macromolecule requires the units referred to as *nucleotides*. A nucleotide is composed of phosphorylated ribose sugar and a nitrogen base.

3. C There are two major macromolecules referred to as *nucleic acids,* deoxyribonucleic acid (DNA) and ribonucleic acid (RNA). Each strand or molecule is composed of an alternating sugar, phosphate backbone attached to nitrogenous bases. DNA is comprised of adenine, cytosine, guanine, and thymine, whereas the thymine is substituted with uracil in RNA.

4. A The two strands of DNA that form the double helix are primarily stabilized by the adenine to thymine double hydrogen bonding and the guanine to cytosine triple hydrogen bonds. The nitrogenous bases are hydrophobic and therefore rotate to the inside of the molecule, whereas the sugar phosphate backbone is very hydrophilic, orienting to the outside. The hydrogen bonds and chemical composition of the molecules work together to stabilize the DNA double helix.

5. Ribonucleic acid differs from DNA in all the following, *except*:

A. RNA molecules are single stranded
B. RNA molecules contain uracil in place of thymine
C. RNA molecules are extremely stable
D. RNA often contains secondary structure or folding of the molecule

Molecular/Nucleic acid chemistry/2

6. The DNA sequence 5′-AGTTACCGATGA-3′ is complementary to which of the following DNA strands?

A. 5′-AGUUACCGAUGA-3′
B. 5′-TCAATGGCTACT-3′
C. 5′-TCATCGGTAACT-3′
D. 5′-UGUGCCUTTGU-3′

Molecular/Nucleic acid chemistry/2

Answers to Questions 5–6

5. C Unlike DNA, RNA molecules are single stranded. RNA contains uracil and not thymine as a nitrogenous base. In addition, RNA molecules are folded into a variety of secondary structures to facilitate binding or interacting with other molecules that support the function of the construct. Because RNA is single stranded it is extremely unstable and degrades easily in the environment.

6. C The complementary strand when written 5′ to 3′ is the opposite of the original strand.

5′-AGTTACCGATGA-3′

3′-TCAATGGCTACT-5′

4.2
Basic Concepts

1. Cloning a human gene into a bacterium to make a molecular probe requires which vector?
- **A.** Plasmid
- **B.** Bacterial microsome
- **C.** 30S bacterial ribosome
- **D.** Single-stranded DNA

Molecular/Basic concepts/1

2. The process of copying a DNA sequence into an RNA molecule is termed:
- **A.** Replication
- **B.** Translation
- **C.** Transcription
- **D.** Transduction

Molecular/Basic concepts/1

3. Extrachromosomal autonomously replicating DNA molecules are termed:
- **A.** Phage
- **B.** Plasmids
- **C.** Virions
- **D.** Chromosomes

Molecular/Basic concepts/1

4. Prokaryotic chromosomes are best described as:
- **A.** Single double-stranded monocistronic macromolecules
- **B.** Linear single-stranded polycistronic sequences
- **C.** Containing exons and introns in tandem and double stranded
- **D.** Single double-stranded polycistronic macromolecules

Molecular/Basic concepts/2

5. Identify the mismatched molecular process with the cellular location in a eukaryotic cell for processing of nucleic acid molecules.
- **A.** Translation—nucleus
- **B.** Replication—nucleus
- **C.** Transcription—nucleus
- **D.** mRNA splicing—nucleus

Molecular/Basic concepts/2

Answers to Questions 1–5

1. A A plasmid is a circular dsDNA molecule. Plasmids can self-replicate separately from the chromosome. To clone a gene or DNA sequence, the fragment must contain the same restriction endonuclease site as the plasmid. Once the plasmid is digested with the endonuclease, the restriction ends of the DNA fragment or sequence pair with the plasmid ends. The two pieces, the gene of interest and the plasmid DNA, are repaired or joined together using ligase enzyme. The plasmid carrying the sequence of interest or cloned gene can then be used to determine the function of the cloned sequence or gene.

2. C A DNA template is required to synthesize a complementary RNA molecule. The process of synthesizing an RNA molecule from a DNA template is referred to as *transcription*. A nucleic acid gene coding sequence of nucleotides must be transcribed before it can be translated into a protein sequence.

3. B Extrachromosomal elements that can be found in both eukaryotic and prokaryotic cells that are capable of self-replicating or autonomous replication separate from the cellular chromosome are termed *plasmids*. Plasmids often carry an accessory function or sequences of genes that provide an evolutionary advantage to the cell harboring the molecule.

4. D Prokaryotic chromosomes are typically double-stranded circular molecules. Because of the small size of the prokaryotic organisms, the chromosomes are polycistronic. A cistron is a gene sequence that codes for a functional product. As a double-stranded molecule, sequences for genes overlap to accommodate the required number of genes in a small molecule. In other words, a single stretch of DNA sequence codes for more than one gene and more than one function product; referred to as *polygenes* or *polycistronic*.

5. A DNA replication in a eukaryotic cell takes place in the nucleus. DNA molecules in the nucleus are also transcribed to RNA in the nucleus. Once a messenger RNA, or mRNA, that codes for a protein is transcribed in the nucleus, it must be spliced to remove the intervening sequences or noncoding regions of the gene prior to being transported out of the nucleus to the cytoplasm, where it can be translated into a protein.

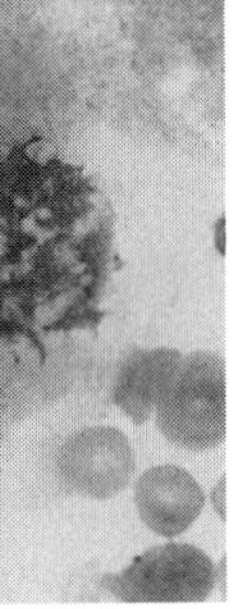

4.3 Biochemical Reagents

1. **Which base pair sequence is *most* likely to serve as a binding site for a restriction endonuclease?**
   A. A-T-T-C-A
   T-A-A-G-T
   B. C-T-A-C-T-G
   G-A-T-G-A-C
   C. C-A-C
   G-T-G
   D. A-A-G-C-T-T
   T-T-C-G-A-A

   Molecular/Biochemical reagents/2

2. **What intercalating agent can be used to visualize DNA that has been separated by electrophoresis?**
   A. Silver nitrate
   B. Nicotinamide adenine dinucleotide
   C. Cationic dye
   D. Ethidium bromide

   Molecular/Biochemical reagents/1

3. **What is the unique characteristic of the enzyme, *Taq* DNA polymerase, used in polymerase chain reaction (PCR)?**
   A. It can be enzyme labeled
   B. It is more efficient than eukaryotic polymerases
   C. It is heat stable
   D. It works with DNA of any species

   Molecular/Biochemical reagents/1

4. **PCR or amplification of nucleic acids requires a reagent master mix, which must contain:**
   A. Reaction buffer, dNTPs, calcium, and DNA polymerase
   B. Water, reaction buffer, dNTPs, probes, fluorophores, and DNA polymerase
   C. Reaction buffer, dNTPs, $MgCl_2$, DNA polymerase, primers, and nuclease-free water
   D. Reaction buffer, reverse transcriptase, dNTPs, DNA polymerase, and a cofactor

   Molecular/Biochemical reagents/2

Answers to Questions 1–4

1. D Restriction endonucleases are enzymes that cut dsDNA into fragments and are important tools used in molecular diagnostics. Each restriction enzyme recognizes a specific oligonucleotide sequence, and the size and number of fragments it produces when DNA is digested depend on the number of times that sequence is repeated in the DNA molecule. Restriction endonucleases recognize palindromic sequences (i.e., the base sequence of complementary strands reads the same from opposite directions). The sequence

A-A-G-C-T-T
T-T-C-G-A-A

is the recognition site for *HindIII*, a restriction endonuclease isolated from *Haemophilus influenzae*.

2. D When ethidium bromide inserts or intercalates between the base pairs of dsDNA, the dye becomes fluorescent, releasing 480 nm light when stimulated by long wavelength ultraviolet (UV) light. Ethidium bromide staining has a sensitivity of approximately 10 ng/mL (1.5 ng per band) DNA. It may be added to molten agarose or capillary electrophoresis (CE) buffer at a concentration of 0.5 µg/mL to visualize and quantify DNA. Ethidium bromide is rarely used outside a research facility because it is carcinogenic and is considered hazardous waste.

3. C Because heat is used to denature dsDNA with every cycle of PCR, the polymerase used must be heat stable. *Taq* polymerase is obtained from *Thermus aquaticus*. It retains its activity even after repeated heating at 95°C. A typical PCR cycle involves heating to 94°C for denaturation, cooling to 64°C for annealing, and heating to 72°C for extension.

4. C A PCR master mix contains a reaction buffer that is a combination of salts and stabilizers along with nuclease-free water to prevent degradation of the sample nucleic acid template and primers or probes during the reaction. In addition, the DNA polymerase enzyme that is required to catalyze the synthesis or amplification of the nucleic acid template requires an enzymatic cofactor, $MgCl_2$. Primers that are small oligonucleotides that bind to the template to facilitate the amplification of the specific sequence are essential for the reaction. The last component that is needed is the building blocks of the nucleic acid or dideoxynucleotide triphosphates (dNTPs), adenine, cytosine, thymine, and guanine.

5. DNA polymerases' primary function is for the polymerization of nucleotides; however, the enzyme also serves as an exonuclease. What is the significance of the DNA polymerase secondary function?

A. The exonuclease activity catalyzes nicks in the strand to facilitate secondary structure of the double helix

B. The exonuclease activity ensures degradation of DNA in both 5′ to 3′ and 3′ to 5′ directions to prevent mutations

C. The exonuclease activity is primarily for editing and attaching the remaining molecules necessary to make of the replication complex

D. The exonuclease activity is only functional when the DNA in the cell has been chemically damaged or altered

Molecular/Biochemical reagents/2

6. The enzyme capable of catalyzing the polymerization of RNA from DNA is:

A. RNA transcriptase

B. Reverse transcriptase

C. RNA polymerase

D. RNase

Molecular/Biochemical reagents/1

7. The enzyme that is necessary to join two DNA fragments together that have been digested using restriction enzymes is:

A. Helicase

B. DNase

C. Topoisomerase

D. Ligase

Molecular/Biochemical reagents/1

8. When isolating genomic DNA from a sample containing cellular material, what is the purpose of adding proteinase K?

A. Remove contaminating nucleic acids such as mRNA

B. Inhibit endogenous nucleases to prevent nucleic acid degradation

C. Remove contaminating cellular proteins that may interfere with upstream analysis

D. Precipitate proteins to facilitate extraction of the nucleic acids in a single phase

Molecular/Biochemical reagents/2

Answers to Questions 5–8

5. B The primary function of DNA polymerases is to polymerize nucleotides creating a DNA strand. Some polymerases have a secondary ability to degrade or remove nucleotides from the growing DNA strand in either the 5′ to 3′ or 3′ to 5′ direction to prevent errors in the sequence or base changes that would result in the placement of an incorrect nucleotide causing a mismatch base-base paired nucleotide in the final double-stranded molecule and a mutation.

6. C RNA polymerase, like DNA polymerase, catalyzes the synthesis of RNA in both prokaryotic and eukaryotic organisms. Prokaryotes typically have one RNA polymerase, whereas eukaryotes have three types that synthesize different RNA molecules within the cell.

7. D Restriction endonucleases are designed to cleave DNA at specific sequences. When a sequence is digested into fragments using an endonuclease, the process creates sticky ends or blunt ends. Sticky ends have one strand that is longer than the second strand, creating an overhand. A second fragment that has been digested with the same restriction endonuclease will have a matching staggered cut, like a puzzle piece. DNA ligase catalyzes the formation of a phosphodiester bond between an adjacent 3′ hydroxyl group and a 5′ phosphoryl nucleotide end. This in essence repairs or connects the two fragments. This technique is widely used to clone or insert DNA fragments from one molecule into another.

8. C Proteinase K is an enzyme that is used to digest the contaminating proteins in a nucleic acid extraction process. Once the protein material is digested, it is typically separated from the nucleic acid in a series of steps that include liquid phase separation or solid matrix that binds the nucleic acids. Both methods require washing of the samples to remove unwanted materials.

9. When isolating RNA from a whole blood sample, the sample must be stored in an appropriate buffer. What type of reagent or buffer is preferred for the storage and preservation of RNA following isolation?

A. Deionized water is sufficient for storage, once the RNA is purified properly
B. DEPC (diethyl pyrocarbonate) and water
C. Vanadyl ribonuclease complexes
D. Tap water containing RNase inhibitors

Molecular/Biochemical reagents/2

10. Modified nucleic acids that are used for the detection of target sequences that are resistant to degradation and can overcome the repelling effects of the charged nucleic acid backbone include which of the following?

A. FRET (fluorescence resonance energy transfer) and PNA (peptide nucleic acid) probes
B. Molecular beacon and scorpion probes
C. Locked nucleic acid and scorpion probes
D. PNA and locked nucleic acid probes

Molecular/Biochemical reagents/2

Answers to Questions 9–10

9. C Vanadyl ribonuclease complexes contain a vanadyl ribonucleoside that is an analog of ribonucleic acid and therefore prevents the binding of RNases to RNA, decreasing the degradation in the samples. DEPC has been historically used in RNA preparations but can adversely affect tris buffers by binding to amine groups and interfering with upstream reactions.

10. D Both PNA and locked nucleic acids are synthetic probes that contain modified nucleic acids that are resistant to degradation by nucleases. In addition, PNA probes do not have a phosphodiester backbone like native nucleic acids and therefore are not easily repelled from hybridizing, improving the binding efficiency to the target molecule.

4.4
Genetics

1. **In humans, which component of a gene is translated into a protein?**
   A. Intron
   B. Exon
   C. Promoter
   D. TATA box

   Molecular/Human genetics/1

2. **Which statement best describes a single nucleotide DNA polymorphism?**
   A. A point mutation arising in a gene
   B. Any change in DNA that is associated with abnormal function
   C. A change in the base sequence of DNA that is translated into an abnormal protein
   D. A variation in DNA that occurs with a frequency of at least 1%

   Molecular/Human genetics/1

3. **Which method is *best* suited to detect resistance mutations to targeted cancer drugs?**
   A. Real-time PCR
   B. Digital PCR
   C. Next-generation sequencing (NGS)
   D. Nested PCR

   Molecular/Human genetics/2

4. **How is the fetal cell-free DNA (cfDNA) differentiated from the mother's DNA in a sample of the mother's plasma?**
   A. The father's DNA is used as a probe
   B. *Hemoglobin F* is used as a reference gene
   C. A heterozygous polymorphism on the fetal chromosome is used as a beacon
   D. Fetal DNA can be isolated by flow cytometry

   Molecular/Human genetics/2

Answers to Questions 1–4

1. B Exons are the components of genes that determine the amino acid sequence of the protein synthesized. Exons are separated by regions called *introns*, which are transcribed and later removed from mRNA before translation.

2. D The human genome contains approximately 3 billion base pairs and approximately 25,000 genes. Post-transcription modification of mRNA enables production of about 100,000 proteins. However, approximately 99.9% of the DNA is homologous. The remaining 0.1% is variable and accounts for individual differences. A *polymorphism* is an individual difference in a single nucleotide within a DNA sequence or length that occurs in at least 1% of the population. Polymorphisms arise from mutation and are transmitted to offspring. They are subject to selection pressures that cause genes to drift in the population.

3. C Mutations occurring in a gene that is the target of therapy, such as the epidermal growth factor receptor (*EGFR*) gene, can render the cancer resistant to that inhibitor or monoclonal antibody molecule. If the mutation is known, then any type of PCR can detect the mutation. However, when a patient stops responding to a targeted cancer drug and the genetic variant is unknown, NGS must be used to identify and characterize the DNA sequence. This information can be used to ensure that the targeted cancer drug is effective for the patient's treatment.

4. C Measurement of fetal cfDNA in maternal plasma is used to screen for 21 trisomy and other aneuploidies. Circulating fetal cfDNA enters maternal plasma by crossing the placenta. Fetal chromosomes are identified during sequencing by a heterozygous polymorphism carried only on the fetal chromosomes (the mother is homozygous). DNA extracted from maternal plasma is sequenced by using NGS. If two copies of the chromosome are present, the ratio of DNA containing the heterozygous fetal and homozygous maternal polymorphisms will be the same as for the other chromosomes. If a trisomy is present, then the ratio of fetal to maternal DNA for the affected chromosome will be higher.

5. Which is the *most* common method used for parentage testing in the United States?
A. STR (short tandem repeats) analysis
B. Nuclear DNA sequencing
C. Human leukocyte antigen (HLA) DNA typing
D. Mitochondrial DNA sequencing

Molecular/Human genetics/2

6. To prove exclusion in DNA paternity testing, why is it important to identify two genes that must come from the biological father?
A. A single exclusion can result from laboratory error
B. A single exclusion can result from germline mutation within one locus being tested
C. The biological father may be a blood relative to the alleged father
D. The purported mother may not be the biological mother

Molecular/Human genetics/3

7. In human genetics, STRs can be amplified and used for different applications, including all the following, *except*:
A. Forensic science using the HLA-DQ alpha system
B. Identification of gender using the Y-STR
C. Gender testing using the amelogenin locus in combination with STRs
D. Identification of specific genes or coding regions

Molecular/Human genetics/3

8. Genetic concordance can best be defined as:
A. 97% identity between two samples in a genome
B. All locus genotypes or alleles from two sources are the same
C. Collection of all peaks or bands in a distribution of a genome are similar
D. The relative frequency of two alleles matching in a population

Molecular/Human genetics/2

Answers to Questions 5–8

5. A DNA testing is the primary method of determining parentage because it has 100% accuracy in exclusion and greater than 99.9% accuracy in inclusion of parentage. DNA testing is at least 10-fold more conclusive than the combination of HLA, blood group, and protein markers, and DNA samples can be tested prenatally, neonatally, and after death. Testing is performed on nuclear DNA because mitochondrial DNA is inherited exclusively from the mother. Rather than testing for base sequence variations within genes, DNA is tested for length polymorphisms. These are short base sequences within the introns that repeat. The number of times the sequence repeats is inherited as a trait. STRs are oligonucleotide sequences of four or five base pairs. Usually, 12 STR loci are amplified by PCR using specific oligonucleotide primers labeled with fluorescent dyes. The products are detected by using capillary electrophoresis. The size of the fragments and their fluorescence determine which alleles are present.

6. B Two exclusions are needed, rather than one, to be 100% certain of nonpaternity because of the rare possibility of a mutation having occurred in one of the loci being tested. Loci used for DNA testing are sufficiently polymorphic that the mother's sample is not necessary to determine paternity. Exclusion is based on the premise that the biological father must have at least one allele in common with the child at each locus.

7. D STRs are blocks of repetitive sequences in the genome that undergo expansion or shortening from one generation to the next. STRs are commonly 4 to 5 bp repeat units. Mutations within these repeats are very rare. When analyzing STRs, at least 8 to more than 20 loci are evaluated to minimize any minor mutations in the data analysis. STRs can be used in forensic analysis and HLA typing, gender identification using the Y chromosome STR system, and gender testing in a fetus using the amelogenin locus, which is located on both the X and Y chromosomes in combination with STRs. It is not useful for the identification of specific genes or coding sequences because they are noncoding regions of the genome.

8. B Genetic concordance occurs when examining two separate samples to match the identity of an individual. It is an expression of all locus genotypes or alleles from two sources being the same. Samples are said to be in concordance if a single individual is determined to be the donor of both genotypes. Exclusion or concordance occurs when at least one locus genotype is different, except for paternity testing. This is due to mutational events that may generate a new allele in an offspring.

9. In the genome of a microorganism including the mobilome, all the following are considered mobile genetic elements (MGEs) *except*:
A. Insertion sequences
B. Chromosomes
C. Plasmids
D. Integrons
Molecular/Microbial genetics/1

10. Eukaryotic organisms contain multiple chromosomes within the nucleus; however, prokaryotes have a single chromosome. An exception to this is:
A. When two cells are in the process of genetic transfer and conjugation with another
B. There is no time when a prokaryotic cell has more than one chromosome
C. When bacteria divide rapidly, such as during active division, and a cell may harbor multiple copies of the chromosome
D. Some bacteria do not have a single chromosome; this is not a common characteristic
Molecular/Microbial genetics/2

11. The structure of the bacterial cell allows microorganisms to rapidly adjust to the surrounding environment. Which of the following explains the mechanism(s) that facilitates this process?
A. The activation and expression of genes occur simultaneously in the cytoplasm of the cell
B. A bacterial cell has three polymerase enzymes, and each catalyzes a unique process
C. Bacterial genes are simpler and do not require splicing or modification
D. Bacterial cells store needed proteins readily in vesicles within the cytoplasm to respond to environmental changes
Molecular/Microbial genetics/2

12. Restriction enzymes (endonucleases) originate in bacteria. What is the function for a restriction endonuclease within the microorganism?
A. Bacterial endonucleases promote mutation and genetic change to enhance evolutionary changes
B. Bacterial endonucleases splice mRNA molecules for processing during translation
C. Bacterial endonucleases are DNA repair enzymes used to prevent severe DNA damage
D. Bacterial endonucleases digest foreign DNA that enters the cell to prevent lethal mutation or damage to the chromosome
Molecular/Microbial genetics/2

Answers to Questions 9–12

9. B The bacterial genome consists of all genetic material within the cell and all genes are not confined to the chromosome. Many genes are located on MGEs and are considered the mobilome within the organisms. This consists of extrachromosomal elements including plasmids, transposable elements (insertion sequences, composite or complex transposons), and integrons. Although pieces of a bacterial chromosome may be transferred to another cell or offspring as a result of the excision of an MGE from the chromosome, the chromosome is not considered an MGE.

10. C Some bacteria such as *Escherichia coli*, divide approximately every 20 minutes. To facilitate this rapid rate of cellular division, the cell must produce multiple copies of the chromosome. This results in a cell having multiple copies of the chromosome during this process. Typically, all prokaryotes are defined by the presence of a single copy of the chromosome that is not inside a nucleus, which distinguishes them from eukaryotic cells.

11. A The major reason prokaryotic cells can rapidly respond to the ever-changing environment is the ability to transcribe RNA and translate functional proteins directly from the DNA without processing and transfer of the molecules to the outside of a nucleus. In addition, mRNA molecules can be translated by multiple ribosomes before the mRNA transcript is fully complete during the process. This permits microorganisms to inhibit or induce the activity of metabolic enzymes or other products to rapidly respond to environmental changes.

12. D Restriction enzymes or bacterial endonucleases are produced by specific microorganisms to digest unwanted invading nucleic acids from bacteriophages or viruses. The restriction endonuclease recognizes a specific sequence to digest or fragment a nucleic acid molecule. The sequences are termed *restriction sites*. However, the organism that produces the enzyme does not contain the restriction site within their own nucleic acids, which prevents the prokaryotic cell from digesting their own nucleic acid while preventing a bacteriophage from replicating or inserting into the cell's chromosome.

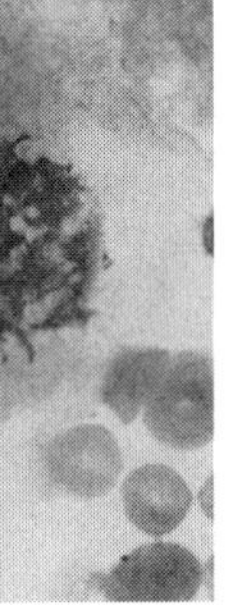

4.5
Molecular Techniques

1. Which double-stranded DNA molecule has the highest melting temperature?

A. An oligonucleotide with a repeating sequence of A-A-A at the 5′ end
B. A molecule of 5,000 base pairs with a high number of A-T base pairs
C. An oligonucleotide with many repeating C-G-C codons
D. A DNA polymer with a high number of A-T-T trinucleotide repeats

Molecular/Techniques/2

2. What process can be used to make a DNA probe produce a fluorescent or chemiluminescent signal?

A. Enzymatic attachment of acridinium esters to terminal ends of the probe
B. Substitution of biotinylated or fluorescent nucleotides into the probe
C. Splicing the gene for β-galactosidase into the probe
D. Heat denaturation of the probe followed by acid treatment

Molecular/Techniques/1

3. What term describes the products produced when DNA is digested by endonucleases?

A. Mosaicisms
B. Chimeras
C. Amplicons
D. Restriction fragments

Molecular/Techniques/1

Answers to Questions 1–3

1. C The melting temperature (T_m) of DNA refers to the temperature required to separate the molecule into single strands. The T_m is the temperature required to convert half of the DNA from double-stranded DNA (dsDNA) to single-stranded DNA (ssDNA). This is performed by breaking the hydrogen bonds between base pairs. A-T base pairs have two hydrogen bonds, whereas C-G base pairs have three. Therefore, molecules with a high proportion of C-G base pairs are more resistant to heat denaturation or melting. It takes 4 degrees Celsius to denature a C-G base pair and 2 degrees Celsius to denature an A-T base pair.

2. B There are several methods that can be utilized to incorporate labeled nucleic acids into a probe. Independent of the method used, a detection molecule that is either a fluorophore or chemiluminescent compound is attached to a nucleotide that is incorporated into the probe sequence using molecular techniques.

3. D When a restriction enzyme cuts two different DNA molecules, the size of some fragments will differ because the number and position of restriction sites differ. Such fragments are called *restriction fragments*.

4. The following figure shows a DNA size standard (ladder) made by restriction enzyme digestion (*PstI*) of lambda phage DNA that has been separated by agarose gel electrophoresis. Which DNA band has the *highest* molecular weight?

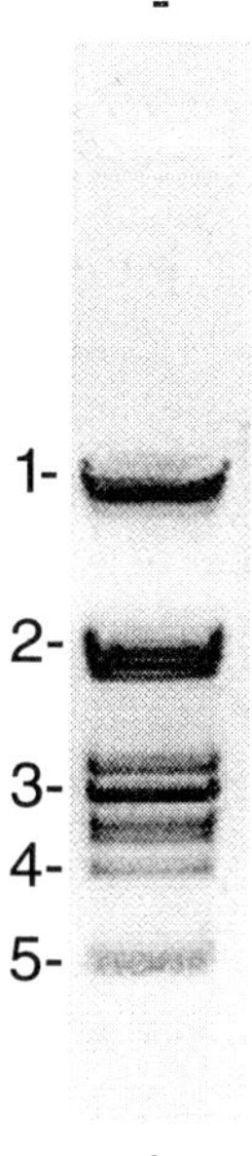

A. 1
B. 2
C. 3
D. 4

Molecular/Techniques/2

5. Which technique is used to detect DNA containing a specific base sequence by applying a labeled probe to DNA bands immobilized onto a nitrocellulose membrane after electrophoresis?

A. Southern blot
B. Northern blot
C. Dot blot
D. Western blot

Molecular/Techniques/1

6. PCR involves three processes. Select the order in which these occur.

A. Extension → annealing → denaturation
B. Annealing → denaturation → extension
C. Denaturation → annealing → extension
D. Denaturation → extension → annealing

Molecular/Techniques/1

7. In the PCR cycle, how is denaturation accomplished?

A. Heat
B. Alkali treatment
C. Addition of sulfonylurea
D. Formamide

Molecular/Techniques/1

Answers to Questions 4–7

4. A Each phosphoric acid subunit within a phosphodiester bond to adjacent deoxyribose molecules has a single negative charge at an alkaline pH. Because the charge is distributed evenly, smaller fragments move more rapidly through the gel. When suspended in an alkaline buffer (pH 8), such as tris-borate-EDTA (TBE) or tris-acetate-EDTA (TAE), the DNA fragments migrate toward the anode at a rate that is inversely proportional to the log10 of molecular size. If the distance traveled is plotted against the log of molecular weight, the plot will be a straight line with a negative slope because the larger the molecule, the more slowly it moves through the pores of the gel. The plot can be calibrated with a DNA size ladder, and the molecular weight of DNA fragments can be determined from the calibration curve.

5. A Southern blot hybridization is a method commonly used to detect genes in both PCR products and restriction endonuclease separation techniques. The DNA fragments or PCR amplicons are electrophoresed, and the DNA fragments are transferred by suction or electrical current and an ionized buffer to a nylon or nitrocellulose membrane. The bands are immobilized and denatured on the membrane, and a solution containing the labeled probe is added. Hybridization is the binding of the complementary base sequence of the probe to the target sequence. This process is highly dependent on temperature, ionic strength of the buffer, and the presence of reagents in the hybridization solution that influence stringency (the degree of exactness of base pairing).

6. C The PCR process results in identical copies of a piece of dsDNA. The process involves three steps that are repeated to double the number of copies produced with each cycle. The first step is denaturation to separate the complementary strands. Annealing occurs when a primer binds upstream to the segment of interest on each strand, called the *template*. Extension involves the enzymatic addition of nucleotides to the primer to complete the new strand.

7. A In PCR, the separation of dsDNA occurs by heating the sample to a temperature between 90°C and 94°C. This breaks the double bonds between the base pairs and is reversible by lowering the temperature. Alkali, high salt, and formamide also denature dsDNA, but they are not used in PCR because they would have to be removed and added with every cycle.

8. What is the composition of the primer used in PCR?

A. A cocktail of enzymes and nucleotide triphosphates that bind to the target
B. An oligonucleotide complementary to bases at the 3′ end of the target
C. A small piece of dsDNA that attaches to the template
D. A probe made of mRNA that binds downstream from the target

Molecular/Techniques/2

9. The master mix solution used for PCR contains which of the following reagents?

A. Deoxyribonucleotide triphosphates
B. Deoxyribonucleotide monophosphates
C. Deoxyribonucleosides
D. Ribonucleotide monophosphates

Molecular/Techniques/1

10. In PCR methods, how can several targets be copied simultaneously and detected?

A. By following the increase in absorbance at 260 nm during melting
B. By labeling multiple primers with different fluorophores
C. By substitution of hybridization probes for primers
D. By analysis of adenosine tail signatures

Molecular/Techniques/1

11. Which formula predicts the number of PCR products that can be produced during amplification?

A. 2^n, where n is the number of cycles
B. N^4, where N is the number of cycles
C. $p^2 + 2pq + q^2 = 1$, where p and q are the numbers of primers
D. $N^2/2$, where N is the number of cycles

Molecular/Techniques/2

12. Which statement *best* describes the method of branched DNA signal amplification?

A. The DNA template is amplified directly by using patented enzymes
B. Multiple primers are used to create branches of the template DNA, permitting multiple extension sites
C. The target DNA is denatured and hybridized to RNA, and the hybrid molecules are amplified by both DNA and RNA polymerases
D. The target DNA is bound by multiple probes, and those are amplified instead of the target DNA

Molecular/Techniques/2

Answers to Questions 8–12

8. B PCR primers are small oligonucleotides, usually 20 to 30 bases, complementary to the base sequence at the 3′ end of the target DNA. Two primers are used, one to the sense strand of DNA (the strand containing the gene) and the other to its complement (the antisense strand). Primers for PCR are made only for the 3′ end of each target sequence because the DNA polymerase that extends the primer does so only by addition of bases in the 5′ → 3′ direction.

9. A The master mix solution contains all the reagents needed to generate new dsDNA. This includes DNA polymerase, the enzyme needed to replicate the target sequence, primers to initiate replication, magnesium (a polymerase cofactor), buffers to maintain pH, and deoxyribonucleotide triphosphates, which are the substrates for DNA polymerase (adenosine triphosphate, guanosine triphosphate, thymidine triphosphate, and cytosine triphosphate).

10. B In PCR, several target sequences can be tested simultaneously using multiple primers (multiplex PCR). Several methods exist for detection and quantitation of possible PCR products. The primers can be labeled with different fluorescent dyes. These can be detected after PCR by capillary electrophoresis using laser-induced fluorescence or using a melt-curve analysis in real-time PCR.

11. A PCR has the potential to double the quantity of PCR products with every cycle. Therefore, 2^n predicts the number of PCR products that can be produced from n cycles. For example, if 30 cycles are programmed, then 2^{30} predicts slightly over 1 billion PCR products. The formula $p^2 + 2pq + q^2 = 1$ describes the distribution of a two-allele gene in a population.

12. D In branched DNA (bDNA) signal amplification, the target DNA is denatured and added to a well containing immobilized probes. One end of each probe hybridizes with the target DNA, capturing it, and the other extender probes contain multiple branches that bind substrate molecules for alkaline phosphatase labeled nucleotides. After washing to remove the unbound labeled probes, dioxetane is added, and chemiluminescence is measured. A thermocycler is not used, and the target DNA is not amplified.

13. A PCR reaction is performed, and the negative control demonstrates the presence of a detectable number of PCR products (amplicons) by capillary electrophoresis. What is the *most* likely cause?

A. False-positive post-PCR hybridization reaction resulting from low stringency
B. Dimerization of PCR primers
C. Contamination of control sample with template DNA
D. Background signal from gel fluorescence or inadequate removal of unbound probe

Molecular/Techniques/3

14. How can a false-negative PCR test caused by the presence of an inhibitor in the reaction in a patient's sample be detected?

A. Using a positive control
B. Using internal control
C. Performing each test in duplicate
D. Performing serial dilutions of the sample

Molecular/Techniques/2

15. All the following are requirements for reducing contamination in DNA amplification methods *except*:

A. Use of aerosol barrier pipette tips when transferring samples or reaction products
B. Preparation of reagents in a dead air box or biological safety cabinet
C. A separate area for performing preamplification, postamplification, and detection steps
D. Pretreatment of samples with high-intensity UV light

Molecular/Techniques/2

Answers to Questions 13–15

13. C PCR and other methods of DNA amplification can result in nonspecific amplification caused by a contaminated sample or reagent with extraneous nucleic acid DNA. The contaminating nucleic acids may be from other samples, positive controls, or amplicons from a previous amplification reaction. Each PCR test run must contain a negative (as well as positive) control. The negative control test contains all PCR reagents and nontemplate DNA, but the template DNA is absent. The negative control should produce no detectable amplicons. This demonstrates that any amplicons produced are a direct result of the primer specifically reacting with the desired template.

14. B Some samples may contain inhibitors in the PCR reaction. For example, a sample in which DNA was extracted by using a cation chelator to prevent DNA degradation may be contaminated with residual chelating reagent. Because DNA polymerase requires magnesium (Mg^{+2}), a cation, this will inhibit amplicon production. An internal control can identify this problem. The sample is mixed with an internal control. Depending on the assay design, the same primers used to amplify the desired target will amplify the internal control, an extrinsic homologous control. Heterologous internal controls are non-target-derived and require a second set of primers that are different from the target primers for amplification. The internal control should always be amplified, but the product can be distinguished from the target amplicons. Failure of a sample to demonstrate the internal control product in an assay where positive and negative control reactions are valid indicates the presence of an inhibitor in the sample.

15. D The laboratory area where manual DNA amplification methods are performed should be organized so that workflow moves from preamplification to amplification and detection. In addition to standard precautions, cotton-plugged tips are used to prevent aerosol contamination of samples. As few as 10 copies of the template introduced into the reaction by accident are likely to cause a false-positive result. UV light causes cross-linking of thymine bases in dsDNA, which prevents replication. This has been used as a post-PCR method of reducing contamination.

16. Which method has been used successfully to reduce contamination in the preamplification stage of PCR?

A. Substitution of deoxyuridine triphosphate for deoxythymidine triphosphate in the master mix
B. Use of low-molecular-size primers
C. Use of a denaturation temperature above 95°C
D. Pretreatment of samples with antisense RNA

Molecular/Techniques/2

17. How are PCR methods adapted to yield quantitative data?

A. Comparing PCR products to an internal standard
B. By applying a conversion factor to the PCR signal that converts it to copies per milliliter
C. By determining the mass of PCR products using UV spectrophotometry
D. By making serial dilutions of the sample

Molecular/Techniques/2

18. In real-time PCR, quantitation can be performed without standards of known copy number. Relative quantitation (estimated concentration) is possible because:

A. Each cycle generates a twofold increase in product
B. Each cycle threshold represents a 10-fold increase in product
C. The fluorescence of two samples can be compared directly
D. Concentration is proportional to fluorescence at the endpoint of the PCR reaction

Molecular/Techniques/3

Answers to Questions 16–18

16. A One method of preventing PCR products from previous assays from contaminating a sample or test in progress is to substitute the RNA base uracil for thymine in the PCR products. *Taq* polymerase will insert deoxyuridine phosphate instead of deoxythymidine phosphate during the primer extension phase of each cycle. The enzyme uracil *N*-glycosylase is added to the master mix along with deoxyuridine triphosphate, which replaces deoxythymidine triphosphate. Prior to the first denaturation, the enzyme hydrolyzes the bond between uracil and deoxyribose. When the sample is heated to separate the strands, the enzyme becomes denatured and any contaminating PCR products fragment into small oligonucleotides that cannot be replicated.

17. A Quantitative PCR can be used to measure viral load and gene expression. However, the PCR process is associated with a high run-to-run variance that can be reduced by simultaneously measuring the PCR products of an internal standard of known concentration (molecules per PCR). For example, in competitive PCR, a DNA template having the same primer-binding region but that is shorter than the native DNA is added to each sample. The signal used to determine concentration is derived from the ratio of the native DNA product to the competitive template product. This value is compared with the signal generated by adding a known amount of DNA from a reference gene (internal standard) and is reported as copies per milliliter or copies per molecule of reference gene. Some quantitative PCR methods use external standards. However, an advantage of the internal standard method is that the calibrator is subject to the same influences as the target DNA by being mixed with DNA from the patient's sample.

18. A Concentration is exponentially related to fluorescence at the start of the PCR reaction, but beyond the early exponential phase, the relationship does not hold. The cycle threshold is in the exponential phase of amplification, which is why the Ct is used for quantification. In theory, because each cycle doubles the amount of PCR product, two samples that differ in Ct by four cycles differ in PCR product by 16-fold. However, this assumes 100% efficiency in the PCR reaction and does not consider the differences in the amount of starting material. A commonly used formula to estimate PCR product is the $\Delta\Delta CT$ method. The sample PCR product is normalized by subtracting the PCR product of a reference gene (e.g., actin). In addition, a control well is also measured, and its product is subtracted from the test sample after subtracting the signal for the same reference gene. Relative concentration = $2^{-\Delta\Delta CT}$, where the $\Delta\Delta CT = \Delta CT$ sample minus ΔCt control.

19. Which real-time PCR parameter can be used to detect the presence of a contaminant?
A. Threshold cycle
B. Baseline
C. Melting temperature
D. Relative fluorescent intensity
Molecular/Techniques/2

20. In real-time PCR, what value is needed to determine the threshold?
A. Background signal
B. Melting temperature
C. Maximum fluorescence
D. Threshold cycle
Molecular/Techniques/2

21. In real-time PCR, which of the following methods is *not* based on using a probe?
A. TaqMan
B. Molecular beacon
C. Scorpion
D. SYBR green
Molecular/Techniques/2

22. Which statement accurately describes the process of fluorescence *in situ* hybridization (FISH)?
A. Hybridization is performed on DNA extracted from cells
B. Hybridization is performed directly on intact chromosomes
C. Hybridization probes are attached to histones associated with the chromosomes
D. Hybridization occurs by attachment to the probe only at the centromere
Molecular/Techniques/1

Answers to Questions 19–22

19. C In real-time PCR, the melting temperature (T_m) corresponds to the temperature at which half of the DNA product separates into single strands. When the negative first derivative ($-\Delta F/\Delta T$) is plotted against temperature, the melting peak for the PCR product is produced. When more than a single melting peak occurs, there is more than a single PCR product. Thus, melting temperature analysis can identify situations in which an unexpected product or a contaminant may be present.

20. A In real-time PCR, the fluorescence of the reporter probe is proportional to the concentration of PCR products. For quantitation of PCR products, a well factor and background fluorescence must be determined. Well factor values are analogous to cuvette blanks. They are used to correct the measurements from each well so that the same concentration of fluorescent dye gives the same signal intensity regardless of the well. The threshold is the lowest signal that indicates the presence of product. It can be calculated manually from a real-time amplification curve by finding the average standard deviation of the fluorescent signal (relative fluorescence unit [RFU]) from cycles 2 to 10. This is multiplied by 10 to give the threshold value in RFUs.

21. D The first three methods are probe-based PCR, whereas SYBR green is not. SYBR green is an intercalating dye that fluoresces when bound to dsDNA. Therefore, it can be used to quantify any PCR product but will also fluoresce with primer dimers that may form in the PCR master mix. This can cause results to be falsely elevated.

22. B FISH is used to detect abnormalities of chromosomes in cells and tissues by facilitating the direct attachment of a fluorescent-labeled oligonucleotide probe or probes to the chromosome. Hybridization of the oligonucleotide probe requires treatment of the cells with proteinase K and other agents, such as nonionic detergent, to increase permeability. Prehybridization may be required to decrease background fluorescence. Denaturation requires controlled temperatures at or near the melting point and the addition of a hybridization solution. This usually contains formamide, sodium chloride and sodium citrate, and EDTA to weaken the hydrogen bonds of the dsDNA target. Hybridization of the fluorescent-labeled probe(s) to the chromosomal DNA also requires highly controlled temperature incubation. After incubating with the cells, any unattached probe is removed by washing, and the cells are examined with a fluorescent microscope containing the appropriate filters to transmit excited light from the specific probe(s).

23. Which type of specimen would be *unsuitable* for FISH analysis?

A. Paraffin-embedded tissue
B. Cells with chromosomes in metaphase
C. Cells with chromosomes in interphase
D. Blood samples submitted for paternity testing

Molecular/Techniques/2

24. FISH can distinguish each of the following chromosomal abnormalities *except*:

A. Aneuploidy
B. Translocation
C. Deletion
D. Trinucleotide repeats

Molecular/Techniques/1

25. In array technology, which molecules are labeled?

A. The immobilized DNA molecules
B. The sample DNA
C. Both target and sample molecules
D. The substrate matrix

Molecular/Techniques/1

Answers to Questions 23–25

23. D FISH can be used with almost any type of cell preparation, including frozen sections, formalin-fixed tissues, embedded tissues, and cell suspensions, such as those derived from amniotic fluid or chorionic villus sampling, provided they are pure. Cells in suspension can be dropped onto glass slides or concentrated by using a cytocentrifuge before processing. Paternity testing is based on comparison of STRs that are identified by fragment analysis.

24. D FISH can detect conditions that are associated with structural chromosomal abnormalities and an abnormal number of chromosomes (aneuploidy). A screening test for aneuploidy employs probes labeled with different fluorescent dyes that simultaneously detect trisomy 21, 18, and 13 and the X and Y chromosomes. Deletions cause the absence of a fluorescent signal when expected, and microdeletions, such as those that occur on the short arm of chromosome 5 in cri du chat ("cat cry") syndrome, can be detected by FISH. Translocations cause two different FISH probes to bind to the same chromosome. Such probes are used to identify *IgH* gene translocations, such as t(11:14) in multiple myeloma, which may be of prognostic value. However, trinucleotide repeats, repetitive sequences of the same three base pairs, are not detected by FISH. This is associated with fragile X syndrome, myotonic dystrophy, Huntington disease, and other genetic diseases. PCR or Southern blotting are used for detection of these repeats, depending on their number.

25. B An array is an organized arrangement of known molecules (either DNA or proteins for proteomic array analysis). DNA arrays are used primarily for studying gene expression and single nucleotide polymorphisms. Commercially prepared arrays use short synthetic oligonucleotides (12–36 bases) of ssDNA immobilized onto a substrate, usually a glass or a silicon chip. These are usually called the *targets*, and a single array can contain hundreds to many thousands of targets. The sample DNA is usually derived by reverse transcriptase PCR of test cells. This produces single-stranded complementary DNA (cDNA) representative of active genes within the cells. These are labeled with one or two fluorescent dyes and, therefore, are usually called *probes*. However, some commercial systems refer to the immobilized (array) DNA as the probe and the labeled DNA as the target.

26. How can all the mRNA within a sample be amplified to prepare microarray probes?

A. A specific primer for each mRNA must be synthesized
B. A primer is made to the poly (A) tail of mRNA
C. Nonspecific attachment of T7 polymerase occurs when the cells are treated with detergent
D. Random primer sets are used under low stringency conditions

Molecular/Techniques/2

27. Protein microarray analysis requires the use of which of the following techniques to generate a protein profile?

A. Electrophoresis
B. Mass spectroscopy
C. Thin-layer chromatography
D. Gas chromatography

Molecular/Techniques/1

Answers to Questions 26–27

26. B When mRNA is transcribed, the enzyme polyA polymerase adds 50 to 250 adenine bases to the 3′ end of the molecule. This poly (A) tail protects the mRNA from enzymatic degradation and promotes its binding to the ribosome. Because almost all eukaryotic mRNA has a poly (A) tail, oligo dT primers are used to initiate reverse transcription, making cDNA copies of the mRNA, and oligo dA primers are used to initiate amplification of the cDNA product.

27. B Protein microarray analysis uses immobilized "bait" to isolate proteins from serum, body fluids, or cell lysates. The array may contain antibodies, antigens, receptor molecules, or protein-binding ligands (e.g., drugs). The proteins can be identified by fluorescent- or enzyme-labeled probes and can be analyzed by mass spectroscopy to produce a fingerprint of the proteins isolated on the array. This can be compared with a learning set, a combination of proteins associated with a specific disease, such as ovarian cancer. If the pattern falls within specified parameters determined by the learning set, then cancer is identified. Mass spectrometry analysis is based on determining the time required for each protein to move through a mass filter. Two related instrument principles are used, matrix-assisted laser desorption ionization–time of flight mass spectrometry (MALDI-TOF), and surface enhanced laser desorption ionization–time of flight mass spectrometry (SELDI-TOF). Both use a laser to ionize the proteins and a mass filter to separate them based on their mass:charge ratio. Because protein expression of cancer cells is altered before morphology changes, the analysis of protein patterns of serum and suspected cells provides an opportunity for diagnosis at an early stage of progression or at a premalignant state.

28. NGS involves four general steps in which order?
A. Bridge amplification → fragmentation → cluster formation → analysis
B. Library preparation → cluster generation → sequencing → data analysis
C. Fragmentation → genome alignment → library formation → sequencing
D. Amplification → surface sequencing → deep sequencing → proofreading
Molecular/Techniques/1

29. Which method uses the process of bridge amplification?
A. Real-time PCR
B. Branched-chain signal amplification
C. NGS
D. Rolling circle amplification
Molecular/Techniques/2

30. Which of the following is a method of sequencing used in NGS?
A. Cyclic reversible dye termination
B. Chain termination using dNTPs
C. Matrix-assisted laser desorption ionization–time of flight mass spectrometry
D. Dye primer sequencing
Molecular/Techniques/2

Answers to Questions 28–30

28. B NGS is a process of massively parallel sequencing of small pieces of DNA. Each sequenced product or amplicon is referred to as a *read*. The first step in NGS is preparation of a library of small templates. This is accomplished by fragmentation of the DNA sample using sonication. The fragments are ligated to adaptors at both ends to form the library of DNA that will be clonally amplified. Cluster generation involves first making exact copies of each fragment composing the library DNA and isolating them from the others so that they are clones of the initial fragments. The clones are separated from each other in separate wells, on separate beads, or on a glass slide. The sequencing reaction requires at least several hundred copies of each clone to do a sequence read; therefore, PCR is carried out again on these separated clones. Sequencing involves making complementary strands to the amplicons of a single clone. These reads are typically 100 to 1,000 base pairs, depending on the platform. Once the sequence of these short strands has been determined, they are assembled by a process called *alignment*, in which the sequence reads are compared with a reference genome.

29. C NGS is a process to rapidly and economically sequence DNA. There are several methodologies for NGS, but all involve parallel amplification of small subunits prior to sequencing. Therefore, each subunit is sequenced rapidly many times, and the data from the fragments are assembled to give a high-fidelity sequence of the starting material. Because amplification is used, NGS requires a much smaller amount of DNA compared with the Sanger method. Bridge amplification is a process used in NGS. The DNA is fragmented, and the pieces are phosphorylated at the 5′ end followed by an enzymatic attachment of adenine to the 3′ end. Fragments anneal to a small double-stranded primer (flow anchor) fixed to a glass surface, well, or bead. One strand of the flow anchor has an extra thymine extending from its 3′ end that is ligated to the adenine of the target fragment. The polymerase copies the fragment forming a loop, a process called *bridge amplification*. Millions of DNA clusters can be made by this process for sequencing.

30. A Reversible dye termination involves the addition of all four dNTPs, each conjugated to a different fluorescent dye at its 3′ end. When a dNTP is added to the template, extension is terminated but, unlike in Sanger sequencing, the blocking moiety is reversible. The slide, well, or bead is washed to remove the unbound dNTPs and UV light or catalyst (tris 2-carboxyethylphosphine) is used to release the dye causing fluorescence and allowing extension to continue. The wavelength of emitted light is used to identify the nucleotide that was added. Master mix is added again, and the process is repeated.

31. Which NGS modality will result in the fewest incidental findings?
A. Whole-genome sequencing (WGS)
B. Whole-exome sequencing (WES)
C. Targeted gene panel
D. Targeted gene sequencing
Molecular/Techniques/2

32. What is the benefit of digital PCR over traditional PCR?
A. It is more efficient when working with a large template
B. Product can be detected prior to the PCR reaction endpoint
C. It quantifies the amount of target sequence without need for external standards
D. It can be multiplexed
Molecular/Techniques/2

33. When the amount of sample is too small, what type of error will be most pronounced in NGS?
A. Amplification bias
B. Signal reads
C. Duplication
D. Contamination
Molecular/Techniques/3

34. Which type of assay constitutes a liquid biopsy?
A. Immunohistochemical detection of a growth factor receptor on breast tissue
B. Tumor cell analysis of blasts by flow cytometry
C. Immunophenotyping of lymphocytes collected by fine-needle aspiration cytology
D. Detection of oncogenes in circulating cell-free tumor DNA from non–small cell lung cancer
Molecular/Techniques/2

Answers to Questions 31–34

31. D WGS sequences the entire genome and is the most comprehensive and expensive modality. WES sequences only the exons of the genome. Both are most useful in those situations in which the location of the mutation is unknown, but they are associated with the most incidental findings. Targeted gene sequencing and gene panels result in the least number of incidental findings but may miss any mutations if the locations are unknown.

32. C Both digital and traditional PCR methods can be multiplexed by using primers labeled with different fluorescent dyes. In digital PCR, several thousand of the same PCR reactions are performed on the sample in parallel. Digital PCR computes the absolute quantity (copies/microliter/sample) of starting template using a Poisson distribution algorithm based on the probability of template duplication and the number of positive reactions (droplets containing amplicons). Copies per droplet = $-\log n(1 - p)$, where p is the percentage of positive droplets divided by 100. The DNA sample is digested with a restriction enzyme and then partitioned in an oil emulsion to separate it into nanoliter droplets. The droplets are so small that there is a very high likelihood that each one will contain only a single copy of the target sequence or none. These droplets become surfaces for PCR. As with real-time PCR, digital PCR uses FRET or fluorescence-generating probes. Unlike in real-time PCR, droplets are transferred to a flow cell at the endpoint. Fluorescence denotes amplicon production. The number of positive reactions is determined by the number of copies of the template in the original sample, but unlike in real-time PCR, it is not dependent on cycle threshold.

33. C PCR in NGS typically produces an error in one out of every 1,000 bases added. *Amplification bias* is a term used to describe the overamplification of smaller fragments in PCR. Contamination occurs when more than a single molecule of DNA is present on the same medium (e.g., on the same bead). Duplication occurs when two or more molecules of DNA from the same clone end up on different beads. When the quantity of starting DNA is too small, more cycles are needed to get sufficient copies for sequencing, and this results in duplication errors, which can be as high as 30%. Such duplicates will appear as identical reads from different parts of the genome.

34. D *Liquid biopsy* refers to analysis of circulating cell-free DNA (cfDNA) released into plasma by a variety of cell types including tumor cells. Although circulating tumor cell DNA is a very small fraction of total cfDNA, it can be measured by using gene-specific primers to oncogenes as an example of the diagnostic utility for liquid biopsy.

35. A tissue sample for PCR was processed for DNA by simple lysis and proteinase K digestion. The lysate was diluted 1:100 and its absorbance measured in a UV spectrophotometer at 260 nm and 280 nm. The absorbance ratio 260:280 was 1.2. What does this indicate?

A. The DNA concentration is too high for PCR
B. The DNA concentration is too low for PCR
C. The sample contains too much protein
D. The sample is optimal for PCR

Molecular/Techniques/2

36. Which component is needed for a thermal cycler to amplify DNA?

A. Programmable heating and cooling unit
B. Vacuum chamber with zero head space
C. Sealed airtight constant-temperature chamber
D. Temperature-controlled ionization chamber

Molecular/Techniques/1

37. What is the recommended threshold cycle (Ct) in real-time PCR?

A. 5 times the standard deviation of the baseline
B. 10 times the standard deviation of the baseline
C. Empirically determined
D. Dependent on the curvature of the cycle

Molecular/Techniques/2

38. The quality of molecular testing depends on the sample. What is the recommended blood collection anticoagulant for extraction of nucleic acids and why?

A. EDTA (ethylene diamine tetra-acetic acid) prevents clotting by binding calcium but does not chelate magnesium, which is used in amplification reactions
B. No anticoagulant; serum is used as a rich source of proteins, lipids, and other molecules
C. Heparin because it does not interfere with the enzymatic activity of the molecular assay
D. Sodium citrate because it forms a covalent bond with nucleic acids, enhancing extraction

Molecular/Techniques/2

Answers to Questions 35–38

35. C The mass and purity of DNA affect the efficiency of DNA amplification. A common way to determine the amount of DNA recovered from a sample is to measure its absorbance at 260 nm, where the nitrogenous bases have an absorbance maximum. Based on the molar absorptivity of DNA at 260 nm, an absorbance of 1.0 equates to 50 ng/μL; thus, multiplying the absorbance by 50 and the dilution factor estimates the DNA concentration in ng/μL. However, proteins also absorb at 260 nm and, if present in sufficient amounts, will cause overestimation of DNA and inhibit amplification. An absorbance maximum for protein is 280 nm because of the phenolic rings of tyrosine and tryptophan. The absorbance ratio of 260:280 is a measure of protein contamination. If the ratio is below 1.7, then too much protein is present, and further purification is needed.

36. A The PCR for DNA amplification consists of three phases. Denaturation requires a temperature of 90°C to 94°C and separates the dsDNA. Annealing requires a temperature of 40°C to 65°C and allows the primers to bind to the target base sequence. Extension requires a temperature of 72°C and allows the heat-stable polymerase to add complementary bases to the primer in the 5′ to 3′ direction. A cycle consists of each temperature stage for a specific number of minutes and most procedures require 20 or more cycles to generate a detectable quantity of target DNA. Rapid heating and cooling are usually achieved using a thermoelectric block that is cooled by forced airflow.

37. C The maximum curvature of the plot approximates the Ct. A line is drawn from the threshold value on the *y*-axis through the curve, and a perpendicular drop to the *x*-axis. The Ct is determined by the intersection point on the *x*-axis. The threshold is usually determined by an algorithm but can be calculated manually as 10 times the average standard deviation of the RFUs (relative fluorescence unit) for cycles 2 to 10.

38. A The most used anticoagulant is EDTA because it prevents clotting by binding calcium and does not interfere with amplification reactions. Although heparin can be utilized in some assays, the assay must be validated for the use of this anticoagulant as it has been known to interfere with amplification reactions.

39. When extracting genomic DNA, all the following external factors can affect the quality of the final nucleic acid sample *except*:

A. Scalability
B. Age
C. Previous handling
D. Storage

Molecular/Techniques/2

40. During nucleic acid isolation or extraction, alcohol is used to precipitate or concentrate the molecules. What is the best alcohol reagent and technique used for precipitation in a liquid extraction that provides the highest yield?

A. Ethanol (90.25% reagent grade) at room temperature
B. Isopropanol at room temperature
C. Ethanol (90.25% reagent grade) at freezer temperatures
D. Isopropanol at freezer temperatures

Molecular/Techniques2

41. Automated nucleic extraction methods utilize what general methodology for the isolation of specific DNA or RNA sequences?

A. Column filtration to bind the nucleic acids followed by a salt precipitation and purification
B. Centrifugation to separate contaminating materials prior to application to a membrane followed by numerous washes
C. Liquid phase reaction followed by a solid phase reaction or mixed method
D. A solid matrix and carrier RNA or DNA to enhance recovery

Molecular/Techniques/2

42. Although many clinical laboratories no longer utilize manual organic extraction methods for the isolation of nucleic acids, the technique provides what advantage over automated methods?

A. Hazardous chemical disposal
B. Improved yield and purity
C. Less labor intensive
D. No fume hood is required

Molecular/Techniques/2

Answers to Questions 39–42

39. A External factors including sample age, previous handling, and storage may affect the yield and quality of extracted nucleic acids. Improper handling and storage may result in degradation or loss of integrity of nucleic acids. Scalability and throughput are important for determining what methodology is useful in a particular laboratory but do not affect the sample integrity.

40. C The choice of reagent alcohol is dependent on the required yield; however, isopropanol precipitates DNA at room temperature and reduces the coprecipitation of salts that may interfere with the assay and may provide lower yield. The optimal yield of precipitation occurs when using reagent-grade ethanol at freezing temperatures. The lower temperatures will result in higher yield but may require an additional purification step to remove unwanted salt precipitation.

41. D In many solid phase extraction methods, the matrix is typically a silica membrane, or beads are used in conjunction with a carrier RNA or DNA molecule that enhances recovery, preventing irreversible binding of the target. This permits removal or extraction of the nucleic acids from the carrier, using buffers to elute and remove only the RNA or DNA for use in subsequent molecular techniques including amplification and detection methods.

42. B Manual organic nucleic extractions have many disadvantages in comparison to automated methods. They are very labor intensive, and require a fume hood and the use and disposal of hazardous chemicals. However, they provide one very important advantage in samples that may contain very small amounts of nucleic acids: they provide a higher yield and purity when performed properly than most automated methods.

43. Separation of nucleic acids in gel electrophoresis is based on size and shape. The following factors may inhibit the normal migration of a DNA molecule during electrophoretic separation *except*:

A. Variation of ionic strength in the buffer concentration

B. Overloading the sample in the initial well of the gel matrix

C. Incorporating a marker dye in the gel matrix or with the sample during loading

D. Overheating or bubbles in the gel matrix

Molecular/Techniques/2

44. Probe to target hybridization depends on optimization of all the following parameters in a molecular assay *except*:

A. The ionic charge of the nitrocellulose membrane

B. Sequence similarity

C. Temperature during the reaction

D. Salt concentration in the hybridization buffer

Molecular/Techniques/2

45. During the optimization of a hybridization assay to locate a new target gene of unknown length, you are willing to identify sequences that contain a few mismatched bases to identify not only the wild type but also potential mutations. Which of the following hybridization reaction conditions would you use?

A. Low salt, low temperature, low urea

B. High salt, high temperature, high urea

C. Low salt, high urea, high temperature

D. High salt, low urea, low temperature

Molecular/Techniques/3

46. Multiple DNA sequencing methods are utilized in different methods. Which of the following methods includes chemical digestion or cleavage of DNA?

A. Pyrosequencing

B. Maxam-Gilbert sequencing

C. Sanger sequencing

D. Edman degradation sequencing

Molecular/Techniques/2

Answers to Questions 43–46

43. C Gel matrixes vary in concentrations to separate different sizes of nucleic acids to improve resolution. In addition, the buffer concentration can increase or decrease migration based on ionic concentrations. Overloading the sample in the gel can result in retardation of the sample or getting stuck at the top of the gel. Finally, overheating can cause artifacts in the migration pattern that result in curving, or what is known as "smiling," and bubbles can simply impede, alter, or stop migration depending on the size and number in the matrix.

44. A The binding of a probe to a specific target nucleic acid is dependent on the sequence similarity, temperature of the reaction, and salt concentration of the buffer or stringency of the reaction. Sequences with low similarity can interact if the temperature of the reaction is significantly lower than the melting temperature of the sequence. In addition, high salt concentrations in the hybridization buffer reduce the electrostatic repulsion between the backbone of the probe and target sequence and can also result in nonspecific binding or hybridization by forcing interactions between a sequence that is mismatched with the probe. If a nitrocellulose membrane is used in a hybridization reaction, the membrane is typically blocked during the assay to prevent nonspecific hybridization, and therefore, the direct binding of a probe to a target sequence is not affected by the charge of the membrane.

45. D The high salt will decrease the electrostatic repulsion between the backbones of the probe and the sequences, allowing nonspecific interactions between the mismatched pairs. In addition, the low temperature will also allow less movement in the reaction, improving hybridization. Urea is a denaturing agent; low urea will also permit hybridization to occur in the reaction.

46. B Maxam-Gilbert sequencing is used to determine the sequence of either double- or single-stranded nucleic acids. The isolated nucleic acid is chemically denatured followed by treatment. The sample is separated into four tubes, once for each different nucleotide, A, T, G, and C. Each individual nucleotide reaction is then treated with a chemical that modifies specific bases such as dimethyl sulfate (guanidine) or hydrazine (cytosine and thymine). Each fragment is then labeled at the 5′ end for detection. The fragments can then be separated by electrophoresis and will migrate differentially based on size in different reactions.

47. All the following are methods that amplify RNA isolated from a sample *except*:

A. NASBA (nucleic-acid sequence-based amplification)
B. TMA (transcription mediated amplification)
C. PCR
D. 3SR (self-sustained sequencing replication)

Molecular/Techniques/1

48. Samples that are appropriate for the application and analysis using microarray technology to identify an inherited or acquired human disease include all the following *except*:

A. Saliva
B. Bone marrow
C. Whole blood
D. Feces

Molecular/Techniques/2

49. There are several methods available to minimize or prevent nonspecific amplification in PCR reactions. Which of the following techniques can minimize nonspecific amplification?

A. Minimizing the PCR master mix contents
B. Isothermal PCR
C. High-fidelity polymerase
D. Reducing the amplification cycles

Molecular/Techniques/2

Answers to Questions 47–49

47. C PCR is a DNA amplification technique. A specialized type of PCR, reverse transcription PCR, requires an additional step or cycle to convert RNA to DNA. Transcription-based methods that can amplify the RNA that is isolated from the sample without a DNA intermediate include TMA, NASBA, and 3SR.

48. D Feces is not an appropriate sample for the detection of human disease because it contains interfering substances as well as a large microbiome that could interfere with the accuracy of the test results.

49. A High-fidelity polymerases are enzymes that have a lower error rate or are less likely to make mistakes when amplifying a complementary strand of nucleic acid. Hot-start PCR prevents nonspecific interactions of the master mix contents prior to the addition of the polymerase, improving the quality and specificity of the amplification. This is also true for optimizing, not minimizing, the master mix components to ensure the correct ratio of primers to template and buffer. This avoids primer dimers and nonspecific binding if there is too much primer in relationship to the template in a reaction. And, finally, reducing the number of amplification cycles avoids nonspecific amplification. This can occur after multiple cycles of PCR because the area or size of the amplification cuvette becomes crowded with nucleic acids, forcing interactions between primers and nucleic acids that are mismatches, resulting in amplification.

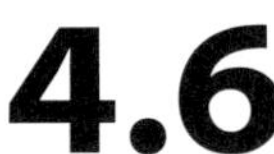

4.6

Molecular Laboratory Practices

1. Molecular laboratories require a very specific workflow to prevent contamination and degradation of nucleic acids. All the following are considered good laboratory practices within a molecular diagnostic laboratory *except*:

A. Use of UV light for decontamination of pipettes and items that cannot be autoclaved

B. One-way workflow from dirty to clean areas

C. Barrier pipettes to minimize or prevent contamination of pipettes during manual processes.

D. Separation of reagents into individual vials of all master mix components to prevent cross contamination

Molecular/Laboratory practices/2

2. In addition to the normal patient identifiers and test information, some molecular tests such as forensics or parentage testing require more information. All the following are required prior to the completion of the tests *except*:

A. Patient consent form

B. Photo identification

C. Chain of custody

D. Transfusion history

Molecular/Laboratory practices/2

3. When an FDA (Food and Drug Administration)-approved molecular test is performed according to the manufacturer's protocol, the implementation of the test requires:

A. Verification of the accuracy and precision

B. Validation of the accuracy, precision, and reference range

C. Verification of the accuracy, precision, and reportable and reference ranges

D. Validation of the accuracy, precision, and reportable and reference ranges

Molecular/Laboratory practices/2

Answers to Questions 1–3

1. D One-way workflow is recommended to prevent cross contamination from dirty areas or sample preparation to clean areas, amplification, and detection to prevent accidental contamination. In addition, barrier pipette tips prevent contamination along with the use of UV light to remove any residual material as most pipettes cannot be autoclaved. However, it is recommended that master mix be prepared and aliquoted to individual assay requirements to avoid repeatedly entering a stock of a single reagent for every use. This minimizes the likelihood of cross contamination of a reagent during each subsequent run, which would require replacing all reagents in a lot or kit.

2. D In complex genetic testing, it is important to always obtain the patient's consent and understanding of the test and the information that it will yield. It is also necessary to determine and confirm the identity of the individual with a validated form of photo identification. In forensic cases, the chain of custody is necessary. Although transfusion history is generally documented in a health record, it is the least likely to be required in forensic or parentage testing of nucleic acids.

3. C An FDA-approved molecular test performed according to the manufacturer's protocols, with no modifications, requires the verification of accuracy, precision, and reportable and reference ranges. If the laboratory changes any manufacturer parameters, then the test must be validated for clinical performance.

4. A new assay for a gene mutation is implemented in the laboratory. In the identification of the mutation, of 100 patients, 95 were identified who had evidence of the associated disease state. What is the measured test performance criterion that is evident from this evaluation?

A. Analytical specificity
B. Clinical sensitivity
C. Analyte measurement range
D. Linearity

Molecular/Laboratory practices/2

5. A new assay for the detection of epidermal growth factor receptor (EGFR) mutations was successfully detected in 34 patients in positive specimens and yielded negative results in 40 normal specimens. What is the measured test performance criterion being evaluated and evident from this information?

A. Analytic sensitivity
B. Analytic specificity
C. Reportable range
D. Clinical sensitivity

Molecular/Laboratory practices/2

6. When determining the analyte's measurable range in the test validation of a molecular assay and demonstrating linearity with calibrators, it is important that the calibrators meet the following criteria:

A. Documented source and quality from the manufacturer
B. Documented source, quality, and preparation but may be provided in an alternate matrix upon receipt
C. Documented source, quality, and preparation but must be provided in the same matrix used in the diagnostic assay
D. Documented lot, quality, and source

Molecular/Laboratory practices/2

7. Analyte specific reagents (ASRs) make up the active part of many homebrew tests and are classified according to risk. Most ASRs are included in which risk classification?

A. Class I
B. Class II
C. Class III
D. Class IV

Molecular/Laboratory practices/1

Answers to Questions 4–7

4. B When 100 patients with a gene mutation are tested and 95 of them demonstrate the disease, the clinical sensitivity is said to be 95%. Clinical sensitivity is the test's ability to predict the presence of a disease state.

5. B When an assay successfully detects mutations in positive specimens or individuals who demonstrate a specific condition or phenotype and yields negative results in normal specimens, or there are no false positives, that is a measure of analytical specificity. The analytical specificity in a molecular assay is the ability of the assay to detect only the intended target and no other nonspecific sequences.

6. C In the test validation of a molecular assay, the analyte's measurable range must be determined using samples of the appropriate type and matrix but can be diluted and dissolved into the appropriate matrix. The source, quality, and preparation of the calibrators must be documented and include a certificate of quality from the manufacturer.

7. A Most manufactured analyte specific reagents (ASRs) are considered Class 1 or low risk and include materials for tests such as FISH, hybrid capture, and microarrays. Class II and III assays typically include the tests that are used in blood banks to screen for infectious diseases and for diagnostics of other infectious diseases such as tuberculosis.

8. When proficiency testing materials are not available commercially for molecular testing, what option can a laboratory utilize to assess the competency of the laboratory personnel?

A. Proficiency testing is not required unless the test is FDA approved
B. Split specimens between two personnel on different days meets the minimum requirement
C. Interlaboratory blinded split specimens is the preferred method
D. Quality control material from a manufacturer can be used as proficiency specimens

Molecular/Laboratory practices/2

9. When reporting sequencing data of mutations, it is important to include a description of the penetrance. Penetrance refers to the:

A. Probability of the presence of a mutation with the disease
B. Probability of the presence of a mutation without disease
C. Probability of the presence of disease with the mutation
D. Probability of the absence of the mutation with the presence of the disease

Molecular/Laboratory practices/2

Answers to Questions 8–9

8. C The availability of proficiency testing samples from manufacturers may be limited with the advancements in molecular diagnostics. Proficiency testing should be completed at least twice a year to evaluate staff competencies. When no commercial material is available, laboratories can exchange blinded split specimens.

9. B The penetrance of a mutation is defined as the probability of having a mutation but not developing or demonstrating the associated disease state.

BIBLIOGRAPHY

1. Buckingham L. *Molecular Diagnostics: Fundamentals, Methods, and Clinical Applications*. 3rd ed. F.A. Davis Company; 2019.
2. Jorde LB, Carey JC, Bamshad MJ. *Medical Genetics.* 6th ed. Elsevier; 2020.
3. Rifai N, Chiu RWK, Young I, Burnham CD, Wittwer CT. *Tietz Textbook of Laboratory Medicine.* 7th ed. Elsevier; 2023.
4. Tille PM. *Bailey and Scott's Diagnostic Microbiology.* 16th ed. Elsevier; 2026.
5. Warford A, Presneau N, eds. *Molecular Diagnostics: Fundamentals of Biomedical Science.* Oxford University Press; 2019.

CHAPTER 5

Urinalysis and Body Fluids

5.1 *Routine Urinalysis*

5.2 *Urine Microscopy and Clinical Correlations*

5.3 *Cerebrospinal, Serous, and Synovial Fluids*

5.4 *Amniotic, Gastrointestinal, Seminal Fluids, and Blood Specimens*

5.1

Routine Urinalysis

1. Urine formation consists of:

A. Filtration, secretion, and reabsorption
B. Filtration, circulation, and absorption
C. Plasma uptake, potassium secretion, and collection
D. Filtration, secretion, and absorption

Urinalysis/Routine/1

2. Regulation of the blood flow to and within the kidneys is under the control of:

A. The renin-angiotensin-aldosterone system
B. The concentration of salt in the vasa recta
C. High plasma sodium content
D. Vasodilation of the renal arterioles

Urinalysis/Routine/1

3. Which statement concerning renal tubular function is true?

A. In salt deprivation, the kidneys will conserve sodium at the expense of potassium
B. Potassium is not excreted when serum concentration is less than 3.5 mmol/L
C. No substance can be excreted into urine at a rate that exceeds the glomerular filtration rate (GFR)
D. When tubular function is lost, the specific gravity (SG) of urine will be below 1.005

Urinalysis/Routine/2

4. Which of the following is *inappropriate* when collecting urine for routine bacteriologic culture?

A. The container must be sterile
B. The clean catch midstream technique must be used
C. The collected sample must be plated within 2 hours unless refrigerated
D. The sample may be held at 2°C to 8°C for up to 48 hours prior to plating

Urinalysis/Routine/2

Answers to Questions 1–4

1. A Urine formation consists of filtration of substances under high pressure from the blood through the glomerulus. Composition is then adjusted by moving additional substances from the blood into the filtrate (secretion) and returning certain substances from the glomerular filtrate to the blood (reabsorption).

2. A Regulation of the blood flow to and within the kidney is under control of the renin-angiotensin-aldosterone system. Low plasma sodium content causes a decrease in water retention within the circulatory system, resulting in decreased overall blood volume and a subsequent decrease in blood pressure. These changes are detected by the juxtaglomerular apparatus. As blood flows through the juxtaglomerular apparatus, blood pressure and sodium levels are monitored. If either the blood pressure or sodium concentration is low, the juxtaglomerular apparatus secretes the enzyme renin. Renin reacts with angiotensinogen in the blood to produce the inert hormone angiotensin I. As angiotensin I passes through the lungs, converting enzymes change it to the active form angiotensin.

3. A Sodium is a threshold substance; that is, no sodium will be excreted in urine until the renal threshold (a plasma sodium concentration of approximately 120 mmol/L) is exceeded. Potassium is not a threshold substance and will be secreted by the tubules even when plasma potassium levels are low. Patients on diuretics or who have hypovolemia become hypokalemic for this reason. Some substances (e.g., penicillin) can be excreted at a rate exceeding glomerular filtration because the tubules secrete them. The tubules are responsible for concentrating the filtrate in conditions of water deprivation and diluting it in conditions of water excess. When tubular function is lost, salt and water equilibrate by passive diffusion, and the SG of urine becomes the same as that of plasma, approximately 1.010.

4. D Urine specimens should be plated and incubated within 2 hours of collection (some laboratories use a 1-hour time limit) and within 24 hours if the sample is refrigerated at 2°C to 8°C immediately after collection. No additives are permitted when urine is collected for culture. Clean catch midstream method is primarily used for specimen collection. A catheter or suprapubic collection may be used in special patient populations that cannot obtain the clean catch midstream.

5. Which statement about sample collection for routine urinalysis is true?
- **A.** Preservative tablets should be used for collecting random urine specimens
- **B.** Containers may be washed and reused if rinsed in deionized H_2O
- **C.** Samples may be stored at room temperature for up to 2 hours
- **D.** A midday sample is preferred when renal disease is suspected

Urinalysis/Routine/2

6. Which urine color correlates correctly with the corresponding pigment-producing substance?
- **A.** Smoky red urine with homogentisic acid
- **B.** Dark amber urine with myoglobin
- **C.** Dark yellow urine and yellow foam with bilirubin
- **D.** Red-brown urine with biliverdin

Urinalysis/Routine/2

7. Which of the following substances cause urine to produce red fluorescence when examined under an ultraviolet lamp (360 nm)?
- **A.** Myoglobin
- **B.** Porphobilinogen (PBG)
- **C.** Urobilin
- **D.** Coproporphyrin

Urinalysis/Routine/2

8. Which of the following conditions could be found with a pale-yellow urine with a high specific gravity?
- **A.** Acute intermittent porphyria
- **B.** Diabetes mellitus
- **C.** Diabetes insipidus
- **D.** Liver disease

Urinalysis/Routine/2

9. Which condition is indicated by a cloudy pink urine?
- **A.** Diabetes mellitus
- **B.** Upper urinary tract infection (UTI)
- **C.** Dehydration
- **D.** Kidney stones

Urinalysis/Routine/2

10. Which of the following specific gravity results correlates with diabetes insipidus?
- **A.** 1.029
- **B.** 1.011
- **C.** 1.020
- **D.** 1.003

Urinalysis/Routine/2

Answers to Questions 5–10

5. C The first morning voided sample is the most sensitive for screening purposes because formed elements are concentrated, but random samples are satisfactory because glomerular bleeding, albuminuria, and cast formation may occur at any time. Preservative tablets should be avoided because they may cause chemical interference with some dry reagent strip and turbidimetric protein tests. Changes in glucose, bilirubin, and urobilinogen can occur within 30 minutes of collection. Therefore, samples should be refrigerated if not tested within 2 hours.

6. C Bilirubin causes urine to turn dark yellow/orange/amber colored. Homogentisic acid causes dark brown or black urine. Myoglobin causes a red to red-brown color in urine, and biliverdin causes a green or yellow-green color. In addition to metabolic diseases and renal diseases, abnormal color can be caused by drugs, dyes excreted by the kidneys, and natural or artificial food coloring.

7. D Myoglobin causes positive tests for blood but does not cause urine to fluoresce. PBG causes urine to become dark (orange to orange-brown) on standing but does not fluoresce. Uroporphyrin and coproporphyrin produce red or orange-red fluorescence at 360 nm. Unlike hemoglobin, porphyrins lack peroxidase activity. Urobilin is an oxidation product of urobilinogen. It turns the urine orange to orange-brown but does not produce fluorescence.

8. B Diabetes mellitus causes polyuria, which will cause the urine to be very pale and dilute and the SG will be elevated due to the presence of glucose. Diabetes insipidus will cause a very pale dilute urine; however, the SG will not be elevated due to glucose. Acute intermittent porphyria produces increased urinary delta-aminolevulinic acid (Δ-ALA) and PBG. The PBG turns urine orange to orange-brown upon standing. Liver disease will cause the urine to be green (bilirubin oxidized to biliverdin) or dark yellow to amber in color.

9. D Kidney stones and other trauma cause injury and the presence of RBCs in urine, which would account for the pink color. Cells could make the urine hazy or cloudy, but hemoglobin would cause it to be clear. In an infection the urine could be cloudy, but not pink. Diabetes and dehydration should not affect turbidity of the urine and would not cause a pink color.

10. D Diabetes insipidus is characterized by a low SG due to the decrease in antidiuretic hormone (ADH).

11. Which of the following methods is used for detecting porphobilinogen (PBG) in urine?
A. Ehrlich reaction
B. Peroxidase
C. Watson-Schwartz test
D. Sodium nitroprusside
Urinalysis/Routine/1

12. A brown or black pigment in urine can be caused by:
A. Pyridium
B. Phenolsulfonphthalein (PSP)
C. Rifampin
D. Melanin
Urinalysis/Routine/1

13. Urine that is amber colored may be caused by:
A. Melanin
B. Bilirubin
C. *Pseudomonas* infection
D. Hemolytic anemia
Urinalysis/Routine/1

14. Which of the following tests is unaffected by standing or improperly stored urine?
A. Glucose
B. Protein
C. pH
D. Bilirubin
Urinalysis/Routine/2

15. Which one of the following characteristics would be an indication that a test result should be reflexed to a microscopic examination of urinary sediment?
A. High volume
B. Pale color
C. Turbidity
D. Clean catch midstream collection
Urinalysis/Routine/2

16. Which of the following is *appropriate* when collecting a 24-hour urine sample?
A. Urine in the bladder is voided at the start of the test and added to the collection container
B. At 24 hours, any urine in the bladder is voided and discarded
C. Urine in the bladder is voided at the start of the test and flushed down the toilet
D. Ten milliliters of 1N sodium hydroxide should be added to the container before collection
Urinalysis/Routine/2

Answers to Questions 11–16

11. A The Ehrlich reaction is the standard method for detecting PBG in urine as well as urobilinogen. The Watson-Schwartz test will detect urobilinogen, but not PBG. Sodium nitroprusside detects ketones in urine, and peroxidase testing is used to detect blood.

12. D Excretion of melanin in malignant melanoma and homogentisic acid in alkaptonuria cause urine to turn black on standing. Other substances that may cause brown or black urine are methemoglobin, PBG, porphobilin, and urobilin. Pyridium, PSP dye, and rifampin are three examples of drugs that cause red or orange-red urine.

13. B Bilirubin causes urine to become dark yellow or amber in color. Melanin (an oxidation product of the colorless pigment melanogen, produced in excess when a malignant melanoma is present) can cause a urine to become brown or black on standing. *Pseudomonas* infection can cause urine to be blue or green as a result of increased urine indican. Hemolytic anemia can cause a red or red-brown color due to the presence of old hemoglobin from RBC breakdown.

14. B Standing urine may become alkaline because of loss of volatile acids and ammonia production. Bilirubin glucuronides may become hydrolyzed to unconjugated bilirubin or oxidized to biliverdin, resulting in a false-negative result on the dry reagent strip test. Glucose can be consumed by glycolysis or oxidation by cells. Protein stays stable in standing urine.

15. C Urine microscopy reflex testing is used by laboratories that do not perform automated microscopic urinalysis because of the low likelihood of significant findings when the microscopic analysis is performed on samples with normal physical characteristics and biochemical results. Urine samples with abnormal clarity are likely to have cells (RBCs, WBCs) or bacteria that would cause a positive strip result and reflex a microscopic.

16. C When collecting a 24-hour urine sample, the bladder must be emptied of urine at the start of the test and the urine discarded. The bladder must be emptied at the conclusion of the test and the urine added to the collection. Refrigeration is the primary method of preservation for most 24-hour collections.

17. Urine production of less than 400 mL/day is:
A. Consistent with normal renal function and H_2O balance
B. Termed isosthenuria
C. Defined as oliguria
D. Associated with diabetes mellitus
Urinalysis/Routine/2

18. Which of the following contributes to SG, but not to osmolality?
A. Protein
B. Salt
C. Urea
D. Glucose
Urinalysis/Routine/1

19. Urine with an SG consistently between 1.002 and 1.003 indicates:
A. Acute glomerulonephritis
B. Renal tubular failure
C. Diabetes insipidus
D. Addison disease
Urinalysis/Routine/1

20. In which of the following conditions is the urine SG *likely* to consistently be below 1.010?
A. Diabetes mellitus
B. Drug overdose
C. Chronic renal failure
D. Prerenal failure
Urinalysis/Routine/2

21. Which statement regarding methods for measuring SG is true?
A. Refractometry is the most accurate way to determine dissolved solute concentration
B. Colorimetric SG test results are falsely elevated when a large quantity of glucose is present
C. Colorimetric SG readings are falsely low when pH is alkaline
D. Refractometry will be falsely decreased when protein is present
Urinalysis/Routine2

22. What is the principle of the colorimetric reagent strip determination of SG in urine?
A. Ionic strength alters the pK_a of a polyelectrolyte
B. Sodium and other cations are chelated by a ligand that changes color
C. Anions displace a pH indicator from a mordant, making it water soluble
D. Ionized solutes catalyze oxidation of an azo dye
Urinalysis/Routine/1

Answers to Questions 17–22

17. C Normal daily urine excretion is usually 600 to 1,600 mL/day. *Isosthenuria* refers to urine of constant SG of 1.010, which is the SG of the glomerular filtrate. Glycosuria causes retention of H_2O within the tubule, resulting in dehydration and polyuria, rather than oliguria. Oliguria is defined as urinary output less than 400 mL/day.

18. A All substances that dissolve in the urine contribute to osmotic pressure or osmolality. This includes non-ionized solutes such as urea, uric acid, and glucose as well as salts, but not colloids, such as protein and lipids.

19. C In severe renal diseases, the tubules fail to concentrate the urine filtrate. Salt and H_2O equilibrate by diffusion, causing an SG of about 1.010. If the SG of urine is below the plasma level, free H_2O is lost. This results from failure to produce antidiuretic hormone (inherited diabetes insipidus) or from failure of the tubules to respond to ADH (nephrogenic diabetes insipidus, which can be caused by drugs, polycystic kidney disease, and hypercalcemia).

20. C Glucose and drug metabolites increase the SG of urine. In prerenal failure, the renal tubules are undamaged. Ineffective arterial pressure stimulates aldosterone release. This increases sodium reabsorption, which stimulates ADH release. Water and salt are retained, and the urine:plasma (U:P) osmolar ratio exceeds 2:1. Chronic renal failure is associated with nocturia, polyuria, and low SG caused by scarring of the collecting tubules.

21. C Cells and undissolved solutes refract light and will cause a falsely high SG reading by refractometry. Colorimetric SG tests are less sensitive to nonionized compounds, such as urea and glucose, and are negatively biased (falsely low) when large quantities of nonelectrolytes are present. Colorimetric SG readings are determined by a pH change on the test pad and are approximately 0.005 lower when pH is 6.5 or higher. Osmometry is the most accurate way to measure the concentration of dissolved solutes in urine.

22. A This test is based on the change in the pK (dissociation constant) of the polyelectrolyte in response to the ionic solutes present in the urine sample. As ionized particles (Na^+ and K^+) in the urine attach to the polyelectrolyte material in the reagent pad, hydrogen ions (H^+) are released from the polyelectrolyte. The released hydrogen ions cause a change in the pH of the pad. The indicator will be blue at low SG and green at higher SG.

23. Which statement regarding urine pH is accurate?
A. A high-protein diet promotes an alkaline urine pH
B. pH tends to decrease as urine is stored
C. Contamination should be suspected if urine pH is less than 4.5
D. Bacteriuria is most often associated with a low urine pH
Urinalysis/Routine/2

24. In renal tubular acidosis, the pH of urine is:
A. Consistently acid
B. Consistently alkaline
C. Neutral
D. Variable, depending on diet
Urinalysis/Routine/1

25. The normal daily urine output for an adult is approximately:
A. 0.2 to 0.5 L
B. 0.6 to 1.6 L
C. 2.7 to 3.0 L
D. 3.2 to 3.5 L
Urinalysis/Routine/1

26. The SG of the urine filtrate in the Bowman space is approximately:
A. 1.000 to 1.002
B. 1.004 to 1.006
C. 1.008 to 1.010
D. 1.012 to 1.014
Urinalysis/Routine/1

27. A patient with partially compensated respiratory alkalosis would have a urine pH of:
A. 4.5 to 5.5
B. 5.5 to 6.5
C. 6.5 to 7.5
D. 7.5 to 8.5
Urinalysis/Routine/2

28. Which of the following is *most* likely to cause a false-positive result on the dry reagent strip test for urinary protein?
A. Urine of high SG
B. Highly buffered alkaline urine
C. Bence-Jones protein
D. Salicylates
Urinalysis/Routine2

Answers to Questions 23–28

23. C Bacteriuria is usually associated with an alkaline pH caused by the production of ammonia from urea. Extended storage may result in loss of volatile acids, causing increased pH. A high-protein diet promotes excretion of inorganic acids resulting in an acidic urine pH. The tubular maximum for hydrogen ion secretion occurs when urine pH reaches 4.5, the lowest urinary pH that the kidneys can produce.

24. B Renal tubular acidosis results from a defect in the renal tubular reabsorption of bicarbonate. Hydrogen ions are not secreted when bicarbonate ions are not reabsorbed. Wasting of sodium bicarbonate ($NaHCO_3$) and potassium bicarbonate ($KHCO_3$) results in alkaline urine and hypokalemia in association with acidosis.

25. B Under conditions of normal fluid intake, the reference range for urine volume is 0.6 to 1.6 L/day. Urine output will vary widely with fluid intake. In cases of fluid deprivation, almost all urine filtrate will be reabsorbed, resulting in daily excretion as low as 500 mL. When fluid intake is excessive, up to 2.0 L of urine may be voided. Urine output beyond these extremes is considered abnormal.

26. C The SG of the filtrate in the Bowman space is 1.010, which approximates the SG of plasma because sodium, chloride, glucose, urea, and other main solutes are completely filtered by the glomeruli. This corresponds to an osmolality of approximately 280 mOsm/kg.

27. D Urine pH is determined by diet, acid–base balance, water balance, and renal function. In partially compensated respiratory alkalosis, the kidneys reabsorb less bicarbonate, which results in lower net acid excretion. The loss of bicarbonate helps compensate for alkalosis and causes urine pH to be alkaline.

28. B Highly buffered alkaline urine will override the buffer system causing a rise in pH and producing a color change that is unrelated to protein. In addition to highly buffered alkaline urine, a false-positive protein result on the dry reagent strip test may be caused by quaternary ammonium compounds, which increase urine pH. Because the dry reagent strip tests are insensitive to globulins, a false-negative result is likely in the case of Bence-Jones proteinuria. Positive interference by drugs is uncommon for dry reagent strip protein tests but is common for turbidimetric tests. High urinary SG will suppress the color reaction of the strip protein tests.

29. When testing for urinary protein with sulfosalicylic acid (SSA), which condition produces a false-positive result?

A. Highly buffered alkaline urine
B. The presence of x-ray contrast medium
C. Increased urinary SG
D. The presence of red blood cells (RBCs)

Urinalysis/Routine/2

30. A discrepancy between the urine SG determined by measuring refractive index and urine osmolality would be *most* likely to occur:

A. After catheterization of the urinary tract
B. In diabetes mellitus
C. After intravenous radiographic dye
D. In uremia

Urinalysis/Routine/2

31. Which of the following is *likely* to result in a false-negative dry reagent strip test for proteinuria?

A. Penicillin
B. Aspirin
C. Amorphous phosphates
D. Bence-Jones protein

Urinalysis/Routine/1

32. Daily loss of protein in urine normally does not exceed:

A. 30 mg/day
B. 50 mg/day
C. 100 mg/day
D. 150 mg/day

Urinalysis/Routine/1

33. Which of the following will not cause a false-positive result on turbidimetric protein tests?

A. Tolbutamide
B. X-ray contrast medium
C. Penicillin or sulfa antibiotics
D. Ascorbic acid

Urinalysis/Routine/2

Answers to Questions 29–33

29. B Turbidimetric assays are used to test urine suspected of giving a false-positive result on the dry reagent strip test for albumin because the urine is highly alkaline (pH greater than or equal to 8.0) or contains pigmentation that interferes with reading the protein test pad. In addition, SSA tests are used when screening urine for an increased concentration of globulins because dry reagent strip tests are far less sensitive to globulins. SSA is less specific but more sensitive for albuminuria than conventional dry reagent strip tests. Iodinated dyes, penicillin, salicylate, and tolbutamide may result in false-positive results. Trace turbidity is difficult to determine when urine is cloudy because of bacteriuria, mucus, or crystals. Alkaline urine may titrate SSA, reducing its sensitivity. For these reasons, the SSA test is not used routinely.

30. C The radiographic dye contains iodine and is highly refractile. This increases the refractive index of urine, causing falsely high measurement of solute concentration. The refractive index is affected by the size and shape of solutes and undissolved solids, such as protein. Osmolality is the most specific measure of total solute concentration because it is affected only by the number of dissolved solutes.

31. D Dry reagent strip tests using tetrabromophenol blue or tetrachlorophenol tetrabromosulfophthalein are most sensitive to albumin and poorly sensitive to globulins and may not detect immunoglobulin light chains. Turbidimetric methods, such as 3% SSA, will often detect Bence-Jones protein but may give a false-positive reaction with penicillin, tolbutamide, salicylates, and x-ray contrast dyes containing iodine. Amorphous phosphates may precipitate in refrigerated urine, making interpretation of turbidimetric tests difficult.

32. D Small amounts of albumin and other low-molecular-weight proteins, such as amylase, β-microglobulins, and immunoglobulin fragments, are excreted in urine. Proteinuria does not normally exceed 30 mg/dL or 150 mg/day. The detection limit of the SSA test to albumin is approximately 1.5 to 2.0 mg/dL, and for dry reagent strip tests, it is approximately 15 mg/dL. Therefore, trace positives by either method may occur in the absence of renal disease.

33. D Ascorbic acid may reduce diazo salts used in the bilirubin and nitrite tests and react with hydrogen peroxide in peroxidase reactions. Therefore, individuals taking megadoses of ascorbic acid (vitamin C) may show negative interference with tests for glucose, blood, bilirubin, and nitrite. Ascorbate does not cause either a false-negative or false-positive reaction for protein.

34. Which statement *best* describes the clinical utility of tests for microalbuminuria?

A. Testing may detect early renal involvement in diabetes mellitus
B. Microalbuminuria refers to a specific subfraction of albumin found only in persons with diabetic nephropathy
C. A positive test result indicates the presence of orthostatic albuminuria
D. Testing should be part of routine urinalysis

Urinalysis/Routine/2

35. Dry reagent strip tests for microalbuminuria that compare albumin to creatinine determine the creatinine concentration based on which principle?

A. Formation of a Cu^{+2}–creatinine complex
B. Enzymatic assay using sarcosine oxidase and peroxidase
C. Reaction of creatinine with alkaline sodium picrate
D. Change in pH as creatinine is converted to creatine

Urinalysis/Routine/2

36. Which of the following conditions is *least* likely to be detected by dry reagent strip tests for proteinuria?

A. Orthostatic albuminuria
B. Chronic renal failure
C. Pyelonephritis
D. Renal tubular proteinuria

Urinalysis/Routine/2

37. The normal renal threshold for glucose is:

A. 70 to 85 mg/dL
B. 100 to 115 mg/dL
C. 130 to 145 mg/dL
D. 165 to 180 mg/dL

Urinalysis/Routine/1

Answers to Questions 34–37

34. A The microalbumin test is an assay for measuring urinary albumin concentration that has an increased sensitivity (detection limit below 15 mg/dL) and is recommended for patients who are at risk for chronic renal disease, especially individuals with diabetes mellitus. In diabetes, an early sign of renal involvement is an increased rate of albumin excretion in the range of 20 to 200 μg/mL or more than 30 mg albumin per gram of creatinine. Results in this range are significant in the at-risk population, even though the dry reagent strip test for protein may yield negative results. Dry reagent strip tests for microalbuminuria are too sensitive for use in routine urinalysis but are useful in screening patients with diabetes and hypertension for increased urinary albumin excretion.

35. A The dry reagent strip test for creatinine contains anhydrous buffered copper (II) sulfate ($CuSO_4$), alcoholic tetramethylbenzidine, and diisopropylbenzene dihydroperoxide. In the presence of creatinine, a copper–creatinine complex forms. This catalyzes the oxidation of a benzidine derivative by an alcoholic peroxide, forming a blue color on the test pad. Color intensity is proportional to creatinine concentration. Negative interference occurs from ascorbate and ethylenediaminetetraacetic acid (EDTA), which chelates the copper. Positive interference occurs from hemoglobin and some drugs (e.g., nitrofurantoin). The microalbumin concentration is determined by the protein error of the indicator effect using a dye with increased sensitivity, tetrabromophenol blue.

36. D The detection limit (sensitivity) of dry reagent strip protein tests is approximately 15 mg/dL albumin and is sufficient to detect urinary albumin levels found in orthostatic albuminuria and renal diseases, except for tubular proteinuria. Renal tubular proteinuria results from failure of damaged tubules to reabsorb small proteins, such as β_2-microglobulin. Dry reagent strip tests for proteinuria are most sensitive to albumin and poorly sensitive to globulins and do not detect small quantities of hemoglobin, myoglobin, or microglobulin. Electrophoresis of urine is used to detect renal tubular proteinuria.

37. D The renal threshold is the concentration of a substance (e.g., glucose) in blood that must be exceeded before it can be detected in urine. Threshold substances require a carrier to transport them from the tubular lumen to the vasa recta. When the carrier becomes saturated, the tubular maximum is reached, causing the substance to be excreted in urine.

38. In which of the following conditions is glycosuria *most* likely?
A. Addison disease
B. Hypothyroidism
C. Pregnancy
D. Hypopituitarism
Urinalysis/Routine/2

39. In addition to ascorbate, the glucose oxidase reaction may be inhibited by which substance?
A. Acetoacetic acid (AAA)
B. Aminocaproic acid
C. Creatinine
D. Azopyridium
Urinalysis/Routine/1

40. A positive glucose oxidase test and a negative test for reducing sugars indicates:
A. True glycosuria
B. The specimen was allowed to sit at room temperature for 6 hours
C. False-negative reducing test result caused by ascorbate
D. Galactosuria
Urinalysis/Routine/2

41. A negative glucose oxidase test and a positive test for reducing sugars in urine indicates:
A. True glycosuria
B. A false-negative glucose oxidase reaction
C. The presence of a non-glucose reducing sugar, such as galactose
D. A trace quantity of glucose
Urinalysis/Routine/2

42. In what condition may urinary ketone tests underestimate ketosis?
A. Acidosis
B. Hemolytic anemia
C. Renal failure
D. Excessive use of vitamin C
Urinalysis/Routine/2

43. Acetoacetic acid (AAA) is detected in urine by reaction with:
A. Sodium nitroprusside
B. *o*-Toluidine
C. *m*-Dinitrobenzene
D. *m*-Dinitrophenylhydrazine
Urinalysis/Routine/1

Answers to Questions 38–43

38. C In addition to diabetes mellitus, glycosuria may occur in other endocrine diseases, in pregnancy, in response to drugs that affect glucose tolerance or renal threshold, and in several other conditions, especially those involving the liver or the central nervous system (CNS). Cushing disease and hyperthyroidism cause impaired glucose tolerance and hyperglycemia. Increased estrogens produced in pregnancy lower the renal threshold for glucose and may impair glucose tolerance. Hyperpituitarism causes hyperglycemia mediated by increased release of growth hormone.

39. A AAA and salicylates may inhibit the glucose oxidase reaction by the same mechanism as ascorbate. These reducing agents compete with the chromogen for hydrogen peroxide. Low SG may increase and high SG may decrease the color reaction for glucose in urine.

40. A Glucose oxidase is specific for β-D-glucose. Therefore, a positive reaction is always considered significant unless contamination is evident. A reducing test should not be used to confirm a positive result on the glucose oxidase test because this test is not as specific or as sensitive. Reducing sugar tests are used to screen infants for inborn errors of carbohydrate metabolism, such as galactosuria, but are not used to screen for glycosuria.

41. C Reducing tests utilize alkaline copper sulfate and heat to oxidize glucose. Other reducing substances, including several sugars and antibiotics, may react, making the test inappropriate as a screening test for glucose. A positive test result for reducing sugars seen with a negative glucose oxidase test result may occur in lactose disorders, galactose disorders, fructosuria, and other disorders of carbohydrate metabolism. Such tests should always be confirmed with chromatography to identify the specific sugar and with assay of the specific enzyme involved.

42. A Tests for urinary ketone bodies are sensitive to acetoacetic acid. They react weakly with acetone and do not react with β-hydroxybutyric acid. Acidosis favors formation of β-hydroxybutyric acid and may cause a falsely low estimate of urine ketones in diabetic ketoacidosis. Ketonuria has many causes other than diabetic ketoacidosis, such as pregnancy, fever, protein calorie malnutrition, and dietary carbohydrate restriction. Trace ketones tend to be more clinically significant when seen in urine with a low SG.

43. A Urinary ketones are detected using alkaline sodium nitroprusside (nitroferricyanide). Mesna and other sulfhydryl compounds may cause a false-positive result on dry reagent strip tests, phenylpyruvic acid, and some antibiotics with the ketonetube test.

44. Nondiabetic ketonuria can occur in all the following *except*:
A. Pregnancy
B. Renal failure
C. Starvation
D. Lactate acidosis
Urinalysis/Routine/2

45. Which of the following statements regarding the classic nitroprusside reaction for ketones is true?
A. The reaction is most sensitive to acetone
B. Nitroprusside reacts with acetone, acetoacetic acid, and β-hydroxybutyric acid
C. It may be falsely positive in phenylketonuria
D. The reaction is recommended for diagnosing ketoacidosis
Urinalysis/Routine/2

46. Hemoglobin in urine can be differentiated from myoglobin by using:
A. 80% ammonium sulfate to precipitate hemoglobin
B. Sodium dithionite to reduce hemoglobin
C. Microscopy
D. The dry reagent strip blood test
Urinalysis/Routine/2

47. Which of the following conditions is associated with a negative blood test result and an increase in urine urobilinogen?
A. Calculi of the kidney or bladder
B. Malignancy of the kidney or urinary system
C. Crush injury
D. Extravascular hemolytic anemia
Urinalysis/Routine/2

48. Which statement about the dry reagent strip blood test is true?
A. The test is based on the reaction of acetoacetic acid
B. It is a pseudoperoxidase reaction
C. A nonhemolyzed trace will cause a solid color pad
D. Ascorbic acid will cause a false-positive reaction
Urinalysis/Routine/2

Answers to Questions 44–48

44. B Ketonuria results from excessive oxidation of fats forming acetyl coenzyme A (CoA). In addition to diabetes mellitus, ketonuria occurs in starvation, carbohydrate restriction, alkalosis, lactate acidosis, and von Gierke disease (glycogen stores cannot be utilized). Ketonuria also occurs in pregnancy, associated with increased vomiting and cyclic fever.

45. C Tests for ketones are less sensitive to acetone than to AAA and do not detect β-hydroxybutyric acid. High levels of phenylpyruvic acid (phenylketonuria) will cause a false-positive reaction in the classic nitroprusside reaction but do not usually interfere with the dry reagent strip test for ketones. Serum ketones can be measured by gas chromatography, and β-hydroxybutyric acid can be measured enzymatically. The enzymatic assay for β-hydroxybutyrate in plasma is the recommended test for diagnosing ketoacidosis because acidosis favors its formation.

46. A Both hemoglobin and myoglobin have peroxidase activity and cause a positive blood test result. However, myoglobin is soluble in 80% weight per volume (w/v) ammonium sulfate in urine, but hemoglobin precipitates. A positive blood reaction with supernatant after addition of ammonium sulfate and sodium hydroxide (NaOH) confirms the presence of myoglobin. The presence of RBCs indicates that hemoglobin, rather than myoglobin, is present; however, the absence of RBCs does not rule out the presence of hemoglobin as the cause of a positive blood test result.

47. D A positive result on the blood test can occur from renal or lower urinary tract bleeding, intravascular hemolytic anemia, and transfusion reaction. Extravascular hemolysis results in increased bilirubin production, rather than in plasma hemoglobin. This may cause increased urobilinogen in urine, but not a positive blood reaction.

48. B The blood reaction is peroxide plus a chromogen reacts with the hemoglobin to produce an oxidized chromogen plus water. Hemoglobin has peroxidase activity and catalyzes the oxidation of tetramethylbenzidine by peroxide. The reaction is sensitive to submilligram levels of free hemoglobin, whereas visible hemolysis does not occur unless free hemoglobin exceeds 20 mg/dL. Nonhemolyzed trace will produce a speckled pad, not a solid pad. A solid pad will be present with hemoglobin.

49. A moderately positive result on the blood test and trace protein test are seen on the dry reagent strip, and 11 to 20 RBCs/high-power field (HPF) are present on microscopic examination. These results are *most* likely caused by which of the following?
- A. Transfusion reaction
- B. Myoglobinuria
- C. Intravascular hemolytic anemia
- D. Recent urinary tract catheterization

Urinalysis/Routine/3

50. Which of the following urinalysis results are discrepant?
- A. Small amount of blood, but negative protein
- B. Moderate amount of blood, but no RBCs in microscopic examination
- C. Negative blood, but 6 to 10 RBCs/HPF
- D. Negative blood, but positive protein

Urinalysis/Routine/3

51. Which of the following statements regarding the dry reagent strip test for bilirubin is true?
- A. A positive test result is seen in prehepatic, hepatic, and posthepatic jaundice
- B. The test detects only conjugated bilirubin
- C. Standing urine may become falsely positive because of bacterial contamination
- D. High levels of ascorbate will cause positive interference

Urinalysis/Routine/2

52. Which of the following reagents is used to detect urobilinogen in urine?
- A. *p*-Dinitrobenzene
- B. Watson-Schwartz reagent
- C. Erlich aldehyde reagent
- D. *p*-Dichloroaniline

Urinalysis/Routine/1

Answers to Questions 49–52

49. D The blood test detects intact RBCs, hemoglobinuria, and myoglobinuria. Causes of hemoglobinuria include intravascular hemolytic anemias, transfusion reactions, and lysis of RBCs in the filtrate or urine caused by alkaline or hypotonic conditions. Causes of hematuria include acute and chronic glomerulonephritis, pyelonephritis, polycystic kidney disease, renal calculi, bladder and renal cancers, and catheterization of the urinary tract.

50. C The blood test detects as little as 0.015 mg/dL free hemoglobin and 4 to 5 RBCs/μL. The protein test detects 15 mg/dL albumin, but substantially more hemoglobin is required to obtain a positive test result. Therefore, a small blood reaction (nonhemolyzed or moderately hemolyzed trace, trace, or small) usually occurs in the absence of positive protein. A positive blood test result often occurs in the absence of RBCs in microscopic examination. This can result from intravascular hemolysis, myoglobinuria, or lysis of RBCs caused by alkaline or hypotonic urine. A positive test result for protein and a negative blood test result occur commonly in such conditions as orthostatic albuminuria, UTI, and diabetes mellitus. However, a negative blood test result should not occur if more than 3 to 4 RBCs/HPF are seen in the microscopic examination. Either the blood test is falsely negative (a missed nonhemolyzed trace), or yeast has been mistaken for RBCs.

51. B Only the conjugated form of bilirubin is excreted into urine. Urinary bilirubin is positive in necrotic and obstructive jaundice but not in prehepatic jaundice, which results in a high level of serum unconjugated bilirubin. The highest levels of urinary bilirubin occur in obstructive jaundice, which causes decreased urinary urobilinogen. Very few drugs have been reported to interfere with urine bilirubin tests, which are based on the formation of azobilirubin by reaction with a diazonium salt. Positive interference by rifampin and chlorpromazine have been reported. Urine must be fresh because sunlight destroys bilirubin. Bacteria may cause hydrolysis of glucuronides, forming unconjugated bilirubin, which does not react with the diazonium reagent. Ascorbate inhibits the reaction by reducing the diazo reagent.

52. C Urobilinogen reacts with the Ehrlich aldehyde reagent (*p*-dimethylaminobenzaldehyde in hydrochloric acid [HCl]) to form a pink color. Dry reagent strips use either *p*-dimethylaminobenzaldehyde or 4-methoxybenzene diazonium tetrafluoroborate to detect urobilinogen. The former reagent may react with porphobilinogen, salicylate, and sulfonamides giving falsely high results. False-positive results may occur in the presence of pyridium and gantrisin, which color urine orange-red. Formalin may cause a false-negative reaction.

53. Which of the following statements regarding urinary urobilinogen is true?

A. Diurnal variation occurs, and the highest levels are seen in the early morning
B. High levels accompanied by a positive bilirubin test result indicate obstructive jaundice
C. Dry reagent strip tests do not detect decreased levels
D. False-positive results may occur if urine is stored for more than 2 hours

Urinalysis/Routine/2

54. Which of the following statements regarding the test for nitrite in urine is correct?

A. It detects more than 95% of clinically significant bacteriuria
B. Formation of nitrite is unaffected by the urine pH
C. The test is dependent on adequate dietary nitrate content
D. A positive test differentiates bacteriuria and *in vitro* bacterial contamination

Urinalysis/Routine/2

55. Which statement about the dry reagent strip test for leukocytes is correct?

A. The test detects only intact white blood cells (WBCs)
B. The reaction is based on the hydrolysis of substrate by WBC esterases
C. Several antibiotics may give a false-positive reaction
D. Strong oxidizing agents will cause a false-negative reaction

Urinalysis/Routine/2

56. Which of the following statements about creatinine clearance is correct?

A. Dietary restrictions are required during the 24 hours preceding the test
B. Fluid intake must be restricted to below 600 mL in the 6 hours preceding the test
C. Creatinine clearance is mainly determined by renal tubular function
D. Creatinine clearance is dependent on lean body mass

Urinalysis/Routine/1

Answers to Questions 53–56

53. C Urobilinogen exhibits diurnal variation, and highest levels are seen in the afternoon. A 2-hour postprandial afternoon sample is the sample of choice for detecting increased urine urobilinogen. Urobilinogen is formed by the bacterial reduction of conjugated bilirubin in the bowel. In obstructive jaundice, delivery of bilirubin into the intestine is blocked, resulting in decreased fecal, serum, and urine urobilinogen. However, the dry reagent strip tests are not sensitive enough to detect abnormally low levels. Urobilinogen is rapidly oxidized to urobilin, which does not react with dry reagent strip tests.

54. C The nitrite test is dependent on the activity of bacterial reductase, and false-negative results have been reported when urine is highly acidic. Nitrite is formed by reduction of diet-derived nitrates and reacts with *p*-arsanilic acid or sulfanilamide to form a diazonium compound. This reacts with benzoquinoline to form pink azo dye. False-negative results also occur in the presence of ascorbate, which reduces the diazonium product. Nitrite is positive in about 70% of clinically significant bacterial infections of the urinary tract. Sensitivity is limited by the requirements for dietary nitrate and 3- to 4-hour storage time in the bladder. In addition, the causative bacteria must be able to reduce nitrate.

55. B Polymorphonuclear neutrophils (PMNs) in urine are detected by the presence of esterases that hydrolyze an acid ester, such as indoxylcarbonic acid. The product reacts with a diazonium salt to give a purple color. The test detects esterases in urine as well as intact WBCs but is not sensitive to less than 5 to 10 WBCs/HPF. Several antibiotics, high protein, and high SG inhibit the esterase reaction. Strong oxidizers will cause a false-positive result.

56. D Body size determines how much creatinine is produced, and clearance must be normalized to eliminate this variable. Because of the difficulty in collecting a valid 24-hour urine sample, the estimated glomerular filtration rate (eGFR) is recommended as the screening test for low GFR. Creatinine clearance should be used when lean body mass may not be accurately represented by the patient's age and gender as used in the Modification of Diet in Renal Disease Study (MDRD) formula for eGFR. Although some creatinine is derived from the diet, it is rapidly filtered by the glomeruli, and time variations are reduced by collection of urine for 24 hours. Creatinine is produced from oxidation of creatine at a constant rate of about 2% per day. It is filtered completely and not significantly reabsorbed. However, creatinine secretion by the tubules is increased when filtrate flow is slow, and patients must be given at least 600 mL of H_2O at the start of the test and kept well hydrated throughout.

57. A male patient's eGFR is 75 mL/min. This indicates:

A. Normal glomerular filtration rate (GFR)
B. The patient is uremic and will be hyperkalemic
C. Renal tubular dysfunction
D. Reduced glomerular filtration

Urinalysis/Routine/2

58. Which of the following substances are used to calculate eGFR?

A. *p*-Aminohippuric acid (PAH)
B. Glycine
C. Cysteine
D. Cystatin C

Urinalysis/Routine/1

59. Which statement regarding urea is correct?

A. Urea is 100% filtered by the glomeruli
B. Blood urea levels are independent of diet
C. Urea is not significantly reabsorbed by the tubules
D. Urea excretion is a specific measure of glomerular function

Urinalysis/Routine/1

60. Given the following data, calculate the creatinine clearance:

Plasma creatinine = 1.2 mg/dL
Urine creatinine = 100 mg/dL
Urine volume = 1.4 L/day
Body surface area = 1.80 m^2

A. 47 mL/min
B. 78 mL/min
C. 100 mL/min
D. 116 mL/min

Urinalysis/Routine/2

61. Given the following dry reagent strip urinalysis results, select the *most* appropriate course of action:

pH = 8.0 Protein = 1+ Glucose = Neg Blood = Neg
Ketone = Neg Nitrite = Neg Bilirubin = Neg

A. Report the results, assuming acceptable quality control
B. Check pH with a pH meter before reporting
C. Perform a turbidimetric protein test, instead of the dipstick protein test, and report
D. Request a new specimen

Urinalysis/Routine/3

Answers to Questions 57–61

57. D The eGFR reference range is 90 to 120 mL/min. Values below the lower reference limit, but greater than 60 mL/min, indicate glomerular damage but not of severity sufficient to cause symptoms or uremia.

58. D Cystatin C is a small protease inhibitor that is produced at a constant rate, is eliminated exclusively by glomerular filtration, and is not dependent on age, gender, or nutritional status. Plasma cystatin C is increased when the GFR is decreased, and levels can be used to give an eGFR in a similar manner to plasma creatinine. PAH is a substance that is completely filtered by the glomerulus and secreted by the tubules. Amino acids are partially reabsorbed by the tubules and are not present in blood at a constant rate.

59. A Blood urea nitrogen (BUN) is a sensitive indicator of renal disease but is not specific for glomerular function. BUN levels are affected by diet, hepatic function, tubular function, and filtrate flow, as well as the GFR. Although urea is completely filtered by the glomerulus, the tubules reabsorb 30% to 40% of the filtered urea, and this is why BUN concentration is higher than plasma creatinine. In prerenal failure, up to 70% of the filtered urea can be reabsorbed because of the slow movement of filtrate through the tubules. This causes BUN to rise much more than plasma creatinine in this condition. A BUN:creatinine ratio of 20:1 is highly suggestive of prerenal failure.

60. B The clearance formula is $U/(P \times V) \times 1.73/A$, where U = urine creatinine (mg/dL), P = plasma creatinine (mg/dL), V = urine volume (mL/min), and 1.73 = mean body surface area (m^2):

100 mg/dL ÷ 1.2 mg/dL × 1.4 L/day × 1,000 mL/L × 1 day/1,440 min × (1.73 m^2 ÷ 1.8 m^2) = 78 mL/min

Note that the creatinine clearance is low (lower reference limit approximately 95 mL/min for males and 85 mL/min for females), although the serum creatinine is still within limits (0.5–1.2 mg/dL). The clearance test is more sensitive if performed properly because as serum creatinine goes up, urine creatinine goes down.

61. C Highly buffered alkaline urine may cause a false-positive result on the dry reagent strip protein test by titrating the acid buffer on the reagent pad. Protein should be measured by an alternate method that is not subject to positive interference by highly buffered alkaline urine. A pH of 8.5 or greater should have a new specimen requested because of the probability of improper handling.

62. Given the following urinalysis results, select the most appropriate course of action:

pH = 8.0	Protein = Trace	Glucose = Neg
Ketone = Small	Blood = Neg	Nitrite = Neg
Microscopic findings:		
RBCs = 0–2/HPF	WBCs = 20–50/HPF	
Bacteria = Large	Crystals = Small, $CaCO_3$	

A. Call for a new specimen because urine was contaminated *in vitro*
B. Recheck pH because $CaCO_3$ does not occur at alkaline pH
C. No indication of error is present; results indicate a UTI
D. Report all results except bacteria because the nitrite test was negative

Urinalysis/Routine/3

63. A biochemical profile gives the following results:

Creatinine = 1.4 mg/dL
BUN = 35 mg/dL
K = 5.5 mmol/L

All other results are considered within proper reference range. Urine from the patient has an osmolality of 975 mOsm/kg. Select the *most* appropriate course of action.

A. Check for hemolysis
B. Repeat the BUN, and report only if normal
C. Repeat the serum creatinine, and report only if elevated
D. Report the results

Urinalysis/Routine/3

64. A 2 p.m. urinalysis shows trace glucose on the dry reagent strip test. Fasting blood glucose drawn 8 hours earlier is 100 mg/dL. No other results are outside of the reference range. Select the *most* appropriate course of action.

A. Repeat the urine glucose, and report if positive
B. Perform a test for reducing sugars, and report the result
C. Perform a quantitative urine glucose; report as trace if greater than 100 mg/dL
D. Request a new urine specimen

Urinalysis/Routine/3

65. A urine sample taken after a suspected transfusion reaction has a positive test for blood, but intact RBCs are not seen on microscopic examination. Which test result would rule out an intravascular hemolytic transfusion reaction?

A. Negative urine urobilinogen
B. Serum unconjugated bilirubin below 1.0 mg/dL
C. Serum potassium below 6.0 mmol/L
D. Normal plasma haptoglobin

Urinalysis/Routine/3

Answers to Questions 62–65

62. C A positive nitrite result requires infection with a nitrate-reducing organism, dietary nitrate, and incubation of urine in the bladder. The test is positive in about 70% of UTI cases. Alkaline pH, bacteriuria, and leukocytes point to UTI.

63. D Patients with prerenal failure usually have a BUN:creatinine ratio greater than 20:1. Reduced renal blood flow causes increased urea reabsorption and high urine osmolality. Patients are usually hypertensive and show fluid retention and hyperkalemia.

64. A Urine glucose concentration depends on blood glucose concentration at the time urine is formed. The postprandial glucose (2 p.m.) level exceeded the renal threshold, resulting in trace glycosuria. Tests for reducing sugars are not used to confirm a positive urine glucose test result.

65. D The plasma free hemoglobin will be increased immediately after a hemolytic transfusion reaction, and the haptoglobin will be decreased. The hemoglobin will be eliminated by the kidneys, but the haptoglobin will remain low or undetectable for 2 to 3 days. Normal urine urobilinogen and serum unconjugated bilirubin help in ruling out extravascular hemolysis but would be elevated in an intravascular hemolytic transfusion reaction. Pretransfusion potassium is needed to evaluate the contribution of hemolysis to the posttransfusion result.

66. Given the following urinalysis results, select the *most* appropriate course of action:

pH = 5.0	Protein = Neg	Glucose = 1,000 mg/dL
Blood = Neg		Bilirubin = Neg
Ketone = Moderate		SSA protein = 1+

A. Report the SSA protein test result instead of the dry reagent strip test result
B. Call for a list of medications administered to the patient
C. Perform a quantitative urinary albumin
D. Perform a test for microalbuminuria

Urinalysis/Routine/3

67. A urine specimen is dark orange and turns brown after storage in the refrigerator overnight. The laboratory professional requests a new specimen. The second specimen is bright orange and is tested immediately. Which test result would differ between the two specimens?

A. Ketone
B. Leukocyte esterase
C. Urobilinogen
D. Nitrite

Urinalysis/Routine/3

68. A patient's random urine sample consistently contains a trace of protein but no casts, cells, or other biochemical abnormality. The first voided morning sample is consistently negative for protein. These findings can be explained by:

A. Normal diurnal variation in protein loss
B. Early glomerulonephritis
C. Orthostatic or postural albuminuria
D. Microalbuminuria

Urinalysis/Routine/3

69. Given the following data for creatinine clearance, select the *most* appropriate course of action:

Volume = 2.8 L/day; surface area = 1.73 m^2;
urine creatinine = 100 mg/dL;
serum creatinine = 1.2 mg/dL

A. Report a creatinine clearance of 162 mL/min
B. Repeat the urine creatinine; results point to a dilution error
C. Request a new 24-hour urine sample
D. Request the patient's age and gender

Urinalysis/Routine/3

Answers to Questions 66–69

66. B False-positive SSA results most often are due to medications and radiographic dyes. The combination of glucose and ketone positivity of urine points to a patient with insulin-dependent diabetes.
A false-positive SSA test result is likely if tolbutamide (Orinase) has been administered.

67. C Urinary urobilinogen is increased in persons with extravascular hemolysis or hepatocellular liver disease. A freshly voided specimen is needed to detect urobilinogen because it is rapidly photo-oxidized to urobilin. This is accompanied by a color change from orange to brown. Urobilin does not react with 2,4-dimethylaminobenzaldehyde or 4-methoxybenzenediazonium tetrafluoroborate, which are used to detect urobilinogen. Consequently, the urobilinogen test in the first sample will be normal but will be increased in the second sample if tested immediately after collection. The best sample for detecting urobilinogen is a 2-hour timed urine sample collected in the midafternoon, when urobilinogen excretion is highest. Ketones and nitrites do not alter the pigment of the urine sample. Leukocytes cause the urine to be turbid but do not cause abnormal color. These three tests are stable for 24 hours when urine is refrigerated within 30 minutes of collection.

68. C Protein and other constituents of urine will often be highest in the first morning void. A normal first-voided sample makes glomerular disease highly unlikely. Orthostatic albuminuria is a benign condition sometimes seen in adolescents who are tall and have a bent posture that puts back pressure on the kidneys. The quantity of albumin excreted into the urine is small. Diagnosis is made by demonstrating a positive test after the person is erect for several hours, and the absence of proteinuria when the person is recumbent. Microalbuminuria seen in individuals with diabetes is usually accompanied by a positive test result for urinary glucose.

69. C A calculated clearance more than 140 mL/min is greater than the upper physiological limit. The high volume per day suggests the addition of H_2O, or urine that should have been voided and discarded at the start of sample collection. The result should be considered invalid.

70. An elevated amylase is obtained on a stat serum collected at 8 p.m. An amylase performed at 8 a.m. that morning was within the expected reference range. The laboratory professional also noted that urine amylase was measured at 6 p.m. Select the *most* appropriate course of action.

A. Repeat the stat amylase; report only if within normal limits
B. Repeat both the morning and afternoon serum amylase, and report only if they agree
C. Request a new specimen; do not report results of the stat sample
D. Review the amylase result on the 6 p.m. urine sample; if elevated, report the stat amylase

Urinalysis/Routine/3

71. A 24-hour urine sample from an adult patient indicated a catecholamine level of 140 μg/day (upper reference limit 150 μg/day). The 24-hour urine creatinine level is 0.6 g/day. Select the *best* course of action.

A. Check the urine pH to verify that it is less than 2.0
B. Report the result in μg catecholamines per milligram of creatinine
C. Request a new 24-hour urine sample
D. Measure the vanillylmandelic acid (VMA), and report the catecholamine result only if elevated

Urinalysis/Routine/3

72. When testing for drugs of abuse in urine, which of the following test results indicate dilution and sample rejection?

A. Temperature at sample submission 92°F
B. SG 1.002; creatinine 15 mg/dL
C. pH 5.8; temperature 94°F
D. SG 1.012; creatinine 25 mg/dL

Urinalysis/Routine/3

73. A urine specimen has an SG of 1.025 and is strongly positive for nitrite. All other dry reagent strip test results are within the expected reference range, and the microscopic examination was unremarkable, showing no WBCs or bacteria. The urine sample was submitted as part of a pre-employment physical examination that also includes drug testing. What *most* likely caused these results?

A. A viral infection of the kidney
B. A urinary tract infection (UTI) in an immunosuppressed person
C. An adulterated urine specimen
D. Error in reading the nitrite pad caused by poor reflectometer calibration

Urinalysis/Routine/3

Answers to Questions 70–73

70. D Serum amylase peaks 2 to 10 hours after an episode of acute pancreatitis, and this may have caused the elevated serum amylase at 8 p.m. Urinary amylase parallels serum amylase; therefore, a positive urine test at 6 p.m. makes sample collection error unlikely.

71. C Urine creatinine of less than 0.8 g/day indicates incomplete sample collection. The patient's daily catecholamine excretion would be misinterpreted from this result.

72. B Tampering with a sample submitted for abuse substance testing can be either by dilution or substitution. Substance Abuse and Mental Health Services Administration (SAMHSA) certified workplace drug testing laboratories are required to test for both, and reject samples based on SAMHSA cutoffs. A specimen is too dilute for testing if the creatinine is less than 20 mg/dL and SG below 1.003. A sample is considered substituted if creatinine is less than 5.0 mg/dL and SG less than 1.002. Values in A and C for pH and temperature are within acceptable limits.

73. C Urine validity testing for drugs of abuse includes tests for nitrite, glutathione, pyridinium dichromate, and peroxide in addition to pH, SG, and creatinine. These substances are known to cause negative interference in the enzyme-multiplied immunoassay technique (EMIT test). A viral infection of the kidney would be associated with high numbers of renal tubular epithelial cells and leukocytes. An infection in an immunosuppressed person would still produce urinary WBCs. Although laboratory errors are possible, a false-positive result caused by reflectometer error would be suspected if the test pad were negative when reading it manually.

5.2

Urine Microscopy and Clinical Correlations

1. **Which of the following dyes are used to differentiate renal tubular cells from transitional epithelium and PMNs?**
   A. Hematoxylin
   B. Sternheimer-Malbin
   C. Methylene blue
   D. Wright

   Urinalysis/Microscopy/1

2. **Which of the following statements regarding WBCs in urinary sediment is correct?**
   A. "Glitter cells" seen in urinary sediment are a sign of renal disease
   B. Bacteriuria in the absence of WBCs indicates lower UTI
   C. WBCs other than PMNs are not found in urinary sediment
   D. WBC casts indicate that pyuria is of renal, rather than lower urinary, origin

   Urinalysis/Microscopy/2

3. **Which description of urinary sediment with the Sternheimer-Malbin stain is correct?**
   A. Transitional epithelium: cytoplasm pale blue, nucleus dark blue
   B. Renal epithelium: cytoplasm light blue, nucleus dark purple
   C. Glitter cells: cytoplasm dark blue, nucleus dark purple
   D. Squamous epithelium: cytoplasm pink, nucleus pale blue

   Urinalysis/Microscopy/2

Answers to Questions 1–3

1. B The Sternheimer-Malbin stain (crystal violet and safranin) is a supravital stain used to differentiate renal tubular epithelium from transitional cells and PMNs. The mononuclear cells are clearly distinguished from both live and dead PMNs. Transitional cells have pale blue cytoplasm, but renal cells take up both dyes, resulting in an azurophilic appearance (orange-purple cytoplasm and dark purple nucleus).

2. D The presence of WBC casts is always significant and, when associated with pyuria and bacteriuria, indicates renal involvement in the infection. Most WBCs in urinary sediment will be PMNs. Eosinophils and mononuclear WBCs will occasionally be seen. High numbers of eosinophils often indicate an allergic drug reaction, causing inflammation in the medullary interstitium and tubules. Mononuclear cells are especially likely in patients with chronic inflammatory diseases and in renal transplant rejection, where they may account for as many as 30% of the WBCs. Glitter cells are PMNs with highly refractile granules exhibiting brownian movement. They are seen only when the urine SG is below 1.020. These cells resist staining with the Sternheimer-Malbin stain and are living (fresh) WBCs. When seen in large numbers, they indicate urinary tract injury (with pseudopod extensions, they point to infection). The presence of bacteria in urine in the absence of PMNs usually results from contamination by vaginal or skin flora that multiply *in vitro*, especially in unrefrigerated specimens.

3. A After staining with the Sternheimer-Malbin stain, transitional epithelium cells are readily differentiated from renal tubular cells because their cytoplasm is pale blue. The effects of this stain on the other types of cells is noted in the following table.

Type of Cell	Color of Nucleus	Color of Cytoplasm
Renal tubular	Dark purple	Orange-purple
Transitional epithelium	Dark blue	Pale blue
Squamous epithelium	Orange-purple	Purple/blue
Live WBCs	Don't stain	Don't stain
Dead WBCs	Deep purple-blue	Pale orange-blue
RBCs	NA	Pale pink

4. A 5-mL urine specimen is submitted for routine urinalysis and is analyzed immediately. The SG of the sample is 1.012, and the pH is 6.5. The dry reagent strip blood test is strongly positive (3+), and the microscopic examination shows 11 to 20 RBCs/HPF. The leukocyte esterase reaction is positive (1+), and the microscopic examination shows 0 to 2 WBCs/HPF. What is the *most* likely cause of these results?

A. Myoglobin is present in the sample
B. Free hemoglobin is present
C. Insufficient volume is causing microscopic results to be underestimated
D. Some WBCs have been misidentified as RBCs

Urinalysis/Clinical correlation/3

5. Which of the following statements regarding epithelial cells in the urinary system is correct?

A. Caudate epithelial cells originate from the upper urethra
B. Transitional cells originate from the upper urethra, ureters, bladder, or renal pelvis
C. Cells from the proximal renal tubule are usually round
D. Squamous epithelia cells line the vagina, urethra, and wall of the urinary bladder

Urinalysis/Microscopy/2

6. Which of the statements regarding examination of unstained urinary sediment is correct?

A. Renal cells can be differentiated reliably from WBCs
B. Large numbers of transitional cells are often seen after catheterization
C. Neoplastic cells from the bladder are not found in urinary sediment
D. RBCs are easily differentiated from nonbudding yeast cells

Urinalysis/Microscopy/2

7. Which of the following statements regarding cells found in urinary sediment is correct?

A. Transitional cells resist swelling in hypotonic urine
B. Renal tubular cells can appear as different shapes and have an eccentric round nucleus
C. Trichomonads have an oval shape with a prominent nucleus and a single anterior flagellum
D. Clumps of bacteria are frequently mistaken for blood casts

Urinalysis/Microscopy/2

Answers to Questions 4–7

4. C Given the SG and pH, most RBCs and WBCs will be intact. Both the RBC and WBC counts are lower than expected from the dry reagent strip test results. Myoglobin or free hemoglobin may account for the poor correlation between the blood reaction and the RBC count, but this does not explain the lower-than-expected WBC count. Microscopic reference ranges are based on concentrating a uniform volume of sediment from 12 mL of urine. When less urine is used, falsely low results will be obtained unless corrective action is taken. The specimen should be diluted with normal saline to 12 mL, then centrifuged at 450 $\times$ *g* for 5 minutes. Urinary sediment should be prepared according to the established procedure and the results multiplied by the dilution factor (in this case, 12 $\div$ 5, or 2.4).

5. B Caudate cells are transitional epithelium that have a sawtooth-shaped tail and are found in the urinary bladder and the pelvis of the kidney. Transitional epithelia line the upper two thirds of the urethra and the ureters as well as the urinary bladder and renal pelvis. Renal tubular cells may be columnar, polyhedral, or oval, depending on the portion of the tubule from which they originate. Cells from the proximal tubule are columnar and have a distinctive brush border. Squamous epithelia line the vagina and lower third of the urethra.

6. B Renal cells and PMNs are about the same size and can be confused in unstained sediment. Catheterization often releases large clumps or sheets of transitional and squamous cells. These should be distinguished from neoplastic cells derived from the urinary bladder. When cells appear atypical (e.g., large cells in metaphase), they should be referred to a pathologist for cytological examination. Nonbudding yeast cells are approximately the same in size and appearance as RBCs. When RBCs are reported in the absence of a positive blood test, the probability of an error in microscopy is high. The microscopic examination should be reviewed for the presence of yeast.

7. B Transitional epithelial cells readily take up H_2O and appear much larger than renal cells or WBCs when urine is hypotonic. Transitional cells are considered a normal component of the sediment unless present in large numbers and associated with signs of inflammation, such as mucus and PMNs, or presenting features of malignant cells. In contrast, renal cells are significant when seen conclusively in the sediment. They are often teardrop-shaped, polyhedral, or elongated cells with a round eccentric nucleus. Conclusive identification requires staining. *Trichomonas vaginalis* displays an indistinct nucleus and two pairs of prominent anterior flagella. Amorphous urate crystals deposited on the slide may be mistaken for granular or blood casts.

8. Which of the following statements regarding RBCs in the urinary sediment is true?

A. Yeast cells will lyse in dilute acetic acid, but RBCs will not
B. RBCs are often swollen in hypertonic urine
C. RBCs of glomerular origin often appear dysmorphic
D. Yeast cells will tumble when the cover glass is touched, but RBCs will not

Urinalysis/Microscopy/2

9. In which of the following diseases are renal tubular epithelial cells not shed in the urine?

A. Malignant renal disease
B. Acute glomerulonephritis
C. Nephrotic syndrome
D. Cytomegalovirus (CMV) infection of the kidney

Urinalysis/Clinical correlations/2

10. The ova of which parasite can be identified in the urinary sediment?

A. *Trichomonas vaginalis*
B. *Entamoeba histolytica*
C. *Schistosoma hematobium*
D. *Trichuris trichiura*

Urinalysis/Microscopy/1

11. Oval fat bodies are often seen in:

A. Chronic glomerulonephritis
B. Nephrotic syndrome
C. Acute tubular nephrosis
D. Renal failure of any cause

Urinalysis/Microscopy/2

12. Which statement regarding urinary casts is correct?

A. Many hyaline casts may appear in urinary sediment after jogging or exercise
B. The finding of even a single cast indicates renal disease
C. Casts can be seen in significant numbers even when protein tests are negative
D. Hyaline casts will dissolve readily in acid urine

Urinalysis/Microscopy/2

13. Which condition promotes the formation of casts in urine?

A. Chronic production of alkaline urine
B. Polyuria
C. Reduced filtrate formation
D. Low urine SG

Urinalysis/Clinical correlations/2

Answers to Questions 8–13

8. C RBCs are difficult to distinguish from nonbudding yeast in unstained sediment. RBCs tumble when the cover glass is touched and will lyse when the sediment is reconstituted in normal saline containing 2% volume per volume (v/v) acetic acid. A nonhemolyzed trace blood reaction confirms the presence of RBCs. RBCs have a granular appearance in hypertonic urine because of crenation. The RBC membrane becomes distorted when passing through the glomerulus, often appearing scalloped, serrated, or invaginated. Such cells are called *dysmorphic RBCs* and are associated with glomerulonephritis.

9. A Although seen in glomerulonephritis and pyelonephritis, the largest numbers of renal tubular cells appear in urine in association with viral infections of the kidney. Renal epithelium may show characteristic viral inclusions associated with CMV and rubella. High numbers of renal epithelium are also found in the sediment of patients with drug-induced tubular nephrosis and in some cases of heavy metal poisoning. Renal tumors do not usually shed cells into urine.

10. C Ova of *S. hematobium* can be recovered from urine because the adult trematodes colonize the blood vessels of the urinary bladder. The eggs are approximately 150 × 60 μm and are nonoperculated. They are yellowish and have a prominent terminal spine.

11. B Oval fat bodies are degenerated renal tubular epithelia that have reabsorbed cholesterol from the filtrate. Although they can occur in any inflammatory disease of the tubules, they are commonly seen in nephrotic syndrome, which is characterized by marked proteinuria and hyperlipidemia.

12. A Proteinuria accompanies casts in the urine (cylindruria) because protein is the principal component of casts. After strenuous exercise, hyaline casts may be present in urinary sediment in significant numbers but will disappear after resting for at least 24 hours. Casts more readily dissolve in alkaline urine. The finding of a single cast, even a cellular cast, is not indicative of renal disease and should be considered a chance occurrence.

13. C Cast formation is promoted by an acid filtrate, high solute concentration, slow movement of filtrate, and reduced filtrate formation. The appearance of a cast is dependent on the location and the time spent in the tubule, as well as the chemical and cellular composition of the filtrate.

14. The mucoprotein that forms the matrix of a hyaline cast is called:
A. Bence-Jones protein
B. β-Microglobulin
C. Uromodulin
D. Arginine-rich glycoprotein
Urinalysis/Microscopy/1

15. "Pseudocasts" are often caused by:
A. A dirty cover glass or slide
B. Bacterial contamination
C. Amorphous urates
D. Many WBCs
Urinalysis/Clinical correlations/2

16. Which of the following statements regarding urinary casts is correct?
A. Fine granular casts are more significant than coarse granular casts
B. Cast formation is always clinically significant
C. The appearance of cylindroids signals the onset of end-stage renal disease
D. Broad casts are associated with severe renal tubular obstruction
Urinalysis/Clinical correlations/2

17. A sediment with moderate hematuria and RBC casts *most* likely results from:
A. Chronic pyelonephritis
B. Nephrotic syndrome
C. Acute glomerulonephritis
D. Lower urinary tract obstruction
Urinalysis/Clinical correlations/2

18. Urine sediment characterized by pyuria with bacterial and WBC casts indicates:
A. Nephrotic syndrome
B. Pyelonephritis
C. Polycystic kidney disease
D. Cystitis
Urinalysis/Clinical correlations/2

19. Which type of casts signals the presence of chronic renal failure?
A. Blood casts
B. Fine granular casts
C. Waxy casts
D. Fatty casts
Urinalysis/Clinical correlations/2

Answers to Questions 14–19

14. C Hyaline casts are composed of a mucoprotein called *uromodulin*, previously called *Tamm-Horsfall protein*. In addition, casts may contain cells, immunoglobulins, light chains, cellular proteins, fat, bacteria, and crystalloids.

15. C Pseudocasts are formed by amorphous urates that may deposit in uniform cylindrical shapes as the sediment settles under the cover glass. They may be mistaken for granular or blood casts. However, they are highly refractile and lack the well-defined borders of true casts.

16. D There is no clinical difference between fine and coarse granular casts. Granular casts may form by degeneration of cellular casts or from inclusion of urinary calculi, but some are of unknown etiology. *Cylindruria* refers to the presence of casts in the urine. Hyaline casts may be seen in small numbers in normal patients and in large numbers following strenuous exercise and long-distance running. Hyaline casts may also be increased in patients taking certain drugs, such as diuretics. Broad casts form in dilated or distal tubules and indicate severe tubular obstruction seen in chronic renal failure. Waxy casts form when there is prolonged stasis in the tubules and signal end-stage renal failure. Cylindroids are casts with tails and have no special clinical significance.

17. C RBC casts indicate the renal origin of hematuria. Urinary tract obstruction may be associated with hematuria from ruptured vessels, but not casts. WBCs and WBC casts predominate in pyelonephritis. Urinary sediment in chronic glomerulonephritis is variable but usually exhibits moderate to severe intermittent hematuria. In addition, pyuria and cylindruria (cast formation) (with granular, blood, broad, waxy, and epithelial casts) are frequent. In nephrotic syndrome, the sediment may be unremarkable except for the presence of oval fat bodies and hyaline casts. In some cases, fatty, waxy, and epithelial cell casts may also be found.

18. B Pyelonephritis results from bacterial infection of the renal pelvis and interstitium. It is characterized by polyuria resulting from failure of the tubules to reabsorb fluid. Compression and obstruction of the tubules by WBCs reduce H_2O reabsorption. The finding of WBC casts helps differentiate pyelonephritis from UTI.

19. C Waxy casts form from the degeneration of cellular casts. Because the casts must remain lodged in the tubule long enough for the granular protein matrix to waxify, they are associated with chronic and end-stage renal failure. Both waxy and broad casts form in chronic renal failure when there is severe stasis, and they are associated with a poor prognosis.

20. Urinalysis of a sample from a patient suspected of having a transfusion reaction reveals small, yellow-brown crystals in the microscopic examination. Dry reagent strip tests are within acceptable limits except for the presence of a moderate amount of blood and trace positive protein. The pH of the urine is 6.5. What test should be performed to identify the crystals?

A. Confirmatory test for bilirubin
B. Cyanide–nitroprusside test
C. Polarizing microscopy
D. Prussian blue stain

Urinalysis/Clinical correlations/3

21. When examining urinary sediment, which of the following is considered an abnormal finding?

A. 2 RBCs/HPF
B. 1 hyaline cast per low-power field (LPF)
C. 1 renal cell cast per LPF
D. 5 WBCs/HPF

Urinalysis/Microscopy/2

22. A urine sample with a pH of 6.0 produces an abundance of pink sediment after centrifugation that appears as densely packed yellow-brown to reddish brown granules. The crystals are so dense that no other formed elements can be evaluated. What is the *best* course of action?

A. Request a new urine specimen
B. Warm the sample at 56°C for 5 minutes then respin
C. Acidify a 12-mL aliquot with 3 drops of glacial acetic acid
D. Add 5 drops of 1N HCl to the sediment and examine

Urinalysis/Microscopy/3

23. How can hexagonal uric acid crystals be distinguished from cystine crystals?

A. Cystine is insoluble in HCl, but uric acid is soluble
B. Cystine gives a positive nitroprusside test after reduction with sodium cyanide
C. Cystine crystals are more highly pigmented
D. Cystine crystals form at neutral or alkaline pH, uric acid forms at neutral to acidic pH

Urinalysis/Microscopy/2

24. The presence of tyrosine and leucine crystals together in urinary sediment usually indicates:

A. Renal failure
B. Chronic liver disease
C. Hemolytic anemia
D. Hartnup disease

Urinalysis/Microscopy/2

Answers to Questions 20–24

20. D A positive blood test result and trace protein occurring with a normal test for urobilinogen and an absence of RBCs are consistent with an intravascular transfusion reaction. Small, yellow-brown granular crystals at an acid pH may be uric acid, bilirubin, or hemosiderin. Bilirubin crystals are ruled out by the negative result on the dry reagent strip test for bilirubin. Potassium ferrocyanide is used in the Prussian blue staining reaction to detect hemosiderin deposits in urinary sediment. Hemosiderin is associated with hemochromatosis and increased RBC destruction. Causes of urinary hemosiderin include transfusion reaction, intravascular hemolytic anemia, and pernicious anemia.

21. C Epithelial casts (casts containing renal tubular epithelial cells) are rarely seen but indicate a disease process affecting the renal tubules. They are associated with diseases causing necrosis of the tubules, such as hepatitis, CMV and other viral infections, and mercury and ethylene glycol toxicity. Even occasional cellular casts are considered clinically significant.

22. B Urates are yellow-brown or reddish brown granules and form in acid or neutral urine. They often form following refrigeration of urine and can be dissolved by mixing the urine, warming at 56°C for 5 minutes, and recentrifuging. Amorphous phosphates are colorless and form in neutral or alkaline urine. They dissolve in diluted acetic acid but precipitate if heated.

23. B Flat, six-sided uric acid crystals may be mistaken for cystine crystals. Both crystals form at an acid to neutral pH. Cystine crystals are colorless, whereas uric acid crystals are pigmented (yellow, reddish brown). Cystine transmits polarized light and is soluble in dilute HCl. Uric acid is insoluble in HCl and is less anisotropic. Cystine is reduced by sodium cyanide, forming cysteine. The –SH group of cysteine reacts with nitroprusside to form a red color.

24. B Tyrosine crystals may occur in tyrosinemia, an inborn error of tyrosine metabolism caused by a deficiency of fumarylacetoacetate hydrolase, *p*-hydroxyphenylpyruvic acid oxidase, or tyrosine aminotransferase (causes of tyrosinuria). However, when seen along with leucine crystals, the cause is chronic liver disease, usually cirrhosis of the liver. Tyrosine usually forms fine brown or yellow needles, and leucine forms yellow spheres with concentric rings.

25. Which of the following crystals is considered nonpathological?
A. Hemosiderin
B. Bilirubin
C. Ammonium biurate
D. Cholesterol
Urinalysis/Clinical correlations/2

26. At which pH are ammonium biurate crystals usually found in urine?
A. Acid urine only
B. Acid or neutral urine
C. Neutral or alkaline urine
D. Alkaline urine only
Urinalysis/Microscopy/1

27. Which of the following crystals is seen commonly in alkaline and neutral urine?
A. Calcium oxalate
B. Uric acid
C. Triple phosphate
D. Cholesterol
Urinalysis/Microscopy/1

28. Which crystal appears in urine as a long, thin hexagonal plate and is linked to ingestion of large amounts of benzoic acid?
A. Cystine
B. Hippuric acid
C. Oxalic acid
D. Uric acid
Urinalysis/Microscopy/2

29. Small, yellow needles are seen in the sediment of a urine sample with a pH of 6.0. Which of the following crystals can be ruled out?
A. Sulfa crystals
B. Bilirubin crystals
C. Uric acid crystals
D. Cholesterol crystals
Urinalysis/Microscopy/2

30. Oval fat bodies are derived from:
A. Renal tubular epithelium
B. Transitional epithelium
C. Degenerated WBCs
D. Mucoprotein matrix
Urinalysis/Clinical correlations/1

31. Oval fat bodies are often associated with:
A. Nephrotic syndrome
B. Acute glomerulonephritis
C. Aminoaciduria
D. Pyelonephritis
Urinalysis/Clinical correlations/2

Answers to Questions 25–31

25. C Abnormal crystals are those that result from a pathological process. Hemosiderin crystals result from intravascular RBC destruction. Bilirubin crystals are found in severe necrotic and obstructive liver diseases, and cholesterol crystals in nephrotic syndrome, diabetes mellitus, and hypercholesterolemia. Ammonium biurate crystals form due to improper specimen handling.

26. D Ammonium biurate is often called a "thornapple" crystal because it forms a dark brown spiny sphere. Calcium carbonate ($CaCO_3$) is another common crystal that is seen only in alkaline urine (often due to improper specimen handling). Sodium urate and uric acid form in acid or neutral urine.

27. C Triple phosphate, also called *magnesium ammonium phosphate*, may be present in neutral or alkaline urine. Most commonly, triple phosphate crystals are six-sided plates that resemble a coffin lid. Crystals containing phosphates do not occur in acid urine.

28. B Hippuric acid forms long, colorless, flat, six-sided plates. It results from the metabolism of benzoic acid and resembles the "coffin lid" appearance of triple phosphate. It may occur normally because of ingestion of vegetables preserved with benzoic acid.

29. D Cholesterol crystals are colorless rectangular plates that often have a notched corner and appear stacked in a stair-step arrangement. Cholesterol crystals are highly anisotropic and can be positively identified by using a polarizing microscope. Bilirubin, sulfa, or uric acid crystals may occur as small yellow or yellow-brown needles or rods in neutral or acid urine. Bilirubin crystals should be suspected when the dry reagent strip test for bilirubin yields a positive result and cells in the sediment are dark yellow (bile stained). Sulfa crystals are soluble in acetone, concentrated HCl, and NaOH.

30. A Oval fat bodies form from degenerated renal epithelial cells that have reabsorbed cholesterol from the filtrate. They stain with Oil Red O or Sudan III. The fat globules within the cells give a Maltese cross effect when examined under polarized light.

31. A Nephrotic syndrome can be caused by several diseases that can result in injury and increased permeability of the glomerular basement membrane. This defect yields proteinuria and hypoalbuminemia. Major hallmarks of this syndrome are hyperlipidemia and lipiduria.

32. Urine of constant SG ranging from 1.008 to 1.010 *most* likely indicates:
A. Addison disease
B. Renal tubular failure
C. Prerenal failure
D. Diabetes insipidus
Urinalysis/Clinical correlations/2

33. Which of the following characterizes prerenal failure and helps to differentiate it from acute renal failure caused by renal disease?
A. BUN:creatinine ratio of 20:1 or higher
B. Urine:plasma osmolal ratio less than 2:1
C. Excess loss of sodium in urine
D. Dehydration
Urinalysis/Clinical correlations/2

34. Which of the following conditions characterizes chronic glomerulonephritis and differentiates it from acute glomerulonephritis?
A. Hematuria
B. Polyuria
C. Hypertension
D. Azotemia
Urinalysis/Clinical correlations/2

35. Which of the following conditions is seen in acute renal failure and differentiates it from prerenal failure?
A. Hyperkalemia and uremia
B. Oliguria and edema
C. Low creatinine clearance
D. Abnormal urinary sediment
Urinalysis/Clinical correlations/2

36. Which of the following conditions characterizes acute renal failure and differentiates it from chronic renal failure?
A. Hyperkalemia
B. Hematuria
C. Cylindruria
D. Proteinuria
Urinalysis/Clinical correlations/2

37. The serum concentration of which analyte is likely to be decreased in untreated cases of acute renal failure?
A. Hydrogen ions
B. Inorganic phosphorus
C. Calcium
D. Uric acid
Urinalysis/Clinical correlations/2

Answers to Questions 32–37

32. B The SG of the filtrate in the Bowman space is approximately 1.010. Urine produced consistently with an SG of 1.010 has the same osmolality of plasma and results from failure of the tubules to modify the urine filtrate.

33. A Prerenal failure is caused by deficient renal blood flow. The tubules are undamaged and will reabsorb more BUN than normal because filtrate flow is slow. Under the influence of aldosterone, they reabsorb sodium and concentrate the urine. The BUN:creatinine ratio and the U:P osmolal ratio are very high, and sodium output is low. In renal disease, the BUN: creatinine ratio is 10 or less, the U:P osmolal ratio approaches 1.0, and the daily sodium excretion is high.

34. B Acute glomerulonephritis results in severe compression of the glomerular vessels. This reduces filtration, causing a progression from oliguria to anuria. In contrast, polyuria is associated with chronic glomerulonephritis, which causes scarring of the collecting tubules. Both acute and chronic glomerulonephritis cause low urine osmolality, azotemia, acidosis, hypertension, proteinuria, and hematuria.

35. D Reduced glomerular filtration as evidenced by low creatinine clearance characterizes both prerenal failure and acute renal failure. This results in retention of fluid, causing edema, reduced urine volume, hypertension, uremia, and hyperkalemia in both prerenal failure and acute renal failure. The kidneys are not damaged in prerenal failure, and therefore, the microscopic examination is usually normal.

36. A In acute renal failure, reduced glomerular filtration coupled with decreased tubular secretion results in hyperkalemia. In chronic renal failure, scarring of the collecting tubules prevents salt and H_2O reabsorption. This can result in normal or low serum potassium despite reduced glomerular filtration. The sediment in chronic renal failure is characterized by intermittent heavy hematuria and proteinuria.

37. C Decreased glomerular filtration in renal failure results in high serum creatinine, BUN, and uric acid. Failure of the tubules results in retention of hydrogen ions and phosphates, causing acidosis and an increased anion gap. The tubules fail to respond to parathyroid hormone, resulting in excessive loss of calcium in urine. Serum sodium is usually normal or slightly increased, whereas hyperkalemia is a constant finding in acute renal failure.

38. Which of the following conditions is associated with the *greatest* proteinuria?
A. Acute glomerulonephritis
B. Chronic glomerulonephritis
C. Nephrotic syndrome
D. Acute pyelonephritis
Urinalysis/Clinical correlations/2

39. Which of the following conditions is often a cause of glomerulonephritis?
A. Hypertension
B. CMV infection
C. Systemic lupus erythematosus (SLE)
D. Heavy metal poisoning
Urinalysis/Clinical correlations/2

40. Acute pyelonephritis is commonly caused by:
A. Bacterial infection of the medullary interstitium
B. Circulatory failure
C. Renal calculi
D. Antigen–antibody reactions within the glomeruli
Urinalysis/Clinical correlations/2

41. Which of the following is associated with nephrotic syndrome?
A. Hyperlipidemia
B. Uremia
C. Hematuria and pyuria
D. Dehydration
Urinalysis/Clinical correlations/2

Answers to Questions 38–41

38. C Although all four conditions are associated with proteinuria, it is greatest in nephrotic syndrome. In nephrotic syndrome, urinary albumin loss is typically more than 4 g/day or 3 mg/mg creatinine, causing dry reagent strip protein tests to give 3+ to 4+ reactions. In contrast to glomerulonephritis and pyelonephritis, the urinary protein is often only 1+ to 2+.

39. C Autoimmune diseases, diabetes mellitus, and nephrotoxic drugs are common causes of acute glomerulonephritis. Autoimmune damage may result from the deposition of antigen–antibody complexes and complement-mediated damage, as occurs in poststreptococcal glomerulonephritis, or from the production of autoantibodies that attack the basement membrane, as in Goodpasture syndrome. Acute glomerulonephritis is often classified by the pattern of injury rather than by the cause. For example, insulin deficiency produces sclerotic vascular damage to glomeruli, often resulting in crescentic glomerulonephritis. Group A *Streptococcus* and SLE result in immunologically mediated damage to the glomeruli, usually causing membranous or membranoproliferative glomerulonephritis. CMV infections and heavy metal poisoning cause damage to the tubules, resulting in nephrosis.

40. A Acute pyelonephritis is caused by infection of the medullary interstitium, usually by coliforms that enter from the lower urinary tract. *Escherichia coli* is often implicated. Because it is focused in the medulla, the disease involves mainly the tubules. As opposed to acute glomerulonephritis, pyelonephritis is not associated with reduced creatinine clearance, azotemia, or oliguria. Reabsorption of salt and water is blocked, resulting in hyperkalemia, acidosis, and polyuria.

41. A Hyperlipidemia is a common feature of nephrotic syndrome due to the increased hepatic lipid production. Although casts may be present, the urinary sediment in nephrotic syndrome in adults is not characterized by RBCs and WBCs or by RBC, blood, and WBC casts. In nephrotic syndrome, unlike renal failure (nephritic syndrome), the creatinine clearance and serum potassium are usually normal. Nephrotic syndrome can be secondary to other renal diseases, infections, and drug treatment. In such cases, it is often transient. When it follows the anuric phase of acute glomerulonephritis, it signals a reversal in the course of the disease.

42. Which of the following conditions is a characteristic finding in patients with obstructive renal disease?
A. Polyuria
B. Azotemia
C. Dehydration
D. Alkalosis

Urinalysis/Clinical correlations/2

43. The most common kidney stones are composed of:
A. Magnesium ammonium phosphate
B. Calcium oxalate
C. Calcium phosphate
D. Calcium carbonate

Urinalysis/Clinical correlations/1

44. Which of the following abnormal crystals is often associated with formation of renal calculi?
A. Cystine
B. Ampicillin
C. Tyrosine
D. Leucine

Urinalysis/Clinical correlations/2

45. Which statement about renal calculi is correct?
A. Calcium oxalate and calcium phosphate account for about three-fourths of all stones
B. Uric acid stones can be seen on radiography
C. Triple phosphate stones are found principally in the ureters
D. Stones are usually composed of single salts

Urinalysis/Clinical correlations/2

Answers to Questions 42–45

42. B Azotemia (elevated levels of nitrogenous waste products in the blood such as urea and creatinine) is characteristic in obstructive renal disease. Obstructive renal disease may result from renal or urinary tract calculi, benign prostatic hypertrophy, chronic UTI, or urogenital malignancy. Obstruction causes the hydrostatic pressure in the Bowman space to increase. This pressure opposes glomerular filtration. If the hydrostatic pressure in the Bowman space equals the hydrostatic pressure in the glomeruli, then filtration will not occur, resulting in anuria. Postrenal failure produces many of the same serum abnormalities as acute renal failure, including hyperkalemia, acidosis, edema, and azotemia. Urinary sediment will often be abnormal as well. Bacteriuria and pyuria are common, and hematuria may result from rupture of the vasa recta or other blood vessels.

43. B Over three-fourths of urinary tract stones are composed of calcium salts, with the largest number being calcium oxalate, and hyperparathyroidism is commonly associated with calcium stones. Stones composed of magnesium ammonium phosphate are called *struvite* and lodge in the renal pelvis, causing a characteristic "staghorn" appearance on radiographic examination. Stones mainly composed of calcium phosphate are called *hydroxyapatite* or *bushite*, depending on the calcium composition. Stones of $CaCO_3$ are called *carbonate apatite*.

44. A Cystinuria is caused by an autosomal recessive defect in the tubular reabsorption of dibasic amino acids (a renal-type aminoaciduria). Cystine crystals are highly insoluble and form kidney stones. Tyrosine crystals form fine dark sheaves or needles and may result from liver disease or tyrosinosis, an overflow of aminoaciduria. Leucine crystals form yellow spheres with concentric rings and are seen in chronic liver disease. Ampicillin (rarely) forms long colorless prisms in sheaves in some patients being treated with high doses.

45. A Three-fourths of all stones contain calcium, and three-fourths of these contain calcium oxalate. Stones are usually composed of several inorganic salts, but calcium oxalate is the most common component of urinary stones. Oxalates are hard, dark, and coarse stones. Uric acid stones are always pigmented yellow to reddish brown. They are small translucent stones not apparent on radiography. Stones made of primarily calcium phosphate (as hydroxyapatite) are light and crumble easily. Stones made of struvite (triple phosphate or ammonium magnesium phosphate) are radiodense and lodge in the renal pelvis, forming an outline of the structures resembling the antlers of a deer (staghorn calculi).

46. A 6-mL pediatric urine sample is processed for routine urinalysis. The sediment is prepared by centrifuging all the urine remaining after performing the biochemical tests. The following results are obtained:

SG = 1.015	Blood = Large	Leukocytes = Moderate
Protein = 2+	RBCs: 5–10/HPF	WBCs: 5–10/HPF

Select the *most* appropriate course of action.

A. Report the results; blood and protein correlate with microscopic results
B. Report biochemical results only; request a new sample for the microscopic examination
C. Request a new sample and report as quantity not sufficient (QNS)
D. Recentrifuge the supernatant and repeat the microscopic examination

Urinalysis/Clinical correlations/3

47. Given the following urinalysis results, select the *most* appropriate course of action:

pH = 6.0	Protein = Neg	Glucose = Neg
Ketone = Trace	Blood = Neg	Bilirubin = Neg
Microscopic findings:		
Mucus = Small	Ammonium urate = Large	

A. Recheck urine pH
B. Report these results, assuming acceptable quality control
C. Repeat the dry reagent strip tests to confirm the ketone result
D. Request a new sample and repeat the urinalysis

Urinalysis/Clinical correlations/3

48. Given the following urinalysis results, select the *most* appropriate first course of action:

pH = 6.0	Protein = Neg	Glucose = Neg
Ketone = Neg	Blood = Neg	Bilirubin = Neg
Other findings:		
Color: Intense yellow	Transparency: Clear	Microscopic: Crystals, Bilirubin granules = Small

A. Repeat the dry reagent strip test for bilirubin
B. Request a new sample
C. Recheck the pH
D. Perform a test for urinary urobilinogen

Urinalysis/Clinical correlations/3

49. Following a transfusion reaction, urine from a patient gives positive test results for blood and protein. The SG is 1.015. No RBCs or WBCs are evident in the microscopic examination of the urine sample. The results:

A. Indicate renal injury induced by transfusion reaction
B. Support the finding of an extravascular transfusion reaction
C. Support the finding of an intravascular transfusion reaction
D. Rule out a transfusion reaction caused by RBC incompatibility

Urinalysis/Clinical correlations/3

Answers to Questions 46–49

46. B This discrepancy between the blood reaction and RBC count resulted from spinning less than 12 mL of urine. When volume is below 12 mL, the sample should be diluted with saline to 12 mL before concentrating. Results are multiplied by the dilution (12 mL/mL urine) to give the correct range.

47. A Ammonium urate crystals occur at alkaline pH only. The pH should be checked, and if it is below 7.0, the crystals should be reviewed for correct identification. The trace ketone does not require confirmation, provided that the quality control of the reagent strips is acceptable.

48. A Bilirubin crystals cannot occur in urine without bilirubin. The dry reagent strip test should be repeated, and if the result is negative, a new specimen should be requested as bilirubin may have degraded due to storage. If a second sample yields a negative result, the crystals should be reviewed before reporting. Abnormal crystals occur only in acid or neutral urine.

49. C RBCs usually remain intact at an SG of 1.015. The absence of RBCs, WBCs, and casts points to hemoglobinuria caused by intravascular hemolysis rather than glomerular injury. A positive protein reaction will occur if sufficient hemoglobin is present.

50. Urinalysis results from a 35-year-old female are as follows:

SG = 1.015	pH = 7.5	Protein = Trace
Glucose = Small	Ketone = Neg	Blood = Neg
Leukocytes = Moderate		
Microscopic findings:		
RBCs: 5–10/HPF	WBCs: 25–50/HPF	

Select the *most* appropriate course of action.
- **A.** Recheck the blood reaction; if negative, look for budding yeast
- **B.** Repeat the WBC count
- **C.** Report all results except that for blood
- **D.** Request the list of medications used

Urinalysis/Clinical correlations/3

51. A routine urinalysis indicates the following results:

pH =6.5	Protein = Neg	Blood = Neg
Glucose= Trace	Ketone = Neg	
Microscopic findings:		
Blood casts: 5–10/LFP	Mucus: Small	Crystals: Large, amorphous

The results are *most* likely explained by:
- **A.** False-negative blood reaction
- **B.** False-negative protein reaction
- **C.** Pseudocasts of urate mistaken for true casts
- **D.** Mucus mistaken for casts

Urinalysis/Clinical correlations/3

52. When examining a urinary sediment under 400× magnification, the medical laboratory scientist noted many RBCs to have cytoplasmic blebs and an irregular distribution of the hemoglobin. This phenomenon is most often caused by:
- **A.** Intravascular hemolytic anemia
- **B.** Glomerular disease
- **C.** Hypotonic or alkaline urine
- **D.** Severe dehydration

Urinalysis/Clinical correlations/2

53. A urine sample with a pH of 8.0 and a specific gravity of 1.005 had a positive blood reaction (1+) but is negative for protein, and no RBCs are present in the microscopic examination of urinary sediment. What *best* explains these findings?
- **A.** High pH and low SG caused a false-positive blood reaction
- **B.** The blood reaction and protein reaction are discrepant
- **C.** Hemoglobin is present without intact RBCs because of hemolysis
- **D.** An error was made in the microscopic examination

Urinalysis/Clinical correlation/3

54. A urine sample has a negative blood reaction and 5 to 10 cells/HPF that resemble RBCs. What is the *best* course of action?
- **A.** Mix a drop of sediment with 1 drop of diluted acetic acid and re-examine
- **B.** Report the results without further testing
- **C.** Repeat the blood test, and if negative, report the results
- **D.** If the leukocyte esterase test is positive, report the cells as WBCs

Urinalysis/Clinical correlations/3

Answers to Questions 50–54

50. A A nonhemolyzed trace may have been overlooked and the blood test should be repeated. A false-negative result (e.g., megadoses of vitamin C) rarely occurs. Yeast cells often accompany pyuria and glycosuria and are easily mistaken for RBCs.

51. C At pH 6.5, amorphous crystals are most often urate. These form yellow-brown or reddish brown refractile deposits, sometimes resembling blood or granular casts. The number of blood casts reported could not have occurred with negative protein and blood test results.

52. B When RBCs pass through the damaged endothelial wall of the glomerulus, they become distorted, and such cells are described as dysmorphic in appearance. They are characterized by uneven distribution of hemoglobin, cytoplasmic blebs, and an asymmetrical membrane distinct from crenation. The cytoplasm may be extruded from the cell and may aggregate at the membrane, giving the cell a wavy appearance. A predominance of dysmorphic RBCs in the microscopic examination points to glomerular bleeding as opposed to hematuria from other causes. Intravascular hemolytic anemia causes hemoglobinuria, rather than hematuria. RBCs lyse in hypotonic and alkaline urine. Severe dehydration is not a cause of hematuria.

53. C RBCs will lyse in alkaline or dilute urine, and this sample displays both. The blood test is sensitive to as little is 0.015 mg/dL hemoglobin, and the protein test is significantly less sensitive. As a result, a trace to small positive blood and negative protein are commonly encountered.

54. A When 5 to 10 RBCs/HPF are seen, the blood test should show a nonhemolyzed trace. Therefore, it is likely that the cells are not RBCs. RBCs are easily confused with nonbudding yeast cells and may also be mistaken for WBCs. RBCs will lyse in dilute acetic acid, but yeast and WBCs will not. If a yeast infection is present, then the leukocyte esterase test result will likely be positive; therefore, the leukocyte esterase test cannot be used to determine the identity of the cells. The Sternheimer-Malbin stain can be used to differentiate WBCs from RBCs and yeast.

5.3

Cerebrospinal, Serous, and Synovial Fluids

1. Cerebrospinal fluid (CSF) is formed by ultrafiltration of plasma through the:
A. Choroid plexus
B. Sagittal sinus
C. Anterior cerebral lymphatics
D. Arachnoid membrane

Body fluids/Cerebrospinal fluid/1

2. Which statement regarding CSF is true?
A. Normal values for mononuclear cells are higher for infants than for adults
B. Absolute neutrophilia is not significant if the total WBC count is less than 25/µL
C. The first aliquot of CSF should be sent to the microbiology laboratory
D. Neutrophils compose most WBCs in normal CSF

Body fluids/Cerebrospinal fluid/2

3. When collecting CSF, the difference between opening and closing fluid pressure greater than 100 mm H_2O indicates:
A. Low CSF volume
B. Subarachnoid hemorrhage
C. Meningitis
D. Hydrocephalus

Body fluids/Cerebrospinal fluid/2

Answers to Questions 1–3

1. A CSF is formed by ultrafiltration of plasma through the choroid plexus, a tuft of capillaries in the pia mater located in the third and fourth ventricles. Endothelia of the choroid plexus vessels and ependymal cells lining the ventricles act as a barrier to the passage of proteins, drugs, and metabolites. Glucose in CSF is about 60% of the plasma glucose. Total protein in CSF is only 15 to 45 mg/dL, while chloride levels are 10% to 15% higher than in plasma. Approximately 500 mL of ultrafiltrate is produced per day, the bulk of which is returned to circulation via the sagittal sinus. The normal volume of CSF in adults is 100 to 160 mL (10–60 mL for small children).

2. A Lymphocytes account for 40% to 80% of WBCs in adults, monocytes and macrophages for 20% to 50%. Neutrophils should be less than 10% of the WBCs. The reference range for WBCs in adults is 0 to 5/µL. A majority of PMNs can be significant even if the WBC count is normal. In infants, monocytes account for 50% to 90% of WBCs, and the upper limit for WBCs is 30/µL. The first aliquot is sent to the chemistry department because it may be contaminated with blood or skin flora.

3. A Normal CSF volume in adults is 100 to 160 mL. When volume is low, an abnormally high difference is observed between the opening and closing pressure. The difference is normally 10 to 30 mm H_2O, after removal of 15 to 20 mL. Low opening pressure is caused by reduced volume or block above the puncture site. High opening pressure may result from high CSF volume, CNS hemorrhage, or malignancy.

4. Which of the following findings is consistent with a subarachnoid hemorrhage rather than a traumatic lumbar puncture?
A. Clearing of the fluid as it is aspirated
B. A clear supernatant after centrifugation
C. Xanthochromia
D. Presence of a protein in the sample
Body fluids/Cerebrospinal fluid/2

5. The term used to denote a high WBC count in the CSF is:
A. Empyema
B. Neutrophilia
C. Pleocytosis
D. Hyperglycorrhachia
Body fluids/Cerebrospinal fluid/1

Answers to Questions 4–5

4. C Xanthochromia is yellow pigmentation of CSF caused by subarachnoid hemorrhage, high CSF protein, free hemoglobin, or bilirubin. The bilirubin may be caused by hepatic disease, CNS hemorrhage, or prior traumatic tap. In subarachnoid hemorrhage, the fluid will be pink if the RBC count is greater than 500/μL. It will turn orange as RBCs lyse in the first few hours and then will turn yellow after about 12 hours. Granulocyte infiltration occurs immediately after a subarachnoid hemorrhage and disappears after 24 hours. It is followed by an increase in macrophages, showing evidence of erythrophagocytosis that remains for up to 2 weeks. After subarachnoid hemorrhage, D-dimer is present in CSF and can be used to distinguish between a traumatic tap and subarachnoid hemorrhage.

5. C Pleocytosis refers to an increase in WBCs within CSF. Bacterial meningitis causes a neutrophilic pleocytosis, viral meningitis a lymphocytic pleocytosis, and tuberculous and fungal meningitis a mixed-cell pleocytosis. Other causes of pleocytosis include multiple sclerosis (MS), cerebral hemorrhage or infarction, and leukemia. Empyema is a collection of pus inside a body cavity. Hyperglycorrhachia is an abnormally high glucose concentration in CSF.

6. Which of the adult CSF values in the following table are consistent with bacterial meningitis?

	WBCs	Lymphocytes	Monocytes	Eosinophils	Neutrophils	Neuroectodermal Cells
A.	50/μL	44%	55%	0%	0%	1%
B.	300/μL	75%	21%	3%	0%	1%
C.	2,000/μL	5%	15%	0%	80%	0%
D.	2,500/μL	40%	50%	0%	10%	0%

Body fluids/Cerebrospinal fluid/2

7. Given the following data, determine the corrected CSF WBC count:

	CSF Values	Peripheral Blood Values
RBCs	6,000/μL	4.0×10^6/μL
WBCs	150/μL	5.0×10^3/μL

A. 8/μL
B. 142/μL
C. 120/μL
D. 145/μL
Body fluids/Cerebrospinal fluid/2

8. What is the *most* likely cause of the following CSF results?

CSF glucose 20 mg/dL; CSF protein 200 mg/dL;
CSF lactate 50 mg/dL (reference range 5–25 mg/dL)

A. Viral meningitis
B. Viral encephalitis
C. Cryptococcal meningitis
D. Acute bacterial meningitis
Body fluids/Cerebrospinal fluid/2

9. Which of the following conditions is *most* often associated with normal CSF glucose and protein?
A. Multiple sclerosis
B. Malignancy
C. Subarachnoid hemorrhage
D. Viral meningitis
Body fluids/Cerebrospinal fluid/2

Answers to Questions 6–9

6. C Normal WBC counts for CSF are 0 to 5/μL for adults and 0 to 30/μL for children. Neutrophils predominate the differential in bacterial meningitis, whereas lymphocytes predominate in viral meningitis. Hemorrhage and traumatic tap will also cause increased PMNs, and WBC counts should be corrected using the CSF RBC count.

7. B Corrected WBC count = WBCs in CSF – [(Blood WBCs × CSF RBCs) ÷ Blood RBCs]

Corrected WBC count = 150/μL – [(5,000/μL WBCs × 6,000/μL RBCs) ÷ 4,000,000/μL RBCs]

Corrected WBC count = 150/μL – 7.5/μL

Corrected WBC count = 142/μL

8. D Acute bacterial meningitis causes increased production of immunoglobulin (Ig) in CSF. Glucose levels are below normal (less than 40 mg/dL) because of consumption by PMNs and bacteria. Lactate levels rise because of increased pressure and hypoxia (greater than 35 mg/dL being correlated with bacterial meningitis). When associated with increased PMNs and lactate dehydrogenase (LDH), these findings point to bacterial meningitis.

9. D In viral (aseptic) meningitis, the CSF glucose is usually above 40 mg/dL and the total protein is normal or slightly increased. Low CSF glucose and elevated total protein are seen in malignancy and subarachnoid hemorrhage and in some patients with MS. Low glucose in malignancy and MS results from increased utilization. Glucose is reduced in subarachnoid hemorrhage because of the release of glycolytic enzymes from the RBCs. All three conditions result in high CSF protein, but MS is associated with an increased IgG index owing to local production of IgG.

10. The diagnosis of MS is suggested by which CSF finding?
A. The presence of elevated protein and low glucose
B. A decreased IgG index
C. The presence of oligoclonal bands by electrophoresis
D. An increased level of CSF β-microglobulin
Body fluids/Cerebrospinal fluid/2

11. Which of the following results is consistent with fungal meningitis?
A. Normal CSF glucose
B. Pleocytosis of mixed cellularity
C. Normal CSF protein
D. High CSF lactate
Body fluids/Cerebrospinal fluid/2

12. In what suspected condition should a wet prep using a warm slide be examined?
A. Cryptococcal meningitis
B. Amoebic meningoencephalitis
C. *Mycobacterium tuberculosis* infection
D. Neurosyphilis
Body fluids/Cerebrospinal fluid/2

13. Which of the following tests could be used to determine if there is damage to the integrity of the blood–brain barrier?
A. Protein
B. Lactate
C. Albumin
D. Ammonia
Body fluids/Cerebrospinal fluid/2

14. Which of the following is an *inappropriate* procedure for performing routine CSF analysis?
A. A differential is done only if the total WBC count is greater than 10/μL
B. A differential should be done on a stained CSF concentrate
C. A minimum of 30 WBCs should be differentiated
D. A Wright-stained slide should be examined, rather than a chamber differential
Body fluids/Cerebrospinal fluid/2

15. Which cell is present in CSF in greater numbers in newborns than in older children or adults?
A. Eosinophils
B. Lymphocytes
C. Monocytes
D. Neutrophils
Body fluids/Cerebrospinal fluid/2

Answers to Questions 10–15

10. C The presence of oligoclonal banding (two or more discrete bands in the gamma zone following electrophoresis) is seen in 90% of persons with MS and in few other diseases. Although not entirely definitive, it is the single most effective laboratory test for the diagnosis of MS. When performing CSF electrophoresis, the serum pattern must be compared with the CSF pattern. At least some of the oligoclonal bands must *not* be found in the serum pattern for the test result to be considered positive. β_2-Microglobulins are increased in CSF in inflammatory diseases (especially malignant diseases). The total CSF protein is increased in less than half of the patients with MS. The IgG index is increased in 80% or more of MS cases. Although the IgG index is sensitive, it is increased in many other disorders.

11. B Fungal meningitis usually produces a pleocytosis (an increased number of cells, typically WBCs, in a body fluid) of mixed cellularity consisting of lymphocytes, PMNs, monocytes, and eosinophils. In some cases, lymphocytes predominate, whereas in others, most of the WBCs are PMNs. In fungal meningitis, glucose is low and the total protein elevated; however, unlike bacterial meningitis, the lactate is usually below 35 mg/dL.

12. B Amoeba in CSF appear very similar to monocytes in stained films but can be differentiated by their characteristic pseudopod mobility in a wet prep on a prewarmed slide. *Naegleria fowleri* and *Acanthamoeba* spp. are causative agents of primary amoebic meningoencephalitis.

13. C Albumin is a protein fraction used to look for damage to the blood–brain barrier. Albumin is not made in the CSF but is transported across the blood–brain barrier. The formula CSF albumin/serum albumin is used, and any index value less than 9 represents an intact blood–brain barrier. A value higher than 9 indicates damage to the blood–brain barrier.

14. A A relative (percent) increase in PMNs may be significant even when the WBC count does not exceed the upper limit of normal. For this reason, a WBC differential using a concentrated CSF sample is always performed on neonates and when the WBC count is greater than 5/μL. Cytocentrifugation should be used to concentrate the cells followed by staining with the Wright stain.

15. C In newborns, the Upper Reference Limit (URL) for WBCs is 30/μL (URL for adults is 5/μL) with most WBCs being monocytes or macrophages. In normal neonates, monocytes (including macrophages and histiocytes) account for about 75% of the WBCs, lymphocytes for about 20%, and PMNs for about 3%. In normal adults, lymphocytes account for about 60% of the WBCs, monocytes for about 35%, and PMNs for about 2%.

16. Neutrophilic pleocytosis is usually associated with all of the following *except*:
A. Cerebral infarction
B. Malignancy
C. Meningitis
D. Neurosyphilis
Body fluids/Cerebrospinal fluid/2

17. Which statement about CSF protein is true?
A. An abnormal serum protein electrophoretic pattern does not affect the CSF pattern
B. The upper reference limit (URL) for CSF total protein in newborns is one half the adult level
C. CSF IgG is increased in panencephalitis, malignancy, and neurosyphilis
D. Antibodies to *Treponema pallidum* disappear after successful antibiotic therapy
Body fluids/Cerebrospinal fluid/2

18. Which of the following statements regarding routine microbiological examination of CSF is correct?
A. A Gram stain is performed on the CSF prior to concentration
B. The Gram stain is positive in fewer than 40% of cases of acute bacterial meningitis
C. India ink and acid-fast stains are indicated if neutrophilic pleocytosis is present
D. All CSF specimens should be cultured using sheep blood agar, chocolate agar, and supplemented broth
Body fluids/Cerebrospinal fluid/2

19. Which organism is the *most* frequent cause of bacterial meningitis in neonates?
A. *Neisseria meningitidis*
B. Group B *Streptococcus*
C. *Haemophilus influenzae*
D. *Klebsiella pneumoniae*
Body fluids/Cerebrospinal fluid/2

20. Following a head injury, which protein will identify the presence of CSF leakage through the nose?
A. Transthyretin
B. Myelin basic protein
C. β-Transferrin
D. C-reactive protein
Body fluids/Cerebrospinal fluid/2

Answers to Questions 16–20

16. D In neurosyphilis, there is usually absolute lymphocytosis and increased total protein and IgG index. Neutrophils may appear in CSF associated with many causes, making it necessary to correlate results of biochemical assays with hematologic findings. Low glucose and high protein levels occur in both malignancy and bacterial meningitis. Tumor markers and lactate may be helpful in distinguishing malignancy from bacterial meningitis. Neutrophils also will accumulate after any brain injury or trauma.

17. C Although the blood–brain barrier excludes most plasma proteins, abnormal serum proteins can cause parallel CSF electrophoretic patterns. Therefore, an abnormal CSF pattern indicates CNS disease only if not duplicated by the serum pattern. Normal CSF total protein in newborns may be up to two times higher than adult levels. Antibodies to *T. pallidum* remain in CSF after treatment, but nontreponemal antibodies disappear. Although the *T. pallidum* particle agglutination (TP-PA) test for specific antibodies is more sensitive, the Venereal Disease Research Laboratory (VDRL) test is often performed concurrently. A positive result for both tests is diagnostic of active tertiary syphilis.

18. D A culture should be performed on the sediment of the third aliquot of CSF after it is centrifuged. Blood and chocolate agar and anaerobic broth should always be used and, if sterile, held for a minimum of 3 days. Blood cultures should be done because septicemia occurs in about one half of bacterial meningitis cases. Gram staining is always performed by using the sediment of the CSF because it is positive in more than 70% of acute bacterial meningitis cases. India ink, acid-fast, and wet preparations may be ordered if an absolute monocytosis is present.

19. B Group B *Streptococcus* and *E. coli* are the two most common isolates in neonates. *H. influenzae, K. pneumoniae*, and *N. meningitidis* are the most common isolates in children. *S. pneumoniae* is the most frequent isolate identified in older adults.

20. C In cases of trauma, it may be necessary to differentiate rhinorrhea from CSF leakage, and this can be done by immunofixation electrophoresis to identify β-transferrin (also called *tau protein*) found in CSF, but not in serum. Transthyretin or prealbumin is present in far greater concentration in CSF than in blood but may not be seen if CSF is diluted with nasal fluid. Myelin basic protein is a component of nerve sheaths and is present in CSF in about 60% of individuals with MS. It is also found in patients with other demyelinating diseases, SLE, stroke, and brain injury. C-reactive protein is elevated in the CSF of approximately two thirds of patients with bacterial meningitis.

21. Which of the following statements regarding serous fluids is correct?

A. The normal volume of pleural fluid is 30 to 50 mL

B. Mesothelial cells, PMNs, lymphocytes, and macrophages may be present in normal fluids

C. Radiography can detect a 10% increase in the volume of a serous fluid

D. Normal serous fluids are colorless

Body fluids/Serous fluid/2

22. The term *effusion* refers to:

A. A chest fluid that is purulent

B. A serous fluid that is chylous

C. Abnormal accumulation of serous fluid

D. An inflammatory process affecting the appearance of a serous fluid

Body fluids/Pleural fluid/1

23. Which of the following laboratory results are characteristic of a transudative fluid?

A. SG = 1.018

B. Total protein = 3.2 g/dL

C. LDH fluid/serum ratio = 0.25

D. Total protein fluid:serum ratio = 0.65

Body fluids/Transudate/2

24. Which observation is *least* useful in distinguishing a hemorrhagic serous fluid from a traumatic tap?

A. Clearing of fluid as it is aspirated

B. Presence of xanthochromia

C. The formation of a clot

D. Diminished RBC count in successive aliquots

Body fluids/Serous fluids/2

25. Which of the following laboratory results on a serous fluid is *most* likely to be caused by a traumatic tap?

A. An RBC count of 8,000/μL

B. A WBC count of 6,000/μL

C. A hematocrit of 35%

D. A neutrophil count of 55%

Body fluids/Serous fluid/2

Answers to Questions 21–25

21. B Serous fluids include pleural, pericardial, and peritoneal fluids. They form from ultrafiltration of plasma through serous membranes, which are lined with specialized epithelium called *mesothelium*. They make up about 5% of the cells in serous fluid and may be difficult to differentiate from malignant cells. Pleural fluid volume is normally less than 10 mL. The volume of pericardial fluid is normally 10 to 50 mL and peritoneal fluid 30 to 50 mL. Radiography can detect an increase in serous fluids of 300 mL or more. Normal serous fluids are clear and range in color from straw to light yellow.

22. C Effusions are classified as either transudates, exudates, or chylous. Transudates result from abnormal hemodynamics (e.g., congestive heart failure, liver disease), and exudates and chylous fluids from local disease. Pleural fluid that is purulent is called *empyemic fluid*. Such fluid has a WBC count of 10,000/μL or greater.

23. C Transudative fluids are distinguished from exudative fluids by the physical appearance, cellularity, SG, total protein, LDH, cholesterol, and bilirubin. Exudative fluids have a fluid:serum LDH ratio greater than 0.6 caused by release of the enzyme from inflammatory or malignant cells. Exudative fluids have a total protein greater than 3.0 g/dL, SG greater than 1.015, fluid:serum total protein ratio greater than 0.6, cholesterol greater than 60 mg/dL (fluid:serum ratio greater than 0.3) and fluid:serum bilirubin ratio greater than 0.6. Exudates are caused by infection, infarction, malignancy, rheumatoid diseases, and trauma.

24. C A clot may form in a hemorrhagic fluid or following a traumatic tap. However, transudative fluid will not clot. Xanthochromia indicates either an exudative process or prior traumatic tap. Hemorrhagic pleural fluids usually have RBC counts greater than 100,000/μL and are usually caused by lung neoplasms. Clearing of fluid or diminished RBC counts in successive tubes favors a diagnosis of a traumatic tap.

25. A Normal fluids have a WBC count less than 1,000/μL but counts between 1,000 and 2,500/μL may be seen in both exudates and transudates. All WBC types are present, but no type should account for greater than 50% of the leukocyte count. A RBC count less than 10,000/μL is usually caused by a traumatic tap. A fluid hematocrit like blood is caused by a hemothorax. Pleural fluids containing greater than 100,000/μL RBCs are associated most often with malignancies but are also seen in trauma and pulmonary infarction.

26. Which condition is commonly associated with an exudative effusion?
A. Congestive heart failure
B. Malignancy
C. Nephrotic syndrome
D. Cirrhosis
Body fluids/Exudate/2

27. A pleural effusion can be associated with:
A. Necrosis
B. Pulmonary infarction or infection
C. Systemic lupus erythematosus (SLE) or rheumatoid arthritis (RA)
D. Lymphatic obstruction
Body fluids/Exudates/2

28. Which of the following conditions is most often associated with a pleural fluid glucose below 30 mg/dL?
A. Diabetes mellitus
B. Pancreatitis
C. Rheumatoid arthritis
D. Bacterial pneumonia
Body fluids/Pleural fluid/2

29. In which condition is the pleural fluid pH likely to be above 7.3?
A. Bacterial pneumonia with parapneumonic exudate
B. Rheumatoid pleuritis
C. Esophageal rupture
D. Pneumothorax
Body fluids/Pleural fluid/2

30. Which of the following hematology values *best* frames the upper reference limits (URLs) for peritoneal fluid?

	WBC Count	Percentage of PMNs	RBC Count
A.	300/µL	25%	100,000/µL
B.	10,000/µL	50%	500,000/µL
C.	50,000/µL	50%	500,000/µL
D.	100,000/µL	75%	1,000,000/µL

Body fluids/Serous fluids/2

31. Which of the following characteristics is higher for synovial fluid than for the serous fluids?
A. Specific gravity
B. Glucose
C. Total protein
D. Viscosity
Body fluids/Synovial fluid/1

Answers to Questions 26–31

26. B Exudative effusions are caused by inflammatory processes and cellular infiltration as seen in malignancy. In addition to an RBC count greater than 100,000/µL, malignancies often involve the lung, colon, breast, or pancreas and often produce carcinoembryonic antigen. In contrast, transudative fluids are caused by circulatory problems, usually decreased oncotic pressure or increased hydrostatic pressure.

27. D Malignancy, pulmonary infarction, SLE, and RA are characterized by inflammation, with increases in protein, WBCs, and LDH. Exudates can also be caused by tuberculosis, pancreatitis, and lymphoma. Lymphatic obstruction is often associated with lymphoma and other malignancies that block the flow of lymph into the azygous vein. This causes pleural (chylous) effusions. Pleural effusions are also caused by traumatic injury to the thoracic duct.

28. C Normal pleural fluid has the same glucose concentration as plasma. Hyperglycemia is the only condition that is associated with a high pleural fluid glucose. Low glucose levels (less than 60 mg/dL) may be seen in infection, malignancy, and rheumatic diseases. However, glucose levels are lowest (often below 30 mg/dL) and are a constant finding when rheumatoid disease affects the lungs. Pancreatitis causes an exudative peritoneal and pleural effusion with an elevated peritoneal fluid amylase (without a low glucose).

29. D The pH of pleural fluid is approximately 7.64, and values below 7.30 are usually associated with a poorer prognosis and usually require drainage. Esophageal rupture produces the lowest pH with values in the range of 6.0 to 6.3. In addition, pleural fluid pH is low in rheumatoid disease involving the lungs and pleura, some malignancies, and SLE. Low pH and glucose in pleural fluid are seen in lung abscesses and exudative bacterial pneumonia (called *parapneumonic effusion*). Pneumothorax results from air entering the pleural space and does not produce a low pH.

30. A Peritoneal fluid normally has a WBC count less than 300/µL. Neutrophils should account for no more than 25% of the WBCs. A majority of PMNs indicate a bacterial infection of the peritoneum. Lymphocytosis suggests malignancy, tuberculosis, cirrhosis, and lymphatic leakage.

31. D Synovial fluid has approximately the same SG and glucose as plasma and the serous fluids but is far more viscous because of a high content of mucoprotein (hyaluronate) secreted by the synovium. Viscosity is estimated by pulling the fluid from the tip of a syringe or pipet. Normal fluid gives a string longer than 4 cm. Low viscosity indicates inflammation.

32. In which type of arthritis is the synovial WBC count likely to be greater than 50,000/μL?
A. Septic arthritis
B. Osteoarthritis
C. Rheumatoid arthritis
D. Hemorrhagic arthritis
Body fluids/Synovial fluid/2

33. What type of cell is a ragocyte?
A. Cartilage cell seen in inflammatory arthritis
B. A polymorphonuclear neutrophil (PMN) with inclusions formed by immune complexes
C. A plasma cell seen in rheumatoid arthritis (RA)
D. A macrophage containing large inclusions
Body fluids/Microscopy/1

34. Which of the following crystals is the most common cause of gout?
A. Uric acid or monosodium urate
B. Calcium pyrophosphate or apatite
C. Calcium oxalate
D. Cholesterol
Body fluids/Synovial fluid/1

35. Which crystal causes "pseudogout"?
A. Oxalic acid
B. Calcium pyrophosphate
C. Calcium oxalate
D. Cholesterol
Body fluids/Synovial fluid/1

36. A synovial fluid sample is examined by using a polarizing microscope with a red compensating filter. Crystals are seen as yellow when the long axis of the crystal is parallel to the slow vibrating light. When the long axis of the crystal is perpendicular to the slow vibrating light, the crystals appear blue. What type of crystal is present?
A. Calcium oxalate
B. Calcium pyrophosphate
C. Uric acid
D. Cholesterol
Body fluids/Synovial fluid/2

37. In which condition is the synovial fluid glucose *most* likely to be within normal limits?
A. Septic arthritis
B. Inflammatory arthritis
C. Hemorrhagic arthritis
D. Gout
Body fluids/Synovial fluid/2

Answers to Questions 32–37

32. A The WBC count is elevated in all types of arthritis but is greatest (50,000–100,000/μL) in septic arthritis. Neutrophils comprise less than 25% of WBCs in normal and noninflammatory arthritis but are greater than 50% in inflammatory and septic arthritis.

33. B Ragocytes are PMNs containing dark granules composed of immunoglobulins, but they may be seen in gout and septic arthritis as well as RA. Lupus erythematosus (LE) cells may be seen in fluid from patients with systemic lupus erythematosus (SLE). Reiter cells, macrophages with ingested globular inclusions, are seen in Reiter syndrome and other inflammatory diseases.

34. A Although all the crystals mentioned can cause crystal-induced arthritis, uric acid and sodium urate crystals cause gout and are seen in about 90% of patients with gout.

35. B Calcium pyrophosphate crystals occur as needles or small rhombic plates and can be confused with uric acid. They rotate planes in polarized light but not as strongly as uric acid. Synovial fluid should never be collected in tubes containing powdered EDTA because it may form crystals that can be mistaken for *in vivo* crystals. The recommended anticoagulant is sodium heparin, although liquid EDTA may be used.

36. C Polarized microscopy with a red compensating filter differentiates uric acid from pseudogout crystals. When the long axis of uric acid needles is parallel to the slow vibrating light, the crystals appear yellow. When the long axis is perpendicular to the slow vibrating light, the crystals appear blue. Calcium pyrophosphate gives the reverse effect.

37. C Synovial fluid glucose is normally less than 10 mg/dL below serum glucose and should be collected after an 8-hour fast to ensure that the fluid and plasma are equilibrated. In septic arthritis, the glucose level is often greater than 40 mg/dL below the serum level and about 25 to 40 mg/dL lower in inflammatory arthritis, which includes gout. Osteoarthritis and hemorrhagic arthritis are not usually associated with low joint fluid glucose.

38. Which statement about synovial fluid in rheumatoid arthritis (RA) is correct?

A. Synovial:serum IgG is usually 1:2 or higher
B. Total hemolytic complement is elevated
C. Ninety percent of RA cases test positive for rheumatoid factor in synovial fluid
D. Demonstration of rheumatoid factor in joint fluid is diagnostic for RA

Body fluids/Synovial fluid/2

39. Which of the following organisms accounts for most septic arthritis cases in young and middle-aged adults?

A. *H. influenzae*
B. *Neisseria gonorrhoeae*
C. *Staphylococcus aureus*
D. *Borrelia burgdorferi*

Body fluids/Synovial fluid/2

40. Which of the following hematology values *best* frames the upper reference limits for synovial fluid?

	WBC Count	Percentage of PMNs	RBC Count
A.	200/µL	25%	2,000/µL
B.	5,000/µL	50%	10,000/µL
C.	10,000/µL	50%	50,000/µL
D.	20,000/µL	5%	500,000/µL

Body fluids/Synovial fluid/2

41. A toluidine blue chamber count on CSF gives the following values:

CSF Counts	Peripheral Blood Counts
WBCs 10×10^6/L	WBCs 5×10^9/L
RBCs $1{,}000 \times 10^6$/L	RBCs 5×10^{12}/L

After correcting the WBC count in CSF, the laboratory professional should:

A. Report the WBC count as 9×10^6/L without additional testing
B. Report the WBC count and number of PMNs identified by the chamber count
C. Perform a differential on a direct smear of the CSF
D. Concentrate the CSF using a cytocentrifuge and perform a differential

Body fluids/Cerebrospinal fluid/3

Answers to Questions 38–41

38. A Normally, IgG in synovial fluid is about 10% of the serum IgG level. CH_{50} levels in serum and synovium are more differential. Both are increased in Reiter syndrome but are often low in SLE; synovial CH_{50} is decreased and serum CH_{50} is normal (or increased) in RA. Rheumatoid factor can be present in both serum and synovial fluids from patients with RA, SLE, and other inflammatory diseases. Rheumatoid factor is present in synovial fluid of approximately 60% of patients with RA.

39. B Synovial fluid is normally sterile, and all the organisms listed may cause septic arthritis. *N. gonorrhoeae* is responsible for about 75% of septic arthritis cases occurring in young and middle-aged adults. *Staphylococcus* is responsible for most cases involving older adults and is the most frequently identified isolate from infected joint replacements. *Haemophilus* spp., *Staphylococcus* spp., and *Streptococcus* spp. are the most common causes of arthritis in young children.

40. A The WBC count of normal joint fluid is 200/µL or less. Values greater than 5,000/µL cause the fluid to be purulent and occur in septic arthritis, RA, and gout. WBC counts greater than 50,000 µL indicate septic arthritis. Most WBCs in normal fluid are monocytes, which usually account for 50% to 65%. Neutrophils and lymphocytes should account for no greater than 25% each. An increase in RBCs occurs in cases of infectious and hemorrhagic arthritis or results from a traumatic tap.

41. D A differential is performed by using CSF concentrate on all neonatal samples and whenever the WBC count is greater than 5/µL. A toluidine blue chamber count of PMNs is not sufficiently sensitive to detect neutrophilic pleocytosis.

42. A blood-tainted pleural fluid sample is submitted for culture. Which test result would be *most* conclusive in classifying the fluid as an exudate?

	Test	Result
A.	LDH fluid/serum	0.65
B.	Total protein	3.2 g/dL
C.	RBC count	10,000/μL
D.	WBC count	1,500/μL

Body fluids/Pleural fluid/3

43. A pleural fluid sample submitted to the laboratory is milky in appearance. Which test would be *most* useful in differentiating between a chylous and pseudochylous effusion?

A. Fluid:serum triglyceride ratio
B. Fluid WBC count
C. Fluid total protein
D. Fluid:serum LDH ratio

Body fluids/Pleural fluid/3

44. A CSF sample from an 8-year-old child with a fever of unknown origin was tested for glucose, total protein, lactate, and IgG index. Glucose was 180 mg/dL, but all other results were within the reference range. The CSF WBC count was 7×10^6/L, and the RBC count was 10×10^6/L. The differential showed 50% lymphocytes, 35% monocytes, 10% macrophages, 3% neutrophils, and 2% neuroectodermal cells. What is the *most* likely cause of these results?

A. Aseptic meningitis
B. Traumatic tap
C. Subarachnoid hemorrhage
D. Hyperglycemia

Body fluids/Cerebrospinal fluid/3

45. A WBC count and differential performed on ascites fluid gave a WBC count of 20,000/μL with 90% macrophages. The gross appearance of the fluid was described by the laboratorian as "thick and bloody." It was noted in the report that several clusters of these cells were observed and that the majority of the cells contained many vacuoles resembling paper-punch holes. What do the observations suggest?

A. Malignant mesothelial cells were counted as macrophages
B. Adenocarcinoma from a metastatic site
C. Lymphoma infiltrating the peritoneal cavity
D. Nodular sclerosing type Hodgkin disease

Body fluids/Serous fluids/3

Answers to Questions 42–45

42. A A traumatic tap makes classification of fluids difficult based on cell counts and protein concentration. The values reported for protein, RBCs, and WBCs can occur in either an exudate or bloody transudate, but the LDH ratio is significant.

43. A Chylous effusions are caused by extravasation of lymphatic fluid into the pleural cavity. Pseudochylous effusions are caused by necrosis. Both fluids often appear white and opalescent, but both effusions can also be bloody, green, or yellow, in addition to being turbid. However, chylous effusions are odorless and have a twofold higher triglyceride compared with plasma. They also usually show lymphocytosis. Pseudochylous effusions are foul smelling and usually have a mixed cellularity and an elevated cholesterol. These effusions may have triglyceride, but the concentration is usually below 50 mg/dL. Chylous effusions are most often caused by lymphoma or other malignancy or trauma and, like pseudochylous effusions, may have an increased LDH fluid:serum ratio, total protein, and WBC count.

44. D CSF glucose is approximately 60% of plasma glucose but may be somewhat lower in a person with diabetes. The reference range is approximately 40 to 70 mg/dL. A CSF glucose level above 70 mg/dL is caused by a high plasma glucose that equilibrates with CSF. Therefore, hyperglycorrhachia is caused by hyperglycemia. The WBC count in a child between 5 and 12 years of age is 0 to 10×10^6/L (0–10/μL). The normal RBC count and protein rule out subarachnoid hemorrhage and traumatic tap. Although aseptic meningitis cannot be ruled out conclusively, it is unlikely given a normal WBC count and IgG index.

45. A Bloody, exudative fluids with a preponderance of a singular cell type are suggestive of malignancy. The cellularity in malignancy is variable but lymphocytosis occurs in about half the cases. Mesothelial cells normally comprise less than 10% of the cells in serous fluid. They may be resting cells, reactive, degenerated, or phagocytic in nonmalignant conditions. In inflammatory conditions, they are often increased and resemble macrophages. However, clusters or balls of such cells and paper-punch vacuoles throughout the cytoplasm and over the nucleus are characteristics of malignant mesothelial cells. Such cells secrete hyaluronic acid, making the fluid highly viscous. The gross appearance of this fluid suggests malignancy. The description of these cells points to mesothelioma, and this specimen should be referred for cytological examination to confirm the diagnosis.

46. A CSF sample submitted for cell counts has a visible clot. What is the *best* course of action?

A. Count RBCs and WBCs manually after diluting the fluid with normal saline
B. Tease the cells out of the clot before counting, then dilute with WBC counting fluid
C. Request a new sample
D. Perform a WBC count without correction

Body fluids/Cerebrospinal fluid/3

47. Total hemolytic complement and glucose are ordered on a synovial fluid sample that is too viscous to pipet. What is the *best* course of action?

A. Dilute the sample in saline
B. Add 1 mg/mL hyaluronidase to the sample, and incubate at room temperature for 30 minutes
C. Warm the sample to 65°C for 10 minutes
D. Request a new specimen

Body fluids/Synovial fluid/3

48. A CSF cytospin smear shows many smudge cells and macrophages with torn cell membranes. What *most* likely caused this problem?

A. Failure to add albumin to the cytospin cup
B. Failure to collect the CSF in EDTA
C. Centrifuge speed too low
D. Improper alignment

Body fluids/Cerebrospinal fluid/3

49. An automated cell counter was used to count RBCs and WBCs in a turbid pleural fluid sample. The WBC count was 5×10^{10}/L (50,000/μL) and the RBC count was 5.5×10^{10}/L (55,000/μL). What is the significance of the RBC count?

A. The RBC count is not significant and should be reported as 5,000/μL
B. The RBC count should be reported as determined by the analyzer
C. A manual RBC count should be performed
D. A manual RBC and WBC count should be performed and reported instead

Body fluids/Cell count/3

Answers to Questions 46–49

46. C Although the sample is still suitable for microbiological analysis, it will not give reliable cell counts or biochemistry results because of extensive contamination with peripheral blood.

47. B Joint fluid too viscous to pipet accurately cannot be diluted accurately. Complement is heat labile, and total hemolytic complement is destroyed when the sample is heated to 56°C for 5 minutes. Joint fluid is difficult to collect, and a new sample is likely to have the same problem.

48. A Cellular distortion caused by centrifugation is a common problem and can be reduced by adding 22% bovine albumin or 10% dextran to the cytospin cup along with the sample. In the absence of a large subarachnoid hemorrhage, CSF does not clot because it contains no fibrinogen, and the sample can be collected and counted without anticoagulant.

49. A Electronic cell counters are validated for body fluid cell counts with specific minimum detection limits. For most counters, this is 50 to 200 total nucleated cells (TNCs)/μL and 10,000 RBC/μL. Specialized counters using fluorescent and image analysis can achieve low end sensitivities for both TNC and RBC counts of 0 to 1/μL. Because the RBCs are lysed in the WBC bath, the WBC count represents the number of nucleated cells present. When cell counters that perform CBCs are used, the WBCs are not lysed in the RBC bath and would be counted as RBCs. In this case, the empyemic fluid would cause the RBC count to be erroneously elevated, and this should be corrected before reporting by subtracting the WBC count from the RBC count.

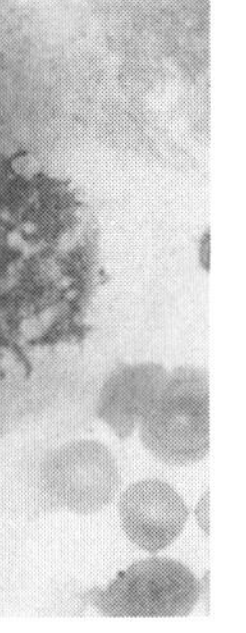

5.4

Amniotic, Gastrointestinal, Seminal Fluids, and Blood Specimens

1. Which of the following statements about amniotic fluid bilirubin measured by scanning spectrophotometry is true?

A. The 410-nm peak is caused by hemoglobin, and the 450-nm peak is caused by bilirubin
B. Baseline correction is not required because a diode array detector is used
C. Chloroform extraction is necessary only when meconium is present
D. In normal amniotic fluid, bilirubin increases with gestational age

Body fluids/Amniotic fluid/2

2. Which test *best* correlates with the severity of hemolytic disease of the fetus and newborn (HDFN)?

A. Rh antibody titer of the mother
B. Lecithin/sphingomyelin (L/S) ratio
C. Amniotic fluid bilirubin
D. Urinary estradiol

Body fluids/Amniotic fluid/2

3. Which is the reference method for determining fetal lung maturity (FLM)?

A. Human placental lactogen
B. Lecithin to sphingomyelin (L/S) ratio
C. Amniotic fluid bilirubin
D. Urinary estriol

Body fluids/Amniotic fluid/2

Answers to Questions 1–3

1. A Amniotic fluid bilirubin reflects the extent of fetal RBC destruction in cases of hemolytic disease of the fetus and newborn (HDFN). The fluid is centrifuged and absorbance measured from 350 to 600 nm simultaneously by using a photodiode array detector. Background absorbance is corrected by constructing a baseline using the absorbances at 365 nm and 550 nm. The delta absorbance (ΔA) of hemoglobin at 410 nm and of bilirubin at 450 nm is determined by subtracting the absorbance of the baseline from the respective peaks. Samples that are not grossly hemolyzed can be corrected for oxyhemoglobin by subtracting 5% of the ΔA at 410 nm from the ΔA at 450 nm. When hemolysis is severe or meconium is present, bilirubin must be extracted in chloroform before measuring absorbance. Bilirubin normally decreases with increasing gestational age because fetal urine contributes more to amniotic fluid volume as the fetus matures. The bilirubin concentration must be correlated with gestational age to correctly evaluate the severity of HDFN.

2. C Amniotic fluid bilirubin is the best index of the severity of HDFN and is measured by diode array spectrophotometry across the 365 to 550 nm range. When hemoglobin produces a positive slope at 410 nm, the bilirubin should be extracted with chloroform prior to scanning. Extraction methods give the best correlation with RBC destruction.

3. B Respiratory distress syndrome (RDS) develops when surfactants are insufficient to prevent collapse of the infant's alveoli during expiration. Tests measuring pulmonary phospholipid surfactants are the most specific and sensitive indicators of RDS. An L/S ratio greater than 2:1 (in some laboratories 2.5:1) is the most widely accepted measure of FLM. Most of the surfactants in the amniotic fluid are present in the form of lamellar bodies. These can be counted using an electronic cell counter at the settings for enumerating platelets. Laboratories must correlate the lamellar body count (LBC) that corresponds to an L/S ratio of 2:1. The LBC cutoff will differ depending on the counter.

4. Which of the following statements regarding the lecithin to sphingomyelin (L/S) ratio is correct?

A. A ratio of 2:1 or greater usually indicates adequate pulmonary surfactant to prevent respiratory distress syndrome (RDS)
B. A ratio of 1.5:1 indicates fetal lung maturity in pregnancies associated with diabetes mellitus
C. Sphingomyelin levels increase during the third trimester, causing the L/S ratio to fall slightly during the last 2 weeks of gestation
D. A phosphatidylglycerol (PG) spot indicates the presence of meconium in the amniotic fluid

Body fluids/Amniotic fluid/2

5. Which of the following conditions is *most* likely to cause a falsely low L/S ratio?

A. The presence of phosphatidylglycerol in amniotic fluid
B. Freezing the specimen for 1 month at –20°C
C. Centrifugation at 1,000 × *g* for 10 minutes
D. Maternal diabetes mellitus

Body fluids/Amniotic fluid/3

6. Which of the following statements accurately describes human chorionic gonadotropin (hCG) levels in pregnancy?

A. Levels of hCG rise throughout pregnancy
B. In ectopic pregnancy, serum hCG doubling time is below expected levels
C. Molar pregnancies are associated with lower levels than expected for the time of gestation
D. hCG returns to nonpregnant levels within 2 days following delivery, stillbirth, or abortion

Body fluids/Blood/2

Answers to Questions 4–6

4. A Pulmonary surfactants are mainly desaturated lecithins produced by type II granular pneumocytes. The L/S ratio increases toward the end of the third trimester because of increased production of lecithin. The concentration of sphingomyelin remains constant throughout gestation and serves as an internal reference. Meconium contains less lecithin than amniotic fluid and will usually decrease the L/S ratio; however, meconium produces a spot that can be misinterpreted as lecithin, leading to a falsely increased L/S ratio. Sufficient PG to produce a spot is seen only when the L/S ratio is 2:1 or higher. PG is not present in either blood or meconium, and therefore, its presence indicates fetal lung maturity. In diabetes, the fetal lungs may mature more slowly than normal, and infants may develop RDS when the L/S ratio is 2:1 or slightly higher. For this reason, an L/S of 3:1 more closely correlates with fetal lung maturity when testing amniotic fluid from mothers with diabetes. As in all other cases, when the amniotic fluid from a diabetic mother is positive for PG, fetal lung maturity is established.

5. C Pulmonary surfactants are largely present in the form of lamellar bodies and can be lost by centrifuging the amniotic fluid at high *g* force. Centrifuge speed should be the minimum required to spin down cells (450 *g* for 10 minutes at 4°C). Samples that cannot be measured immediately should be refrigerated or frozen. Samples are stable for up to 3 days at 2°C to 8°C and for months when frozen at –20°C or lower. Meconium and blood may also introduce errors when measuring the L/S ratio. Blood has an L/S ratio of approximately 2:1 and will falsely raise the L/S ratio when fetal lungs are immature and depress the L/S ratio when fetal lungs are mature.

6. B In normal pregnancy, hCG levels rise exponentially following implantation and peak at weeks 9 to 12, reaching more than 100,000 mIU/mL. The hCG doubling time averages 2.2 days. In ectopic pregnancy, the expected increase between consecutive days is below normal. Levels fall after the first trimester to about 20,000 mIU/mL and then remain at about that level through term. Hydatiform moles are associated with greatly elevated levels of hCG. Serum hCG can take up to 4 weeks to return to nonpregnant (less than 25 mIU/mL) or baseline (less than 5 mIU/mL) levels following delivery, stillbirth, or abortion.

7. Which of the following statements regarding pregnancy testing is true?

A. β-Subunits of hCG, thyroid-stimulating hormone (TSH), and follicle-stimulating hormone (FSH) are identical
B. Antibodies against the β-subunit of hCG cross-react with luteinizing hormone (LH)
C. A false-positive result may occur in patients with heterophile antibodies
D. Serum should not be used for pregnancy tests because proteins interfere

Body fluids/Blood/2

8. A pregnant person was seen by their physician, who suspected a molar pregnancy. An hCG test was ordered, and the levels were found to be low. The sample was diluted 10-fold and the assay was repeated. The level following dilution was grossly elevated. What *best* explains this situation?

A. The wrong specimen was diluted
B. A pipeting error was made in the first analysis
C. Antigen excess caused a falsely low result in the undiluted sample
D. An inhibitor of the antigen–antibody reaction was present in the sample

Body fluids/Blood/3

9. Which assay result is often *approximately* 25% below the expected level in pregnancies associated with Down syndrome?

A. Serum unconjugated estriol
B. Lecithin to sphingomyelin (L/S) ratio
C. Amniotic fluid bilirubin
D. Urinary chorionic gonadotropin

Body fluids/Clinical correlations/2

Answers to Questions 7–9

7. C The α-subunit of hCG is very similar to the α-subunit of TSH and FSH and identical to LH. Although the β-subunits of hCG and LH are very similar, antibodies can be made to the β-subunit of hCG that do not cross-react with LH or other pituitary hormones. Most enzyme immunoassay (EIA) methods utilize two monoclonal antibodies against different sites of the hCG molecule. One antibody is specific for the carboxy terminal end of the β-chain, and the other reacts with the α-chain, resulting in a positive test only when intact hCG is present. Because monoclonal antibodies are usually derived from mouse hybridomas, rare false-positive results may occur in patients who have anti-mouse immunoglobulin antibodies. Although the test can detect lower levels of hCG, 25 mIU/mL is the positive cutoff for pregnancy. Serum is preferred over urine because serum levels are more consistently above the cutoff compared with random urine in very early pregnancy.

8. C Assays of intact hCG are double antibody sandwich immunoassays. One antibody reacts with the α-subunit and the other with the β-subunit. In assays when both antibodies are added together; a process called the "hook effect" is known to occur. In extreme antigen excess, the hCG saturates both antibodies, preventing sandwich formation. This results in measurement of falsely low levels of hCG.

9. A Estriol is produced by the placenta as well as the fetal and maternal adrenal glands and liver. Free estriol produced by the placenta is rapidly conjugated by the maternal liver. Almost all maternal serum unconjugated (free) estriol is derived from the fetus and is a direct reflection of current fetal placental function. Serum unconjugated estriol (uE_3) measured during the second trimester is used along with serum alpha fetoprotein (AFP), hCG, and dimeric inhibin A as part of the quad marker screening test for Down syndrome. AFP and uE_3 are decreased by approximately 25%, inhibin A is increased by a factor of approximately 1.8, and hCG is increased by a factor of approximately 2.5 in Down syndrome pregnancies. When all four assays are combined with adjustments for maternal age, gestational age, race, maternal weight, and diabetes, the detection rate is approximately 70% to 80% and the false-positive rate 7%.

10. Which of the following statements about alpha fetoprotein (AFP) is correct?
- **A.** Maternal serum may be used to screen for open neural tube defects
- **B.** Levels above 4 ng/mL are considered positive
- **C.** Elevated levels in amniotic fluid are specific for spina bifida
- **D.** AFP levels increase in pregnancies associated with Down syndrome

Body fluids/Blood/2

11. First-trimester screening for Down syndrome can be performed using which markers?
- **A.** AFP and unconjugated estriol
- **B.** Free β-hCG and pregnancy-associated plasma protein A
- **C.** Intact hCG and dimeric inhibin A
- **D.** Dimeric inhibin B and AFP

Body fluids/Clinical correlations/1

12. When performing marker screening tests for Down syndrome, why are results expressed in multiples of the median (MoM), rather than in concentration?
- **A.** Concentration is not normally distributed
- **B.** MoM normalizes for gestational age
- **C.** Some tests cannot be reported in mass units
- **D.** Mean cannot be determined accurately for these analytes

Body fluids/Clinical correlations/1

Answers to Questions 10–12

10. A Maternal serum AFP increases steadily until 2 months prior to full term as AFP passes from the fetal urine into the amniotic fluid. Because serum levels are dependent on gestational age, URLs depend on the date of the last menstrual period. AFP is measured between 14-and 18 weeks' gestation, and levels are reported as multiples of the median to permit interlaboratory comparison. When serum levels are high, ultrasonography is used to determine fetal age and rule out twins. Increased maternal serum AFP levels (greater than 2.5 multiples of the mean [MoM]) may result from many diseases in addition to open neural tube defects, such as spina bifida. These include anencephaly, ventral wall defects, congenital hypothyroidism, and Turner syndrome. Decreased levels (less than 0.75 MoM) may be seen in approximately 25% of Down syndrome pregnancies.

11. B Maternal serum AFP levels are too low to measure accurately during the first trimester, and intact hCG and estriol do not discriminate well between 21 trisomy pregnancy and normal pregnancy before the second trimester. First trimester screening for Down syndrome (and trisomy 18) can be performed between weeks 10 and 13 by using free β-hCG (almost twofold higher in Down syndrome) and pregnancy-associated plasma protein A (PAPP-A), which has a median in Down syndrome less than half of that seen in normal pregnancy. These two markers used together with high-resolution ultrasonography to determine nuchal fold thickness (swelling at the base of the neck) have a sensitivity of 85% to 90%. Nuchal fold thickness (NT) in Down syndrome averages 1.5 MoM compared with 1.0 MoM for normal pregnancy.

12. B Reporting of screening markers as MoM has two advantages: (1) It eliminates interlaboratory variation in reference ranges seen when concentration units are reported. Laboratories using different methods (antibodies or calibrators) may have significantly different mass unit results for the same sample, necessitating different reference ranges. (2) The reference range in concentration units is also dependent on the gestational age at the time of sample collection; however, the average result that is not a concern is always 1.0 MoM, regardless of the gestational age of the cohort. Use of MoM obviates the need to report specific reference ranges based on method or gestational age and makes calculation of risk less complicated.

13. Which test for 21 trisomy is *not* recommended for people who are carrying twins?
A. First trimester triple marker screening
B. Maternal plasma cell-free fetal DNA
C. Chorionic villus sampling
D. Second trimester quad marker screening
Body fluids/Clinical correlations/2

14. Which statement regarding the fetal fibronectin test is true?
A. A positive test is correlated with a low probability of delivery within 14 days
B. The test should not be performed before week 24 or after the end of week 34
C. The test is performed on amniotic fluid
D. The test is used to identify amniotic fluid after rupture of the fetal membranes
Body fluids/Clinical correlations/1

15. What is the term for spermatozoa in which the anterior portion of the headpiece is smaller than normal?
A. Azoospermia
B. Microcephaly
C. Acrosomal deficiency
D. Necrozoospermia
Body fluids/Seminal fluid/1

16. What is the *most* common cause of male infertility?
A. Mumps
B. Klinefelter syndrome
C. Varicocele
D. Malignancy
Body fluids/Seminal fluid/2

17. Which of the following values is the lower limit for sperm concentration?
A. 15 million per milliliter
B. 40 million per milliliter
C. 60 million per milliliter
D. 100 million per milliliter
Body fluids/Seminal fluid/2

Answers to Questions 13–17

13. B Down syndrome can result from a 14–21 translocation or isochromosome formation, but most cases arise from nondisjunction of chromosome 21 during meiosis. Plasma cell-free DNA testing can be performed as early as week 10 and detects fetal DNA released from fetal cells that have crossed the placenta. The test measures the ratio of fetal DNA:maternal DNA from chromosomes X, Y, 13, 18, and 21 with use of single nucleotide polymorphisms on the respective chromosomes to distinguish fetal DNA from maternal DNA. This ratio can be misinterpreted if more than one fetus is present. If any screening test is positive, amniocentesis or chronic villus sampling is performed, and trisomy is investigated by using chromosome karyotyping, microarray, or fluorescence *in situ* hybridization (FISH) on fetal cells.

14. B The fetal fibronectin test is used mainly to rule out the likelihood of preterm delivery in high-risk pregnancies or in females with signs of preterm labor between weeks 24 and 34 of pregnancy. Fetal fibronectin is a basement membrane protein produced by the amnion and chorion. It is present in cervical secretions in early pregnancy but disappears by about week 20. When there is inflammation to the membranes preceding delivery, fibronectin is released and can be found in cervicovaginal secretions. A positive test (greater than 50 ng/mL) has a sensitivity of about 60% in predicting preterm birth. However, a negative test has a 92% negative predictive value for the likelihood of preterm delivery and effectively rules out preterm delivery within the next 2 weeks.

15. C Spermatozoa have a well-defined headpiece consisting of the acrosome and nucleus. The acrosome comprises the anterior portion of the head and contains nutrients and enzymes needed for penetration of the ovum. A thin filament, the neckpiece, connects the head and tail. The tail is divided into the midpiece, principal piece (main piece), and endpiece.

16. C Varicocele is the hardening of veins that drain the testes. This causes blood from the adrenal vein to flow into the spermatic vein. Adrenal corticosteroids retard the development of spermatozoa. Mumps, Klinefelter syndrome, and malignancy cause testicular failure, which accounts for about 10% of infertility cases in males.

17. A The reference range for spermatozoa is 15 to 150 $\times$ 10^6/mL. Concentrations below 15 $\times$ 10^6/mL are considered abnormal. The sperm concentration is multiplied by the seminal fluid volume to determine the sperm count. The lower limit of normal for the sperm count is 40 $\times$ 10^6 per ejaculate. This often results from obstruction of the ejaculatory duct or testicular failure.

18. In which of the following conditions are sperm count, shape, and motility involved?
A. Oligozoospermia
B. Asthenozoospermia
C. Azoospermia
D. Hyperspermia
Body fluid/Seminal fluid/2

19. Which of the following stains is used to determine sperm viability?
A. Eosin
B. Hematoxylin
C. Papanicolaou
D. Methylene blue
Body fluids/Seminal fluid/1

20. Which of the following semen analysis results are considered abnormal?
A. Volume 1.0 mL
B. Liquefaction 40 minutes at room temperature
C. pH 7.6
D. Motility 50% progressive movement
Body fluids/Seminal fluid/2

21. Which of the following sample collection and processing conditions will lead to *inaccurate* seminal fluid analysis results?
A. Sample stored at room temperature for 1 hour before testing
B. Sample collected in a condom following coitus
C. Sample collected without an anticoagulant
D. Sample collected without use of a condom
Body fluids/Seminal fluid/2

22. When performing a seminal fluid analysis, what is the upper limit of normal for WBCs?
A. 1×10^6/mL
B. 5×10^6/mL
C. 10×10^6/mL
D. 20×10^6/mL
Body fluids/Seminal fluid/2

Answers to Questions 18–22

18. A In oligozoospermia, there may be a low sperm count as well as abnormal sperm shape and movement. Azoospermia describes semen containing no sperm, and asthenozoospermia involves sperm that do not move correctly.

19. A Eosin is excluded by living sperm and is used to determine the percentage of living cells. Papanicolaou, Giemsa, and hematoxylin stains are used to evaluate sperm morphology. The viability test should be performed whenever the results of the motility test are subnormal.

20. A The normal volume of seminal fluid is 1.5 to 5.0 mL. A lower volume than 1.5 mL causes a low sperm count (sperm/mL × volume) and can be caused by absence of the seminal vesicles or prostate, ductal obstruction, or retrograde ejaculation of seminal fluid into the urinary bladder. The seminal fluid should coagulate within 5 minutes after ejaculation because of secretions of the seminal vesicles. Proteases, such as prostate-specific antigen (PSA), hydrolyze semenogelin and fibronectin, causing liquefaction to occur within 1 hour at room temperature. The seminal fluid pH should be between 7.2 and 8.0. Motility is evaluated by grading the movement of two replicates of 200 sperm in 5 HPFs. It is normal when 32% or greater show progressive movement or when 40% or greater demonstrates progressive and nonprogressive movement.

21. B A seminal fluid sample should not be collected following coitus. The patient should abstain from ejaculation for at least 2 days but no more than 7 days prior to submitting the sample. A condom should not be used because it may contain spermicides. The sample should be collected at the testing site in a sterile jar with a wide opening and stored at room temperature. The specimen should be analyzed as soon as possible. The time between collection and delivery to the laboratory must be documented. Motility should be determined as soon as the fluid has liquefied (maximum storage time is 1 hour). Anticoagulants are not used; if the sample fails to liquefy, it can be treated with chymotrypsin before analysis.

22. A When evaluating sperm morphology, the number of round cells (immature spermatozoa and WBCs) should also be determined. The number of each cell type is counted along with 200 mature sperm and then divided by 2 to determine their percentage. This is multiplied by the sperm concentration to give the absolute count per milliliter. An increased number of WBCs is an indicator of infection and is usually associated with prostatitis. Round cells are also estimated by noting their number per high-power field. Each round cell per field counted with the 40× objective corresponds to 1 million per milliliter. The upper limit of normal for WBCs is 1×10^6/mL and for immature sperm 5×10^6/mL.

23. Which carbohydrate measurement is clinically useful when performing a seminal fluid analysis?
A. Glucose
B. Galactose
C. Fructose
D. Maltose
Body fluids/Seminal fluid/1

24. Which condition is *most* often associated with gastric ulcers?
A. Cancer of the stomach
B. *Helicobacter pylori* infection
C. Zollinger-Ellison (Z-E) syndrome
D. Pernicious anemia
Body fluids/Clinical correlations/2

25. In which condition is the *highest* level of serum gastrin usually seen?
A. Atrophic gastritis
B. Pernicious anemia
C. Zollinger-Ellison syndrome
D. Cancer of the stomach
Body fluids/Clinical correlations/2

26. How does the stomach protect itself from digestion?
A. Produces insulin to break down carbohydrates
B. Secretes bile to neutralize the acid
C. Produces mucus and bicarbonate
D. Stimulates gastric base production
Body fluids/Clinical correlations/1

27. What is the role of gastrin in gastric functions?
A. Stimulate gastric acid secretion and enhance gastric motility
B. Regulate nutrient absorption
C. Produce cholecystokinin–pancreozymin
D. Promote bile production
Body fluids/Clinical correlations/2

28. Which of the following tests would be normal in pancreatic insufficiency?
A. Secretin stimulation
B. D-Xylose absorption
C. 24-hour fecal fat
D. β-Carotene absorption
Body fluids/Clinical correlations/2

Answers to Questions 23–28

23. C Fructose is the primary nutrient in the seminal fluid and is needed for motility. It is supplied by the seminal vesicles and is low when the vas deferens or seminal vesicles are absent. The lower limit of normal is 150 mg/dL, or 13 μmol, per ejaculate.

24. B Peptic ulcer disease may be caused by either gastric or duodenal ulcers, which are associated with discomfort, hyperacidity, and bleeding. Hyperacidity is most often caused by *H. pylori* infection, which can cause both gastric and duodenal ulcers. In the absence of a positive test for *H. pylori* (e.g., endoscopic biopsy, breath test, enzyme-linked immunosorbent assay [ELISA], polymerase chain reaction [PCR]) and no history of drug-induced ulcers, Z-E syndrome (gastrinoma) should be suspected, and can usually be identified by a plasma gastrin assay. Cancer of the stomach is associated with increased gastric fluid volume but not hyperacidity. Pernicious anemia is associated with gastric hypoacidity, and not ulcers.

25. C Z-E syndrome results from a gastrin-secreting tumor, gastrinoma, usually originating in the pancreas. It is characterized by very high levels of plasma gastrin which in turn will cause the stomach to form too much acid. In duodenal ulcers, increased gastric acidity occurs, but fasting plasma gastrin levels are normal. In stomach cancer, gastric volume is increased but acidity is not, and plasma gastrin levels are variable.

26. C The columnar epithelial cells in the stomach, known as *surface mucous cells* or *foveolar cells*, secrete a thick layer of mucus that covers and protects the stomach lining from its own digestive juices. These cells are also responsible for producing bicarbonate ions that are mixed into the mucus layer to protect the stomach.

27. A Gastrin, a hormone produced by the stomach, has a primary function of stimulating secretion of the gastric acid HCl. Secondarily it will regulate gastric motility by stimulating muscle contractions. Cholecystokinin–pancreozymin is produced in the duodenum and will cause the release of digestive enzymes and bile from the pancreas and gallbladder.

28. B The xylose absorption test differentiates pancreatic insufficiency from malabsorption syndrome (both cause deficient fat absorption). Xylose is absorbed by the small intestine without the aid of pancreatic enzymes. It is not metabolized and is excreted into urine. Low levels indicate gastrointestinal malabsorption. A 24-hour fecal fat results would be elevated, and β-carotene (fat-soluble vitamin) absorption will be decreased.

29. Which of the following is commonly associated with occult blood?

A. Colon cancer
B. Atrophic gastritis
C. Pernicious anemia
D. Pancreatitis

Body fluids/Clinical correlations/2

30. Which test is *most* sensitive in detecting chronic pancreatitis?

A. Fecal trypsin
B. Fecal chymotrypsin
C. Fecal elastin-1
D. Plasma lipase

Body fluids/Clinical correlations/2

31. Results of a fetal lung maturity (FLM) study from a patient with diabetes mellitus are as follows:

L/S ratio = 2.0; Phosphatidyl glycerol (PG) = Neg; Creatinine = 2.5 mg/dL

Given these results, the laboratory professional should:

A. Report the result and recommend repeating the L/S ratio in 24 hours
B. Perform scanning spectrophotometry on the fluid to determine if blood is present
C. Repeat the L/S ratio after 4 hours and report those results
D. Report the results as invalid

Body fluids/Amniotic fluid/3

32. A sperm motility test was performed, and 200 sperm were evaluated in each of two duplicates. The first sample demonstrated progressive movement in 50% and nonprogressive movement in 35%, and 15% were nonmotile. The second demonstrated progressive movement in 35% and nonprogressive movement in 35%, and 30% were nonmotile. What is the *best* course of action?

A. Report the average of the two values for progressive movement
B. Report the higher of the two values
C. Repeat the motility test
D. Call for a new specimen

Body fluids/Seminal fluid/3

33. A quantitative serum hCG is ordered on a male patient. The technologist should:

A. Perform the test and report the result
B. Request that the order be canceled
C. Perform the test and report the result if negative
D. Perform the test and report the result only if greater than 25 IU/L

Body fluids/Blood/3

Answers to Questions 29–33

29. A Blood in feces is a very sensitive indicator of gastrointestinal bleeding and is an excellent screening test to detect asymptomatic ulcers and malignancy of the gastrointestinal tract. However, the test is nonspecific and contamination with vaginal blood is a frequent source of error.

30. C Digestive enzyme tests are used to identify infants and children with pancreatic insufficiency associated with cystic fibrosis, and adults who have chronic pancreatitis. Such tests include fecal trypsin and chymotrypsin, serum immunoreactive trypsin, serum lipase, and fecal elastase-1. Fecal chymotrypsin is somewhat more sensitive in diagnosing pancreatic insufficiency and chronic pancreatitis than fecal trypsin or serum immunoreactive trypsin, but the most sensitive and specific enzyme test is fecal elastase-1, which is low in about 90% of patients with cystic fibrosis as well as pancreatic insufficiency and in greater than 75% of adults with moderate to severe chronic pancreatitis. Lipase is neither sensitive nor specific for chronic pancreatitis.

31. A In patients with poorly controlled diabetes, lung maturity may be delayed and an L/S ratio of 2:1 may be associated with respiratory distress syndrome. A positive PG spot correlates with an L/S ratio of 2:1 or higher and rules out a falsely increased result caused by blood contamination. However, the appearance of PG in amniotic fluid is often delayed in diabetes. The best course of action is to wait an additional 24 hours and perform another L/S ratio on a fresh sample of amniotic fluid because an L/S ratio of 3:1 would indicate a high probability of lung maturity.

32. C Sperm motility should be performed in duplicate and 200 cells per sample in several fields should be evaluated for movement. Agreement between duplicates must be within a specified percentage based on the category with the highest percentage. In this case, progressive movement is highest at 50%, and the difference between replicates should be no greater than 10%.

33. A hCG may be produced in men by tumors of trophoblastic origin, such as teratoma and seminoma, and is an important marker for nontrophoblastic tumors as well.

34. A lamellar body count (LBC) was performed on an amniotic fluid sample that was slightly pink within 1 hour of specimen collection. The sample was stored at 4°C prior to analysis. The result was 25,000/µL, classified as intermediate risk of respiratory distress syndrome. The provider waited 24 hours and collected a new sample that was counted within 2 hours of collection on the same instrument. The LBC of the new sample was 14,000/µL and the patient was reclassified as high risk for delivery. Which statement *best* explains these results?

A. Loss of lamellar bodies occurred in the second sample because of storage
B. Blood caused a falsely elevated result for the first sample
C. The fetal status changed in 24 hours because of respiratory illness
D. The difference in counts is the result of day-to-day physiological and instrument variance

Body fluids/Clinical correlations/3

Answer to Question 34

34. B Lamellar bodies are small particles containing pulmonary surfactants that are made by type II pneumocytes, and their number in amniotic fluid increases as the concentration of phospholipids increases. They are about the same size as platelets and are counted in the platelet channel of cell counters. If the amniotic fluid sample is contaminated with blood, platelets will falsely raise the LBC. Amniotic fluid samples for LBC are stable for several days when stored at 4°C. However, cutoffs for FLM need to be established by each laboratory because there are significant differences in LBCs between different counters.

BIBLIOGRAPHY

1. Bishop M, Fody E, Van Siclen C, Mistler JM, Moy M. *Clinical Chemistry: Principles, Techniques, and Correlations*. 9th ed. Jones & Bartlett Learning; 2023.
2. King-Strasinger S, Schaub Di Lorenzo M. *Urinalysis and Body Fluids*. 6th ed. F.A. Davis Company; 2014.
3. Tanck E, Ulalulae A. *Quick Compendium of Medical Laboratory Sciences*. 2nd ed. ASCP Press; 2023.

CHAPTER 6

Clinical Chemistry

6.1 *Instrumentation and Methodology*

6.2 *Blood Gases, pH, Electrolytes, and Vitamins*

6.3 *Carbohydrates, Hemoglobin, Iron, and Bilirubin*

6.4 *Creatinine, Uric Acid, BUN, and Ammonia*

6.5 *Proteins, Electrophoresis, and Lipids*

6.6 *Enzymes and Cardiac Markers*

6.7 *Clinical Endocrinology*

6.8 *Toxicology, Therapeutic Drug Monitoring, and Trace Metals*

6.9 *Tumor Markers*

6.1

Instrumentation and Methodology

1. **Which formula correctly describes the relationship between absorbance (A) and percent transmittance (%T)?**
   A. A = 2 – log %T
   B. A = log T
   C. A = –log %T
   D. A = 2 – %T

   Chemistry/Instrumentation and methodology/Spectrophotometry/1

2. **A solution that has a transmittance of 1.0%T would have an absorbance of:**
   A. 1.0
   B. 2.0
   C. 1.0%
   D. 99.0%

   Chemistry/Instrumentation and methodology/Spectrophotometry/2

3. **Which of two instruments can be assumed to have the narrower bandpass? Assume that wavelength is accurately calibrated.**
   A. The instrument giving the highest absorbance for a solution of 0.1 mmol/L NADH at 340 nm
   B. The instrument giving the lowest %T for a solution of nickel sulfate at 700 nm
   C. The instrument giving the highest %T reading for 1.0% volume per volume (v/v) HCl at 350 nm
   D. The instrument giving the most linear plot of absorbance versus concentration

   Chemistry/Instrumentation and methodology/Spectrophotometry/3

4. **An analyzer measures light scatter at a 90° angle to the light source, and the amount of scattered light is proportional to the analyte concentration. Which spectrophotometric principle is being described?**
   A. Fluorometry
   B. Nephelometry
   C. Potentiometry
   D. Electrochemistry

   Chemistry/Instrumentation and methodology/Spectrophotometry/1

Answers to Questions 1–4

1. A Absorbance is proportional to the inverse log of transmittance:

$$A = -\log T \times \log 1/T$$

Multiplying the numerator and denominator by 100 gives:

$$A = \log (100/100 \times T)$$

$$100 \times T = \%T \text{ substituting } \%T \text{ for } 100 \times T \text{ gives:}$$

$$A = \log 100/\%T$$

$$A = \log 100 - \log\%T$$

$$A = 2.0 - \log\%T$$

2. B Absorbance is proportional to the inverse log of transmittance:

$$A = -\log T = \log 1/T$$

$$A = 2.0 - \log\%T$$

$$A = 2.0 - \log 1.0$$

$$\text{The log of } 1.0 = 0$$

$$A = 2.0$$

3. A Bandpass is defined by the range of wavelengths passed through the sample at the specified wavelength setting. It can be measured using any solution having a narrow absorbance peak (e.g., NADH at 340 nm). The instrument producing the purest monochromatic light will have the highest absorbance reading.

4. B Nephelometry is the spectrophotometric principle in which the detector measures the light scatter at a 90° angle as compared to the light source, and the amount of scattered light is proportional to the concentration of the analyte in the solution.

5. A single-point calibration is performed between each blood gas sample to:
A. Correct the electrode slope
B. Correct electrode and instrument drift
C. Compensate for temperature variance
D. Prevent contamination by the previous sample
Chemistry/Instrumentation and methodology/2

6. The determination of the O_2 saturation of hemoglobin (Hgb) is *best* accomplished by:
A. Polychromatic absorbance measurements of a whole blood hemolysate
B. Near infrared transcutaneous absorbance measurement
C. Treatment of whole blood with alkaline dithionite prior to measuring absorbance
D. Calculation using Po_2 and total Hgb by direct spectrophotometry
Chemistry/Instrumentation and methodology/1

7. Which of the following provides the most accurate measurement of inorganic phosphorus (P_i) in serum?
A. Rate of unreduced phosphomolybdate formation at 340 nm
B. Measurement of phosphomolybdenum blue at 680 nm
C. Use of aminonaptholsulfonic acid to reduce phosphomolybdate
D. Formation of a complex with malachite green dye
Chemistry/Instrumentation and methodology/2

8. When measuring calcium with the complexometric dye *o*-cresolphthalein complexone, magnesium is kept from interfering by:
A. Using an alkaline pH
B. Adding 8-hydroxyquinoline
C. Measuring at 450 nm
D. Complexing to ethylenediaminetetraacetic acid (EDTA)
Chemistry/Instrumentation and methodology/1

9. Which stationary phase is used for the measurement of HgbA1c by HPLC?
A. Octadecylsilane (C18)
B. Cation exchanger
C. Anion exchanger
D. Polystyrene divinylbenzene
Chemistry/Instrumentation and methodology/Chromatography/2

10. Which of the following is the reference method for measuring serum glucose?
A. Somogyi-Nelson
B. Hexokinase
C. Glucose oxidase
D. Glucose dehydrogenase
Chemistry/Instrumentation and methodology/1

Answers to Questions 5–10

5. B Calibration using a single standard corrects the instrument for error at the labeled value of the calibrator but does not correct for analytic errors away from the set point. A two-point calibration adjusts the slope response of the electrode, eliminating proportional error caused by poor electrode performance.

6. A Measurement of oxyhemoglobin, deoxyhemoglobin (reduced Hgb), carboxyhemoglobin, methemoglobin, and sulfhemoglobin can be accomplished by using direct spectrophotometry at multiple wavelengths and the absorptivity coefficients of each pigment at those wavelengths.

7. A Inorganic phosphorus is proportional to the rate of absorbance increase at 340 nm when it combines with ammonium molybdate. Colorimetric methods suffer from interferences resulting from the reduction of ammonium phosphomolybdate.

8. B *o*-Cresolphthalein complexone can be used to measure either magnesium or calcium. Interference in calcium assays is prevented by addition of 8-hydroxyquinoline, which chelates magnesium.

9. B The high-pressure liquid chromatography (HLPC) method used for HgbA1c quantitation is a form of ion exchange chromatography. Elution is accomplished by increasing the ionic strength of the mobile phase. Cations in the buffer displace the Hgb pigments from the column.

10. B The hexokinase method is considered more accurate than glucose oxidase methods because the coupling reaction using glucose-6-phosphate dehydrogenase (G-6-PD) is highly specific.

11. Polarographic methods for glucose analysis are based on which principle of measurement?
A. Nonenzymatic oxidation of glucose
B. The rate of O_2 depletion
C. Chemiluminescence caused by formation of adenosine triphosphate (ATP)
D. The change in electrical potential as glucose is oxidized

Chemistry/Instrumentation and methodology/Polarography/1

12. In addition to polarography, what other electrochemical method can be used to measure glucose in plasma?
A. Conductivity
B. Potentiometry
C. Anodic stripping voltammetry
D. Amperometry

Chemistry/Instrumentation and methodology/Polarography/1

13. Select the enzyme that is *most* specific for β-D-glucose in glucose determination.
A. Hexokinase
B. Glucose-6-phosphate dehydrogenase (G-6-PD)
C. Phosphohexisomerase
D. Glucose oxidase

Chemistry/Instrumentation and methodology/1

14. Select the coupling enzyme used in the hexokinase method for glucose.
A. G-6-PD
B. Peroxidase
C. Glucose dehydrogenase
D. Glucose-6-phosphatase

Chemistry/Instrumentation and methodology/1

15. Which glucose method is subject to falsely low results caused by ascorbate?
A. Hexokinase
B. Glucose dehydrogenase
C. Trinder glucose oxidase
D. Polarography oxygen consumption

Chemistry/Instrumentation and methodology/1

16. Oxygen consumption electrode method for glucose measurement is also referred to as:
A. Amperometric measurement
B. Hexokinase reaction
C. Trinder reaction
D. Polarography measurement

Chemistry/Instrumentation and methodology/Polarography/1

17. Which of the following methods of measurement for glycated hemoglobin is the preferred method of use in the clinical laboratory and is not affected by temperature or hemoglobin variants?
A. Cation-exchange chromatography
B. Affinity chromatography
C. Electrophoresis
D. Thin-layer chromatography (TLC)

Chemistry/Instrumentation and methodology/Chromatography/1

Answers to Questions 11–17

11. B Polarographic glucose electrodes measure the consumption of O_2 as glucose is oxidized. Glucose oxidase in the reagent catalyzes the oxidation of glucose by O_2 forming H_2O_2. As the dissolved O_2 decreases, less is reduced at the cathode, resulting in a decrease in current proportional to glucose concentration

12. D In some critical care analyzers, amperometric measurement of glucose is used.

13. D Glucose oxidase is the most specific enzyme reacting with only β-D-glucose.

14. A Hexokinase catalyzes the phosphorylation of glucose using ATP as the phosphate donor. Glucose 6-phosphate (glucose $6PO_4$) is oxidized to 6-phosphogluconate and NAD^+ is reduced to NADH using G-6-PD.

15. C Although glucose oxidase is specific for β-D-glucose, the coupling (indicator) reaction is prone to negative interference from ascorbate, uric acid, acetoacetic acid, and other reducing agents.

16. D *Polarography* refers to the analytical process whereby a polarographic oxygen sensor is modified to measure the rate of oxygen consumption as a means to prevent interference in the glucose oxidase measurement.

17. B Affinity chromatography is the preferred method of measurement, where the glycosylated hemoglobin attaches to the boronate group of the resin and is preferentially eluted.

18. Identify the reference method for total calcium (Ca^{2+}).
A. Orthocresolphthalein complexone
B. Arsenazo II dye
C. Atomic absorption spectrometry
D. Ion-selective electrode
Chemistry/Instrumentation and methodology/1

19. Which reagent is used to extract amphetamine, an alkaline drug, from urine?
A. Neutral solution of ethyl acetate
B. Chloroform and sodium acetate
C. Alkali and organic solvent
D. Acid and sodium chloride
Chemistry/Instrumentation and methodology/1

20. Which reagent is used to extract morphine, an alkaline drug, from urine?
A. Neutral solution of ethyl acetate
B. Chloroform and sodium acetate
C. Alkali and organic solvent
D. Acid and sodium chloride
Chemistry/Instrumentation and methodology/1

21. The determination of the carboxyhemoglobin is *best* accomplished by:
A. Polychromatic absorbance measurements of a whole blood hemolysate
B. Near infrared transcutaneous absorbance measurement
C. Treatment of whole blood with alkaline dithionite prior to measuring absorbance
D. Calculation using Po_2 and total Hgb by direct spectrophotometry
Chemistry/Instrumentation and methodology/1

22. The determination of the methemoglobin is *best* accomplished by:
A. Near infrared transcutaneous absorbance measurement
B. Polychromatic absorbance measurements of a whole blood hemolysate
C. Treatment of whole blood with alkaline dithionite prior to measuring absorbance
D. Calculation using Po_2 and total Hgb by direct spectrophotometry
Chemistry/Instrumentation and methodology/1

Answers to Questions 18–22

18. C While orthocresolphthalein complexone (CPC) or arsenazo III dye are methodologies commonly incorporated into large analyzers, atomic absorption spectrometry (AAS) remains the reference method for total Ca^{2+} and is rarely used in the clinical setting.

19. C Alkaline drugs, such as amphetamine, are extracted at alkaline pH. Ideally, the pH for extracting alkaline drugs into an organic solvent should be 2 pH units greater than the negative log of the dissociation constant (pKa) of the drug.

20. C Alkaline drugs, such as amphetamine, are extracted at alkaline pH. Ideally, the pH for extracting alkaline drugs into an organic solvent should be 2 pH units greater than the negative log of the dissociation constant (pKa) of the drug.

21. A Measurement of oxyhemoglobin, deoxyhemoglobin (reduced Hgb), carboxyhemoglobin, methemoglobin, and sulfhemoglobin can be accomplished by using direct spectrophotometry at multiple wavelengths and the absorptivity coefficients of each pigment at those wavelengths.

22. B Measurement of oxyhemoglobin, deoxyhemoglobin (reduced Hgb), carboxyhemoglobin, methemoglobin, and sulfhemoglobin can be accomplished by using direct spectrophotometry at multiple wavelengths and the absorptivity coefficients of each pigment at those wavelengths.

23. Which statement *best* describes the principle of nephelometry?
- **A.** Nephelometry measures light intensity that is reflected from a solid surface
- **B.** Nephelometry measures light by atoms in solution that, when excited by short wavelength light, emit longer wavelength low-energy light
- **C.** Nephelometry measures light of a specific wavelength produced when a molecule returns from an excited state to an unexcited state
- **D.** Nephelometry measures light scatter as light passes through a turbid solution

Chemistry/Instrumentation and methodology/Nephelometry/2

24. The purpose of the nebulizer in an atomic absorption spectrophotometer that uses a flame is to:
- **A.** Uniformly distribute the sample in the flame
- **B.** Cause ejection of an outer shell electron
- **C.** Reduce evaporation of the sample
- **D.** Burn off organic impurities

Chemistry/Instrumentation and methodology/Atomic absorption/2

25. A flameless atomic absorption spectrophotometer dehydrates and atomizes a sample using:
- **A.** A graphite capillary furnace
- **B.** An electron gun
- **C.** A thermoelectric semiconductor
- **D.** A thermospray platform

Chemistry/Instrumentation and methodology/Atomic absorption/1

26. When measuring lead (Pb) in whole blood using atomic absorption spectrophotometry, what reagent is required to obtain the needed sensitivity and precision?
- **A.** Lanthanum
- **B.** Lithium
- **C.** Triton X-100
- **D.** Chloride

Chemistry/Instrumentation and methodology/Atomic absorption/1

27. Interference in atomic absorption spectrophotometry caused by differences in viscosity is called:
- **A.** Absorption interference
- **B.** Matrix effect
- **C.** Ionization interference
- **D.** Quenching

Chemistry/Instrumentation and methodology/Atomic absorption/1

Answers to Questions 23–27

23. D In nephelometry, scattered light is measured at a specific wavelength as it passes through a turbid solution in relation to a reference solution. Reflectance photometry measures light intensity that is reflected off a solid surface as used in dry slide technology. Fluorometry is the measurement of light by molecules that emit long wavelength, short energy light when excited by short wavelength, high energy light. AAS measures light at a specific wavelength that is returning from an excited state to a resting state.

24. A The nebulizer in atomic absorption spectrophotometry disperses the sample into a fine aerosol, distributing it evenly into the flame. Heat from the flame is used to evaporate water and break the ionic bonds of salts, forming ground state atoms. The flame also excites a small percentage of the atoms, which release a characteristic emission line.

25. A Flameless atomic absorption uses a hollow tube of graphite with quartz ends. The tube is heated in stages by an electric current to successively dry, ash, and atomize the sample. During the ash and atomization steps, argon is injected into the tube to distribute the atoms. The furnace is slower than a flame atomizer because it must cool down before introduction of the next sample.

26. C A graphite furnace is utilized for measuring lead where the matrix modifier consists of Triton X-100, ammonium phosphate, and nitric acid.

27. B Significant differences in aspiration and atomization result when the matrix of the sample and unknowns differ. Differences in viscosity and protein content are major causes of matrix error.

28. When measuring calcium by atomic absorption spectrophotometry, which is required?

A. An organic extraction reagent to deconjugate calcium from protein
B. An internal standard
C. A magnesium chelator
D. Lanthanum oxide to chelate phosphates

Chemistry/Instrumentation and methodology/Atomic absorption/1

29. Ion-selective analyzers using undiluted samples provide an advantage over analyzers that use a diluted sample. Which item is correct?

A. Can measure over a wider range of concentration
B. Are not subject to pseudohyponatremia caused by high lipids
C. Do not require temperature equilibration
D. Require less maintenance

Chemistry/Instrumentation and methodology/Ion selective/1

30. Select the equation describing the potential that develops at the surface of an ion-selective electrode (ISE).

A. van Deemter equation
B. van Slyke equation
C. Nernst equation
D. Henderson–Hasselbalch equation

Chemistry/Instrumentation and methodology/Ion selective/1

31. The reference potential of a silver–silver chloride electrode is determined by the:

A. Concentration of the potassium chloride filling solution
B. Surface area of the electrode
C. Activity of total anion in the paste covering the electrode
D. The concentration of silver in the paste covering the electrode

Chemistry/Instrumentation and methodology/Ion selective/1

32. The term *RT/nF* in the Nernst equation defines the:

A. Potential at the ion-selective membrane
B. Slope of the electrode
C. Decomposition potential
D. Isopotential point of the electrode

Chemistry/Instrumentation and methodology/Electrochemistry/1

Answers to Questions 28–32

28. D Lanthanum oxide is required in atomic absorption spectrophotometry to displace calcium, forming lanthanum phosphate and eliminating interference from phosphates.

29. B Ion-selective analyzers measure the electrolyte dissolved in the fluid phase of the sample in millimoles per liter of plasma water. When undiluted blood is assayed, the measurement is independent of colloids, such as protein and lipid. Hyperlipemic samples cause falsely low sodium measurements when assayed by ion-selective analyzers requiring dilution because lipids displace plasma water containing the electrolytes.

30. C The Nernst equation describes the potential that develops at the surface of an ISE. The van Deemter equation describes the relation between the velocity of mobile phase to column efficiency in gas chromatography (GC). The Henderson-Hasselbalch equation is used to determine the pH of a solution containing a weak acid and its salt. van Slyke developed an apparatus to measure carbon dioxide (CO_2) and oxygen (O_2) content by using a manometer.

31. A Because silver and silver chloride have an activity of 1.0, and all components except chloride are constants, the potential of the reference electrode is determined by the chloride concentration of the filling solution.

32. B In the Nernst equation, the term *RT/nF* defines the slope of the electrode. R = the molar gas constant, T = temperature in kelvins, F = Faraday's constant, and n = the number of electrons donated per atom of reductant. The slope depends on the temperature of the solution and the valence of the reductant.

33. The ion-selective membrane used to measure potassium is made of:
A. High-borosilicate glass membrane
B. Polyvinyl chloride dioctylphenyl phosphonate ion exchanger
C. Valinomycin gel
D. Calomel

Chemistry/Instrumentation and methodology/Ion selective/1

34. The response of a sodium electrode to a 10-fold increase in sodium concentration should be:
A. A 10-fold drop in potential
B. An increase in potential of approximately 60 mV
C. An increase in potential of approximately 10 mV
D. A decrease in potential of approximately 10 mV

Chemistry/Instrumentation and methodology/Ion selective/2

35. Which of the electrodes below is a current-producing (amperometric) rather than a voltage-producing (potentiometric) electrode?
A. Clark electrode
B. Severinghaus electrode
C. pH electrode
D. Ionized calcium electrode

Chemistry/Instrumentation and methodology/Amperometry/1

36. Which of the following would cause a "response" error from an ISE for sodium when measuring serum but not the calibrator?
A. Interference from other electrolytes
B. Protein coating the ion-selective membrane
C. An over-range in sodium concentration
D. Protein binding to sodium ions

Chemistry/Instrumentation and methodology/Ion selective/2

37. In polarography, the voltage needed to cause depolarization of the cathode is called the:
A. Half-wave potential
B. Isopotential point
C. Decomposition potential
D. Polarization potential

Instrumentation and methodology/Polarography/1

38. Persistent noise from an ISE is *most* often caused by:
A. Contamination of the sample
B. Blocked junction at the salt bridge
C. Over-range from high concentration
D. Improper calibration

Chemistry/Instrumentation and methodology/Ion selective/1

Answers to Questions 33–38

33. C The ion-selective membrane used to measure potassium is made of valinomycin gel. Valinomycin is an antibiotic with a highly selective reversible-binding affinity for potassium ions.

34. B The Nernst equation predicts an increase of approximately 60 mV per 10-fold increase in sodium activity. For sodium:

$$E = E° + RT/nF \times 2.3 \log_{10}[Na^+]$$
$$RT/nF \times 2.3 = 60 \text{ mV at } 37°C$$

Therefore:

$$E = E° + 60 \text{ mV} \times \log_{10}[Na^+]$$

If sodium concentration is 10 mmol/L, then:

$$E = E° + 60 \text{ mV} \times \log_{10}[10] = E° + 60 \text{ mV}$$

If sodium concentration increases from 10 mmol/L to 100 mmol/L, then:

$$E = E° + 60 \text{ mV} \times \log_{10}[100]$$
$$= E° + 60 \text{ mV} \times 2$$
$$= E° + 120 \text{ mV}$$

35. A The Clark electrode is current producing (amperometric) and is composed of two half-cells that generate current, not voltage. It is used to measure partial pressure of oxygen (Po_2) and is based on an amperometric method called *polarography.*

36. B Ion-selective analyzers use a microprocessor to monitor electrode response, slope, drift, and noise. When an electrode gives an acceptable response time when measuring an aqueous calibrator, but not when measuring serum, the cause is often protein buildup on the membrane.

37. C In polarography, the decomposition potential is the difference in the electrode potential between the cell's cathode and anode.

38. B Electrode noise from an ISE most often results from an unstable junction potential. Most reference electrodes contain a high concentration of the potassium chloride (KCl) internal solution used to produce reference potential. This forms a salt bridge with the measuring half-cell by contacting sample but is kept from equilibrating via a barrier, called a *junction.* When this junction becomes blocked by salt crystals, the reference potential will be unstable, resulting in fluctuation in the analyzer readout.

39. Which element is reduced at the cathode of a Clark polarographic electrode?
A. Silver
B. Oxygen
C. Chloride
D. Potassium

Chemistry/Instrumentation and methodology/ Polarography/1

40. Which of the following statements accurately characterizes the coulometric titration of chloride?
A. The indicator electrodes generate voltage
B. Constant current must be present across the generator electrodes
C. Silver ions are formed at the generator cathode
D. Chloride concentration is inversely proportional to titration time

Chemistry/Instrumentation and methodology/ Coulometry/1

41. In the coulometric chloride titration:
A. Acetic acid in the titrating solution furnishes the counter ion for reduction
B. The endpoint is detected by amperometry
C. The titrating reagent contains a phosphate buffer to keep pH constant
D. Nitric acid (HNO_3) is used to lower the solubility of AgCl

Chemistry/Instrumentation and methodology/ Coulometry/1

42. Which of the following compounds can interfere with the coulometric chloride assay?
A. Bromide
B. Ascorbate
C. Acetoacetate
D. Nitrate

Chemistry/Instrumentation and methodology/ Coulometry/1

43. Which of the following compounds contributes to the osmolality of plasma?
A. Cholesterol
B. Protein
C. Drug metabolites
D. Triglyceride

Chemistry/Instrumentation and methodology/ Osmolality/1

44. One mole per kilogram water (H_2O) of any solute will cause which of the following?
A. Lower the freezing point by 1.86°C
B. Raise vapor pressure by 0.3 mm Hg
C. Lower the boiling point by 0.52°C
D. Lower osmotic pressure by 22.4 atm

Chemistry/Instrumentation and methodology/ Osmolality/1

Answers to Questions 39–44

39. B The Clark electrode is designed to measure oxygen. O_2 diffuses through a gas-permeable membrane covering the electrode and is reduced at the platinum cathode. Electrons are supplied by the anode, which is made of silver.

40. B In the coulometric titration of chloride, charge or titration time is directly proportional to chloride concentration as long as the rate of oxidation remains constant at the generator. Charge in the form of silver ions is generated by oxidation of silver wire at the generator anode. Silver ions react with chloride ions, forming insoluble silver chloride (AgCl).

41. B The principle of coulometric titration with amperometric detection is found in the chloride titration. Reduction of Ag^+ back to Ag^0 generates the current, which signals the endpoint. Acetic acid lowers the solubility of AgCl, preventing dissociation back to Ag^+. Gelatin or polyvinyl alcohol is needed to prevent pitting of the generator anode. The titrating reagent contains HNO_3, acetic acid, H_2O, and either gelatin or polyvinyl alcohol.

42. A Chloride assays based on either coulometric or chemical titration are subject to positive interference from other anions and electronegative radicals that may be titrated instead of chloride ions. These include other halogens, such as bromide, cyanide, and cysteine.

43. C Osmolality is the concentration (in moles [mol]) of dissolved solute per kilogram solvent. Drug metabolites, in their dissociated salt form, contribute 1 Osm/mol of each dissociated ion or radical. Proteins and lipids are not in solution, and do not contribute to osmolality.

44. A Both freezing point and vapor pressure are lowered by increasing solute concentration. Boiling point and osmotic pressure are raised by increasing solute concentrations, where the solute concentration of a solution opposes a change in its physical state and lowers the concentration of H_2O molecules.

45. What component of a freezing point osmometer measures the sample temperature?
A. Thermistor
B. Thermocouple
C. Capacitor
D. Electrode

Chemistry/Instrumentation and methodology/1

46. What type of measuring circuit is used in a freezing point osmometer?
A. Electrometer
B. Potentiometer
C. Wheatstone bridge
D. Thermal conductivity bridge

Chemistry/Instrumentation and methodology/ Osmolality/1

47. In peroxidase-coupled glucose methods, which reagent complexes with the chromogen?
A. Nitroprusside
B. Phenol
C. Tartrate
D. Hydroxide

Chemistry/Instrumentation and methodology/1

48. Point-of-care tests (POCTs) for whole blood glucose monitoring are based mainly on the use of:
A. Glucose oxidase as the enzyme
B. Amperometry detection
C. Immunochromatography
D. Peroxidase coupling reactions

Chemistry/Instrumentation and methodology/POCT/1

49. The method for measuring iron or lead by plating the metal and then oxidizing it is called:
A. Polarography
B. Coulometry
C. Anodic stripping voltammetry
D. Amperometry

Chemistry/Instrumentation and methodology/ Voltammetry/1

50. The term *isocratic* is used in HPLC to mean that the:
A. Mobile phase is at constant temperature
B. Stationary phase is equilibrated with the mobile phase
C. Mobile phase consists of a constant solvent composition
D. Flow rate of the mobile phase is regulated

Chemistry/Instrumentation and methodology/ Chromatography/1

51. The term *reverse phase* is used in HPLC to indicate that the mobile phase is:
A. More polar than the stationary phase
B. Liquid and the stationary phase is solid
C. Organic and the stationary phase is aqueous
D. A stronger solvent than the stationary phase

Chemistry/Instrumentation and methodology/ Chromatography/1

Answers to Questions 45–51

45. A A thermistor is a temperature-sensitive resistor. The resistance to current flow increases as temperature falls. The temperature at which a solution freezes can be determined by measuring the resistance of the thermistor, where resistance is directly proportional to the osmolality of the sample.

46. C The resistance of the thermistor is measured using a network of resistors called a *Wheatstone bridge.*

47. B The coupling step in the Trinder glucose oxidase method uses peroxidase to catalyze the oxidation of a dye by H_2O_2. Dyes, such as 4-aminophenozone or 4-aminoantipyrine, are coupled to phenol to form a quinoneimine dye that is red and is measured at about 500 nm.

48. B All POCT devices for monitoring blood glucose use either glucose dehydrogenase (GDH) or glucose oxidase and are amperometric.

49. C Anodic stripping voltammetry is used to measure lead. The cation of the metal is plated onto a mercury cathode by applying a negative charge. The voltage of this electrode is reversed until the plated metal is oxidized back to a cation. The current produced by oxidation of the metal is proportional to concentration.

50. C An isocratic separation used in HPLC uses a single mobile phase of constant composition, pH, and polarity, and requires a single pump.

51. A In reverse-phase HPLC, the separation takes place using a nonpolar sorbent (stationary phase), such as octadecylsilane (C18). Solutes that are nonpolar are retained longer compared with polar solutes.

52. What is the primary means of solute separation in HPLC using a C18 (octadecylsilane) column?
A. Anion exchange
B. Size exclusion
C. Partitioning
D. Cation exchange

Chemistry/Instrumentation and methodology/Chromatography/1

53. The *most* commonly used detector for clinical gas–liquid chromatography (GLC) is based on:
A. Ultraviolet (UV) light absorbance at 254 nm
B. Flame ionization
C. Refractive index
D. Thermal conductance

Chemistry/Instrumentation and methodology/Chromatography/1

54. What type of detector is used in HPLC with electrochemical detection (ECD)?
A. Calomel electrode
B. Conductivity electrode
C. Glassy carbon electrode
D. Polarographic electrode

Chemistry/Instrumentation and methodology/Chromatography/1

55. In gas chromatography (GC), the elution order of volatiles is usually based on the:
A. Boiling point
B. Molecular size
C. Carbon content
D. Polarity

Chemistry/Instrumentation and methodology/Chromatography/1

56. Select the chemical that is used in *most* HPLC procedures to decrease solvent polarity.
A. Hexane
B. Nonane
C. Chloroform
D. Acetonitrile

Chemistry/Instrumentation and methodology/Chromatography/1

57. In TLC, the distance the solute migrates divided by the distance the solvent migrates is the:
A. *tR*
B. K_d
C. *Rf*
D. *pK*

Chemistry/Instrumentation and methodology/Chromatography/1

58. Which reagent is used in GC to extract alkaline drugs, such as cocaine metabolites, from urine?
A. Acid and sodium chloride
B. Alkali and organic solvent
C. Chloroform and sodium acetate
D. Neutral solution of ethyl acetate

Chemistry/Instrumentation and methodology/Chromatography/1

Answers to Questions 52–58

52. C In reverse-phase HPLC using C18, the relative solubility between the mobile phase and stationary phase depends on solvent polarity, pH, and ionic strength. The polarity of the compound determines which phase the compound is more attracted to, partitioning between the mobile phase and the stationary phase.

53. B Volatile solutes can be detected in GLC using flame ionization where energy from a flame is used to excite the analytes as they elute from the column.

54. C HPLC with ECD uses a glassy carbon-measuring electrode and a silver–silver chloride reference. The analyte is oxidized or reduced by holding the glassy carbon electrode at a positive voltage (oxidization) or negative voltage (reduction). The resulting current flow is directly proportional to concentration.

55. A In gas chromatography (GC) the order of elution is dependent on the velocity of the analyte. Usually, the lower the boiling point of the compound, the greater the velocity or solubility in carrier gas.

56. D All of the compounds mentioned have nonpolar properties. Because most HPLC is reverse phase in which a polar solvent is used, acetonitrile is used because it is less toxic than chloroform. Hexane and nonane are too nonpolar.

57. C In TLC, *Rf* (retention factor) is the distance migrated by the solute divided by the distance migrated by the solvent. The *tR* refers to the retention time of the solute in HPLC or GC. The K_d is the partition coefficient and is a measure of the relative affinity of solutes for the stationary phase. The pK is the negative logarithm of K, the ionization constant and is a measure of ionization.

58. B Alkaline drugs, such as cocaine, amphetamine, and morphine, are extracted at alkaline pH. Ideally, the pH for extracting alkaline drugs into an organic solvent should be 2 pH units greater than the negative log of dissociation constant (pKa) of the drug.

59. What is the purpose of an internal standard in HPLC and GC methods?
- **A.** To compensate for variation in extraction and injection
- **B.** To correct for background absorbance
- **C.** To compensate for changes in flow rate
- **D.** To correct for coelution of solutes

Chemistry/Instrumentation and methodology/ Chromatography/1

60. What is the confirmatory method for measuring drugs of abuse?
- **A.** HPLC
- **B.** Enzyme-multiplied immunoassay technique (EMIT)
- **C.** Gas chromatography with mass spectroscopy (GC-MS)
- **D.** TLC

Chemistry/Instrumentation and methodology/ Chromatography/1

61. The fragments typically produced and analyzed in methods employing mass spectroscopy are:
- **A.** Of low molecular size ranging from 10 to 100 daltons
- **B.** Cations caused by electron loss or proton attachment
- **C.** Anions caused by bombarding the molecule with an electron source
- **D.** Neutral species formed after excited molecules form a stable resonance structure

Chemistry/Instrumentation and methodology/ Chromatography/1

62. What component is used in a GC-MS but *not* used in an LC-MS?
- **A.** Electron source
- **B.** Mass filter
- **C.** Detector
- **D.** Vacuum

Chemistry/Instrumentation and methodology/ Chromatography/1

63. What process is *most* often used in LC-MS to introduce the sample into the mass filter?
- **A.** Electrospray ionization (ESI)
- **B.** Chemical ionization
- **C.** Electron impact ionization
- **D.** Fast atom bombardment

Chemistry/Instrumentation and methodology/ Chromatography/1

64. In mass spectroscopy, the term *base peak* typically refers to:
- **A.** The peak with the lowest mass
- **B.** The peak with the most abundance
- **C.** A natural isotope of the molecular ion
- **D.** The first peak to reach the mass detector

Chemistry/Instrumentation and methodology/ Chromatography/1

65. Which of the following is the *most* useful method when screening for errors of amino acid and organic acid metabolism?
- **A.** Two-dimensional TLC
- **B.** GC
- **C.** ESI tandem mass spectroscopy (MS/MS)
- **D.** Inductively coupled plasma mass spectroscopy (ICP-MS)

Chemistry/Instrumentation and methodology/ Chromatography/1

Answers to Questions 59–65

59. A The purpose of an internal standard in HPLC and GC methodology reduces error caused by variation in extraction recovery and injection volume.

60. C GC-MS determines the mass spectrum of the compounds eluting from the analytic column. Each substance has a unique and characteristic spectrum of mass fragments. This spectrum is compared with spectra in a library of standards to determine the percent match. A match of greater than 95% is considered confirmatory.

61. B In most MS applications, cations of the molecule are measured. Cations can be formed by electron bombardment (electron ionization).

62. A Most GC-MS instruments utilize electron ionization. Electrons are produced by applying 70 electron volts to a filament of tungsten or rhenium under vacuum. The electrons collide with the neutral molecules coming from the GC, splitting them into fragments.

63. A In LC-MS, the sample is converted into a gaseous state by ESI before it enters the mass filter.

64. B In mass spectrometry, the base peak is typically the "molecular ion" or parent ion. It is the most abundant and most stable ion and gives the best sensitivity for quantitative analysis.

65. C ESI allows a small alcohol-extracted whole blood sample to be analyzed by two mass spectrometers without prior separation by LC or GC. Disorders of both organic and fatty acid metabolism are identified by the specific pattern of acylcarnitine ions produced.

66. In MS/MS, the first mass filter performs the same function as:
- **A.** The ion source
- **B.** The chromatography column
- **C.** Extraction
- **D.** The vacuum system

Chemistry/Instrumentation and methodology/Mass spectrometry/1

67. A GC-MS analysis using nitrogen as the carrier gas shows an extensively noisy baseline. A sample of the solvent (ethyl acetate) used for the extraction procedure was injected and showed the same noise. Results of an Autotune test showed the appearance of a base peak at 16 with two smaller peaks at 17 and 18. These results indicate that:
- **A.** The solvent is contaminated
- **B.** The carrier gas is contaminated
- **C.** There is electrical noise in the detector
- **D.** The ion source is dirty

Chemistry/Instrumentation and methodology/Chromatography/3

68. Why is vacuum necessary in the mass filter of a GC-MS?
- **A.** Ionization does not occur at atmospheric pressure
- **B.** It prevents collision between fragments
- **C.** It removes electrons from the ion source
- **D.** It prevents contamination

Chemistry/Instrumentation and methodology/Chromatography/1

69. Which statement about iron methods is correct?
- **A.** Interference from Hgb can be corrected by a serum blank
- **B.** Colorimetric methods measure binding of Fe^{2+} to a ligand, such as ferrozine
- **C.** Atomic absorption is the method of choice for measurement of serum iron
- **D.** Serum iron can be measured by potentiometry

Chemistry/Instrumentation and methodology/2

70. Which of the following statements regarding the total iron-binding capacity (TIBC) assay is correct?
- **A.** All TIBC methods require addition of excess iron to saturate transferrin
- **B.** All methods require the removal of unbound iron
- **C.** Measurement of TIBC is specific for transferrin-bound iron
- **D.** The chromogen used must be different from the one used for measuring serum iron

Chemistry/Instrumentation and methodology/2

71. When calibrating a pH meter, unstable readings occur for both pH 7.00 and 4.00 calibrators, although both can be set to within 0.1 pH unit. Select the *most* appropriate course of action.
- **A.** Measure the pH of the sample and report to the nearest 0.1 pH
- **B.** Replace both calibrators with unopened buffers and recalibrate
- **C.** Examine the reference electrode junction for salt crystals
- **D.** Move the electrodes to another pH meter and calibrate

Chemistry/Instrumentation and methodology/pH/2

Answers to Questions 66–71

66. B A tandem mass spectrometer (MS/MS) uses two or more mass filters in sequence. The first filter functions as an ion trap to select an ion of interest, similar to a chromatography column separating ionic and nonionic samples.

67. B All of these situations are sources of baseline noise in GC-MS. However, the peak at 16 indicates the presence of O_2 in the carrier gas. O_2 in the atmosphere also contains small quantities of two isotopes with molecular weights of 17 and 18 because of the presence of one and two extra neutrons, respectively.

68. B Vacuum is needed in the mass filter of GC-MS instruments to prevent random collisions between ions that would alter their trajectory or time of flight. The vacuum prevents collision between the carrier gas molecules and the ions.

69. B Most methods use HCl to deconjugate Fe^{3+} from transferrin followed by reduction to Fe^{2+}. This reacts with a neutral ligand, such as ferrozine, tripyridyltriazine (TPTZ), or bathophenanthroline to give a blue complex. Atomic absorption is not the method of choice for serum iron because matrix error and variation of iron recovered by extraction causes bias and poor precision. Hemolysis must be avoided because red blood cells (RBCs), compared with plasma, contain a much higher concentration of iron.

70. A All TIBC methods require addition of excess iron to saturate transferrin. Excess iron is removed by ion exchange or alumina gel columns or precipitation with magnesium carbonate ($MgCO_3$) and the bound iron is measured by the same procedure as is used for serum iron.

71. C Noise in pH measurements often results from a blocked junction between the reservoir of the reference electrode and the test solution. This occurs when salt crystals collect at the junction or when KCl concentration in the reservoir increases because of evaporation of water.

72. A method calls for extracting an acidic drug from urine with an anion exchange column. The pK_a of the drug is 6.5. Extraction is enhanced by adjusting the sample pH to:
A. 8.5
B. 6.5
C. 5.5
D. 4.5
Chemistry/Instrumentation and methodology/pH/3

73. Which reagent is used in the Jendrassik-Grof method to solubilize unconjugated bilirubin?
A. 50% methanol
B. *n*-Butanol
C. Caffeine
D. Acetic acid
Chemistry/Instrumentation and methodology/1

74. Which statement about colorimetric bilirubin methods is true?
A. Direct bilirubin must react with diazo reagent under alkaline conditions
B. Most methods are based upon reaction with diazotized sulfanilic acid
C. Ascorbic acid can be used to eliminate interference caused by Hgb
D. The color of the azobilirubin product is independent of pH
Chemistry/Bilirubin analytical methods/2

75. Which statement regarding the measurement of bilirubin by the Jendrassik-Grof method is correct?
A. The same diluent is used for both total and direct assays to minimize differences in reactivity
B. Positive interference by Hgb is prevented by the addition of HCl after the diazo reaction
C. The color of the azobilirubin product is intensified by the addition of ascorbic acid
D. Fehling reagent is added after the diazo reaction to reduce optical interference by Hgb
Chemistry/Instrumentation and methodology/2

76. After staining a silica gel plate to determine the lecithin:sphingomyelin (L/S) ratio, the medical laboratory scientist notes that the lipid standards both migrated 1 cm faster than usual. What is the *best* course of action?
A. Repeat the separation on a new silica gel plate
B. Check the pH of the developing solvent
C. Prepare fresh developing solvent and repeat the assay
D. Reduce solvent migration time for all subsequent runs
Chemistry/Instrumentation and methodology/3

Answers to Questions 72–76

72. A Extraction of a negatively charged drug onto an anion exchange (positively charged) column is optimal when greater than 99% of the drug is in the form of anion. The extraction pH should be 2 pH units above the pK_a of an acidic drug. When pH = pK_a, the drug will be 50% ionized, and when pH is 2 units higher than the pK_a, almost all the drug is anionic.

73. C A polarity modifier is required to make unconjugated bilirubin soluble in diazo reagent. Caffeine is used in the Jendrassik-Grof method. The Malloy-Evelyn method used 50% methanol to reduce the polarity of the diazo reagent.

74. B Unconjugated bilirubin is poorly soluble in acid, and therefore, direct bilirubin is assayed using diazotized sulfanilic acid diluted in weak HCl. The direct diazo reaction should be measured after no longer than 3 minutes to prevent reaction of unconjugated bilirubin, or the diazo group can be reduced using ascorbate or hydroxylamine, preventing any further reaction.

75. D After addition of diazotized sulfanilic acid and incubation, the diazo group is reduced by ascorbic acid, and the Fehling reagent is added to alkalinize the diluent. The Jendrassik-Grof method uses HCl as the diluent for the measurement of direct bilirubin because unconjugated bilirubin is poorly soluble at low pH. At an alkaline pH, the azobilirubin products change from pink to blue, shifting the absorbance maximum to 600 nm where Hgb does not contribute significantly to absorbance.

76. C Higher retention factor (*Rf*) values indicate greater solubility of lipids in the developing solvent. This may be caused by evaporation of H_2O, lowering the polarity of the solvent.

77. The following chart compares the monthly total bilirubin mean and coefficient of variation (CV) of Laboratory A to the monthly mean and CV of Laboratory B, which uses the same control materials, analyzer, and method:

	Level 1 Control		Level 2 Control	
	Mean	CV	Mean	CV
Lab A	1.1 mg/dL	2.1%	6.7 mg/dL	3.2%
Lab B	1.4 mg/dL	2.2%	7.0 mg/dL	3.6%

Both laboratories performed controls at the beginning of each shift using commercially prepared liquid quality control (QC) sera stored at –20°C. Which of the following conditions would explain these differences?

A. Improper handling of the control material by Laboratory A resulted in loss of bilirubin because of photodegradation
B. The laboratories used a different source of bilirubin calibrator
C. Laboratory B obtained higher results because its precision was poorer
D. Carryover from another reagent falsely elevated the results of Laboratory B

Chemistry/Instrumentation and methodology/3

78. After installing a new analyzer and reviewing the results of patients for 1 month, the lead laboratory scientist notices a greater frequency of patients with abnormally high triglyceride results. Analysis of all chemistry profiles run the next day indicated that triglyceride results are abnormal whenever the test is run immediately after any sample that is measured for lipase. These observations point to which type of error?

A. Specificity of the triglyceride reagents
B. Precision in pipetting of lipemic samples
C. Bias caused by sequence of analysis
D. Reagent carryover

Chemistry/Instrumentation and methodology/3

Answers to Questions 77–78

77. B Interlaboratory variation in bilirubin results is often caused by differences in the assigned value of the calibrator used. Bilirubin calibrators are either serum-based materials that have been reference assayed or unconjugated bilirubin stabilized by addition of alkali and albumin. Calibrator differences result in bias and should be suspected when the laboratory's mean differs significantly from the peer group's mean. The bias in this example is caused by a constant error, rather than a proportional error. Photodegradation generally results in a greater loss of bilirubin at higher concentration and also contributes to random error.

78. D Carryover errors are usually attributed to interference caused by a sample with a very high concentration of analyte preceding a normal sample. However, reagent carryover may also occur on automated systems that use common reagent delivery lines or reusable cuvettes.

79. The digoxin level for a stable patient with a normal ECG result was reported as 7.4 ng/mL (upper reference limit [URL] 2.6 ng/mL) by using a particle-enhanced immunoturbidimetric inhibition method. Renal function test results were normal, and the patient was not taking any other medications. The assay was repeated, and the results were the same. The sample was frozen and sent to a reference laboratory for confirmation. The result was 1.6 ng/mL measured by a competitive chemiluminescent procedure. Which of the following *best* explains the discrepancy in results?

A. The immunoturbidimetric inhibition method was performed improperly
B. Digoxin was lower by the chemiluminescent method because it is less sensitive
C. An interfering substance was present that cross-reacted with the antibody in the immunoturbidimetric inhibition assay
D. Freezing the specimen caused lower results by converting the digoxin to an inactive metabolite

Chemistry/Instrumentation and methodology/3

Answer to Question 79

79. C An error was suspected because there was a discrepancy between the test result and the patient's clinical status. Some substances, called *digoxin-like immunologic factors* (DLIFs) can cross-react with the antibodies used to measure digoxin. The extent of interference varies with the source of antidigoxin used.

Na	K	Cl	HCO_3	BUN	Glucose	Creatinine	Uric Acid
140 mmol/L	3.6 mmol/L	100 mmol/L	28 mmol/L	130 mg/dL	110 mg/dL	1.2 mg/dL	4.8 mg/dL
148 mmol/L	4.2 mmol/L	110 mmol/L	24 mmol/L	135 mg/dL	86 mg/dL	0.8 mg/dL	3.9 mg/dL
138 mmol/L	4.0 mmol/L	105 mmol/L	22 mmol/L	142 mg/dL	190 mg/dL	1.0 mg/dL	4.6 mg/dL

80. The results shown in the preceding table are obtained from three consecutive serum samples using an automated random-access analyzer that samples directly from a bar-coded tube. Calibration and QC performed at the start of the shift are within the acceptable range, and no error codes are reported by the analyzer for any tests on the three samples. Upon results verification, what is the *most* appropriate course of action?

A. Report the results, and proceed with other tests because no analytical problems have been noted
B. Repeat the controls before continuing with further testing, but report the results
C. Check sample identification prior to reporting
D. Do not report blood urea nitrogen (BUN) results for these patients or continue BUN testing

Chemistry/Instrumentation and methodology/3

Answer to Question 80

80. D In three consecutive patients, BUN is found to be elevated five- to 10-fold in the absence of any other laboratory evidence of renal disease. The BUN results must be caused by a systematic error and should not be reported. Further testing for BUN should be withheld until the analytical components of the BUN assay are completely evaluated and the cause of these results are identified and corrected. The glucose results show conclusively that the samples are not from the same patient.

6.2

Blood Gases, pH, Electrolytes, and Vitamins

1. Which of the following represents the Henderson-Hasselbalch equation as applied to blood pH?
A. $pH = 6.1 + \log HCO_3^-/Paco_2$
B. $pH = 6.1 + \log HCO_3^-/(0.03 \times Paco_2)$
C. $pH = 6.1 + \log Dco_2/HCO_3^-$
D. $pH = 6.1 + \log (0.03 \times Paco_2)/HCO_3^-$
Chemistry/pH/1

2. What is the blood pH when the partial pressure of carbon dioxide ($Paco_2$) is 60 mm Hg and the bicarbonate (HCO_3^-) concentration is 18 mmol/L?
A. 6.89
B. 7.00
C. 7.10
D. 7.30
Chemistry/pH/2

3. Which of the following *most closely* represents the reference range for arterial pH?
A. 7.35 to 7.45
B. 7.42 to 7.52
C. 7.38 to 7.68
D. 6.85 to 7.56
Chemistry/pH/1

4. What is the normal ratio of bicarbonate to dissolved carbon dioxide ($HCO_3^-:Dco_2$) in arterial blood?
A. 1:10
B. 10:1
C. 20:1
D. 30:1
Chemistry/Blood gases/1

5. What is the $Paco_2$ if the Dco_2 is 1.8 mmol/L?
A. 24 mm Hg
B. 35 mm Hg
C. 60 mm Hg
D. 72 mm Hg
Chemistry/Blood gases/2

6. In the Henderson-Hasselbalch expression $pH = 6.1 + \log HCO_3^-/Dco_2$, the 6.1 represents:
A. The combined hydration and dissociation constant for CO_2 in blood at 37°C
B. The solubility constant for CO_2 gas
C. The dissociation constant of H_2O
D. The ionization constant of $NaHCO_3$
Chemistry/Blood gases/1

Answers to Questions 1–6

1. B The Henderson-Hasselbalch equation describes the pH of a buffer comprising a weak acid and its salt. pH = pKa+ log salt/acid, where pKa is the negative logarithm of the dissociation constant of the acid. In this case, the salt is sodium bicarbonate ($NaHCO_3$) and the acid is the dissolved CO_2 (Dco_2), which is equal to 0.03 (mmol/L per mm Hg) × Pco_2. The pKa includes both the hydration and dissociation constant for dissolved CO_2 in blood, 6.1.

2. C Solve using the Henderson-Hasselbalch equation. $pH = pK' + \log HCO_3^-/(0.03 \times Pco_2)$, where pK′, the negative logarithm of the combined hydration and dissociation constants for dissolved CO_2 and carbonic acid, is 6.1, and the solubility coefficient for CO_2 gas is 0.03.

$$pH = 6.1 + \log 18/(0.03 \times 60) = 6.1 + \log 18/1.8$$
$$pH = 6.1 + \log 10. \text{ Because } \log 10 = 1, pH = 7.10$$

3. A The reference range for arterial blood pH is 7.35 to 7.45.

4. C The normal ratio of $HCO_3^-:Dco_2$ is 20:1. Acidosis results when this ratio is decreased and alkalosis when it is increased.

5. C Dissolved CO_2 is calculated from the measured Pco_2 × 0.0306, the solubility coefficient for CO_2 gas in blood at 37°C.

$$Dco_2 = Pco_2 \times 0.03$$

Therefore, $Pco_2 = Dco_2/0.03$.

$$Pco_2 = 1.8 \text{ mmol/L} \times 0.03 \text{ mmol/L per mm Hg}$$
$$= 60 \text{ mm Hg}$$

6. A The negative logarithm of K′ is the pK′, which is 6.103 in blood at 37°C.

7. Which of the following contributes the *most* to serum total CO_2 (Tco_2)?
A. $Paco_2$
B. Dco_2
C. HCO_3^-
D. H_2CO_3
Chemistry/Blood gases/1

8. In addition to $NaHCO_3$, what other substance contributes the *most* to the amount of base in blood?
A. Hgb concentration
B. Dissolved O_2 concentration
C. Inorganic phosphorus
D. Organic phosphate
Chemistry/Blood gases/1

9. Which of the following effects results from exposure of a normal arterial blood sample to room air?

A.	Po_2 increased	$Paco_2$ decreased	pH increased
B.	Po_2 decreased	$Paco_2$ increased	pH decreased
C.	Po_2 increased	$Paco_2$ decreased	pH decreased
D.	Po_2 decreased	$Paco_2$ decreased	pH decreased

Chemistry/Blood gases/3

10. Identify the formula for determining O_2 content.
A. O_2 content = % O_2 saturation/100 × Hgb g/dL × 1.39 mL/g + (0.0031 × Po_2)
B. O_2 content = Po_2 × 0.0306 mmol/L/mm
C. O_2 content = O_2 saturation × Hgb g/dL × 0.003 mL/g
D. O_2 content = O_2 capacity × 0.003 mL/g
Chemistry/Blood gases/1

11. Correction of pH for a patient with a body temperature of 38°C would require:
A. Subtraction of 0.015
B. Subtraction of 0.01%
C. Addition of 0.020
D. Subtraction of 0.020
Chemistry/pH/2

12. Select the anticoagulant of choice for blood gas studies.
A. Sodium citrate 3.2%
B. Lithium heparin
C. Sodium citrate 3.8%
D. Ammonium oxalate
Chemistry/Blood gases/1

Answers to Questions 7–12

7. C The total CO_2 is the sum of the Dco_2, H_2CO_3 (carbonic acid or hydrated CO_2), and bicarbonate (as mainly $NaHCO_3$). The serum total CO_2 is primarily equivalent to the bicarbonate concentration, HCO_3^-.

8. A The primary blood buffer bases preventing acidosis, in order of concentration, are bicarbonate, deoxyhemoglobin, albumin, and monohydrogen phosphate.

9. A The Po_2 of air at sea level (21% O_2) is about 150 mm Hg. The Pco_2 of air is only about 0.3 mm Hg. Consequently, blood releases CO_2 gas and gains O_2 when exposed to air. Loss of CO_2 shifts the equilibrium of the bicarbonate buffer system to the right, decreasing hydrogen ion (H^+) concentration and blood becomes more alkaline.

10. A Oxygen content is the sum of O_2 bound to Hgb and O_2 dissolved in the plasma. It is dependent on the Hgb concentration and the percentage of Hgb bound to O_2 (O_2 saturation). Each gram of Hgb binds 1.39 mL of O_2. The dissolved O_2 is determined from the solubility coefficient of O_2 (0.0031 mL per dL/mm Hg) and the Po_2.

$$O_2\ content = \%\ Sat/100 \times Hgb\ in\ g/dL \times 1.39\ mL/g + (0.031 \times Po_2)$$

11. A The pH decreases by 0.015 for each degree Celsius above 37°C. Because the blood gas analyzer measures pH at 37°C, the *in vivo* pH would be 0.015 pH units below the measured pH.

12. B Heparin is the only anticoagulant that does not alter the pH of blood.

13. What is the maximum recommended storage time and temperature for an arterial blood gas sample drawn in a plastic syringe?

	Storage Time	Temperature
A.	10 min	2°C–8°C
B.	20 min	2°C–8°C
C.	30 min	2°C–8°C
D.	30 min	22°C

Chemistry/Blood gases/1

14. A patient's blood gas results are as follows:

pH = 7.26 Dco_2= 2.0 mmol/L HCO_3^-= 29 mmol/L

These results would be classified as:

A. Metabolic acidosis
B. Metabolic alkalosis
C. Respiratory acidosis
D. Respiratory alkalosis

Chemistry/Blood gases/Acid–base status/3

15. A patient's blood gas results are:

pH = 7.50 $Paco_2$ = 55 mm Hg HCO_3^-= 40 mmol/L

These results indicate:

A. Respiratory acidosis
B. Metabolic alkalosis
C. Respiratory alkalosis
D. Metabolic acidosis

Chemistry/Blood gases/Acid–base status/3

16. Which set of results is consistent with uncompensated respiratory alkalosis?

A. pH 7.70 HCO_3^- 30 mmol/L Pco_2 25 mm Hg
B. pH 7.66 HCO_3^- 22 mmol/L Pco_2 20 mm Hg
C. pH 7.46 HCO_3^- 38 mmol/L Pco_2 55 mm Hg
D. pH 7.36 HCO_3^- 22 mmol/L Pco_2 38 mm Hg

Chemistry/Blood gases/Acid–base status/3

17. Which of the following will shift the O_2 dissociation curve to the left?

A. Anemia
B. Hyperthermia
C. Hypercapnia
D. Alkalosis

Chemistry/Blood gases/2

18. In which circumstance will the reporting of calculated O_2 saturation of Hgb based on Po_2, Pco_2, pH, temperature, and Hgb be in error?

A. Carbon monoxide (CO) poisoning
B. Diabetic ketoacidosis
C. Oxygen therapy
D. Assisted ventilation for respiratory failure

Chemistry/Blood gases/3

Answers to Questions 13–18

13. D Arterial blood gas samples collected in plastic syringes should be stored at room temperature because cooling the sample allows O_2 to enter the syringe. Storage time should be no more than 30 minutes because longer storage results in a significant drop in pH and Po_2 and increased Pco_2.

14. C To calculate the Pco_2, the formula $Pco_2 = Dco_2/0.03$ gives a value of ~66 mm Hg (normal 35–45 mm Hg). The cause of this acidosis is CO_2 retention (respiratory acidosis), and it is partially compensated for by renal retention of bicarbonate. Increased Pco_2 will increase H^+ concentration, causing acidosis.

15. B A pH above 7.45 corresponds with alkalosis. Both bicarbonate and $Paco_2$ are elevated. Increased bicarbonate (but not increased CO_2) results in alkalosis; therefore, the classification is metabolic alkalosis, partially compensated for by increased $Paco_2$.

16. B Respiratory alkalosis is caused by hyperventilation, inducing low Pco_2. Very often, in the early phase of an acute respiratory disturbance, the kidneys have not had time to compensate, and the bicarbonate is within normal limits. In option A, the bicarbonate is high and Pco_2 low; thus, both are contributing to alkalosis, and this would be classified as a combined acid–base disturbance. In answer C, the pH is almost normal, and both bicarbonate and Pco_2 are increased. This can occur in the early stage of a metabolic acid–base disturbance when full respiratory compensation occurs or in a combined acid–base disorder. In answer D, both bicarbonate and Pco_2 are within normal limits (22–26 mmol/L, 35–45 mm Hg, respectively), as is the pH.

17. D A left shift in the oxyhemoglobin dissociation curve signifies an increase in the affinity of Hgb for O_2. This occurs in alkalosis, hypothermia, and in those hemoglobinopathies, such as Hgb Chesapeake, which increase the binding of O_2 to heme.

18. A Carbon monoxide (CO) has about 200 times the affinity as O_2 for Hgb and will displace O_2 from Hgb at concentrations that have no significant effect on the Pao_2. Consequently, calculated O_2 saturation will be erroneously high.

19. Which condition results in metabolic acidosis with severe hypokalemia and chronic alkaline urine?
A. Diabetic ketoacidosis
B. Phenformin-induced acidosis
C. Renal tubular acidosis
D. Acidosis caused by starvation
Chemistry/Blood gases/Acid–base status/2

20. Which of the following mechanisms is responsible for metabolic acidosis?
A. Bicarbonate deficiency
B. Excessive retention of dissolved CO_2
C. Accumulation of volatile acids
D. Hyperaldosteronism
Chemistry/Blood gases/Acid–base status/1

21. Which of the following is the primary mechanism of compensation for metabolic acidosis?
A. Hyperventilation
B. Release of epinephrine
C. Aldosterone release
D. Bicarbonate excretion
Chemistry/Blood gases/Acid–base status/2

22. Which condition is associated with *respiratory* (rather than metabolic) alkalosis?
A. Anxiety
B. Hypovolemia
C. Hyperaldosteronism
D. Hypoparathyroidism
Chemistry/Blood gases/Acid–base status/2

23. Which of the following conditions is associated with both metabolic and respiratory alkalosis?
A. Hyperchloremia
B. Hypernatremia
C. Hyperphosphatemia
D. Hypokalemia
Chemistry/Blood gases/Acid–base status/2

24. Which of the following conditions is classified as normochloremic acidosis?
A. Diabetic ketoacidosis
B. Chronic pulmonary obstruction
C. Uremic acidosis
D. Diarrhea
Chemistry/Blood gases/Acid–base status/2

25. Which Pco_2 value would be seen in maximally compensated metabolic acidosis?
A. 15 mm Hg
B. 30 mm Hg
C. 40 mm Hg
D. 60 mm Hg
Chemistry/Blood gases/Acid–base status/3

Answers to Questions 19–25

19. C Metabolic acidosis can be caused by any condition that lowers bicarbonate. In renal tubular acidosis (RTA), an intrinsic defect in the tubules prevents bicarbonate reabsorption. This causes alkaline instead of acidic urine.

20. A Metabolic acidosis is caused by bicarbonate deficiency and metabolic alkalosis by bicarbonate excess. Renal excretion of bicarbonate as potassium bicarbonate ($KHCO_3$) results in metabolic acidosis.

21. A In metabolic acidosis, the respiratory center is stimulated by chemoreceptors in the carotid sinus, causing hyperventilation, an immediate compensatory mechanism. This results in increased release of CO_2.

22. A Respiratory alkalosis is caused by hyperventilation, which leads to decreased Pco_2. Anxiety is a common cause of respiratory alkalosis. Hypovolemia increases the relative concentration of bicarbonate. Excess aldosterone increases net acid excretion by the kidneys. Low levels of parathyroid hormone (PTH) cause increased bicarbonate reabsorption, resulting in alkalosis.

23. D Hypokalemia is both a cause and result of alkalosis. In alkalosis, hydrogen ions may move from the cells into the extracellular fluid and potassium into the cells.

24. A In diabetic ketoacidosis (DKA), acetoacetate and other ketoacids replace bicarbonate. Bicarbonate deficit will lead to hyperchloremia unless the bicarbonate is replaced by an unmeasured anion. In DKA, the chloride remains normal or low, and there is an increased anion gap.

25. A In metabolic acidosis, hyperventilation increases the ratio of bicarbonate to dissolved CO_2. The extent of compensation is limited by the rate of both gas diffusion and diaphragm contraction. The lower limit is between 10 and 15 mm Hg Pco_2, which is the maximum compensatory effect.

26. A patient has the following arterial blood gas results:

pH = 7.56	Pco_2 = 25 mm Hg
Po_2 = 100 mm Hg	HCO_3^- = 22 mmol/L

These results are *most* likely the result of which condition?

A. Improper specimen collection
B. Prolonged storage
C. Hyperventilation
D. Hypokalemia

Chemistry/Blood gases/Acid–base status/3

27. Which of the following values is representative of a patient showing no signs of respiratory distress?

A. pH 7.41, $Paco_2$ 34 mm Hg, HCO_3^- 23 mmol/L
B. pH 7.46, $Paco_2$ 28 mm Hg, HCO_3^- 23 mmol/L
C. pH 7.47, $Paco_2$ 37 mm Hg, HCO_3^- 20 mmol/L
D. pH 7.34, $Paco_2$ 51 mm Hg, HCO_3^- 18 mmol/L

Chemistry/Blood gases/Acid–base status/3

28. What is the expected bicarbonate to dissolved carbon dioxide ratio at pH 7.4 for arterial blood?

A. 10:1
B. 15:1
C. 20:1
D. 25:1

Chemistry/Blood gases/1

29. The Henderson-Hasselbalch equation expressing the relationship of a weak acid, conjugate base, and pH is represented by this formula:

A. $pH = \log pK_a + A^-/HA$
B. $pH = pK_a + \log HA/A^-$
C. $pH = pK_a + \log A^-/HA$
D. $pH = \log pK_a + \log A^-/HA$

Chemistry/Blood gases/1

30. A patient breathing room air has the following arterial blood gas and electrolyte results:

pH = 7.54	Pco_2 = 18.5 mm Hg	Po_2 = 145 mm Hg
HCO_3^- = 18 mmol/L	Na = 135 mmol/L	K = 4.6 mmol/L
Cl = 98 mmol/L	Tco_2 = 20 mmol/L	

The *best* explanation for these results is:

A. Blood for electrolytes was drawn above an IV site
B. Serum sample was hemolyzed
C. Venous blood was sampled for arterial blood gases
D. Blood gas sample was exposed to air

Chemistry/Arterial blood gas/3

31. The following laboratory results are reported. Which result is *most* likely to be erroneous?

Arterial blood gases:	
pH =7.42	Po_2= 90 mm Hg
Pco_2 = 38.0 mm Hg	HCO_3^- = 24 mmol/L
Plasma electrolytes:	
Na = 135 mmol/L	Cl = 98 mmol/L
K = 4.6 mmol/L	Tco_2 = 33 mmol/L

A. pH
B. Na
C. K
D. Tco_2

Chemistry/Arterial blood gas/3

Answers to Questions 26–31

26. C The pH is alkaline (reference range 7.35–7.45) and this can be caused by either low Pco_2 or increased bicarbonate. This patient has a normal bicarbonate (reference range 22–26 mmol/L) and a low Pco_2 (reference range 35–45 mm Hg). Low Pco_2 is always caused by hyperventilation, and therefore, this is a case of uncompensated respiratory alkalosis.

27. A Recall the reference values for pH (7.35–7.45), $Paco_2$ (35–45 mm Hg), and HCO_3^- (22–26 mmol/L) to evaluate the set of values that would be expected under conditions in which no respiratory distress is present.

28. C When the ratio of HCO_3^-:Dco_2 is 20:1, the log of base/acid becomes 1.3. Substituting this in the Henderson-Hasselbalch equation and solving for pH gives pH = 6.1 + log 20; pH = 6.1 + 1.3 = 7.4. Acidosis results when this ratio is decreased and alkalosis when it is increased.

29. C The Henderson-Hasselbalch equation reflects the acid–base relationship in the formula $pH = pK_a + \log [A^-]/[HA]$ where A^- is the base (or proton acceptor), HA is the weak acid (or proton donor), and pK_a is the pH when there is equilibrium of protonated and unprotonated concentrations for the buffer system.

30. D A patient breathing room air cannot have an arterial Po_2 greater than 105 mm Hg because alveolar Po_2 is 110 mm Hg when breathing 20% O_2. Exposure to air caused loss of CO_2 gas and increased pH.

31. D The electrolytes are normal but the Tco_2 is increased significantly. The reference range for venous Tco_2 is 22 to 28 mmol/L. pH, Pco_2, and HCO_3^- are normal, and therefore agree.

32. Given the following serum electrolyte data, determine the anion gap:

Na = 132 mmol/L	K = 4.0 mmol/L
Cl = 90 mmol/L	HCO_3^- = 22 mmol/L

A. 12 mmol/L
B. 24 mmol/L
C. 64 mmol/L
D. Cannot be determined from the information provided

Chemistry/Electrolytes/Anion gap/3

33. Which of the following conditions will cause an increased anion gap?
A. Diarrhea
B. Hypoaldosteronism
C. Hyperkalemia
D. Renal failure

Chemistry/Electrolytes/Anion gap/1

34. Which of the following conditions is associated with an increase in ionized calcium (Ca_i) in blood?
A. Alkalosis
B. Hypoparathyroidism
C. Hyperalbuminemia
D. Malignancy

Chemistry/Electrolytes/Calcium/1

35. Which of the following laboratory results is consistent with primary hypoparathyroidism?
A. Low calcium; high inorganic phosphorus (P_i)
B. Low calcium; low P_i
C. High calcium; high P_i
D. High calcium; low P_i

Chemistry/Electrolytes/Calcium/2

36. Which of the following conditions is associated with hypophosphatemia?
A. Rickets
B. Multiple myeloma
C. Renal failure
D. Hypervitaminosis D

Chemistry/Electrolytes/Phosphate/2

37. Which of the following tests is consistently abnormal in osteoporosis?
A. High urinary calcium
B. High serum P_i
C. Low serum calcium
D. High urine or serum N-telopeptide (NTx) of type 1 collagen

Chemistry/Electrolytes/Calcium/2

38. Which of the following is a marker for bone formation?
A. Osteocalcin
B. Tartrate-resistant acid phosphatase (TRAP)
C. Urinary pyridinoline and deoxypyridinoline
D. Urinary C-telopeptid (CTx) e and NTx crosslinks

Chemistry/Electrolytes/Calcium/2

Answers to Questions 32–38

32. B The anion gap is defined as unmeasured anions minus unmeasured cations in the plasma or serum. It is calculated by subtracting the measured anions (bicarbonate and chloride) from the measured cations (sodium plus potassium, although some laboratories ignore the potassium). A normal anion gap is approximately 12 to 20 mmol/L (8–16 mmol/L when potassium is not included).

$$\text{Anion gap} = (Na + K) - (HCO_3 + Cl)$$
$$= (132 + 4) - (90 + 22) = 24 \text{ mmol/L}$$

33. D An increased anion gap occurs when there is production or retention of anions other than bicarbonate or chloride (measured anions). In renal failure, retention of phosphates and sulfates (as sodium salts) increases the anion gap.

34. D Increased Ca_i occurs in hyperparathyroidism, malignancy, and acidosis.

35. A Hypoparathyroidism with a PTH deficiency causes reduced resorption of calcium from bone, increased renal excretion of calcium, and decreased renal excretion of phosphorus.

36. A Rickets can result from dietary phosphate deficiency, vitamin D deficiency, or an inherited disorder of either vitamin D or phosphorus metabolism.

37. D Serum markers for osteoporosis include both N-telopeptide of type 1 collagen (NTx) and C-telopeptide of type 1 collagen (CTx). Commonly used markers for other bone diseases (e.g., serum or urinary calcium, inorganic phosphorus, total ALP, and vitamin D) are neither sensitive nor specific for osteoporosis. Calcium and phosphorus are usually within normal limits.

38. A Biochemical markers for osteoporosis are classified as either for bone formation or for resorption. Osteocalcin is a protein hormone that stimulates osteoblasts and increases bone mineralization.

39. What role do urinary CTx and NTx play in the management of osteoporosis?
A. Increased urinary excretion is diagnostic of early-stage disease
B. Increased levels indicate a low risk of developing osteoporosis
C. Decreased urinary excretion indicates a positive response to treatment
D. The rate of urinary excretion correlates with the stage of the disease
Chemistry/Electrolytes/Calcium/2

40. Which of the following conditions is associated with a decreased binding of calcium to protein, increasing the proportion of free calcium?
A. Acidosis
B. Hyperalbuminemia
C. Hypoparathyroidism
D. Renal dysfunction
Chemistry/Electrolytes/Calcium/2

41. Thyrocalcitonin, a thyroid hormone, affects serum calcium concentration by:
A. Increasing the amount of calcium absorbed from the gastrointestinal (GI) tract
B. Increasing calcium excretion in the urine
C. Blocking bone resorption of calcium
D. Decreasing phosphorus excretion in urine
Chemistry/Electrolytes/Calcium/2

42. What is the percentage of serum calcium that is ionized?
A. 30%
B. 45%
C. 60%
D. 80%
Chemistry/Electrolytes/Calcium/1

43. Which of the following conditions will cause erroneous Ca_i results? Assume that the samples are collected and stored anaerobically, kept at 4°C until measurement, and stored for no longer than 1 hour.
A. Slight hemolysis during venipuncture
B. Assay of whole blood collected in sodium oxalate
C. Analysis of serum in a barrier gel tube stored at 4°C until the clot has formed
D. Analysis of whole blood collected in sodium heparin
Chemistry/Electrolytes/Calcium/3

44. What role does vitamin D measurement play in the management of osteoporosis?
A. Vitamin D deficiency must be demonstrated to establish the diagnosis
B. Vitamin D is consistently elevated in osteoporosis
C. A vitamin D level within the correct reference range rules out osteoporosis
D. Vitamin D deficiency is a risk factor for developing osteoporosis
Chemistry/Electrolytes/Vitamin D/2

Answers to Questions 39–44

39. C Markers for both bone formation and resorption are used to monitor treatment for osteoporosis. Serum and urinary measurements of CTx and NTx and urinary deoxypyridinoline are used to monitor medications that inhibit bone resorption (e.g., bisphosphonates). CTx, NTx, and deoxypyridinoline decrease with successful treatment.

40. A Acidosis decreased the binding of calcium to albumin. PTH regulates calcium, and if PTH is low, calcium levels would be decreased, which in turn would cause a high level of calcium to be excreted (hypercalciuria).

41. C Thyrocalcitonin, a thyroid hormone, is an antagonist to PTH, and serves to block bone resorption of calcium through inhibiting the actions of PTH and vitamin D.

42. B Calcium exists in serum in three forms: protein bound, ionized, and complexed (as undissociated salts). Only Ca_i is physiologically active. Protein-bound Ca and Ca_i each account for approximately 45% of total calcium, and the remaining 10% is complexed.

43. B Blood collected with heparin and stored on ice no longer than 2 hours is the sample of choice for Ca_i. Citrate, oxalate, and EDTA must not be used because they chelate calcium. Serum may be used provided that the sample is iced, kept capped while clotting, and assayed within 2 hours; barrier gel tubes may be stored longer.

44. D Vitamin D assay is not used to diagnose osteoporosis. Vitamin D deficiency is a cause of secondary osteoporosis, and low levels of PTH, calcium, and estrogen are additional important risk factors. If one or more of these are abnormal, then bone resorption or remodeling may be abnormal, predisposing the individual to osteoporosis.

45. Which statement *best* describes testing recommendations for vitamin D?
- **A.** Vitamin D testing should be reserved only for individuals who demonstrate hypercalcemia of an undetermined cause
- **B.** Vitamin D testing should be specific for the $1,25(OH)D_3$ form
- **C.** Testing should be for total vitamin D when screening for deficiency
- **D.** Vitamin D testing should not be performed if the patient is receiving vitamin D supplementation

Chemistry/Electrolytes/Vitamin D/2

46. Which of the following is considered a water-soluble vitamin?
- **A.** Vitamin A
- **B.** Vitamin B_6
- **C.** Vitamin D
- **D.** Vitamin K

Chemistry/Vitamins/1

47. Which of the following is considered a fat-soluble vitamin?
- **A.** Thiamine
- **B.** Folic acid
- **C.** Cholecalciferol
- **D.** Riboflavin

Chemistry/Vitamins/1

48. The role of this vitamin is to protect the erythrocyte membrane from oxidative stress.
- **A.** Vitamin A
- **B.** Vitamin K
- **C.** Vitamin C
- **D.** Vitamin E

Chemistry/Vitamins/1

49. A biochemical profile routinely performed bimonthly on a patient receiving renal dialysis showed decreased serum calcium and decreased PTH levels. Such a laboratory result may be explained by which of the following circumstances?
- **A.** Malignancy
- **B.** Aluminum toxicity
- **C.** Hypervitaminosis D
- **D.** Acidosis

Chemistry/Electrolytes/Calcium/3

50. The effect of hyperparathyroidism with increased PTH may present with these changes:
- **A.** Decreased circulating serum calcium with increased serum phosphate
- **B.** Increased circulating serum calcium with increased serum phosphate
- **C.** Decreased circulating serum calcium with decreased serum phosphate
- **D.** Increased circulating serum calcium with decreased serum phosphate

Chemistry/Electrolytes/Phosphate/1

Answers to Questions 45–50

45. C The majority of circulating vitamin D is in the 25-hydroxylated form of D_2 and D_3, called 25(OH)D. The plasma 25(OH)D concentration is an expression of both dietary and endogenous vitamin D and is the most appropriate test for detecting nutritional vitamin D deficiency.

46. B Water-soluble vitamins include the B vitamins and vitamin C. Fat-soluble vitamins include vitamins A, D, E, and K.

47. C Cholecalciferol, or vitamin D_3, is a fat-soluble vitamin along with vitamins A, E, and K.The B vitamins thiamine (B_1), folic acid (B_9), and riboflavin (B_2) are water soluble.

48. D Vitamin E is a powerful antioxidant and protects the erythrocyte by strengthening cell membranes.

49. B Excess aluminum causes osteomalacia by inhibiting release of PTH. Malignancy, hypervitaminosis D, and acidosis are associated with high serum calcium. The finding of low PTH would not be expected with low serum calcium unless aluminum poisoning was present. Aluminum present in medications and dialysis bath fluid can cause aluminum toxicity in patients receiving dialysis.

50. D Excess PTH results in increased serum calcium with decreased serum phosphate, and an increased chloride/phosphate ratio.

51. A 2_{2s} QC error occurs for serum calcium by atomic absorption. Fresh standards prepared in 5% weight per volume (w/v) albumin are found to be linear, but repeating the controls with fresh material does not improve the QC results. Select the *most* likely cause of this problem.
A. Matrix effect caused by a viscosity difference between the standards and QC sera
B. Chemical interference caused incomplete atomization
C. Incomplete deconjugation of protein-bound calcium
D. Ionization interference caused by excessive heat
Chemistry/Electrolytes/Calcium/3

52. A physician asks the laboratory to use the serum from a clot tube left over from a chemistry profile run at 8 a.m. for a stat ionized calcium (Ca_i) at 11 a.m. What is the *best* course of action?
A. Perform the assay on the 8 a.m. sample
B. Perform the test only if the serum container was tightly capped
C. Perform the assay on the 8 a.m. sample only if it was refrigerated
D. Request a new sample
Chemistry/Electrolytes/Calcium/3

53. Which electrolyte measurement is least affected by hemolysis?
A. Potassium
B. Calcium
C. Inorganic phosphorus
D. Magnesium
Chemistry/Electrolytes/2

54. Which of the following conditions is associated with hypokalemia?
A. Addison disease
B. Hemolytic anemia
C. Digoxin intoxication
D. Alkalosis
Chemistry/Electrolytes/Potassium/1

55. Which of the following conditions is *most* likely to produce an elevated plasma potassium?
A. Hypoparathyroidism
B. Cushing syndrome
C. Diarrhea
D. Digitalis overdose
Chemistry/Electrolytes/Potassium/2

56. Which of the following values is the threshold critical value (alert or action level) for low plasma potassium?
A. 1.5 mmol/L
B. 2.0 mmol/L
C. 2.5 mmol/L
D. 3.5 mmol/L
Chemistry/Electrolytes/Potassium 1

Answers to Questions 51–56

51. B Poor recovery of calcium by atomic absorption is often caused by failure to break thermostable bonds between calcium and phosphate (a form of chemical interference). The use of 5% w/v albumin in the calibrator produces viscosity and protein-binding characteristics similar to those of plasma, helping to eliminate matrix interference.

52. D Request a new sample. Ca_i is pH dependent. After 3 hours, the Ca_i will be inaccurate, changing in response to a change in pH. Heparinized blood is preferred because it can be assayed immediately. Serum may be used, but the specimen must remain tightly capped while clotting and centrifuging and analyzed immediately thereafter.

53. B Of the choices, calcium is least affected by hemolysis. Potassium, phosphorus, and magnesium are the major intracellular ions, and even slight hemolysis will cause falsely elevated results.

54. D Alkalosis causes potassium to move from the extracellular fluid into the cells as H^+ moves from the cells into the extracellular fluid to compensate for alkalosis. Addison disease (adrenocortical insufficiency) results in low levels of adrenocorticosteroid hormones, including aldosterone and cortisol. Because these hormones promote reabsorption of sodium and secretion of potassium by the collecting tubules, patients with Addison disease display hyperkalemia and hyponatremia. Hemolytic anemia and digoxin intoxication cause release of intracellular potassium.

55. D Digitalis toxicity causes potassium to leave the cells and enter the extracellular fluid, resulting in hyperkalemia. Hypoparathyroidism indirectly causes hypokalemia by inducing alkalosis via increased renal retention of phosphate and bicarbonate. Cushing syndrome (adrenocortical hyperfunction) results in low potassium and elevated sodium. Diarrhea causes loss of sodium and potassium.

56. C The reference range for potassium is 3.6 to 5.4 mmol/L. However, values below 2.5 mmol/L require immediate intervention because below that level there is a grave risk of cardiac arrhythmia, which can lead to cardiac arrest.

57. Which electrolyte is *least* likely to be elevated in renal failure?
A. Potassium
B. Magnesium
C. Inorganic phosphorus
D. Sodium
Chemistry/Electrolytes/Potassium/2

58. Which of the following is the primary mechanism for vasopressin (antidiuretic hormone [ADH]) release?
A. Hypovolemia
B. Hyperosmolar plasma
C. Renin release
D. Reduced renal blood flow
Chemistry/Electrolytes/ADH/2

59. Which of the following conditions is associated with hypernatremia?
A. Diabetes insipidus
B. Hypoaldosteronism
C. Burns
D. Diarrhea
Chemistry/Electrolytes/Sodium/1

60. Which of the following values is the threshold critical value (alert or action level) for high plasma sodium?
A. 150 mmol/L
B. 160 mmol/L
C. 170 mmol/L
D. 180 mmol/L
Chemistry/Electrolytes/Sodium/1

61. Which of the following conditions is associated with total body sodium excess?
A. Renal failure
B. Hyperthyroidism
C. Hypoparathyroidism
D. Diabetic ketoacidosis
Chemistry/Electrolytes/Sodium/1

62. Which of the following conditions is associated with hyponatremia?
A. Diuretic therapy
B. Cushing syndrome
C. Diabetes insipidus
D. Nephrotic syndrome
Chemistry/Electrolytes/Sodium/1

63. Which of the following laboratory results is usually associated with cystic fibrosis?
A. Sweat chloride greater than 60 mmol/L
B. Elevated serum sodium and chloride
C. Elevated fecal trypsin activity
D. Low glucose
Chemistry/Electrolytes/Chloride/1

Answers to Questions 57–63

57. D Poor tubular reabsorption of sodium offsets reduced glomerular filtration. In renal disease, serum sodium is often normal, although total body sodium is increased owing to fluid and salt retention. Reduced glomerular filtration coupled with decreased tubular secretion causes accumulation of potassium, magnesium, and inorganic phosphorus.

58. B Vasopressin/ADH is released by the posterior pituitary in response to increased plasma osmolality.

59. A Diabetes insipidus results from failure to produce ADH. Because the collecting tubules are impermeable to water in the absence of ADH, severe hypovolemia and dehydration result. Hypovolemia stimulates aldosterone release, causing sodium reabsorption, which worsens the hypernatremia. Burns, hypoaldosteronism, diarrhea, and diuretic therapy are common causes of hyponatremia.

60. B The adult reference range for plasma sodium is approximately 135 to 145 mmol/L. Levels in excess of 160 mmol/L are associated with severe dehydration, hypovolemia, and circulatory and heart failure.

61. A When water is retained along with sodium, the result is total body sodium excess, rather than hypernatremia. Renal failure results in poor glomerular filtration and isosmotic equilibration of salt and water.

62. A Diuretics lower blood pressure by promoting water loss. This is accomplished by causing sodium loss from the proximal tubule and/or loop. Cushing syndrome causes hypernatremia by promoting sodium reabsorption in the collecting tubule in exchange for potassium. Diabetes insipidus and nephrotic syndrome promote hypernatremia by causing water loss.

63. A Cystic fibrosis causes obstruction of the exocrine glands, including the sweat glands, mucous glands, and pancreas. Sweat chloride more than 60 mmol/L confirms the clinical diagnosis. Serum sodium and chloride levels are low. Newborns with pancreatic involvement demonstrate fecal trypsin deficiency. Some people with the disease have insulin deficiency and elevated blood glucose.

64. When performing a sweat chloride collection, which of the following steps will result in analytical error?

A. Using unweighed gauze soaked in pilocarpine nitrate on the inner surface of the forearm to stimulate sweating
B. Collecting greater than 75 mg of sweat in 30 minutes
C. Leaving the preweighed gauze on the inside of the arm exposed to air during collection
D. Rinsing the collected sweat from the gauze pad using chloride titrating solution

Chemistry/Electrolytes/Chloride/3

65. Which formula provides an approximate plasma osmolality value?

A. Na + 2(Cl) + BUN + glucose
B. 2(Na) + 2(Cl) + glucose + urea
C. 2(Na) + (glucose/18) + (BUN/2.8)
D. Na + Cl + K + HCO_3^-

Chemistry/Electrolytes/Osmolality1

66. A serum osmolality measured in the emergency department (ED) is 326 mOsm/kg. Two hours later, chemistry results are:

Na = 135 mmol/L	BUN = 18 mg/dL
Glucose = 72 mg/dL	Measured osmolality = 318 mOsm/kg

What do these results suggest?

A. Laboratory error in electrolyte or glucose measurement
B. Drug or alcohol intoxication
C. Specimen misidentification
D. Successful rehydration of the patient

Chemistry/Electrolytes/Osmolality/3

67. A lipemic sample gives a sodium of 130 mmol/L on an analyzer that uses a 1:50 dilution of serum or plasma before introducing it to the ISE. The same sample gives a sodium of 142 mmol/L using a direct (undiluted) ISE. Assuming acceptable quality control, which of the following is the *most* appropriate course of action?

A. Report a sodium result of 136 mmol/L
B. Ultracentrifuge the sample and repeat by ISE
C. Dilute the sample 1:4 and repeat by ISE
D. Report a sodium result of 142 mmol/L

Chemistry/Electrolytes/ISE/3

Answers to Questions 64–67

64. C The sweat chloride procedure requires the application of pilocarpine to stimulate sweating, and the use of iontophoresis to bring the sweat to the surface. During the 30-minute collection of sweat, the gauze must be completely covered to prevent contamination and loss of sweat by evaporation.

65. C Calculated plasma osmolality is based on measurement of sodium, glucose, and urea. Because sodium associates with a counter ion, two times the sodium estimates the millimoles per liter of electrolytes. Some laboratories multiply by 1.86 instead of 2 to correct for undissociated salts. Dividing glucose by 18 converts from milligrams per deciliter to millimoles per liter. Dividing BUN by 2.8 converts from milligrams per deciliter BUN to millimoles per liter urea.

66. B In samples from ED patients, a significant osmolal gap usually results from alcohol or drug consumption. The difference in osmolality between the two samples is 8 mOsm/kg and can be explained by alcohol metabolism during the 2 hours between samples.

67. D Lipemic samples give lower results for sodium (pseudohyponatremia) when diluted prior to measurement because the H_2O phase is mostly diluent, and a significant component of the sample volume is displaced by lipid.

68. Laboratory results on a patient from the ED are:

Glucose = 1,100 mg/dL	Na = 155 mmol/L
K = 1.2 mmol/L	Cl = 115 mmol/L
Tco_2 = 3.0 mmol/L	

What is the *most* likely explanation of these results?

A. Sample drawn above an IV site
B. Metabolic acidosis with increased anion gap
C. Diabetic ketoacidosis
D. Laboratory error measuring electrolytes caused by hyperglycemia

Chemistry/Electrolytes/3

69. A patient has the following electrolyte results:

Na = 130 mmol/L	K = 4.8 mmol/L
Cl = 105 mmol/L	Tco_2 = 26 mmol/L

Assuming acceptable QC, select the *best* course of action.

A. Report the results
B. Check the albumin, total protein, calcium, phosphorus, and magnesium results; if normal, repeat the sodium test
C. Request a new sample
D. Recalibrate and repeat the potassium test

Chemistry/Electrolytes/3

70. A patient's biochemistry results are:

Na = 125 mmol/L	Cl = 106 mmol/L
K = 4.5 mmol/L	Tco_2 = 19 mmol/L
Cholesterol = 240 mg/dL	Triglyceride = 640 mg/dL
Glucose = 107 mg/dL	
Aspartate aminotransferase (AST) = 16 IU/L	
Alanine aminotransferase (ALT) 11 IU/L	
Amylase = 200 U/L	

Select the *most* likely cause of these results.

A. The sample is hemolyzed
B. Serum was not separated from cells in sufficient time
C. Lipemia is causing *in vitro* interference
D. The specimen is contaminated

Chemistry/Electrolytes/3

Answers to Questions 68–70

68. A These results are consistent with dilution of venous blood by the IV fluid containing 5% dextrose and normal saline. The IV fluid is free of potassium and HCO_3^-, accounting for the low level of these electrolytes (incompatible with life).

69. B The anion gap of this sample is less than 4 mmol/L. This may result from laboratory error, retention of an unmeasured cation (e.g., calcium), or low level of unmeasured anion, such as phosphorus or albumin. The sodium is inappropriately low for the chloride and HCO_3^- and should be repeated if no biochemical cause is apparent.

70. C The triglyceride level is about five times normal, causing the sample to be lipemic. This will cause pseudohyponatremia. Lipemia may cause a falsely high rate reaction when amylase is measured by using turbidimetry; however, the high amylase level may be associated with pancreatitis, which results in hyperlipidemia.

6.3

Carbohydrates, Hemoglobin, Iron, and Bilirubin

1. Which of the following biochemical processes is promoted by insulin?
A. Glycogenolysis
B. Gluconeogenesis
C. Lipolysis
D. Uptake of glucose by cells
Chemistry/Carbohydrates/1

2. Which of the following hormones promotes hyperglycemia?
A. Calcitonin
B. Growth hormone
C. Aldosterone
D. Renin
Chemistry/Carbohydrates/1

3. This hormone, from the delta cells of the pancreas, acts to increase circulating plasma glucose while inhibiting other endocrine hormones such as thyroid-stimulating hormone (TSH).
A. Insulin
B. Glucagon
C. Somatostatin
D. Growth hormone
Chemistry/Carbohydrates/2

4. The first step in glucose metabolism is the conversion of glucose to this, using ATP in a reaction catalyzed by hexokinase.
A. Glycogen
B. Glucose-6-phosphate
C. Pyruvate
D. Lactate
Chemistry/Carbohydrates/2

5. Which statement corresponds to the action of growth hormone (GH) on circulating glucose?
A. GH decreases lipolysis
B. GH increases glucose entry into cells
C. GH stimulates insulin
D. GH decreases glycolysis
Chemistry/Carbohydrates/2

Answers to Questions 1–5

1. D Insulin reduces blood glucose levels by increasing glucose uptake by cells. It promotes lipid and glycogen production, induces synthesis of glycolytic enzymes, and inhibits formation of glucose from pyruvate and Krebs cycle intermediates.

2. B Growth hormone (GH) promotes gluconeogenesis to increase glycemic levels. The other hormones are not directly involved in glucose homeostasis. Calcitonin opposes the action of PTH. Aldosterone is the primary mineralocorticoid hormone and stimulates sodium reabsorption and potassium secretion by the kidneys. Renin is released from the kidney as a result of ineffective arterial pressure and promotes activation of angiotensinogen and aldosterone secretion.

3. C The primary function of somatostatin is to regulate hormones and hormone secretions. Produced by the pancreas, it inhibits pancreatic hormones glucagon and insulin, and inhibits TSH and GH release from the pituitary gland.

4. B All three glycolytic pathways (Embden-Meyerhof pathway, aerobic pathway [TCA cycle], anaerobic pathway), include the first step of glucose conversion to glucose-6-phosphate (G6P) using ATP and catalyzed by hexokinase.

5. D The release of GH is stimulated by a decrease in circulating glucose and cortisol levels, and increases plasma glucose by preventing glucose entry into cells and decreasing glycolysis.

6. Which statement regarding sample collection and processing of a fasting blood glucose sample is true?

A. Fasting should be for at least 8 hours before the sample is collected
B. Blood can be allowed to clot at room temperature for up to 60 minutes before measuring
C. Heparin-barrier gel tubes interfere with enzymatic methods
D. Antiglycolytic agents, such as sodium fluoride, cause negative interference

Chemistry/Carbohydrates/1

7. Which of the following is characteristic of type 1 diabetes mellitus?

A. Requires an oral glucose tolerance test (OGTT) for diagnosis
B. Is the most common form of diabetes mellitus
C. Usually occurs after age 40 years
D. Requires insulin replacement to prevent ketosis

Chemistry/Carbohydrates/Disorders and disease/1

8. Which of the following is characteristic of type 2 diabetes mellitus?

A. Insulin levels are consistently low
B. Most cases require a 3-hour OGTT for diagnosis
C. Hyperglycemia is often controlled without insulin replacement
D. The condition is associated with unexplained weight loss

Chemistry/Carbohydrates/Disorders and disease/2

9. Which of the following results falls within the diagnostic criteria for diabetes mellitus?

A. Fasting plasma glucose of 120 mg/dL
B. 2-hour postprandial plasma glucose of 160 mg/dL
C. 2-hour plasma glucose of 180 mg/dL following a 75-g oral glucose challenge
D. Random plasma glucose of 250 mg/dL and presence of symptoms

Chemistry/Carbohydrates/Disorders and disease/2

10. Select the *most* appropriate adult reference range for fasting blood glucose.

A. 40–105 mg/dL (2.22–5.82 mmol/L)
B. 60–140 mg/dL (3.33–7.77 mmol/L)
C. 65–99 mg/dL (3.61–5.50 mmol/L)
D. 75–150 mg/dL (4.16–8.32 mmol/L)

Chemistry/Carbohydrates/1

Answers to Questions 6–10

6. A An 8-hour fast is required for a fasting blood glucose test. Water and most medications are permitted. Sodium fluoride, heparin, EDTA, citrate, and oxalate are acceptable for enzymatic methods. Samples collected in tubes without barrier gel should be stored no longer than 30 minutes at room temperature. Serum and plasma in tubes with barrier gel are stable for several hours at room temperature if centrifuged immediately after collection.

7. D Type 1 is called *insulin-dependent diabetes* because patients must be given insulin to prevent ketosis. Type 2 diabetes is considered *late onset* and is the most common type of diabetes.

8. C Type 2, or *late-onset diabetes*, is associated with a defect in the receptor site for insulin. Patients do not require insulin to prevent ketosis, and hyperglycemia can be controlled in most patients with diet and medication that promote insulin release or glucose loss via the kidneys.

9. D The American Diabetes Association (ADA) recommends the following criteria for diagnosing diabetes mellitus:

- Fasting glucose 126 mg/dL or greater
- Casual (random) glucose 200 mg/dL or greater in the presence of symptoms (polyuria, increased thirst, weight loss)
- Glucose 200 mg/dL or greater at 2 hours after an oral dose of 75 g of glucose
- HgbA1c $\geq$6.5%

A diagnosis of diabetes mellitus is indicated if any one criterion or a combination of these four criteria is met on more than a single testing event.

10. C Reference ranges vary slightly depending on the method and the specimen type. The cutoff value for impaired fasting plasma glucose (prediabetes) recommended by the ADA is 99 mg/dL.

11. When preparing a patient for an OGTT, which of the following conditions will lead to erroneous results?
- **A.** The patient remains ambulatory for 3 days prior to the test
- **B.** Carbohydrate intake is restricted to below 150 g/day for 3 days prior to the test
- **C.** No food, coffee, tea, or smoking is allowed 8 hours before and during the test
- **D.** Administration of 75 g of glucose is given to an adult patient after a 10- to 12-hour fast

Chemistry/Carbohydrates/2

12. Which of the following 2-hour glucose challenge results would be classified as impaired glucose tolerance (IGT)?
- **A.** 130 mg/dL
- **B.** 135 mg/dL
- **C.** 150 mg/dL
- **D.** 204 mg/dL

Chemistry/Carbohydrates/Disorders and disease/2

13. Which statement regarding gestational diabetes mellitus (GDM) is correct?
- **A.** Diagnosed using the same oral glucose tolerance criteria as in nonpregnancy
- **B.** Converts to diabetes mellitus after pregnancy in 60% to 75% of cases
- **C.** Presents no increased health risk to the fetus
- **D.** Is defined as glucose intolerance originating during pregnancy

Chemistry/Carbohydrates/Disorders and disease/1

14. Which of the following findings is characteristic of all forms of clinical hypoglycemia?
- **A.** A fasting blood glucose value less than 55 mg/dL
- **B.** High fasting insulin levels
- **C.** Neuroglycopenic symptoms at the time of low blood sugar
- **D.** Decreased serum C peptide

Chemistry/Carbohydrates/Disorders and disease/2

15. According to the ADA criteria, which result is consistent with a diagnosis of impaired fasting glucose?
- **A.** 99 mg/dL
- **B.** 117 mg/dL
- **C.** 126 mg/dL
- **D.** 135 mg/dL

Chemistry/Carbohydrates/Disorders and disease/2

16. Which statement regarding glycosylated Hgb is true?
- **A.** Has a sugar attached to the C-terminal end of the β-chain
- **B.** Is a highly reversible aminoglycan
- **C.** Reflects the extent of glucose regulation in the 8- to 12-week interval prior to sampling
- **D.** Will be abnormal within 4 days following an episode of hyperglycemia

Chemistry/Carbohydrates/Glycosylated Hb/2

17. Which HgbA1c value equates to an average blood glucose of less than 100 mg/dL?
- **A.** 5%
- **B.** 6.5%
- **C.** 9.5%
- **D.** 11%

Chemistry/Carbohydrates/Glycosylated Hb/2

Answers to Questions 11–17

11. B Standardized OGTTs require that patients receive at least 150 g of carbohydrate per day for 3 days prior to the test to stabilize the synthesis of inducible glycolytic enzymes.

12. C Except in pregnancy, IGT is defined by the ADA as a serum or plasma glucose at 2 hours following a 75-g oral glucose load of 140 mg/dL or greater and less than 200 mg/dL.

13. D Gestational diabetes is considered any degree of glucose intolerance first recognized during the second or third trimester of pregnancy. Control of GDM reduces perinatal complications, such as respiratory distress syndrome, high birth weight, and neonatal jaundice.

14. C Hypoglycemia is characterized by a decrease in plasma glucose concentration such that there may be altered mental status. High fasting insulin levels (usually greater than 6 μg/L) are seen in insulinoma. C peptide is a subunit of proinsulin that is hydrolyzed when insulin is released.

15. B Impaired fasting glucose is defined as a plasma glucose 100 mg/dL or greater but less than 126 mg/dL.

16. C Glycosylated Hgb results from the nonenzymatic attachment of a carbohydrate, such as glucose, to the N-terminal valine of the β-chain of the hemoglobin molecule. The reaction is nonreversible and is related to the time-averaged blood glucose concentration over the life span of the RBCs, or about 12 weeks.

17. A The time-averaged blood glucose is approximated by the formula: (28.7 × HbA1c) - 46.7 = estimated average glucose. An HgbA1c level of 5.0% equates to an average blood glucose of approximately 97 mg/dL.

18. Which statement regarding measurement of HgbA1c is true?

A. Levels do not need to be done fasting
B. Both the labile and stable HgbA1c fractions are measured
C. Samples should be measured within 2 hours of collection
D. The assay must be done by liquid chromatography

Chemistry/Carbohydrates/Glycosylated Hb/2

19. Quantitation of this substance can be used in place of HgbA1c for individuals with hemoglobin variants:

A. Fructosamine
B. Lactose
C. Galactose
D. Sucrose

Chemistry/Carbohydrates/Glycosylated Hb/2

20. A patient who has a positive urinalysis result for glucose and ketones has a glycated Hgb of 4.0%. The fasting glucose performed the previous day was 180 mg/dL. Assuming acceptable QC, you would:

A. Report the glycosylated Hgb
B. Request a new specimen and repeat the glycosylated Hgb
C. Perform an Hgb electrophoresis on the sample
D. Perform a glucose measurement on the sample

Chemistry/Carbohydrates/Glycosylated Hb/3

21. Which statement *best* describes the use of the HgbA1c test?

A. Should be used for monitoring glucose control only
B. May be used for both diagnosis and monitoring
C. Should be used only to monitor individuals with type 1 diabetes
D. May be used only to monitor individuals with type 2 diabetes

Chemistry/Carbohydrates/Glycosylated Hb/2

22. Which HgbA1c value equates to an average blood glucose of approximately 130 mg/dL?

A. 5%
B. 6.5%
C. 9.5%
D. 11%

Chemistry/Carbohydrates/Glycosylated Hb/2

23. What is the recommended cutoff for the early detection of chronic kidney disease in diabetics using the test for albuminuria?

A. Greater than 30 mg/g creatinine
B. Greater than 80 mg/g creatinine
C. Greater than 200 mg/g creatinine
D. Greater than 80 mg/L creatinine

Chemistry/Carbohydrates/Disorders and disease/1

Answers to Questions 18–23

18. A Since HgbA1c represents the average blood glucose 2 to 3 months prior to blood collection, the dietary status of the patient on the day of the test has no effect on the results.

19. A Fructosamine, or glycosylated albumin, measures the amount of sugar attached to albumin over a 2- to 3-week period.

20. B The glycated Hgb is at the lowest normal limit (4%–5.5%), but the fasting glucose indicates frank diabetes mellitus. Although the glycosylated Hgb reflects the average blood glucose 2 to 3 months earlier, the value reported is inconsistent with the other laboratory results. A high probability of sample misidentification or analytical error necessitates that the test be repeated.

21. B The ADA recommends that the HgbA1c test be used both for diagnosis and for monitoring blood glucose levels.

22. B The time-averaged blood glucose is approximated by the formula: (28.7 x HbA1c) - 46.7 = estimated average glucose. An HgbA1c level of 6.5% equates to an average blood glucose of approximately 140 mg/dL.

23. A Albuminuria is the excretion of small quantities of albumin in urine. In those with diabetes, excretion of albumin that is within allowable limits for healthy people may signal the onset of chronic kidney disease.

24. In addition to measuring blood glucose, HgbA1c, and albuminuria, which test should be done on individuals with diabetes once per year?
A. Urine glucose
B. Urine ketone
C. Plasma fructosamine
D. Estimated glomerular filtration rate (eGFR)
Chemistry/Carbohydrates/2

25. Which testing situation is appropriate for the use of point-of-care whole blood glucose methods?
A. Screening for type 2 diabetes mellitus
B. Diagnosis of diabetes mellitus
C. Monitoring of blood glucose control in those with type 1 and type 2 diabetes
D. Monitoring patients with diabetes for hyperglycemic episodes only
Chemistry/Carbohydrates/POCT/2

26. What effect does hematocrit have on point-of-care tests (POCTs) for whole blood glucose monitoring?
A. Low hematocrit decreases glucose readings on all devices
B. High hematocrit raises glucose readings on all devices
C. The effect is variable and dependent on the enzyme/coenzyme system
D. Low hematocrit raises readings, and high hematocrit lowers readings unless corrected
Chemistry/Carbohydrates/POCT/2

27. What is the purpose of C-peptide level testing in a patient with type 1 diabetes?
A. Is an indicator of pancreatic β-cell function
B. Is an indicator of pancreatic α-cell function
C. Is an early marker for renal nephropathy
D. Is an indicator of albuminuria
Chemistry/Carbohydrates/2

28. A sample was collected in a serum-separator tube (SST) at the physician's office for a fasting serum glucose. The sample was transported to the reference lab, unspun, 6 hours later. What effect, if any, is expected on the glucose value upon testing at the reference lab?
A. There is no effect as long as the SST remained closed
B. The serum glucose will decrease 5% to 7% each hour due to glycolysis
C. The serum glucose will increase 5% to 7% over 4 hours due to RBC lysis
D. The serum glucose will be 10% greater than a plasma sample
Chemistry/Carbohydrates/2

Answers to Questions 24–28

24. D Per the ADA, at least annually, an estimated glomerular filtration rate (eGFR) should be performed on all individuals with type 1 diabetes of ≥5 years, and in all individuals with type 2 diabetes, regardless of treatment. Although urinary glucose can identify people who may have diabetes, it is not sensitive enough to manage glucose control on a daily basis. The urinary ketone test is a useful screening test for diabetic and other forms of ketosis. Fructosamine is a useful adjunct to HgbA1c to identify poor control of blood glucose in the past 2 to 4 weeks, but it has not been recommended for routine use for all patients with diabetes.

25. C The ADA does not recommend the use of whole blood glucose monitors for establishing a diagnosis of or screening for diabetes. Whole blood glucose meters should be used by patients with diabetes and caregivers to monitor glucose control.

26. D High hematocrit lowers glucose because RBC glucose concentration in whole blood is lower than in plasma concentration when using POCT glucose monitoring. The hematocrit is calculated and used to mathematically correct the glucose measurement.

27. A C peptide is secreted from the β-cells of the Langerhans cells of the pancreas and is released in circulation along with insulin. It is used to assess β-cell function.

28. B Each hour that the RBCs remain viable, the glucose value is expected to decrease 5% to 7% due to erythrocytic glycolysis. If a delay in analysis is expected for a glucose assay, it is recommended to collect the sample in the gray-top sodium fluoride/potassium oxalate tube to inhibit glycolysis.

29. In a patient with a plasma glucose of 126 mg/dL, the expected cerebrospinal fluid (CSF) glucose value is:
A. 49 mg/dL
B. 63 mg/dL
C. 76 mg/dL
D. 126 mg/dL
Chemistry/Carbohydrates/CSF/2

30. Which statement about glucose in CSF is correct?
A. Levels below 40 mg/dL occur in septic meningitis, cancer, and multiple sclerosis
B. CSF glucose is normally the same as the plasma glucose level
C. Hyperglycorrhachia is caused by dehydration
D. In some clinical conditions, CSF glucose can be greater than plasma glucose
Chemistry/Carbohydrates/CSF/2

31. Which of the following is classified as a mucopolysaccharide storage disease?
A. Pompe disease
B. von Gierke disease
C. Hers disease
D. Hurler syndrome
Chemistry/Carbohydrates/1

32. Identify the enzyme deficiency responsible for type I glycogen storage disease (GSD1 or von Gierke disease).
A. Glucose-6-phosphatase
B. Glycogen phosphorylase
C. Glycogen synthetase
D. β-Glucosidase
Chemistry/Carbohydrates/2

33. Which of the following abnormal laboratory results is found in von Gierke disease?
A. Hyperglycemia
B. Increased glucose response to epinephrine administration
C. Metabolic alkalosis
D. Hyperlipidemia
Chemistry/Carbohydrates/2

34. Which of the following statements about carbohydrate intolerance is true?
A. Galactosemia results from deficiency of galactose-1-phosphate (galactose-1-PO_4) uridine diphosphate (UDP) transferase
B. Galactosemia results in a positive glucose oxidase test for glucose in urine
C. Urinary galactose is seen in both galactosemia and lactase deficiency
D. A galactose tolerance test is used to confirm a diagnosis of galactosemia
Chemistry/Carbohydrates/2

35. Which of the following statements regarding iron metabolism is correct?
A. Iron absorption is decreased by alcohol ingestion
B. Normally, 40% to 50% of ingested iron is absorbed
C. The daily requirement is higher for pregnant and menstruating women
D. Absorption increases with the amount of iron in the body stores
Chemistry/Iron/1

Answers to Questions 29–35

29. C The glucose value in CSF is approximately 60% of the circulating serum glucose value.

30. A A low level of glucose in CSF is significant and is most often associated with bacterial or fungal meningitis, malignancy in the central nervous system (CNS), and some cases of subarachnoid hemorrhage, rheumatoid arthritis, and multiple sclerosis.

31. D Hurler syndrome is an autosomal recessive disease resulting from a deficiency of iduronidase. Glycosaminoglycans (mucopolysaccharides) accumulate in the lysosomes.

32. A Type 1 glycogen storage disease (von Gierke disease) is an autosomal recessive deficiency of glucose-6-phosphatase. Glycogen accumulates in tissues, causing hypoglycemia, ketosis, and fatty liver.

33. D von Gierke disease (Type 1 glycogen storage disease) results from a deficiency of glucose-6-phosphatase. This blocks the hydrolysis of glucose-6-PO_4 to glucose and P_i, preventing degradation of glycogen to glucose. The disease is associated with increased triglyceride levels because fats are mobilized for energy. Lactate acidosis would be present, caused by increased glycolysis.

34. A Galactose is metabolized to galactose-1-PO_4 by the action of galactokinase. Galactose-1-PO_4 UDP transferase converts galactose-1-PO_4 to glucose. Deficiency of either enzyme causes elevated blood and urine galactose.

35. C For adult men and nonmenstruating women, approximately 1 to 2 mg/day of iron is needed to replace the small amount lost mainly by exfoliation of cells. Menstruating women have an additional requirement of 1 mg/day and pregnant women 2 mg/day. Absorption efficiency will increase iron deficiency and decrease iron overload. Iron absorption is enhanced by low gastric pH and is increased by alcohol ingestion.

36. Which of the following processes occurs when iron is in the oxidized (Fe^{3+}) state?
A. Absorption by intestinal epithelium
B. Binding to transferrin and incorporation into ferritin
C. Incorporation into protoporphyrin IX to form functional heme
D. Reaction with chromogens in colorimetric assays
Chemistry/Iron/Analytical methods/1

37. Which of the following is associated with low serum iron and high TIBC?
A. Iron-deficiency anemia
B. Hepatitis
C. Nephrosis
D. Non–iron-deficiency anemias
Chemistry/Iron/Disorders and disease/2

38. Which condition is associated with the lowest percent saturation of transferrin?
A. Hemochromatosis
B. Anemia of chronic infection
C. Iron-deficiency anemia
D. Non–iron-deficiency anemia
Chemistry/Iron/Disorders and disease/2

39. Which condition is *most* often associated with a high serum iron level?
A. Nephrosis
B. Chronic infection or inflammation
C. Polycythemia vera
D. Non–iron-deficiency anemias
Chemistry/Iron/Disorders and disease/2

40. Which of the following is likely to occur *first* in iron-deficiency anemia?
A. Decreased serum iron
B. Increased TIBC
C. Decreased serum ferritin
D. Increased transferrin
Chemistry/Iron/Disorders and disease/2

41. Which formula provides the *best* estimate of serum TIBC?
A. Serum transferrin in mg/dL × 0.70 = TIBC (μg/dL)
B. Serum transferrin in mg/dL × 1.25% saturation= TIBC (μg/dL)
C. Serum iron (μg/dL)/1.2 + 0.06 = TIBC (μg/dL)
D. Serum Fe (μg/dL) × 1.43= TIBC (μg/dL)
Chemistry/Iron/2

Answers to Questions 36–41

36. B Intestinal absorption occurs only if the iron is in the reduced state (Fe^{+2}). Transferrin and ferritin bind iron efficiently only when in the oxidized state, Fe^{+3}.

37. A Iron-deficiency anemia is the principal cause of low serum iron and high TIBC because it promotes increased transferrin. Hepatitis causes increased release of storage iron, resulting in high levels of iron and transferrin. Nephrosis causes low iron and TIBC as a result of loss of both iron and transferrin by the kidneys. Non–iron-deficiency anemias may cause high iron and usually show low TIBC and normal or high ferritin.

38. C Percent saturation can be calculated using the formula %Sat = Serum Fe × 100/TIBC. Normally, transferrin is one-third saturated with iron. In iron-deficiency states, serum iron falls, but transferrin rises. The opposite occurs in hemochromatosis and sideroblastic anemia, resulting in an increased percent saturation.

39. D Non–iron-deficiency anemias, such as pernicious anemia and sideroblastic anemia, produce high serum iron and low TIBC. Nephrosis causes iron loss by the kidneys. Anemia associated with chronic infection causes a low serum iron but, unlike iron deficiency, causes a low (or normal) TIBC and does not cause low ferritin. Polycythemia is associated with increased iron within the RBCs and depletion of iron stores.

40. C Body stores must be depleted of iron before serum iron falls. Thus, serum ferritin falls in the early stages of iron deficiency, making it a more sensitive test than serum iron in uncomplicated cases. Ferritin levels are low only in iron deficiency. However, concurrent illnesses such as malignancy, infection, and inflammation may promote ferritin release from the tissues, causing the serum ferritin to be normal in iron deficiency.

41. B Transferrin is the principal iron transport protein, and TIBC is determined by the serum transferrin concentration. One mole of transferrin binds two moles of Fe^{+3}, so the transferrin concentration can be used to predict the TIBC. The formula TIBC (μg/dL) = serum transferrin (mg/dL) × 1.25 % transferrin saturation can be used for the calculation.

42. Which statement regarding the diagnosis of iron deficiency is correct?

A. Serum iron levels are always higher at night than during the day
B. Serum iron levels begin to fall before the body stores become depleted
C. A normal level of serum ferritin rules out iron deficiency
D. A low serum ferritin is diagnostic of iron deficiency

Chemistry/Iron/Disorders and disease/2

43. Iron overload due to a genetic defect is considered:

A. Thalassemia
B. Hemosiderosis
C. Hemochromatosis
D. Hemodilution

Chemistry/Iron/Disorders and disease/1

44. Iron-deficiency anemia can be characterized by the following laboratory values:

A. Decreased serum iron, increased ferritin, increased transferrin, and increased TIBC
B. Decreased serum iron, decreased ferritin, decreased transferrin, decreased TIBC
C. Decreased serum iron, decreased ferritin, increased transferrin, increased TIBC
D. Decreased serum iron, decreased ferritin, decreased transferrin, increased TIBC

Chemistry/Iron/Disorders and disease/3

45. Results of an iron profile are:

Serum Fe = 40 μg/dL	TIBC = 400 μg/dL
Ferritin = 40 μg/L (reference range 15–200 μg/L)	Transferrin = 300 mg/dL (reference range 200–360 mg/dL)

These results indicate:

A. Error in calculation of TIBC
B. Serum iron falls before ferritin in iron deficiency
C. A defect in iron transport and not iron deficiency
D. Iron deficiency but increased release of ferritin

Chemistry/Iron/3

46. Results of an iron profile are:

Serum Fe = 40 μg/dL TIBC = 400 μg/dL
Ferritin = 50 μg/L

All of the following tests are useful in establishing a diagnosis of iron deficiency *except*:

A. Reticulocyte Hgb content
B. Erythrocyte zinc protoporphyrin
C. Serum transferrin
D. Hgb electrophoresis

Chemistry/Iron/Disorders and disease/3

47. Which of the following statements regarding the metabolism of bilirubin is true?

A. It is formed by hydrolysis of the α-methene bridge of urobilinogen
B. It is reduced to biliverdin prior to excretion
C. It is a by-product of porphyrin production
D. It is produced from the destruction of RBCs

Chemistry/Bilirubin/1

Answers to Questions 42–47

42. D A low ferritin is specific for iron deficiency. Serum iron levels are falsely elevated by hemolysis and subject to diurnal variation. Levels are highest in the morning and lowest at night.

43. C Hemochromatosis is iron accumulation due to a genetic defect that leads to increased iron absorption by the intestines. Hemosiderosis is iron accumulation due to excess iron intake due to multiple blood transfusions or dietary overload.

44. C Iron-deficiency anemia is a reduction of iron stores (ferritin) and a reduction of circulating iron, with increased TIBC and increased transport capacity of transferrin.

45. D Although this patient's serum ferritin is within reference limits, serum iron is low and percent saturation is only 10%. These results point to iron deficiency.

46. D Hemoglobin variants, such as hemoglobinopathies and thalassemias, are not associated with iron deficiency and hemoglobin electrophoresis would not be of value. Reticulocyte Hgb indicates the availability of iron for RBC production and will be low in iron deficiency before serum iron falls. Transferrin is elevated in iron deficiency. Zinc protoporphyrin is elevated in iron deficiency and in lead poisoning.

47. D Reticuloendothelial cells in the spleen digest Hgb and release the iron from heme. The tetrapyrrole ring is opened at the α-methene bridge by heme oxygenase, forming biliverdin. Bilirubin is formed by reduction of biliverdin at the γ-methene bridge. It forms a complex with albumin and is transported to the liver. Synthesis of porphyrins results in production of heme and metabolism of porphyrins other than protoporphyrin IX yields uroporphyrins and coproporphyrins, not bilirubin.

48. Bilirubin is transported from reticuloendothelial cells to the liver by:
- **A.** Albumin
- **B.** Bilirubin-binding globulin
- **C.** Haptoglobin
- **D.** Transferrin

Chemistry/Bilirubin/1

49. In the liver, bilirubin is conjugated by addition of:
- **A.** Vinyl groups
- **B.** Methyl groups
- **C.** Hydroxyl groups
- **D.** Glucuronyl groups

Chemistry/Bilirubin/1

50. Which enzyme is responsible for the conjugation of bilirubin?
- **A.** β-Glucuronidase
- **B.** UDP-glucuronyl transferase
- **C.** Bilirubin oxidase
- **D.** Biliverdin reductase

Chemistry/Bilirubin/1

51. The delta bilirubin fraction refers to:
- **A.** Water-soluble bilirubin
- **B.** Free unconjugated bilirubin
- **C.** Conjugated bilirubin tightly bound to albumin
- **D.** Direct-reacting bilirubin

Chemistry/Bilirubin/1

52. Which of the following processes is part of the normal metabolism of bilirubin?
- **A.** Both conjugated and unconjugated bilirubin are excreted into bile
- **B.** Methene bridges of bilirubin are reduced by intestinal bacteria, resulting in formation of urobilinogen
- **C.** Most of the bilirubin delivered into the intestine is reabsorbed
- **D.** Bilirubin and urobilinogen reabsorbed from the intestine are mainly excreted by the kidneys

Chemistry/Bilirubin/1

53. Which of the following is a characteristic of conjugated bilirubin?
- **A.** It is water soluble
- **B.** It reacts more slowly than unconjugated bilirubin
- **C.** It is more stable than unconjugated bilirubin
- **D.** It has the same absorbance properties as unconjugated bilirubin

Chemistry/Bilirubin/1

54. Which of the following statements *best* defines urobilinogen?
- **A.** It is formed in the intestines by bacterial reduction of bilirubin
- **B.** It consists of a single water-soluble bile pigment
- **C.** It is measured by its reaction with *p*-aminosalicylate
- **D.** In hemolytic anemia, it is decreased in urine and feces

Chemistry/Bilirubin/1

Answers to Questions 48–54

48. A Albumin transports bilirubin, haptoglobin transports free Hgb, and transferrin transports ferric iron.

49. D The esterification of glucuronic acid to the propionyl side chains of the inner pyrrole rings (I and II) makes bilirubin water soluble.

50. B UDP-glucuronyl transferase esterifies glucuronic acid to unconjugated bilirubin, making it water soluble. β-Glucuronidase hydrolyzes glucuronide from bilirubin, hormones, or drugs. Bilirubin oxidase is used in an enzymatic bilirubin assay in which bilirubin is oxidized back to biliverdin and the rate of biliverdin formation is measured at 410 nm. Biliverdin reductase forms bilirubin from biliverdin (and heme oxygenase forms biliverdin from heme).

51. C δ-Bilirubin is a separate fraction from the unconjugated bilirubin, which is bound loosely to albumin.

52. B Most of the conjugated bilirubin delivered into the intestine is deconjugated by β-glucuronidase and then reduced by intestinal flora to form three different reduction products collectively called *urobilinogens*.

53. A *Conjugated bilirubin* refers to bilirubin mono- and diglucuronides. Conjugated bilirubin reacts almost immediately with the aqueous diazo reagent without need for a nonpolar solvent. Conjugated bilirubin is excreted in both bile and urine.

54. A *Urobilinogen* is a collective term given to the reduction products of bilirubin formed by the action of enteric bacteria. Urobilinogen is measured using the Ehrlich reagent, an acid solution of *p*-dimethylaminobenzaldehyde. Urobilinogen excretion is increased in extravascular hemolytic anemias.

55. Which statement *best* defines bilirubin metabolism?

A. Bilirubin undergoes rapid photo-oxidation when exposed to daylight
B. Bilirubin excretion is inhibited by barbiturates
C. Bilirubin excretion is increased by chlorpromazine
D. Bilirubin is excreted only as the diglucuronide

Chemistry/Bilirubin/2

56. Which condition is caused by deficient secretion of bilirubin into the bile canaliculi?

A. Gilbert disease
B. Neonatal hyperbilirubinemia
C. Dubin-Johnson syndrome
D. Crigler-Najjar syndrome

Chemistry/Bilirubin/2

57. In hepatitis, the rise in serum conjugated bilirubin can be caused by:

A. Secondary renal insufficiency
B. Failure of the enterohepatic circulation
C. Enzymatic conversion of urobilinogen to bilirubin
D. Extrahepatic conjugation

Chemistry/Bilirubin/Disorders and disease/2

58. Which of the following is a characteristic of obstructive jaundice?

A. The ratio of direct to total bilirubin is greater than 1:2
B. Conjugated bilirubin is elevated, but unconjugated bilirubin is normal
C. Urinary urobilinogen is increased
D. Urinary bilirubin is normal

Chemistry/Bilirubin/Disorders and disease/2

59. Which of the following would cause an increase in only the unconjugated bilirubin fraction?

A. Hemolytic anemia
B. Obstructive jaundice
C. Hepatitis
D. Hepatic cirrhosis

Chemistry/Bilirubin/Disorders and disease/2

60. Which form of hyperbilirubinemia is caused by an inherited absence of UDP-glucuronyl transferase?

A. Gilbert syndrome
B. Rotor syndrome
C. Crigler-Najjar syndrome
D. Dubin-Johnson syndrome

Chemistry/Bilirubin/Disorders and disease/1

Answers to Questions 55–60

55. A Samples for bilirubin analysis must be protected from direct sunlight. Barbiturates lower serum bilirubin by increasing excretion. Other drugs that cause cholestasis, such as chlorpromazine, increase the serum bilirubin. Although most conjugated bilirubin is in the form of diglucuronide, some monoglucuronide and other glycosides are excreted.

56. C Dubin-Johnson syndrome is an autosomal recessive condition arising from mutation of an *ABC* (ATP-binding cassette) transporter gene. It produces mild jaundice from accumulation of conjugated bilirubin that is not secreted into the bile canaliculi. Direct (and total) bilirubin is elevated, but other liver function is normal.

57. B Conjugated bilirubin is increased in hepatitis and other causes of hepatic necrosis as a result of failure to re-excrete conjugated bilirubin reabsorbed from the intestine. Increased direct bilirubin can also be attributed to accompanying intrahepatic obstruction, which blocks the flow of bile.

58. A Obstruction prevents conjugated bilirubin from reaching the intestine, resulting in decreased production, excretion, and absorption of urobilinogen. Conjugated bilirubin regurgitates into sinusoidal blood and enters the general circulation via the hepatic vein. The level of serum direct (conjugated) bilirubin becomes greater than unconjugated bilirubin. The unconjugated form is also increased because of accompanying necrosis, deconjugation, and inhibition of UDP-glucuronyl transferase.

59. A Hemolytic anemia (prehepatic jaundice) presents a greater bilirubin load to a normal liver, resulting in increased bilirubin excretion. When the rate of bilirubin formation exceeds the rate of excretion, the unconjugated bilirubin rises. Conjugated bilirubin increases because of obstructive processes within the liver or biliary system or from failure of the enterohepatic circulation.

60. C Crigler-Najjar syndrome is a rare condition that occurs in two forms. Type 1 is inherited as an autosomal recessive trait and causes a total deficiency of UDP-glucuronyl transferase. Gilbert syndrome is an autosomal recessive condition characterized by decreased bilirubin uptake and decreased formation of bilirubin diglucuronide. Dubin-Johnson and Rotor syndromes are autosomal recessive disorders associated with defective delivery of bilirubin into the biliary system.

61. Which statement regarding total and direct bilirubin levels is true?
A. Total bilirubin level is a less sensitive and specific marker of liver disease compared with the direct level
B. Direct bilirubin exceeds 3.5 mg/dL in most cases of hemolytic anemia
C. Direct bilirubin is normal in cholestatic liver disease
D. The ratio of direct to total bilirubin exceeds 0.40 in hemolytic anemia

Chemistry/Bilirubin/Disorders and disease/2

62. Which statement *best* characterizes newborn serum bilirubin levels in the first week following delivery?
A. Serum bilirubin 24 hours after delivery should not exceed the URL for adults
B. Jaundice is usually first seen 48 to 72 hours after delivery in neonatal hyperbilirubinemia
C. Serum bilirubin above 5.0 mg/dL occurring 2 to 5 days after delivery indicates hemolytic or hepatic disease
D. Conjugated bilirubin accounts for about 50% of the total bilirubin in neonates

Chemistry/Bilirubin/2

63. Which rare form of newborn jaundice occurs within days of delivery and usually lasts 1 to 3 weeks and is caused by a maternal UDP-glucuronyl transferase inhibitor that crosses the placenta?
A. Gilbert syndrome
B. Lucey-Driscoll syndrome
C. Rotor syndrome
D. Dubin-Johnson syndrome

Chemistry/Bilirubin/Disorders and disease/2

64. A laboratory measures total bilirubin by the Jendrassik-Grof bilirubin method with sample blanking. What would be the effect of moderate hemolysis on the test result?
A. Falsely increased because of optical interference
B. Falsely increased because of release of bilirubin from RBCs
C. Falsely low because of inhibition of the diazo reaction by Hgb
D. No effect because of correction of positive interference by sample blanking

Chemistry/Bilirubin/Analytical methods/2

65. The primary transport protein for bilirubin in circulation is:
A. Transferrin
B. Albumin
C. Ceruloplasmin
D. Ligandin

Chemistry/Bilirubin/1

Answers to Questions 61–65

61. A Direct bilirubin measurement is a sensitive and specific marker for hepatic and posthepatic jaundice because it is not elevated by hemolytic anemia. In hemolytic anemia, the total bilirubin does not exceed 3.5 mg/dL, and the direct:total ratio is less than 0.20. Unconjugated bilirubin is elevated along with direct bilirubin in cholestasis because some necrosis takes place, and some conjugated bilirubin is hydrolyzed back to unconjugated bilirubin.

62. B Neonatal hyperbilirubinemia occurs 48 to 72 hours (2 to 3 days) after birth as a result of increased hemolysis at birth and transient deficiency of the microsomal enzyme, UDP-glucuronyl transferase. Normally, levels rise to about 5 to 10 mg/dL but may be greater than 15 mg/dL, requiring therapy with UV light to photo-oxidize the bilirubin. Neonatal jaundice can last up to 1 week in a mature neonate and up to 2 weeks in premature babies. Neonatal bilirubin is almost exclusively unconjugated.

63. B Lucey-Driscoll syndrome is a rare form of jaundice caused by unconjugated bilirubin that presents within 2 to 4 days of birth and can last several weeks. It is caused by an inhibitor of UDP-glucuronyl transferase in maternal plasma that crosses the placenta.

64. C The sample blank measures the absorbance of the sample and reagent in the absence of azobilirubin formation and corrects the measurement for optical interference caused by Hgb absorbing the wavelength of measurement. However, Hgb is an inhibitor of the diazo reaction and will cause falsely low results in a blank corrected sample. For this reason, direct bichromatic spectrophotometric methods are preferred when measuring bilirubin in neonatal samples, which are often hemolyzed.

65. B Bilirubin is bound by albumin and transported to the liver as unconjugated or indirect bilirubin. Transferrin is an iron transport molecule, ceruloplasmin is associated with copper utilization, and ligandin is a binding protein in the hepatocyte for transport of bilirubin within the liver for conjugation.

66. This disorder, the most common hereditary cause of increased unconjugated bilirubin, is due to a reduction in the activity of the glucuronyl transferase enzyme and is often untreated.
A. Dubin-Johnson syndrome
B. Gilbert syndrome
C. Rotor syndrome
D. Crigler-Najjar syndrome
Chemistry/Bilirubin/Disorders and disease/2

67. At what bilirubin concentration is overt jaundice, or physiological jaundice, observed?
A. 0.5 mg/dL
B. 1.2 mg/dL
C. 2.0 mg/dL
D. 3.0 mg/dL
Chemistry/Bilirubin/Disorders and disease/2

68. A neonatal bilirubin assay performed by bichromatic direct spectrophotometry is 4.1 mg/dL. Four hours later, a second sample assayed for total bilirubin by the Jendrassik-Grof method gives a result of 3.5 mg/dL. Both samples are reported to be hemolyzed. What is the *most* likely explanation for these results?
A. Hgb interference in the second assay
B. δ-Bilirubin contributing to the result of the first assay
C. Falsely high results from the first assay caused by direct bilirubin
D. Physiological variation owing to premature hepatic microsomal enzymes
Chemistry/Bilirubin/Disorders and disease/3

69. Which statement regarding porphyria is accurate?
A. Porphyria is exclusively inherited
B. All types cause an increase in urinary porphyrins
C. All types are associated with anemia
D. Serum, urine, and fecal tests may be needed for diagnosis
Chemistry/Hemoglobin/Porphyria/2

70. Which is the most common form of porphyria?
A. Erythropoietic porphyria
B. Acute intermittent porphyria
C. Variegate porphyria
D. Porphyria cutanea tarda
Chemistry/Hemoglobin/Porphyria/1

Answers to Questions 66–70

66. B Gilbert syndrome is the most common hereditary cause of increased bilirubin and is due to a reduction in the activity of the enzyme glucuronyl transferase. This syndrome does not require treatment and does not result in kernicterus.

67. D Although the upper limit reference range for bilirubin is up to 1.5 mg/dL, jaundice is not noticeable as a clinical sign until the bilirubin concentration is >3.0 mg/dL.

68. A Direct spectrophotometric bilirubin methods employing bichromatic optics correct for the presence of Hgb. The Jendrassik-Grof method is based on a diazo reaction that may be suppressed by Hgb. Because serum blanking and measurement at 600 nm correct for positive interference from Hgb, the results may be falsely low when significant hemolysis is present. In a bichromatic optics assay, a commonly used approach is to measure absorbance at 454 nm and 540 nm. The absorbance contributed by Hgb at 540 nm is equal to the absorbance contributed by Hgb at 454 nm. Therefore, the absorbance difference will correct for free Hgb.

69. D Porphyria may be inherited because of an enzyme defect in heme synthesis or may be acquired as a result of lead poisoning, liver failure, or drug toxicity. They are divided clinically into three groups: neuropsychiatric, cutaneous, or mixed. No one sample type can be used to identify all subgroups.

70. D Porphyria is a rare condition, although most of the inherited forms are autosomal dominant. Porphyria cutanea tarda results from a deficiency of uroporphyrinogen decarboxylase; the enzyme in hepatocytes is susceptible to drugs, alcohol, and hepatitis, which trigger the disease, which is often considered an acquired form of porphyria.

6.4

Creatinine, Uric Acid, BUN, and Ammonia

1. Creatinine is formed from the:
A. Oxidation of creatine
B. Oxidation of protein
C. Deamination of dibasic amino acids
D. Metabolism of purines
Chemistry/Creatinine/1

2. Creatinine is considered one of the substances of choice to measure endogenous renal clearance because:
A. The rate of formation per day is independent of body size
B. It is completely filtered by the glomeruli
C. Plasma levels are highly dependent upon diet
D. Clearance is the same for both men and women
Chemistry/Creatinine/1

3. Which statement *best* describes creatinine?
A. Serum levels are elevated in early renal disease
B. High serum levels result from reduced glomerular filtration
C. Serum creatine has the same diagnostic utility as serum creatinine
D. Serum creatinine is a more sensitive measure of renal function than creatinine clearance
Chemistry/Creatinine/2

4. Which of the following formulas is the correct expression for creatinine clearance?
A. Creatinine clearance = U/P ×V× 1.73/A
B. Creatinine clearance = P/V × U × A/1.73
C. Creatinine clearance = P/V × U × 1.73/A
D. Creatinine clearance = U/V × P ×1.73/A
Chemistry/Creatinine/1

5. Which of the following conditions is *most* likely to cause a falsely high creatinine clearance result?
A. The patient uses the midstream voiding procedure when collecting their urine
B. The patient adds tap water to the urine container because the patient forgot to save one of the urine samples
C. The patient does not include the last void at the conclusion of the test
D. The patient voids at the start of the test and adds the urine to the collection
Chemistry/Creatinine/Disorders and disease/3

6. The modification of diet in renal disease (MDRD) formula for calculating eGFR requires which four parameters?
A. Urine creatinine, serum creatinine, height, weight
B. Serum creatinine, age, gender, race
C. Serum creatinine, height, weight, age
D. Urine creatinine, gender, weight, age
Chemistry/Creatinine/1

Answers to Questions 1–6

1. A Creatinine is produced at a rate of approximately 2% daily from the oxidation of creatine mainly in skeletal muscle.

2. B Creatinine is 100% filtered by the glomeruli. Concentration is dependent on muscle mass but varies by less than 15% per day. Creatinine is not metabolized by the liver or dependent on diet.

3. B Serum creatinine is a specific but not a sensitive measure of glomerular function. About 60% of the filtration capacity of the kidneys is lost when serum creatinine becomes elevated. Because urine creatinine diminishes as serum creatinine increases in renal disease, the creatinine clearance is more sensitive than serum creatinine in detecting glomerular disease.

4. A Creatinine clearance is calculated as the ratio of urine creatinine (U) to plasma creatinine (P) in milligrams per deciliter. This is multiplied by the volume of urine (V) produced per minute and corrected for lean body mass by multiplying by 1.73/A, where A is the patient's body surface area in square meters.

5. D Urine in the bladder should be eliminated and not saved at the start of the test because it represents urine formed prior to the test period. Error is introduced by incomplete emptying of the bladder when short times are used to measure clearance. A 24-hour timed urine collection is the specimen of choice.

6. B The National Kidney Foundation recommends that eGFR be reported each time along with serum creatinine results. eGFR is usually calculated by using the MDRD formula:

$$eGFR\ (mL/min/1.73\ m^2) = 186 \times Plasma\ Cr^{-1.154} \times Age^{-0.203} \times 0.742\ (if\ Female) \times 1.21\ (if\ Black)$$

7. What substance may be measured as an alternative to creatinine for evaluating GFR?
A. Plasma urea
B. Cystatin C
C. Uric acid
D. Potassium
Chemistry/Creatinine/1

8. Which of the following enzymes allows creatine to be measured by coupling to a peroxidase reaction?
A. Glucose-6-phosphate dehydrogenase (G-6-PD)
B. Creatinine deaminase
C. Creatinine amidohydrolase
D. Creatine kinase (CK)
Chemistry/Creatinine/Analytical methods/1

9. Select the primary reagent used in the Jaffe method for creatinine.
A. Alkaline copper II sulfate
B. Saturated picric acid and sodium hydroxide (NaOH)
C. Sodium nitroprusside and phenol
D. Phosphotungstic acid
Chemistry/Creatinine/Analytical methods/1

10. Interference from other reducing substances can be partially eliminated in the Jaffe reaction by:
A. Measuring the product at 340 nm
B. Measuring the product with an electrode
C. Measuring the timed rate of product formation
D. Performing a sample blank
Chemistry/Creatinine/Analytical methods/2

11. Which of the following statements is true?
A. Cystatin C is measured immunochemically
B. The calibrator used for cystatin C is traceable to the National Bureau of Standards calibrator
C. Cystatin C assays have a lower CV compared with plasma creatinine
D. Enzymatic and rate Jaffe reactions for creatinine give comparable results
Chemistry/Creatinine/Cystatin C/3

12. In which case would eGFR derived from the plasma creatinine likely give a more accurate measurement of GFR compared with measurement of plasma cystatin C?
A. Diabetes
B. Chronic renal failure
C. After renal transplantation
D. Chronic hepatitis
Chemistry/Creatinine/Disorders and disease/2

Answers to Questions 7–12

7. B Although all of the analytes listed are increased in chronic kidney disease as a result of low GFR, potassium, urea, and uric acid are not specific for glomerular function. Cystatin C is an inhibitor of cysteine proteases and is completely filtered by the glomerulus then reabsorbed by the tubules. Plasma levels are not influenced by diet, age, gender, or nutritional status. Low GFR causes retention of cystatin C in plasma and levels become abnormally high at clearance rates below 90 mL/min, making the test more sensitive than creatinine.

8. C The peroxidase-coupled enzymatic assay of creatinine is based on the conversion of creatinine to creatine by creatinine amidohydrolase (creatininase). The enzyme then hydrolyzes creatine to produce sarcosine and urea.

9. B The Jaffe method uses saturated picric acid, which oxidizes creatinine in alkali, forming creatinine picrate. The reaction is nonspecific; ketones, ascorbate, proteins, and other reducing agents contribute to the final color.

10. C The Jaffe reaction is nonspecific; proteins and other reducing substances, such as pyruvate, protein, and ascorbate, cause positive interference. Reading the absorbance at 20 and 80 seconds and using the absorbance difference minimizes the effects of those compounds.

11. A Cystatin C can be measured by enzyme immunoassay, immunonephelometry, and immunoturbidimetry. However, there is no standardized calibrator as for cystatin C, and therefore, results vary considerably among laboratories.

12. C Cystatin C is eliminated almost exclusively by the kidneys, and plasma levels are not dependent on age, gender, or nutritional status. However, plasma levels are affected by some drugs, including those used to prevent renal transplant rejection. Increased plasma levels have been reported in chronic inflammatory diseases and cancer.

13. A sample of amniotic fluid collected for fetal lung maturity studies from a female whose pregnancy was compromised by hemolytic disease of the fetus and newborn (HDFN) has a creatinine level of 88 mg/dL. What is the *most* likely cause of this result?
A. The specimen is contaminated by blood
B. Bilirubin has interfered with the measurement of creatinine
C. A random error occurred when the absorbance signal was being processed by the analyzer
D. The fluid is urine from accidental puncture of the urinary bladder
Chemistry/Creatinine/3

14. Which analyte should be reported as a ratio using creatinine concentration as a reference?
A. Albumin
B. Urinary estriol
C. Urinary sodium
D. Urinary urea
Chemistry/Creatinine/1

15. Urea is produced from:
A. The catabolism of proteins and amino acids
B. Oxidation of purines
C. Oxidation of pyrimidines
D. The breakdown of complex carbohydrates
Chemistry/BUN/1

16. Urea concentration is calculated from the BUN by multiplying by a factor of:
A. 0.5
B. 2.14
C. 6.45
D. 14
Chemistry/BUN/2

17. Which of the following statements about serum urea is true?
A. The levels are independent of diet
B. Urea is not reabsorbed by the renal tubules
C. High BUN levels can result from necrotic liver disease
D. BUN is elevated in prerenal as well as renal failure
Chemistry/BUN/2

18. A patient's BUN is 60 mg/dL and serum creatinine is 3.0 mg/dL. These results suggest:
A. Laboratory error measuring BUN
B. Renal failure
C. Prerenal failure
D. Patient was not fasting
Chemistry/BUN/3

19. BUN is determined electrochemically by coupling the urease reaction to the measurement of:
A. H_2O_2
B. The timed rate of increase in conductivity
C. The oxidation of ammonia
D. CO_2
Chemistry/BUN/Analytical methods/2

Answers to Questions 13–19

13. D Creatinine levels in this range are found only in urine specimens.

14. A Measurement of urinary albumin (or albuminuria, formerly called *microalbumin*) concentration should be reported as a ratio of albumin to creatinine (e.g., milligram of albumin per gram of creatinine).

15. A Urea is generated by deamination of amino acids. Uric acid is produced by the catabolism of purines. Oxidation of pyrimidines produces orotic acid.

16. B BUN is multiplied by 2.14 to give the urea concentration in mg/dL.

$$(1\ mg\ urea\ N \div dL) \times (1\ mol\ N \div 14\ mg\ N) \times (1\ mmol\ urea \div 2\ mmol\ N) \times (60\ mg\ urea \div 1\ mmol\ urea) = 2.14\ mg\ urea/dL$$

17. D Urea levels are a sensitive indicator of renal disease, becoming elevated by glomerular injury, tubular damage, or poor blood flow to the kidneys (prerenal failure). Serum urea (and BUN) levels are influenced by diet and are low in necrotic liver disease. Urea is completely filtered by the glomeruli but reabsorbed by the renal tubules at a rate dependent on filtrate flow and tubular status.

18. C BUN is affected by renal blood flow as well as by glomerular and tubular function. When blood flow to the kidneys is diminished by circulatory insufficiency (prerenal failure), glomerular filtration decreases, and tubular reabsorption increases because of slower filtrate flow. As urea is reabsorbed, BUN levels rise higher than plasma creatinine. This causes the BUN:creatinine ratio to be greater than 10:1 in prerenal failure.

19. B A conductivity electrode is used to measure the increase in conductance of the solution as urea is hydrolyzed by urease in the presence of sodium carbonate.

$$Urea + H_2O \rightarrow 2NH_3 + CO_2$$
$$2NH_3 + 2H_2O + Na_2CO_3 \rightarrow 2NH_4^+ + CO_3^{-2} + 2NaOH$$

Ammonium ions increase the conductance of the solution. The timed rate of current increase is proportional to BUN concentration. Alternatively, the ammonium ions produced can be measured by using an ISE.

20. In the UV enzymatic method for BUN, the urease reaction is coupled to a second enzymatic reaction using:
A. AST
B. Glutamate dehydrogenase (GLD)
C. Glutamine synthetase
D. ALT
Chemistry/BUN/Analytical methods/2

21. Which product is measured in the coupling step of the urease-UV method for BUN?
A. CO_2
B. Dinitrophenylhydrazine
C. Diphenylcarbazone
D. NAD^+
Chemistry/BUN/Analytical methods/2

22. Which enzyme deficiency is responsible for phenylketonuria (PKU)?
A. Phenylalanine hydroxylase
B. Tyrosine transaminase
C. *p*-Hydroxyphenylpyruvic acid oxidase
D. Homogentisic acid oxidase
Chemistry/Amino acids/Disorders and disease/1

23. Which of the following conditions is classified as a renal-type aminoaciduria?
A. Fanconi syndrome
B. Wilson disease
C. Hepatitis
D. Homocystinuria
Chemistry/Amino acids/Disorders and disease/2

24. Which aminoaciduria results in the overflow of branched chain amino acids?
A. Hartnup disease
B. Alkaptonuria
C. Homocystinuria
D. Maple syrup urine disease
Chemistry/Amino acids/1

25. In addition to PKU, maple syrup urine disease, and homocystinuria, what other aminoaciduria can be detected by MS/MS?
A. Alkaptonuria
B. Hartnup disease
C. Citrullinemia
D. Cystinuria
Chemistry/Amino acids/Disorders and disease/2

26. Of the methods used to measure amino acids, which is capable of measuring fatty acids simultaneously?
A. MS/MS
B. HPLC
C. Capillary electrophoresis
D. Two-dimensional TLC
Chemistry/Amino acids/Analytical methods/1

Answers to Questions 20–26

20. B BUN is most frequently measured by the urease-UV method in which the urease reaction is coupled to the GLD reaction, generating NAD^+.

$$Urea + H_2O \xrightarrow{Urease} 2NH_3 + CO_2$$
$$2\text{-}Oxoglutarate + NH_3 + NADH + H^+ \xrightarrow{GLD} Glutamate + NAD^+ + H_2O$$

When the urease reaction is performed under first-order conditions, the decrease in absorbance at 340 nm is proportional to the urea concentration.

21. D In the urease-UV method, urease is used to hydrolyze urea, forming CO_2 and ammonia. GLD catalyzes the oxidation of NADH, forming glutamate from 2-oxoglutarate and ammonia. The GLD reaction is used for measuring both BUN and ammonia.

22. A PKU is an overflow aminoaciduria resulting from the accumulation of phenylalanine. It is caused by a deficiency of phenylalanine hydroxylase, which converts phenylalanine to tyrosine.

23. A Fanconi syndrome is an inherited disorder characterized by anemia, mental retardation, rickets, and aminoaciduria. Because the aminoaciduria results from a defect in the renal tubule, it is classified as a renal-type aminoaciduria. Wilson disease (inherited ceruloplasmin deficiency) causes hepatic failure. Hepatitis is classified as a secondary-acquired aminoaciduria. Homocystinuria is a primary-inherited aminoaciduria and is caused by a deficiency of cystathionine synthase.

24. D Valine, leucine, and isoleucine, the branched chain amino acids, accumulate as a result of decarboxylase deficiency in maple syrup urine disease. Alkaptonuria is caused by homogentisic acid oxidase deficiency, causing homogentisic aciduria. Homocystinuria is an overflow-type aminoaciduria, which results from cystathionine synthase deficiency. Hartnup disease is an impaired absorption and increased secretion of tryptophan and other amino acids.

25. C Most states use tandem-mass spectroscopy (MS/MS), which can detect greater than 30 inborn errors of metabolism from a single blood spot. This includes tyrosinemia, citrullinemia, argininosuccinate acidemia, argininemia, and hypermethioninemia.

26. A All four methods are able to separate each amino acid (up to 40 species); however, MS/MS can measure amino acids; organic acids, such as methylmalonic acid; and fatty acids.

27. Blood ammonia levels are usually measured to evaluate:
A. Renal failure
B. Acid–base status
C. Hepatic coma
D. GI malabsorption
Chemistry/Ammonia/Disorders and disease/1

28. Enzymatic measurement of ammonia requires which of the following substrates and coenzymes?
A. 2-Oxogluterate/NADH
B. Glutamate/NADH
C. Glutamine/ATP
D. Glutamine/NAD^+
Chemistry/Ammonia/Analytical methods/1

29. Which statement *best* describes ammonia?
A. Most plasma ammonia is derived from peripheral blood deamination of amino acids
B. Ammonia-induced coma can result from salicylate poisoning
C. Hepatic coma can result from Reye syndrome
D. High plasma ammonia is usually caused by respiratory alkalosis
Chemistry/Ammonia/2

30. A sample for ammonia assay is taken from an IV line that had been capped and injected with lithium heparin (heparin lock). The sample is drawn in a syringe containing lithium heparin and immediately capped and iced. The plasma is separated and analyzed within 20 minutes of collection, and the result is 50 µg/dL higher than one measured 4 hours before. What is the *most* likely explanation of these results?
A. Significantly greater physiological variation is seen with patients with systemic, hepatic, and GI diseases
B. The syringe was contaminated with ammonia
C. One of the two samples was collected from the wrong patient
D. Stasis of blood in the line caused increased ammonia
Chemistry/Ammonia/3

31. Uric acid is derived from:
A. Oxidation of proteins
B. Catabolism of purines
C. Oxidation of pyrimidines
D. Reduction of catecholamines
Chemistry/Uric acid/1

32. Which of the following conditions is associated with hyperuricemia?
A. Renal failure
B. Chronic liver disease
C. Xanthine oxidase deficiency
D. Paget disease of the bone
Chemistry/Uric acid/Disorders and disease/2

Answers to Questions 27–32

27. C Hepatic coma is caused by accumulation of ammonia in the brain as a result of liver failure. The ammonia increases CNS pH.

28. A Enzymatic assays of ammonia utilize glutamate dehydrogenase (GLDH). This enzyme forms glutamate from 2-oxoglutarate and ammonia, resulting in oxidation of NADPH.

29. C Blood ammonia levels will rise in any necrotic liver disease, including hepatitis, Reye syndrome, and drug-induced injury, such as acetaminophen poisoning. Ammonia crosses the blood–brain barrier, which accounts for the frequency of CNS complications and, if severe, hepatic coma.

30. D Falsely elevated blood ammonia levels are commonly caused by improper specimen collection. Venous stasis and prolonged storage cause peripheral deamination of amino acids, causing a falsely high ammonia level.

31. B Uric acid is the principal product of purine (adenosine and guanosine) metabolism.

32. A Excessive retention of uric acid results from renal failure and diuretics (or other drugs) that block uric acid excretion. Xanthine oxidase converts xanthine to uric acid; therefore, a deficiency of this enzyme results in low serum levels of uric acid. Paget disease of bone causes cyclic episodes of bone degeneration and regeneration and is associated with very high serum alkaline phosphatase (ALP) and urinary calcium levels.

33. Orders for uric acid are permitted to be ordered as a *stat* request because:
A. Levels above 10 mg/dL cause urinary tract calculi
B. Uric acid is hepatotoxic
C. High levels induce aplastic anemia
D. High levels cause joint pain
Chemistry/Uric acid/2

34. Which uric acid method is associated with negative bias caused by reducing agents?
A. Uricase coupled to the Trinder reaction
B. UV uricase reaction coupled to catalase and alcohol dehydrogenase reactions
C. Measurement of the rate of absorbance decrease at 290 nm after addition of uricase
D. Amperometry
Chemistry/Uric acid/Analytical methods/2

35. Quality control results for uric acid are as follows:

	Run 1	Run 2	Run 3	Run 4	Mean	s
QC1	3.5	3.8	4.1	4.2	3.6	0.40
QC2	6.8	7.2	7.4	7.5	7.0	0.25

Results should be reported from:
A. Run 1 only
B. Runs 1 and 2
C. Runs 1, 2, and 3
D. Runs 1, 2, 3, and 4
Chemistry/Uric acid/Problem solving/3

Answers to Questions 33–35

33. A Uric acid calculi (translucent compact stones that often lodge in the ureters) form quickly when the serum uric acid level reaches 10 mg/dL and may cause postrenal failure.

34. A The peroxidase-coupled uricase reaction forms allantoin, CO_2, and H_2O_2 from the oxidation of uric acid. When peroxide is used to oxidize a Trinder dye (e.g., a phenol derivative and 4-aminoantipyrine), some negative bias may occur when high levels of ascorbate or other reducing agents are present. Rate UV methods are free from this interference. As with other reactions that generate H_2O_2, the uricase reaction can be used to measure uric acid by using either polarography or amperometry.

35. C Although no single result exceeds the 2s limit, the 4_{1s} rule is broken on Run 4. This means that both QC1 and QC2 exceeded +1s on Run 3 and Run 4.

6.5 *Proteins, Electrophoresis, and Lipids*

1. The Kjeldahl procedure for total protein is based on the premise that:
A. Proteins are negatively charged
B. The pK_a of proteins is the same
C. The nitrogen content of proteins is constant
D. Proteins have similar tyrosine and tryptophan content
Chemistry/Proteins/Analytical methods/1

2. The biuret method is based on which principle?
A. The reaction of phenolic groups with $CuSO_4$
B. Coordinate bonds between Cu^{+2} and carbonyl and imine groups of peptide bonds
C. The protein error of indicator effects producing color when dyes bind protein
D. The reaction of phosphomolybdic acid with protein
Chemistry/Proteins/Analytical methods/1

3. Which statement is the *best* description for the biuret reaction used in total protein determination?
A. It is sensitive to protein levels below 0.1 mg/dL
B. It is suitable for urine, exudates, and transudates
C. Polypeptides and compounds with repeating imine groups react
D. Hemolysis will not interfere
Chemistry/Proteins/Analytical methods/2

4. How much nitrogen by weight, on average, is contained in proteins?
A. 5%
B. 16%
C. 24%
D. 40%
Chemistry/Proteins/2

5. Which of the following statements regarding proteins is true?
A. Total protein and albumin are about 10% higher in ambulatory patients
B. Plasma total protein is about 20% higher than serum levels
C. Albumin normally accounts for about one third of the CSF total protein
D. Transudative serous fluid protein is about two-thirds of the total serum protein
Chemistry/Proteins/2

Answers to Questions 1–5

1. C The Kjeldahl method for total protein measures the nitrogen content of proteins as ammonium ion by back titration after oxidation of proteins by sulfuric acid and heat.

2. B Biuret is a compound with two carbonyl groups and three amino groups and forms coordinate bonds with Cu^{+2} in the same manner as protein.

3. C The reagent reacts with peptides containing at least two peptide bonds, but because of the high concentration of proteins in plasma relative to peptides present, this reactivity causes insignificant bias. The biuret reaction is not sensitive to protein levels below 0.1 g/dL and, therefore, is not sensitive enough for assays of total protein in CSF, urine, or transudates. Slight hemolysis does not cause falsely high results; however, grossly hemolyzed samples contain sufficient globin to cause positive interference.

4. B On average, proteins have 16% nitrogen by weight.

5. A Water pools in the vascular bed in nonambulatory patients, lowering the total protein, albumin, hematocrit, and calcium. Plasma levels of total protein are 0.2 to 0.4 g/dL higher than those in serum (about 5%) because of fibrinogen. CSF albumin levels are approximately two-thirds of the CSF total protein. Transudates have a total protein less than 50% of the serum total protein.

6. Hyperalbuminemia is caused by:
A. Dehydration syndromes
B. Liver disease
C. Burns
D. Gastroenteropathy
Chemistry/Albumin/Disorders and disease/2

7. High serum total protein but low albumin is usually seen in:
A. Multiple myeloma
B. Hepatic cirrhosis
C. Glomerulonephritis
D. Nephrotic syndrome
Chemistry/Albumin/Disorders and disease/2

8. Which of the following conditions is *most* commonly associated with an elevated level of total protein?
A. Glomerular disease
B. Starvation
C. Liver failure
D. Malignancy
Chemistry/Proteins/Disorders and disease/2

9. Which of the following dyes is the *most* specific for measurement of albumin?
A. Bromcresol green (BCG)
B. Bromcresol purple (BCP)
C. Tetrabromosulfophthalein
D. Tetrabromphenol blue
Chemistry/Proteins/Analytical methods/1

10. Which of the following factors is *most* likely to cause a falsely low result when using the BCG dye–binding assay for albumin?
A. The presence of penicillin
B. An incubation time of 120 seconds
C. The presence of bilirubin
D. Lipemia
Chemistry/Proteins/Analytical methods/2

11. At pH 8.6, proteins are______charged and migrate toward the _______.
A. Negatively, anode
B. Positively, cathode
C. Positively, anode
D. Negatively, cathode
Chemistry/Electrophoresis/1

12. Electrophoretic movement of proteins toward the anode will decrease by increasing the:
A. Buffer pH
B. Ionic strength of the buffer
C. Current
D. Voltage
Chemistry/Electrophoresis/2

Answers to Questions 6–12

6. A A high serum albumin level is caused only by dehydration or administration of albumin. Liver disease, burns, gastroenteropathy, nephrosis, starvation, and malignancy cause hypoalbuminemia.

7. A In multiple myeloma, synthesis of large quantities of monoclonal immunoglobulin by plasma cells often results in decreased synthesis of albumin. In glomerulonephritis and nephrotic syndrome, both total protein and albumin are low because of loss of proteins through the glomeruli. In hepatic cirrhosis, decreased hepatic production of protein results in low total protein and albumin.

8. D Malignant disease is usually associated with increased production of immunoglobulin and acute-phase proteins. Glomerular damage causes albumin and other low-molecular-weight proteins to be lost through the kidneys. Liver failure and starvation result in decreased protein synthesis.

9. B BCG and BCP are anionic dyes that undergo a spectral shift when they bind albumin at acid pH. BCP is more specific for albumin compared with BCG. Tetrabromphenol blue and tetrabromosulfophthalein are dyes that have greater affinity for albumin than for globulins and are not sufficiently specific to be used for the measurement of serum albumin.

10. A Penicillin and some other anionic drugs bind to albumin at the same site as the BCG dye, causing falsely low results. Incubation times as long as 2 minutes result in positive interference from globulins, which react with the dye. BCG and BCP are not significantly affected by bilirubin. Lipemic samples may cause positive interference.

11. A When the pH of the solution is above the pI, the protein will have a net negative charge, and therefore migrate to the anode, the positive pole.

12. B In electrophoresis, increasing ionic strength decreases the migration of proteins. Increasing the strength of the field by increasing voltage (or current) increases migration of the charged molecules in electrophoresis.

13. At pH 8.6, the cathodal movement of γ-globulins is caused by:
A. Electroendosmosis
B. Wick flow
C. A net positive charge
D. Cathodal sample application
Chemistry/Electrophoresis/2

14. Which of the following conditions will prevent any migration of proteins across an electrophoretic support medium, such as agarose?
A. Using too high a voltage
B. Excessive current during the procedure
C. Loss of contact between a buffer chamber and the medium
D. Evaporation of solvent from the surface of the medium
Chemistry/Electrophoresis/3

15. Which of the following proteins has the highest isoelectric point (pI)?
A. Albumin
B. Transferrin
C. Ceruloplasmin
D. Immunoglobulin G (IgG)
Chemistry/Electrophoresis/1

16. Which of the following proteins migrates in the β region at pH 8.6?
A. Haptoglobin
B. Orosomucoprotein
C. Antichymotrypsin
D. Transferrin
Chemistry/Electrophoresis/1

17. Which of the following is one advantage of high-resolution (HR) agarose electrophoresis over lower-current electrophoresis?
A. HR procedures detect monoclonal and oligoclonal bands at a lower concentration
B. A smaller sample volume is used
C. Results are obtained more rapidly
D. Densitometric scanning of HR gels is more accurate
Chemistry/Electrophoresis/2

18. Which of the following conditions is associated with "β-γ bridging"?
A. Multiple myeloma
B. Malignancy
C. Hepatic cirrhosis
D. Rheumatoid arthritis
Chemistry/Electrophoresis/Disorders and disease/2

Answers to Questions 13–18

13. A Agarose and cellulose acetate contain fixed anions (e.g., acetate) that attract counter ions when hydrated with buffer. When voltage is applied, the cations migrate to the cathode, creating an osmotic force that draws H_2O with them. This force, called *electroendosmosis,* opposes protein migration toward the anode and may cause some γ-globulins to be displaced toward the cathode.

14. C Movement of proteins is dependent upon the presence of a salt bridge that allows current to flow via transport of ions to the electrodes across the support medium. If the salt bridge is not intact, there will be no migration, even if voltage is maintained across the electrodes.

15. D γ-Globulins are predominantly immunoglobulins and have the highest pI (about 7.2). Albumin has the greatest net negative charge and lowest pI (about 4.6) and is the fastest migrating protein toward the anode at pH 8.6 followed by α_1-, α_2-, β-, and γ-globulins.

16. D Transferrin, β-lipoprotein, C3, and C4 are the dominant proteins in the β-globulin region. Haptoglobin is a protein in the α_2-fraction. Antichymotrypsin and α_1-acid glycoprotein (orosomucoprotein) make up most of the α_1-fraction.

17. A HR agarose procedures use higher current and a cooling device to resolve 12 or more bands. Its disadvantage is that densitometric scans of HR gels usually underestimate albumin.

18. C Hepatic cirrhosis produces a polyclonal gammopathy associated with a high IgA level. This overtakes the valley between β- and γ-zones. Multiple myeloma produces a zone of restricted mobility usually in the γ-region although sometimes in the β- or α_2-region. Malignancy and rheumatoid arthritis produce polyclonal gammopathies classified as chronic inflammatory patterns.

19. Which support medium can be used to determine the molecular weight of a protein?
A. Cellulose acetate
B. Polyacrylamide gel
C. Agar gel
D. Agarose gel
Chemistry/Electrophoresis/2

20. Serum protein and immunofixation electrophoresis (IFE) are ordered. The former is performed, but there is no evidence of monoclonal protein. Select the *best* course of action.
A. Perform quantitative IgG, IgA, and IgM
B. Perform the IFE on the serum
C. Report the result; request a urine sample for protein electrophoresis
D. Perform IFE on the serum and request a urine sample for IFE
Chemistry/Problem solving/3

21. Protein electrophoresis is performed, and all of the proteins have greater anodal mobility than usual. A fast protein is at the edge of the gel, and the bands are blurred. The voltage is set correctly, but the current reading on the ammeter is too low. Select the course of action that would correct this problem.
A. Reduce the voltage
B. Dilute the buffer and adjust the pH
C. Prepare fresh buffer and repeat the test
D. Reduce the running time
Chemistry/Problem solving/3

22. Which of the following stains is used for lipoprotein electrophoresis?
A. Oil Red O
B. Coomassie Brilliant Blue
C. Amido Black
D. Ponceau S
Chemistry/Electrophoresis/1

23. Which of the following serum protein electrophoresis results suggests an acute inflammatory process?

	Albumin	α_1	α_2	β	γ
A.	Decreased	Increased	Decreased	Normal	Normal
B.	Normal	Increased	Normal	Increased	Increased
C.	Decreased	Increased	Increased	Normal	Normal
D.	Increased	Increased	Increased	Increased	Increased

Chemistry/Electrophoresis/Disorders and disease/2

24. Which of the following conditions is usually associated with an acute inflammatory pattern?
A. Myocardial infarction (MI)
B. Malignancy
C. Rheumatoid arthritis
D. Hepatitis
Chemistry/Electrophoresis/Disorders and disease/2

Answers to Questions 19–24

19. B Polyacrylamide gels separate by molecular sieving as well as charge. Polyacrylamide gel electrophoresis (PAGE) after treating with sodium dodecyl sulfate (SDS) separates proteins on the basis of molecular size.

20. C About one of four patients with multiple myeloma have monoclonal free λ- or κ-chains in urine only, and therefore, urine electrophoresis should be included in initial testing.

21. C Increased mobility, decreased resolution, and low current result from low ionic strength. Reducing voltage will slow migration but will not improve resolution. Diluting the buffer will reduce the current, resulting in poorer resolution.

22. A Oil Red O and Sudan Black B stain neutral fats and are used to stain lipoproteins as well as fat in urine or stool. The other stains, Ponceau S, Coomassie Brilliant Blue, and Amido Black, are used for proteins.

23. C Acute inflammation is characterized by increased production of acute-phase proteins. These include α_1-antitrypsin, α_1-acid glycoprotein, α_1-antichymotrypsin, and haptoglobin. Albumin is slightly decreased. γ- and β-fractions are normal.

24. A MI produces a pattern of acute inflammation usually associated with tissue injury. This pattern results from production of acute-phase proteins, including α_1-antitrypsin, α_1-antichymotrypsin, and haptoglobin. Malignancy, rheumatoid arthritis, and hepatitis are associated with a chronic inflammatory pattern.

25. The electrophoretic pattern shown in the following densitometric tracing (shaded gray area) *most* likely indicates:

A. α_1-Antitrypsin deficiency
B. Infection
C. Nephrosis
D. Systemic sclerosis

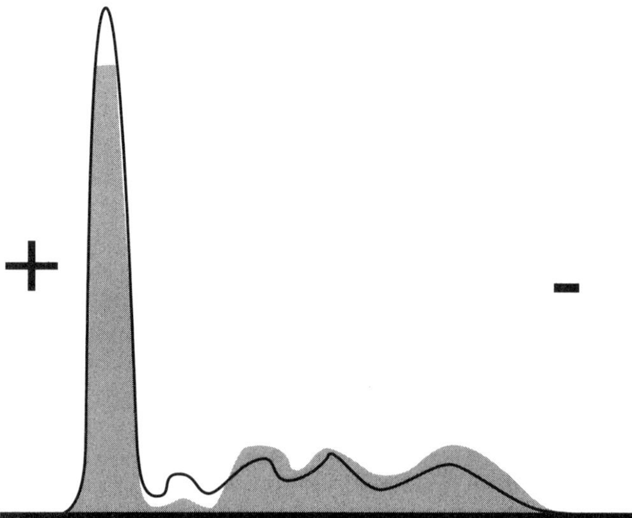

Chemistry/Electrophoresis/Disorders and disease/2

26. What is the clinical utility of testing for serum prealbumin?

A. Low levels are associated with increased free cortisol
B. High levels are an indicator of acute inflammation
C. Serial low levels indicate compromised nutritional status
D. Levels correlate with glomerular injury in patients with diabetes mellitus

Chemistry/Proteins/Prealbumin/1

27. Which serum protein should be measured in a patient suspected of having Wilson disease?

A. Hemopexin
B. α_1-Antitrypsin
C. Haptoglobin
D. Ceruloplasmin

Chemistry/Proteins/Ceruloplasmin/2

28. A patient with hemolytic–uremic syndrome associated with septicemia has a haptoglobin level that is normal, although the plasma free Hgb is elevated, and hemoglobinuria is present. Which test would be more appropriate than haptoglobin to measure this patient's hemolytic episode?

A. Hemopexin
B. α_1-Antitrypsin
C. C-reactive protein (CRP)
D. Transferrin

Chemistry/Proteins/Hemopexin/3

29. Which of the following proteins migrates in the β region at pH 8.6?

A. Haptoglobin
B. Orosomucoprotein
C. Antichymotrypsin
D. Complement C3

Chemistry/Electrophoresis/1

Answers to Questions 25–29

25. A This pattern shows a marked decrease in the α_1-globulin (slightly less than one-fifth of the expected peak area). Staining of the α_1-globulin fraction is predominately determined by the α_1-antitrypsin level.

26. C Prealbumin (also called *transthyretin*) serum levels fall rapidly in patients with deficient protein nutrition. As a result, prealbumin is used to detect malnutrition and to measure the patient's response to dietary supplementation.

27. D Ceruloplasmin is an α_2-globulin that binds most of the serum copper. Levels are low in almost all patients with Wilson disease, an autosomal recessive disorder caused by accumulation of copper in liver, brain, kidney, and other tissues. α_1-Antitrypsin, and haptoglobin are acute-phase proteins and will be increased in inflammatory diseases. Hemopexin is a hemoglobin scavenger.

28. A Hemopexin is a small β-globulin that binds to free heme. Haptoglobin is an acute-phase protein, and hepatic production and release are also increased in response to acute infections.

29. D Transferrin, β-lipoprotein, C3, and C4 are the dominant proteins in the β-globulin region. Haptoglobin is a protein in the α_2-fraction. Antichymotrypsin, and α_1-acid glycoprotein (orosomucoprotein) make up most of the α_1-fraction.

30. Given the serum protein electrophoresis patterns shown, which transaminase results would you expect?

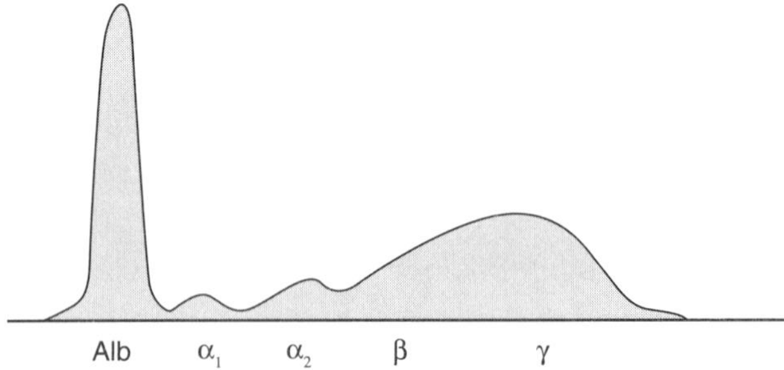

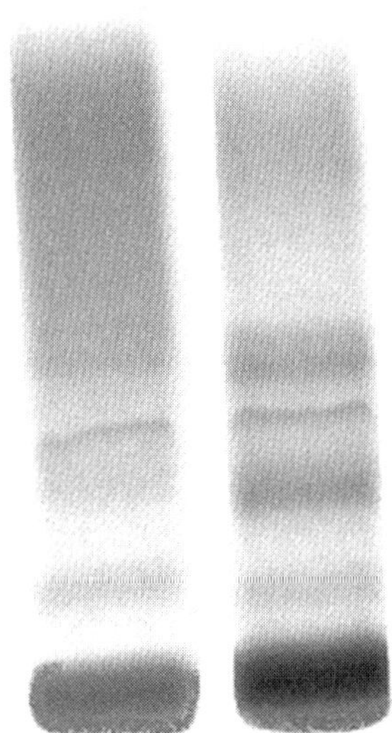

A. Within normal limits for both
B. Marked elevation of both (20–50-fold normal)
C. Mild elevations of both (two- to fivefold normal)
D. Marked elevation of AST but normal ALT

Chemistry/Problem solving/2

31. Alpha fetal protein (AFP) measured in the serum of a 30-year-old pregnant woman at approximately 12 weeks' gestation is 2.5 multiples of the median (MOM). What course of action is *most* appropriate?

A. Repeat the serum AFP in 2 weeks
B. Recommend AFP assay on amniotic fluid
C. Repeat the AFP using the same sample by another method
D. Repeat the AFP using the same sample by the same method

Chemistry/Problem solving/3

32. The reference method of cholesterol determination is:

A. Electrophoresis using polyacrylamide gel
B. GC-MS
C. Isotope dilution mass spectrometry (IDMS)
D. LC-MS

Chemistry/Cholesterol/1

33. This substance is classified as a glycolipid:

A. Chylomicron
B. Lecithin
C. Sphingomyelin
D. Cerebroside

Chemistry/Cholesterol/1

Answers to Questions 30–33

30. C The densitometric scan shows β–γ bridging that supports a diagnosis of hepatic cirrhosis. In this condition one would expect two- to fivefold increases of both transaminases with an ALT:AST ratio below 1.0. The protein electrophoresis and densitometric scan show a significantly reduced albumin and polyclonal gammopathy.

31. A To achieve the needed sensitivity, the test should be repeated at 14 weeks. The analytical sensitivity of immunochemical AFP tests is approximately 5.0 ng/mL. The maternal serum AFP at 12 weeks' gestation is barely above the analytical detection limit. AFP normally first becomes detectable in maternal serum at week 12 and increases by 15% per week through the 26th week of pregnancy.

32. B The GC-MS method involves the hydrolysis of fatty acids on triglycerides and the measurement of glycerol without detection of related sterols. This method agrees with the gold standard of IDMS as applied at the U.S. NIST (National Institute of Standards and Technology).

33. D Cerebroside is a simple glycolipid, also called a *monoglycosylceramide*, necessary for muscles and nerve cell membranes. Chylomicron is a lipoprotein, while lecithin and sphingomyelin are both phospholipids.

34. Identify the order of migration (migration toward the anode from the origin) for lipoprotein electrophoresis in polyacrylamide gel.

A. At the anode, chylomicrons, followed by β-, pre-β-, and α-lipoproteins
B. At the anode, chylomicrons, followed by α-, pre-β-, and β-lipoproteins
C. At the anode, α-lipoproteins followed by pre-β- and β-lipoproteins, then chylomicrons at the cathode origin
D. At the anode, pre-β- and β-lipoproteins, followed by α-lipoproteins, then chylomicrons at the origin near the cathode

Chemistry/Lipoproteins/Analytical methods/1

35. Apolipoprotein (apo) A-I is primarily located within this lipoprotein:

A. Chylomicrons
B. Very low-density lipoprotein (VLDL)
C. Lipoprotein X
D. High-density lipoprotein (HDL)

Chemistry/Lipoproteins/1

36. Which statement *best* describes IFE?

A. Proteins are separated by electrophoresis followed by overlay of monospecific anti-immunoglobulins
B. Proteins react with monospecific antisera followed by electrophoresis
C. Antisera are electrophoresed and then diffused against the patient's serum
D. Serum is electrophoresed; the separated immunoglobulins diffuse against specific antisera placed into troughs

Chemistry/Electrophoresis/2

37. Electrophoresis was performed on both serum and spinal fluid from a patient. The CSF showed distinct oligoclonal banding in the γ region, while the serum of the same patient did not exhibit the same banding. What is the significance of the banding in the CSF electrophoretic pattern?

A. IgG is present in the CSF due to multiple sclerosis
B. The serum electrophoresis is inconclusive and should be repeated
C. This is not significant as the amount of IgG in CSF is typically higher than that in serum
D. This CSF is most likely mislabeled

Chemistry/Electrophoresis/Disorders and disease/2

38. Which of the following statements regarding the identification of monoclonal proteins by IFE is true?

A. The monoclonal band must be present in the γ region
B. When testing for a monoclonal gammopathy, both serum and urine must be examined
C. A diagnosis of monoclonal gammopathy is based upon quantitation of IgG, IgA, and IgM
D. A monoclonal band always indicates a malignant disorder

Chemistry/Electrophoresis/2

39. Which of the following statements regarding paraproteins is true?

A. Oligoclonal banding is seen in the CSF of greater than 90% of patients with multiple sclerosis
B. The Bence-Jones protein heat test is confirmatory for monoclonal light chains
C. Light chains found in urine are always derived from monoclonal protein
D. The IgA band is usually cathodal to the IgG precipitin band

Chemistry/Proteins/2

Answers to Questions 34–39

34. C On electrophoresis, migration occurs toward the anode, with α-lipoproteins, followed by pre-β- and β-lipoproteins, then chylomicrons near or at the origin.

35. D HDL contains two molecules of apolipoprotein A-I in a ring form around the central phospholipid and cholesterol bilayer.

36. A Immunofixation electrophoresis (IFE) is performed on the serum or urine sample in the same manner as for protein electrophoresis. After the proteins are separated, a monospecific antiserum is applied across the surface to form immune complexes.

37. A In the electrophoretic pattern of CSF from patients with a multiple sclerosis diagnosis, multiple oligoclonal bands may be present in the γ region, indicating a production of IgG in the CSF.

38. B Because monoclonal light chains are filtered by the glomerulus, the procedure must be performed on urine as well as serum. Quantitation of IgG, IgA, and IgM indicates the concentration of each class of immunoglobulin but does not distinguish monoclonal gammopathies from polyclonal gammopathies.

39. A Oligoclonal banding is seen in the CSF of more than 90% of patients with multiple sclerosis.

40. Which statement regarding IFE is true?
A. Serum containing a monoclonal protein should have a κ:λ ratio of 0.5
B. A monoclonal band seen with monospecific antiserum should not be visible in the lane where polyvalent antiserum or sulfosalicylic acid was added
C. CSF should be concentrated 50- to 100-fold before performing IFE
D. When oligoclonal bands are seen in CSF, they must also be present in serum to indicate multiple sclerosis
Chemistry/Electrophoresis/2

41. Which test is the *most* sensitive in detecting early monoclonal gammopathies?
A. HR serum protein electrophoresis
B. Urinary electrophoresis for monoclonal light chains
C. Capillary electrophoresis of serum and urine
D. Serum-free light chain immunoassay
Chemistry/Proteins/Disorders and disease/2

42. Which test is the *most* useful way to evaluate the response to treatment for multiple myeloma?
A. Measure of total immunoglobulin
B. Measurement of 24-hour urinary light chain concentration (Bence-Jones protein)
C. Capillary electrophoresis to detect M-protein recurrence
D. Measurement of serum-free light chains
Chemistry/Proteins/Disorders and disease/2

43. Which of the following is more commonly associated with a monoclonal gammopathy of undetermined significance (MGUS)?
A. Bone marrow plasma cells comprise 20% of nucleated cells
B. Monoclonal protein (M-protein) concentration is 3.5 g/dL
C. M-protein is IgG
D. Age greater than 60 at the time of monoclonal protein discovery
Chemistry/Proteins/Disorders and disease/2

44. Select the order of mobility of lipoproteins electrophoresed on agarose at pH 8.6.
A. – Chylomicrons → pre-β → β → α +
B. – β → pre-β → α → chylomicrons +
C. – Chylomicrons → β → pre-β → α +
D. – α → β → pre-β → chylomicrons +
Chemistry/Lipids/Lipoproteins/1

45. Following ultracentrifugation of plasma, which fraction correlates with pre-β-lipoprotein?
A. VLDL
B. Low-density lipoprotein (LDL)
C. HDL
D. Chylomicrons
Chemistry/Lipids/Lipoprotein/2

46. Select the lipoprotein fraction that carries most of the endogenous triglycerides.
A. VLDL
B. LDL
C. HDL
D. Chylomicrons
Chemistry/Lipids/Lipoproteins/2

47. Which lipoprotein accumulates in familial β-dyslipoproteinemia?
A. Chylomicrons
B. VLDL
C. Intermediate-density lipoprotein (IDL)
D. HDL
Chemistry/Lipids/Disorders and disease/1

Answers to Questions 40–47

40. C CSF is usually concentrated 50 to 100 times to increase sensitivity.

41. D Measurement of free light chains is recommended along with protein electrophoresis when testing for myeloma. Immunonephelometric free light chain assays will be positive only in cases where monoclonal light chain production occurs.

42. D Serum-free light chain assays are quantitative and an increase in free light chain production with an abnormal κ:λ ratio occurs earliest in recurrence of myeloma.

43. D About 3% of the U.S. population at age 50 years and 5% at age 70 years have MGUS.

44. C β-Lipoprotein migrates faster on agarose or cellulose acetate because of its more negative apoprotein composition.

45. A VLDL migrates in the pre-β-lipoprotein zone.

46. A VLDL transports the majority of endogenous triglycerides, whereas the triglycerides of chylomicrons are derived entirely from dietary absorption.

47. C IDL has roughly equal amounts of cholesterol and triglyceride. Familial dysbetalipoproteinemia is, in part, caused by a polymorphism of apo E (apo E_2) that has poor affinity for the apo E receptor on hepatocytes.

48. Which of the following mechanisms accounts for the elevated plasma level of β-lipoproteins seen in familial hypercholesterolemia?
A. Hyperinsulinemia
B. ApoB-100 receptor defect
C. ApoC-II activated lipase deficiency
D. ApoE$_3$ deficiency
Chemistry/Lipids/Disorders and disease/2

49. Which enzyme deficiency is *most* commonly associated with familial hypertriglyceridemia associated with fasting plasma chylomicrons?
A. β-Glucocerebrosidase deficiency
B. Lipoprotein lipase deficiency
C. Apo B deficiency
D. Apo C-III deficiency
Chemistry/Lipids/Disorders and disease/2

50. Which of the following conditions is *most* consistently associated with secondary hypercholesterolemia?
A. Hypothyroidism
B. Pancreatitis
C. Oral contraceptive therapy
D. Diabetes mellitus
Chemistry/Lipids/Cholesterol/2

51. Which of the following is associated with Tangier disease?
A. Apo C-II deficiency
B. Homozygous apo B-100 deficiency
C. Apo C-II activated lipase
D. Apo A-I deficiency
Chemistry/Lipids/Disorders and disease/2

52. Which of the following statements describes the endogenous metabolic pathway for lipids?
A. Intestinal enzymes catabolize cholesterol and triglyceride to enter the mucosal cells as micelles
B. Chylomicrons are secreted into the lymph for systemic circulation
C. Dietary triglycerides are hydrolyzed to free fatty acids by lipase and bile acids
D. VLDL and LDL are synthesized in the liver then re-enter peripheral circulation
Chemistry/Lipids/2

53. What is the lipid testing protocol for adults recommended by the National Cholesterol Education Program (NCEP) to evaluate risk for atherosclerosis beginning at age 20 years?
A. Total cholesterol every year
B. Total cholesterol every 2 years
C. Lipid profile every 5 years
D. LDL cholesterol every 2 years
Chemistry/Lipids/1

Answers to Questions 48–53

48. B The production of excess insulin leads to hypertriglyceridemia and is one mechanism responsible for familial endogenous hypertriglyceridemia. Hypercholesterolemia occurs as a result of a mutation of the apo B-100. Apo C-II is an activator of lipoprotein lipase, and a homozygous deficiency results in high plasma chylomicrons and VLDL. Apo E$_3$ deficiency can lead to β-dyslipoproteinemia.

49. B Deficiency of capillary endothelial lipase is the most common cause of fasting chylomicronemia. β-Glucocerebrosidase deficiency results in accumulation of glucocerebrosides. Apo C-II is associated with hypertriglyceridemia. Apo B deficiency is responsible for hypobetalipoproteinemia.

50. A The conditions listed are very commonly encountered causes of secondary hyperlipoproteinemia. Hypothyroidism is usually associated with secondary hypercholesterolemia. Oral contraceptives, pregnancy, and estrogens may cause secondary hypertriglyceridemia. Diabetes mellitus and chronic pancreatitis may produce hypertriglyceridemia.

51. D Deficiency of apo A-I is seen in Tangier disease, a familial hypocholesterolemia. Heterozygotes have about half of the normal level of HDL (familial hypoalphalipoproteinemia), and homozygotes have almost no detectable HDL.

52. D In the endogenous pathway of lipid metabolism, hepatic lipoprotein synthesis converts chylomicrons to VLDL. Through enzymatic processes, VLDL transfers phospholipids and apolipoproteins to other lipoprotein particles, resulting in the conversion of VLDL, ultimately producing LDL.

53. C The NCEP recommends a lipid profile that includes triglycerides, total cholesterol, HDL cholesterol, and LDL cholesterol should be performed every 5 years beginning at age 20 years.

54. What is the *most* appropriate procedure when a fasting lipid study of triglyceride, total cholesterol, HDL cholesterol, and LDL cholesterol tests are ordered?

A. 8 hours; nothing but water allowed
B. 10 hours; water, smoking, coffee, tea (no sugar or cream) allowed
C. 12 hours; nothing but water allowed
D. 16 hours; water, smoking, coffee, tea (no sugar or cream) allowed

Chemistry/Lipids/1

55. Treatment recommendations for patients with coronary heart disease are based on the measurement of which analyte?

A. HDL cholesterol
B. Apo B-100
C. LDL cholesterol
D. Total cholesterol

Chemistry/Lipids/1

56. What is the HDL cholesterol cutoff that constitutes a risk factor for coronary artery disease (CAD) as recommended by NCEP?

A. Less than 30 mg/dL
B. Less than 40 mg/dL
C. Less than 30 mg/dL for males and less than 40 mg/dL for females
D. Less than 45 mg/dL for males and less than 50 mg/dL for females

Chemistry/Lipids/Lipoproteins/1

57. An EDTA blood sample is collected at the physician's office from a nonfasting person for a complete blood count (CBC). Someone from the office called the laboratory 15 minutes after the sample arrived from the courier and requested a lipid study, including triglyceride, total cholesterol, HDL cholesterol, and LDL cholesterol. Which test results should be used to evaluate the patient's risk for CAD?

A. Total cholesterol and LDL cholesterol
B. LDL cholesterol and triglyceride
C. Total cholesterol and HDL cholesterol
D. All four lipid results can be used if the nonfasting triglyceride level is less than 200 mg/dL

Chemistry/Lipids/3

58. Which mutation results in high levels of LDL cholesterol?

A. Lipoprotein lipase (*LPL*)
B. Apoprotein A1 (*APOA1*)
C. Proprotein convertase subtilisin/kexintype 9 (*PCSK9*)
D. Lipin1 (*LPIN1*)

Chemistry/Lipids/Lipoproteins/2

59. Which of the following diseases is caused by a deficiency of sphingomyelinase?

A. Gaucher disease
B. Fabry disease
C. Niemann-Pick disease
D. Tay-Sachs disease

Chemistry/Lipids/Disorders and disease/2

Answers to Questions 54–59

54. C Lipid orders that include fasting triglyceride and LDL cholesterol should be performed by using a plasma or serum specimen whenever possible. A 12- to 14-hour fast is preferred, especially when nonfasting lipids are high. The patient should be instructed to drink nothing but water during this period. Fasting specimens are preferred for total cholesterol and HDL cholesterol as well, but nonfasting specimens may be used for initial screening purposes.

55. C The NECP has identified LDL cholesterol as the target of therapy for reducing the risk of heart attack because lowering LDL cholesterol has proved to be an effective intervention.

56. B The HDL cholesterol cutoff recommended by NCEP is less than 40 mg/dL, regardless of gender. A result below 40 mg/dL counts as a risk factor for CAD.

57. D The American Heart Association (AHA) prefers a 12-hour fasting sample when screening persons for risk of CAD. However, if a fasting sample is unavailable, the AHA recommends performing the lipid panel with a nonfasting sample, provided the triglyceride levels are less than 200 mg/dL.

58. C Mutations of *PCSK9* can result in overexpression of the PCSK9 protein, which binds to the LDL receptor on cells and downregulates it. This results in an accumulation of LDL cholesterol in plasma. *LPL* mutations cause hypertriglyceridemia. *APOA1* mutations cause low HDL. Homozygous *LPIN1* mutations are very rare and cause childhood rhabdomyolysis.

59. C Niemann-Pick disease results from a deficiency of sphingomyelinase; Gaucher disease from β-glucocerebrosidase; Fabry disease (sex-linked) from α-galactosidase A; and Tay-Sachs from N-acetylglucosaminidase A.

60. Which of the following enzymes is common to all enzymatic methods for triglyceride measurement?
A. Glycerol phosphate oxidase
B. Glycerol phosphate dehydrogenase
C. Glycerol kinase
D. Pyruvate kinase
Chemistry/Lipids/Analytical methods/2

61. What is the purpose of the saponification step used in the Abell-Kendall method for cholesterol measurement?
A. Remove phospholipids
B. Reduce sterol molecules structurally similar to cholesterol
C. Convert cholesterol esters to free cholesterol
D. Remove proteins that can interfere with color formation
Chemistry/Lipids/Analytical methods/2

62. Which of the following methods for HDL cholesterol is the reference method?
A. Electrophoresis in polyacrylamide gel
B. Magnesium–phosphotungstate precipitation
C. Magnesium–dextran precipitation
D. Manganese-heparin-chloride precipitation
Chemistry/Lipids/Analytical methods/1

63. Cholesterol esterase is used in enzymatic assays to:
A. Oxidize cholesterol to form peroxide
B. Hydrolyze fatty acids bound to the third carbon atom of cholesterol
C. Separate cholesterol from apo A-I and apo A-II by hydrolysis
D. Reduce NAD^+ to NADH
Chemistry/Lipids/Analytical methods/2

64. Which of the following reagents is used in the homogeneous HDL cholesterol method?
A. Sulfated α-cyclodextrin
B. Magnesium sulfate and dextran sulfate
C. Anti-apo A-I
D. Manganese heparin
Chemistry/Lipids/Analytical methods/2

65. What do direct methods for LDL cholesterol assay have in common?
A. They are inaccurate when plasma triglyceride is above 250 mg/dL
B. All use a detergent to facilitate selective reactivity with reagent enzymes
C. All use monoclonal antibodies to apo A-I and apo C
D. All are free of interference from abnormal lipoproteins
Chemistry/Lipids/Analytical methods/2

66. Lipoprotein (a), or Lp(a), is significant when elevated in serum because it:
A. Is an independent risk factor for atherosclerosis
B. Blocks the clearance of VLDLs
C. Displaces apo A-I from HDLs
D. Is linked closely to a gene for obesity
Chemistry/Lipids/Lipoproteins/1

Answers to Questions 60–66

60. C All enzymatic triglyceride methods require lipase to hydrolyze triglycerides, and glycerol kinase to phosphorylate glycerol, forming glycerol-3-phosphate and adenosine diphosphate (ADP). The most common method couples glycerol kinase (GK) with glycerol phosphate oxidase (GPO) and peroxidase (Px) via the following reactions:
1. Triglyceride + $H_2O \xrightarrow{\text{Lipase}}$ glycerol + fatty acids
2. Glycerol + ATP $\xrightarrow{\text{GK}}$ glycerol-3-phosphate + ADP
3. Glycerol-3-phosphate + $O_2 \xrightarrow{\text{GPO}}$ dihydroxyacetone phosphate + H_2O_2
4. H_2O_2 + phenol + 4-aminophenazone $\xrightarrow{\text{PX}}$ quinoneimine dye + H_2O

61. C The Abell–Kendall method utilizes saponification to hydrolyze the fatty acid esters of cholesterol, forming free cholesterol.

62. D Ultracentrifugation of plasma is used first to remove VLDL that can block the complete precipitation of LDL. This is followed by precipitation of LDL and other non-HDL lipoproteins in the bottom layer with manganese-heparin-chloride.

63. B Cholesterol esterase hydrolyzes fatty acids and is required because cholesterol oxidase cannot utilize esterified cholesterol as a substrate.

64. A The homogeneous HDL cholesterol method uses cholesterol esterase and oxidase enzymes conjugated to polyethylene glycol (PEG). In the presence of sulfated α-cyclodextrin, the enzymes do not react with non-HDL cholesterol molecules.

65. B The direct LDL cholesterol assays are all detergent-based methods.

66. A Lp(a) is a complex of apo B-100 and protein (a) and is thought to promote coronary heart disease by interfering with the normal fibrinolytic process.

67. Which type of dietary fatty acid is *not* associated with an increase in serum LDL cholesterol production?

A. Monounsaturated *trans* fatty acids
B. Saturated fatty acids
C. Monounsaturated *cis* fatty acids
D. Monounsaturated *trans* omega-9 fatty acids

Chemistry/Lipids/1

68. A lipemic specimen collected from an adult after a 12-hour fast was assayed for total cholesterol, triglycerides, and HDL cholesterol by using a direct HDL method. Following are the results:

Total cholesterol = 220 mg/dL
HDL cholesterol = 40 mg/dL
Triglyceride = 420 mg/dL

The physician requests an LDL cholesterol assay after receiving the results. How should the LDL cholesterol be determined?

A. Dilute the specimen 1:10 and repeat all tests. Calculate LDL cholesterol using the Friedewald equation
B. Perform a direct LDL cholesterol assay
C. Ultracentrifuge the sample and repeat the HDL cholesterol on the infranatant. Use the new result to calculate the LDL cholesterol
D. Repeat the HDL cholesterol using the manganese–heparin precipitation method. Use the new result to calculate the LDL cholesterol

Chemistry/Lipids/3

69. A person has a fasting triglyceride level of 240 mg/dL. The physician wishes to know the patient's non-HDL cholesterol level. What cholesterol fractions should be measured?

A. Total cholesterol and HDL cholesterol
B. Total cholesterol and LDL cholesterol
C. HDL cholesterol and LDL cholesterol
D. Total cholesterol and chylomicrons

Chemistry/Lipids/3

Answers to Questions 67–69

67. C Monounsaturated *cis* fatty acids are not associated with increased production of LDL cholesterol. Saturated and *trans* monounsaturated fatty acids are both associated with increased LDL.

68. B An accurate LDL cholesterol can be reported if the direct method for LDL cholesterol is employed. These methods are not subject to interference by triglycerides at a concentration below 700 mg/dL.

69. A When HDL cholesterol is subtracted from total cholesterol, the result is called *non-HDL cholesterol*. This result includes LDL cholesterol, VLDL cholesterol, and atherogenic remnant lipoproteins.

6.6

Enzymes and Cardiac Markers

1. An international unit (IU) of enzyme activity is the quantity of enzyme that:
A. Converts 1 µmol of substrate to product per liter
B. Forms 1 mg of product per deciliter
C. Converts 1 µmol of substrate to product per minute
D. Forms 1 µmol of product per deciliter
Chemistry/Enzymes/1

2. Which of the following measurement modes does *not* allow continuous monitoring of enzyme activity?
A. Initial absorbance is measured followed by a second reading after 5 minutes
B. Absorbance is measured at 10-second intervals for 100 seconds
C. Absorbance is monitored continuously for 1 minute using a chart recorder
D. Reflectance is measured from a xenon source lamp pulsing at 60 Hz
Chemistry/Enzymes/Enzyme kinetics/2

3. Which of the following statements regarding enzymatic reactions is true?
A. The enzyme shifts the equilibrium of the reaction to the right
B. The enzyme alters the equilibrium constant of the reaction
C. The enzyme increases the rate of the reaction
D. The enzyme alters the energy difference between reactants and products
Chemistry/Enzymes/Enzyme kinetics/1

4. Which statement about enzymes is true?
A. An enzyme alters the free energy of the reaction
B. Enzymes cause a reaction with positive free energy to occur spontaneously
C. An enzyme's natural substrate has the highest K_m
D. A competitive inhibitor will alter the apparent K_m of the reaction
Chemistry/Enzymes/2

5. Of the following, which is an example of an enzyme classified as an oxidoreductase?
A. LDH
B. AST
C. Aldolase
D. ALP
Chemistry/Enzymes/1

Answers to Questions 1–5

1. C The international unit is a rate expressed in micromoles per minute. Activity is reported as international units per liter (IU/L) or milli–international units per milliliter (mIU/mL).

2. A A kinetic assay uses several evenly spaced absorbance measurements to calculate the change in absorbance per unit time.

3. C An enzyme will accelerate the rate of a reaction, reducing the time required to reach equilibrium. The concentration of reactants and products at equilibrium will be the same with or without the enzyme.

4. D Competitive inhibitors bind to the active site where the enzyme binds substrate and are overcome by increasing the substrate concentration. Enzymes alter the energy of activation by forming the enzyme substrate complex. Enzymes do not alter the free energy or direction of a reaction.

5. A Lactate dehydrogenase, LDH, is classified as an oxidoreductase. It is a hydrogen transfer enzyme that uses the coenzyme NAD+ to catalyze lactate to pyruvate. The enzyme AST is classified as a transferase, aldolase is classified as a lyase, and ALP is an example of a hydrolase enzyme.

6. Which of the following enzymes is classified as a hydrolase enzyme?
A. ALP
B. LD
C. CK
D. AST

Chemistry/Enzymes/1

7. Which of the following statements is true?
A. Apoenzyme + prosthetic group = holoenzyme
B. A coenzyme is an inorganic molecule required for activity
C. Cofactors are as tightly bound to the enzyme as prosthetic groups
D. All enzymes have optimal activity at pH 7.00

Chemistry/Enzymes/2

8. Which of the following statements about enzymatic reactions is true?
A. NADH has absorbance maxima at 340 and 366 nm
B. Enzyme concentration must be in excess to achieve zero-order kinetics
C. Rate is proportional to substrate concentration in a zero-order reaction
D. Accumulation of the product increases the reaction rate

Chemistry/Enzymes/Enzyme kinetics/2

9. The increase in the level of serum enzymes used to detect cholestatic liver disease is caused mainly by:
A. Enzyme release from dead cells
B. Leakage from cells with altered membrane permeability
C. Decreased perfusion of the tissue
D. Increased production and secretion by cells

Chemistry/Enzymes/Disorders and disease/2

10. How would you classify NADH in terms of enzymatic properties?
A. NADH is a coenzyme in enzymatic reactions
B. NADH is a cofactor in enzymatic reactions
C. NADH is an apoenzyme in enzymatic reactions
D. NADH is an activator in enzymatic reactions

Chemistry/Enzymes/1

11. Which statement describes the effect of temperature on enzymatic activity?
A. For each 5-degree increase in temperature, the rate of enzymatic reaction increases threefold
B. For each 10-degree increase in temperature, the rate of enzymatic reaction will double
C. Denaturation of enzymes is significant after 4 hours at 6°C
D. Denaturation of enzymes is significant at temperatures below 4°C

Chemistry/Enzymes/1

Answers to Questions 6–11

6. A ALP catalyzes the hydrolysis of various phosphomonoesters at an alkaline pH. The enzymes AST and CK are classified as transferase enzymes, while LD is considered an oxidoreductase enzyme.

7. A A holoenzyme is a complete and active system in which the apoenzyme (the protein portion) is bound to the prosthetic group (the coenzyme that is tightly bound to the enzyme). A coenzyme is an organic molecule required for full enzyme activity. Cofactors are inorganic atoms or molecules needed for full catalytic activity. Enzymes can have diverse pH (and temperature) optima.

8. A Most enzymes are measured by monitoring the rate of absorbance change at 340 nm as NADH is produced or consumed. This rate will be proportional to enzyme activity when substrate is in excess. When the enzyme is present in excess, the initial reaction rate will be proportional to substrate concentration.

9. D The amount of enzyme in the serum can be increased by necrosis, altered permeability, secretion, or synthesis.

10. A A coenzyme is an organic cofactor in enzymatic reaction and includes nicotinamide adenine dinucleotide, NADH. Cofactors are nonprotein molecules. An apoenzyme includes the protein portion of an enzyme and its cofactor, while an activator binds to the enzyme to increase enzymatic activity.

11. B For each 10-degree rise in temperature the rate of the enzymatic reaction will approximately double, until denaturation occurs at between 40°C to 50°C. Low temperatures inactivate enzymes and serum or plasma samples can be refrigerated or frozen until analyzed.

12. Which of the following enzymes is activated by calcium ions?
A. CK
B. Amylase
C. ALP
D. LDH
Chemistry/Enzymes/2

13. Which of the following enzymes is a transferase?
A. ALP
B. CK
C. Amylase
D. LDH
Chemistry/Enzymes/2

14. Which statement about methods for measuring LDH is true?
A. The formation of pyruvate from lactate (forward reaction) generates NAD^+
B. The pyruvate-to-lactate reaction proceeds at about twice the rate as the forward reaction
C. The lactate-to-pyruvate reaction is optimized at pH 7.4
D. The negative-rate reaction is preferred
Chemistry/Enzymes/LDH/2

15. Which condition produces the highest elevation of serum LD?
A. Pernicious anemia
B. MI
C. Acute hepatitis
D. Muscular dystrophy
Chemistry/Enzymes/Disorders and disease/LD/2

16. In which condition is the LD *most* likely to be within normal limits?
A. Hepatic carcinoma
B. Pulmonary infarction
C. Acute appendicitis
D. Crush injury
Chemistry/Enzymes/Disorders and disease/LD/2

17. The LD pleural fluid:serum ratio for a transudative fluid is usually:
A. 3:1 or higher
B. 2:1
C. 1:1
D. 1:2 or less
Chemistry/Enzymes/Disorders and disease/LD/2

18. Which disorder would produce the greatest increase in both LD-4 and LD-5?
A. Hemolytic anemia
B. Pulmonary embolism
C. Hepatocellular carcinoma
D. Acute myocardial infarction (AMI)
Chemistry/Enzymes/Disorders and disease/LD/2

19. Which of the following conditions will interfere with the measurement of LD?
A. Slight hemolysis during sample collection
B. Storage at 4°C for 3 days
C. Storage at room temperature for 16 hours
D. Use of plasma collected in heparin
Chemistry/Enzymes/Analytical methods/3

Answers to Questions 12–19

12. B The enzyme amylase requires Ca^{+2}. CK and ALP require Mg^{+2} for full activity.

13. B CK, creatine kinase, along with transaminases, are transferase enzymes.

14. B Although the rate of the reverse reaction (pyruvate → lactate) is faster, the lactate → pyruvate reaction is more popular because it produces a positive rate (generates NADH), is not subject to product inhibition, and is highly linear. The optimal pH for the forward reaction is approximately 8.8.

15. A Serum LD levels are highest in pernicious anemia, reaching 10 to 50 times the URL as a result of intramedullary hemolysis. Moderate elevations (5–10 × URL) usually are seen in acute myocardial infarction (AMI), necrotic liver disease, and muscular dystrophy. Slight increases (2–3 × URL) are sometimes seen in obstructive liver disease.

16. C LD-3 may be only slightly elevated with acute appendicitis. The greatest increase for LD is seen in hepatic carcinoma. LD is also increased in crush injury and muscular dystrophies because of skeletal muscle damage, and in pulmonary infarction resulting from embolism formation.

17. D The LD activity of body fluids is normally less than half that of serum, and a fluid:serum LD ratio greater than 1:2 is highly suggestive of an exudative process.

18. C Liver disease produces an elevated LD-4 and LD-5 with levels reaching up to 10 times the URL in toxic hepatitis and in hepatocellular carcinoma. RBCs are rich in LD-1 and LD-2, and an increased concentration is present in both hemolytic processes and MI. LD-3 increases would be associated with conditions with pulmonary involvement.

19. A RBCs are rich in LD-1 and LD-2, and even slight hemolysis will falsely elevate results. LD is stable for 2 days at room temperature or 1 week at 4°C; however, freezing causes deterioration of LD-5. The activity of LD is inhibited by EDTA; serum or heparinized plasma should be used.

20. A plasma sample from an adult male in a coma as a result of an automobile collision gave the following results:

Total CK = 480 IU/L	CK-MB = 8 μg/L
Myoglobin = 800 μg/L	Troponin I = 2.1 ng/L

What is the *best* interpretation of these results?

A. The person had a heart attack that caused the collision
B. The collision caused traumatic injury, but no heart attack occurred.
C. A heart attack occurred in addition to a stroke
D. It is not possible to tell whether a heart attack has occurred because of the extensive trauma

Chemistry/Enzymes/Disorders and disease/3

21. A specimen for CK performed on an automated analyzer using an optimized Oliver-Rosalki method gives an error flag indicating substrate depletion. The sample is diluted 1:2 and 1:4 by the serial dilution technique and reassayed. After correcting for the dilution, the results are as follows:

1:2 dilution = 3,000 IU/L	1:4 dilution = 3,600 IU/L

Dilutions are made a second time and assayed again but give identical results. What is the *most* likely explanation?

A. The serum became contaminated prior to making the 1:4 dilution
B. The wrong pipet was used to make one of the dilutions
C. An endogenous competitive inhibitor is present in the serum
D. An error has been made in calculating the enzyme activity of one of the two dilutions

Chemistry/Enzymes/CK/3

22. A physician calls to request a CK on a sample already sent to the laboratory for coagulation studies. The sample is 2-hour-old citrated blood and has been stored at 4°C. The plasma shows a hemolytic index of 0.5% hemolysis. The sample was determined to be inadequate, and a new specimen was requested. What is the primary reason for the recollection?

A. The sample could not be used because it was too old
B. The sample could not be used because it is slightly hemolyzed
C. The sample could not be used because it has been stored refrigerated
D. The sample could not be used because the citrate will interfere with testing

Chemistry/Enzymes/CK/3

23. Which of the following statements regarding total CK is true?

A. Levels are unaffected by strenuous exercise
B. Levels are unaffected by repeated intramuscular injections
C. Highest levels are seen in Duchenne muscular dystrophy
D. The enzyme is highly specific for heart injury

Chemistry/Enzymes/CK/2

Answers to Questions 20–23

20. B The automobile collision caused skeletal muscle damage (myoglobin and total CK increases). The CK relative index is 1.6, which is lower than would be expected if the CK-MB were derived from heart damage. Because the TnI is within normal limits, the slight increase in CK-MB is attributed to the gross increase in release of CK from skeletal muscle.

21. C When a competitive inhibitor is present in serum, a dilution of the sample will cause an increase in the reaction rate by reducing the concentration of the inhibitor. Dilution of serum frequently increases the activity of CK and amylase. The same effect will occur when a smaller volume of serum is used in the assay because less inhibitor will be present in the reaction mixture.

22. D The plasma sample was rejected because of being collected in a blue-top sodium citrate tube, which chelates both calcium and magnesium. CK in serum is stable at room temperature for about 4 hours and up to 1 week at 4°C. Slight hemolysis does not interfere; however, significant hemolysis may cause positive interference by contributing adenylate kinase to the serum.

23. C Crush injuries and muscular dystrophy can increase the total CK up to 50 times the URL. Total CK is neither sensitive nor specific for AMI, and an infarct can occur without causing an elevated total CK. Exercise and intramuscular injections can cause a significant increase in total CK.

24. A patient's CK-MB isoenzyme concentration is reported as 18 μg/L and the total CK as 560 IU/L. What is the CK relative index (CKI)?

A. 0.10%
B. 3.2%
C. 10.0%
D. 30.0%

Chemistry/Enzymes/CK/2

25. In a nonmyocardial condition such as muscular dystrophy causing an increased serum CK-MB, which would be expected?

A. An increase in CK-MB that is persistent
B. An increase in the percent CK-BB with an increase in CK-MB
C. The presence of increased troponin I (TnI)
D. A pronounced increase in total CK than CK-MB

Chemistry/Enzymes/Disorders and disease/2

26. Which statement *best* describes the clinical utility of plasma or serum myoglobin?

A. Assessment of nephrotic syndrome
B. Assessment of cardiac injury
C. Assessment of hemolytic anemia
D. Assessment of pulmonary infarction

Chemistry/Cardiac markers/Myoglobin/2

27. Which statement *best* describes cardiac troponin I and T?

A. An enzyme embedded in the endocardium released after MI
B. Two polypeptides that regulate the sliding of contractile proteins in cardiac muscle
C. A peptide that is released in response to ventricular stretching
D. A prohormone released from the pericardium in response to injury

Chemistry/Cardiac markers/Troponin/1

28. What requirements must be met for a troponin assay to be considered a high-sensitivity test?

A. Must have a detection limit of 30 ng/L
B. Must be able to give a value for 100% of the healthy population who have a concentration above the limit of detection
C. Must have a coefficient of variation (CV) of less than 10% at the 99th percentile of the healthy population
D. Must have a clinical specificity of 99% or greater

Chemistry/Cardiac markers/Troponin/2

29. What is the typical time course for high-sensitivity cardiac troponin I (cTnI) or cardiac troponin T (cTnT) following an AMI?

A. Abnormal within 1 hour; peak within 24 hours; return to normal in 7 to 10 days
B. Abnormal within 4 hours; peak within 18 hours; return to normal in 48 hours
C. Abnormal within 4 hours; peak within 24 hours; return to normal in 3 days
D. Abnormal within 6 hours; peak within 36 hours; return to normal in 5 days

Chemistry/Cardiac markers/Troponin/2

Answers to Questions 24–29

24. B The CKI is an expression of the portion of the total CK that is attributed to CK-MB.

$$CKI = \frac{CK-MB\ in\ \mu g/L}{Total\ CK\ in\ IU/L} \times 100$$

$$CKI = \frac{18\ \mu g/L}{560\ IU/L} \times 100\% = 3.2\%$$

25. A In some noncardiac causes of elevated plasma CK-MB, such as muscular dystrophy, there is a persistent elevation of both total CK and CK-MB. TnI and troponin T (TnT) are cardiac-specific markers and are not increased in muscular dystrophy.

26. B Plasma myoglobin is a sensitive marker for AMI; however, it is nonspecific, being present in both skeletal and cardiac muscle cells, and is considered an adjunct marker for troponin or CK-MB. However, specificity is approximately 75% to 85% as a result of skeletal muscle injury or renal insufficiency.

27. B Troponin is a complex of three polypeptides that function as a regulator of actin and tropomyosin, contractile proteins in striated muscle. The three subunits are designated TnC, TnI, and TnT.

28. C A troponin test qualifies as high sensitivity (guideline compliant) if it has a CV less than 10% at the 99th percentile of healthy individuals and gives a measurable result in at least 50% of the healthy population who have a troponin concentration above the limit of detection (LoD).

29. A High-sensitivity cTnI and cTnT exceed the 99th percentile of a healthy population within 1 hour after a heart attack and remain elevated for about 1 week.

30. The following results are reported on an adult male patient being evaluated for chest pain:

	Troponin I (Cutoff = 0.018 µg/L)	CK-MB (Cutoff = 4 µg/L)
Admission	0.21 µg/L	18 µg/L
1-hour postadmission	0.015 µg/L	3 µg/L
2-hours postadmission	0.24 µg/L	20 µg/L

What is the *most* likely cause of these results?

A. The wrong patient was drawn for the 1-hour postadmission sample
B. The patient did not suffer an MI until after admission
C. Hemolysis caused interference with the 1-hour sample
D. The patient is experiencing unstable angina

Chemistry/Cardiac markers/Disorders and disease/3

31. The laboratory reports a very high cardiac troponin level, and the attending physician questions the result because it does not correlate with the patient's condition. The laboratory scientist suspects a false-positive result caused by a heterophile antibody. Which course of action might confirm this?

A. Have the sample assayed on a different platform
B. Dilute the specimen with saline and repeat the test
C. Call for a new specimen, and compare results
D. Ultracentrifuge the sample, and perform the test on the supernatant

Chemistry/Cardiac markers/Disorders and disease/3

32. Serial high-sensitivity cTnI assays were performed on a patient at admission and at 1 hour and 3 hours later. The samples were collected in EDTA tubes. Following are the results (reference range 0–18 ng/L):

Admission = 34 ng/L   1 hour = 32 ng/L
3 hours = 33 ng/L

These results *most* likely indicate:

A. A positive test for AMI
B. Non-MI cause of high cTnI
C. Transmural reinfarction
D. Random error with the 3-hour sample

Chemistry/Cardiac markers/Disorders and disease/3

33. Which of the following cardiac markers is *most* often increased in persons who exhibit unstable angina?

A. Troponin C
B. cTnT
C. CK-MB
D. Myoglobin

Chemistry/Cardiac markers/2

Answers to Questions 30–33

30. A The likely explanation is that the 1-hour postadmission sample was drawn from the wrong patient, or the wrong specimen was analyzed. The admission TnI and CK-MB are both elevated, and above the diagnostic cutoff for MI. Both assays are within normal limits 1 hour after admission, making an analytical error highly unlikely. The rise and fall of both markers take significantly longer than 1 hour after AMI, so the normal result at 1 hour cannot be explained by the pathophysiology of cardiac injury.

31. A Heterophile antibodies (e.g., human anti-mouse antibodies [HAMAs]) may cross-link the two antibodies used in a cardiac troponin immunoassay, causing very high results. Although manufacturers may add blocking agents to neutralize them, high-titer antibodies to mouse immunoglobulins may still interfere. Binding of heterophile antibodies will differ, depending on the source of antibodies used in the assay; thus, other manufacturers' reagents may give very different results. Serial dilution of the sample will give less than an expected reduction in the result and is another means to support that this type of interference is present.

32. B AMI is unlikely because serial measurements do not show increasing cTnI. Three serial cTnI results near the upper normal limit are also near the limit of detection for the test. This can be caused by both noncardiac conditions and cardiac conditions other than AMI, including CHF, left ventricular hypertrophy, pulmonary edema, unstable angina, ischemia, myocarditis, and others.

33. B Persons with unstable angina (angina at rest) who have an elevated cTnT or cTnI are at eight times greater risk of having an MI within the next 6 months. CK-MB and myoglobin have not been useful in the risk assessment of unstable angina.

34. A patient has a plasma cTnT of 10 ng/L at admission. One hour later, the cTnT is 34 ng/L, and 3 hours later 120 ng/L. Electrocardiography (ECG) showed no change over this time. These results are consistent with which condition?

A. Skeletal muscle injury
B. Acute myocardial infarction
C. Unstable angina
D. No evidence of myocardial or skeletal muscle injury

Chemistry/Cardiac markers/Disorders and disease/2

35. A single heparinized plasma sample measured for troponin was found to have a concentration exceeding the laboratory's upper reportable limit. However, the patient had a normal ECG result and was stable without showing any classic signs of MI and had no history of arteriosclerotic cardiovascular disease. What is the *most* likely cause?

A. Chronic renal failure
B. Recent angioplasty
C. Nontransmural MI
D. False-positive troponin

Chemistry/Cardiac markers/Disorders and disease/3

36. An EDTA sample for cTnI assay gives a result of 40 ng/L (reference range 0–13 ng/L). The test is repeated 30 minutes later on a new specimen, and the result is 4 ng/L. A third sample collected 1 hour later gives a result of 5 ng/L. What is the *most* likely explanation?

A. A false-positive result occurred as a result of matrix interference
B. Heparin should have been used instead of EDTA
C. The patient has suffered a heart attack
D. The patient has had an ischemic episode without cardiac injury

Chemistry/Cardiac markers/3

37. When evaluating CK isoenzymes by electrophoresis, which isoenzyme migrates the fastest toward the anode when using agarose gel at pH 8.6?

A. CK1-BB
B. CK2-MB
C. CK3-MM
D. Mitochondrial CK

Chemistry/Cardiac markers/3

38. A patient's biochemistry results are:

ALT = 55 IU/L	AST = 165 IU/L
Glucose = 87 mg/dL	LD = 340 IU/L
Na = 142 mmol/L	K = 6.8 mmol/L
Ca = 8.4 mg/dL	P_i = 7.2 mg/dL

Select the *best* course of action.

A. Report results along with an estimate of the degree of hemolysis
B. Repeat LD, but report all other results
C. Request a new sample
D. Dilute the serum 1:2, and repeat AST and LD

Chemistry/Enzymes/3

Answers to Questions 34–38

34. B These results are consistent with a type 2 heart attack. These are characterized by a serial rise in cardiac troponin with clinical signs of ischemia but the absence of typical ECG changes, such as ST-segment elevation or Q wave.

35. D False-positive troponins have been caused by heterophile antibodies, microfibrin clots in the sample, autoantibodies such as rheumatoid factor, immune complexes, microparticles, and a markedly increased ALP. Although chronic kidney disease, recent angioplasty, and nontransmural MI (necrosis involving only part of the heart wall) can cause a positive cTnI result, they would not cause a level that exceeds the reportable range of the assay.

36. A EDTA is the additive of choice for troponin assays because it avoids microclots that can lead to false-positive results when serum or heparinized plasma is used. False-positive results caused by matrix effects usually revert to normal when the test is repeated on a new sample. An AMI will cause cTnI to increase in serial tests. Although cTnI can be high as a result of cardiac injury and noncardiac conditions, the level should remain elevated in samples taken so closely together.

37. A CK1, or the BB fraction found primarily in the brain, migrates the fastest from the cathode to the anode. CK2-MB migrates between CK1 and CK3. CK3-MM remains near the origin with the mitochondrial CK presents as a band nearest the cathode.

38. A Results indicate a moderately hemolyzed sample. Because sodium, calcium, and glucose are not significantly affected, results should be reported along with an estimate of visible hemolysis.

39. Which test becomes abnormal *earliest* in the progression of acute coronary syndrome?

A. Proprotein convertase subtilisin/kexin type 9 (PCSK9)
B. B-type natriuretic peptide (BNP)
C. Myoglobin
D. High-sensitivity CRP

Chemistry/Cardiac markers/2

40. Which statement *best* describes the clinical utility of BNP?

A. Abnormal levels greater than 100 pg/mL may be caused by obstructive lung disease
B. A test result greater than 100 pg/mL indicates prior myocardial damage caused by AMI that occurred within the last 3 months
C. A test result of less than 100 pg/mL helps rule out congestive heart failure in persons with symptoms associated with coronary insufficiency
D. A level greater than 100 pg/mL is not significant if evidence of congestive heart failure is absent

Chemistry/Cardiac markers/2

41. Which statement *best* describes the clinical utility of plasma homocysteine?

A. Levels are directly related to the quantity of LDL cholesterol in plasma
B. High plasma levels are associated with atherosclerosis and increased risk of thrombosis
C. Persons who have an elevated plasma homocysteine will also have an increased plasma Lp(a)
D. Plasma levels are increased only when there is an inborn error of amino acid metabolism

Chemistry/Cardiac markers/2

42. Which of the following cardiac markers is derived from neutrophils and predicts an increased risk for MI?

A. Lipoprotein-associated phospholipase A_2 (Lp-PLA_2)
B. Glycogen phosphorylase-BB (GP-BB)
C. Cystatin C
D. Myeloperoxidase (MPO)

Chemistry/Cardiac markers/2

43. Which statement accurately describes serum transaminase levels in AMI?

A. ALT is increased 5- to 10-fold after an AMI
B. AST peaks 24–48 hours after an AMI and returns to normal within 4–6 days
C. AST levels are usually 20–50 times the upper limit of normal after an AMI
D. Isoenzymes of AST are of greater diagnostic utility than the total enzyme level

Chemistry/Enzymes/Cardiac markers/2

44. Which of the following statements describes the aminotransferases (AST and ALT)?

A. Isoenzymes of AST and ALT are not found in humans
B. Both transfer an amino group to 2-oxogluterate (α-ketoglutarate)
C. Both require $NADP^+$ as a coenzyme
D. Both utilize four carbon amino acids as substrates

Chemistry/Enzymes/Transaminases/2

Answers to Questions 39–44

39. D High-sensitivity C-reactive protein (hs-CRP) is an acute-phase protein that is increased in inflammation. Such inflammation occurs when coronary artery plaques become disrupted, and therefore, individuals with CAD who have mildly increased CRP are at high risk of disease progression.

40. C Both BNP and N-terminal pro-B-type natriuretic peptide (NT-proBNP) are increased in individuals with congestive heart failure. Levels are not increased in pulmonary obstruction and other conditions that cause physical limitation and symptoms that overlap CHF.

41. B Plasma homocysteine levels are measured as an independent risk factor for CAD. High levels of homocysteine are toxic to vascular endothelium and promote inflammation and plaque formation. Plasma levels are independent of LDL and other cholesterol fractions. Increased plasma homocysteine occurs when there is a block in the conversion of methionine to cysteine.

42. D All of the answer choices are markers for acute coronary syndrome and increased risk of AMI. MPO is released from neutrophils and is thought to destabilize the arterial plaque. Lp-PLA_2 is produced by the arterial wall. GP-BB is released from cardiac myocytes. Cystatin C is a marker for early-stage glomerular disease.

43. B AST rises within 8 hours, peaks at 24 to 48 hours, and returns to normal within 5 days following an AMI, with levels up to 5 to 10 times the URL. ALT may be slightly elevated after an AMI.

44. B Both ALT and AST are classified as aminotransferases. ALT catalyzes the transfer of an amino group from alanine to 2-oxogluterate (α-ketoglutarate), forming pyruvate. AST catalyzes the transfer of an amino group from aspartate (to 2-oxogluterate), forming oxaloacetate.

45. Select the products formed from the forward reaction for measurement of AST.
A. Alanine and α-ketoglutarate
B. Oxaloacetate and glutamate
C. Aspartate and glutamine
D. Glutamate and NADH

Chemistry/Enzymes/Transaminases/1

46. Select the products formed from the forward reaction for measurement of ALT.
A. Aspartate and alanine
B. Alanine and α-ketoglutarate
C. Pyruvate and glutamate
D. Glutamine and NAD^+

Chemistry/Enzymes/Transaminases/1

47. Select the statement to describe analysis for AST and ALT?
A. Hemolysis will cause positive interference in both AST and ALT assays
B. Loss of activity occurs if samples are frozen at –20°C
C. The absorbance at the start of the reaction should not exceed 1.0 A
D. Reaction rates are unaffected by addition of pyridoxal-5′-phosphate (P-5′-P) to the substrate

Chemistry/Enzymes/Transaminases/2

48. Select the coupling enzyme used in the coupled AST analytical measurement.
A. LD
B. Malate dehydrogenase (MD)
C. GLD
D. G-6-PD

Chemistry/Enzymes/Transaminases/1

49. Of the following, which liver condition produces the highest levels of transaminases?
A. Hepatic cirrhosis
B. Obstructive jaundice
C. Hepatic cancer
D. Acute hepatitis

Chemistry/Enzymes/Disorders and disease/Transaminases/1

50. Which condition gives rise to the highest serum level of transaminases?
A. Acute hepatitis
B. Alcoholic cirrhosis
C. Obstructive biliary disease
D. Diffuse intrahepatic cholestasis

Chemistry/Enzymes/Disorders and disease/Transaminases/2

51. In which liver disease is the De Ritis ratio (AST:ALT) usually less than 1.0?
A. Acute hepatitis
B. Chronic hepatitis
C. Hepatic cirrhosis
D. Hepatic carcinoma

Chemistry/Enzymes/Disorders and disease/Transaminase/2

Answers to Questions 45–51

45. B AST forms oxaloacetate and glutamate from aspartate and 2-oxoglutarate.

46. C ALT forms pyruvate and glutamate from the transamination reaction between alanine and 2-oxoglutarate.

47. A RBCs are rich in AST and to a lesser extent in ALT. Hemolysis causes positive interference in both assays, although the effect on AST is greater. Samples are stable for up to 24 hours at room temperature and up to 3 days at 4°C and should be frozen if kept longer. The starting absorbance should be at least 1.5 A for both assays. When P-5′-P is added, a significant increase in activity sometimes occurs.

48. B The coupled analytical measurement for AST uses malate dehydrogenase (MD) to reduce oxaloacetate to malate.

$$\text{Aspartate} + \alpha\text{-ketoglutarate} \xrightarrow{AST} \text{Oxaloacetate} + \text{glutamate}$$
$$\text{Oxaloacetate} + \text{NADH} + H^+ \xrightarrow{MD} \text{Malate} + \text{NAD}^+$$

49. D Elevation of transaminases is greatest in acute hepatitis (20–50 × URL). Levels are moderately elevated (5–10 × URL) in hepatic cancer. They are slightly elevated (2–5 × URL) in chronic hepatitis, hepatic cirrhosis, alcoholic hepatitis, and obstructive jaundice.

50. A The transaminases usually reach 20–50 times the URL in acute viral and toxic hepatitis. Both transaminases are moderately increased (5–10 × URL) in diffuse intrahepatic obstruction and slightly increased (2–5 × URL) in cirrhosis and extrahepatic obstruction.

51. A The De Ritis ratio, or AST:ALT ratio, is used to assess liver function and disease severity. ALT prevails over AST in hepatitis; however, AST is greater than ALT in carcinoma, alcoholic liver disease, and cirrhosis of the liver.

52. Of the following, which liver condition produces the highest levels of transaminases?
A. Hepatic cirrhosis
B. Obstructive jaundice
C. Hepatic cancer
D. Alcoholic hepatitis

Chemistry/Enzymes/Disorders and disease/ Transaminase/2

53. Which of the following statements best describes ALT?
A. ALT is often increased in muscular disease, pancreatitis, and lymphoma
B. ALT is increased in infectious mononucleosis, but AST is usually normal
C. ALT is more specific for liver diseases than is AST
D. ALT levels are increased in pulmonary embolism

Chemistry/Enzymes/Transaminases/2

54. Select the *most* sensitive marker for alcoholic liver disease.
A. GLD
B. ALT
C. AST
D. γ-Glutamyltransferase (GGT)

Chemistry/Enzymes/GGT/2

55. Which enzyme is a useful indicator in both hepatobiliary disease and biliary obstruction?
A. AST
B. ALT
C. 5′-Nucleotidase
D. LD

Chemistry/Enzymes/Disorders and disease/2

56. Which of the following statements best describes the phosphatase enzymes?
A. They hydrolyze ATP and related compounds
B. They are divided into two classes based upon pH needed for activity
C. They exhibit a high specificity for substrate
D. They are activated by P_i

Chemistry/Enzymes/Phosphatase/1

57. Which of the following statements *best* describes the enzyme ALP?
A. In normal adults, the primary tissue source is fast-twitch skeletal muscle
B. Geriatric patients have a lower serum ALP than other adults
C. Serum ALP levels are lower in children than in adults
D. Pregnant women have a higher level of serum ALP than other adults

Chemistry/Enzymes/ALP/2

Answers to Questions 52–57

52. C Levels are moderately elevated (5–10 × URL) in hepatic cancer. They are slightly elevated (2–5 × URL) in chronic hepatitis, hepatic cirrhosis, alcoholic hepatitis, and obstructive jaundice.

53. C ALT is more specific for liver disease than AST. High ALT may result from nonhepatic causes such as AMI, muscle injury or disease, and severe hemolysis. AST is increased in muscle disease, MI, pancreatitis, pulmonary embolism, and lymphoma.

54. D GGT is a more sensitive indicator of alcoholic liver disease, although AST and ALT are elevated in alcoholic hepatitis. Levels of GGT can reach in excess of 25 times the URL in alcoholic hepatitis.

55. C 5′-Nucleotidase is markedly elevated in both intra- and posthepatic obstruction. ALT and AST may be slightly elevated in obstructive jaundice but are markedly in elevated hepatocellular conditions such as hepatitis. LD is usually greater in necrotic jaundice than in obstructive jaundice.

56. B Phosphatases are classified as either alkaline or acid depending upon the pH needed for optimal activity.

57. D Serum ALP levels are often two- or threefold higher than the URL in the third term of pregnancy. Elevations may also be present in pregnancy complications such as hypertension, preeclampsia, and threatened abortion. ALP is higher in children than in adults because of bone growth.

58. Which isoenzyme of ALP is *most* heat stable?
A. Bone
B. Liver
C. Intestinal
D. Placental
Chemistry/Enzymes/ALP/1

59. Which isoenzyme of ALP migrates farthest toward the anode when electrophoresed at pH 8.6?
A. Placental
B. Bone
C. Liver
D. Intestinal
Chemistry/Enzymes/ALP/1

60. This ALP isoenzyme resembles placental ALP and may be re-expressed in tumor cells:
A. Biliary isoenzyme
B. Bone isoenzyme
C. Regan isoenzyme
D. Intestinal isoenzyme
Chemistry/Enzymes/ALP/1

61. Elevated ALP, in the presence of elevated GGT, is suggestive of this type of disorder.
A. Acute hepatitis
B. Hepatocellular disorder
C. Biliary tract obstruction
D. Paget disease
Chemistry/Enzymes/Disorders and disease/ALP/1

62. In which condition would an elevated serum ALP be likely to occur?
A. Small cell lung carcinoma
B. Hemolytic anemia
C. Prostate cancer
D. AMI
Chemistry/Enzymes/Disorders and disease/ALP/2

63. Which condition is *least* likely to be associated with increased serum ALP?
A. Osteomalacia
B. Biliary obstruction
C. Hyperparathyroidism and hyperthyroidism
D. Osteoporosis
Chemistry/Enzymes/Disorders and disease/ALP/2

64. Which substrate is used in the Bowers-McComb method for ALP?
A. *p*-Nitrophenyl phosphate
B. β-Glycerophosphate
C. Phenylphosphate
D. α-Naphthylphosphate
Chemistry/Enzymes/Analytical methods/2

Answers to Questions 58–64

58. D Placental ALP and tumor-associated isoenzymes such as the Regan isoenzyme associated with lung cancer are the only isoenzymes that retain activity when serum is heated to 65°C for 10 minutes. Heat inactivation is used primarily to distinguish liver ALP from bone ALP.

59. C Liver ALP isoenzymes migrate farthest toward the anode, followed by bone, placental, and intestinal fractions.

60. C The Regan isoenzyme, also considered the tumor isoenzyme, resembles placental ALP and considered a carcino-placental alkaline phosphatase. It is observed in individuals with malignant disease.

61. C When the increase in GGT is twofold higher than the increase in ALP, the liver is assumed to be the source of the elevated ALP. Serum ALP is a sensitive marker for extrahepatic obstruction. GGT in serum is derived from the hepatobiliary system and is increased in alcoholic hepatitis, hepatobiliary obstruction, and hepatic cancer. It is not increased in diseases of bone.

62. A ALP is a tumor marker in conditions such as hepatoma, small cell carcinoma of the lung, and ovarian cancer, and resembles placental ALP in most cases.

63. D Total ALP is high in less than 30% of osteoporosis patients; ALP is elevated in osteomalacia (rickets), bone cancer, and bone disease secondary to hyperthyroidism and hyperparathyroidism.

64. A The method of Bowers-McComb is the International Federation of Clinical Chemistry (IFCC)–recommended method for ALP. This method uses 2-amino-2-methyl-1-propanol, pH 10.15, and measures the increase in absorbance at 405 nm as p-nitrophenyl phosphate is hydrolyzed to p-nitrophenol.

65. A serum ALP level greater than twice the elevation of GGT suggests:
A. Misidentification of the specimen
B. Focal intrahepatic obstruction
C. Acute alcoholic hepatitis
D. Bone disease or malignancy
Chemistry/Enzymes/Disorders and disease/ALP/2

66. Which condition is associated with a decrease in ALP activity?
A. Pregnancy
B. Vitamin D–dependent rickets (VDDR)
C. Hypophosphatasia
D. Bone fracture
Chemistry/Enzymes/Disorders and disease/ALP/2

67. In which condition is the measurement of acid phosphatase clinically useful?
A. Measuring the prostatic isoenzyme to screen for prostate cancer
B. Measuring the enzyme in a vaginal swab extract
C. The diagnosis of hemolytic anemia
D. As a marker for bone regeneration
Chemistry/Enzymes/ACP/3

68. Which definition describes the catalytic activity of amylase?
A. Hydrolyzes second α-1-4-glycosidic linkages of starch and glycogen
B. Hydrolyzes all polyglucans completely to produce glucose
C. Oxidatively degrades polysaccharides containing glucose
D. Splits polysaccharides and disaccharides by addition of water
Chemistry/Enzymes/Amylase/1

69. Which of the following amylase substrates is recommended by the IFCC?
A. Starch
B. Maltodextrose
C. Maltotetrose
D. Blocked maltohepatoside
Chemistry/Enzymes/Amylase/1

70. The amylase result is 550 units/L. A 1/4 dilution of the specimen in 9% NaCl gives 180 units/L (before mathematical correction for dilution). The dilution is repeated with the same results. Select the *best* course of action.
A. Report the amylase as 550 units/L
B. Report the amylase as 720 units/L
C. Report the amylase as 900 units/L
D. Dilute the sample 1:10 in distilled water and repeat
Chemistry/Enzymes/Amylase/3

71. How soon following acute abdominal pain due to pancreatitis is the serum amylase expected to peak?
A. 1–2 hours
B. 2–12 hours
C. 3–4 days
D. 5–6 days
Chemistry/Enzymes/Amylase/2

Answers to Questions 65–71

65. D A disproportionate increase in ALP points to a nonhepatic source of ALP, often bone disease. In obstructive jaundice, GGT is elevated more than ALP. GGT is the most sensitive marker of acute alcoholic hepatitis, rising about fivefold higher than ALP.

66. C Hypophosphatasia is a rare genetic disease caused by a mutation in the *TNSALP* gene causing diminished expression of tissue-nonspecific ALP.

67. B The clinical use of prostatic acid phosphatase is confined to the investigation of sexual assault.

68. A Amylase in humans is a hydrolase that splits the second α-1-4-glycosidic bonds of polyglucans forming maltose.

69. D In the IFCC-recommended method, *p*-nitrophenyl maltoheptaoside is used.

70. B A 1/4 dilution refers to one part serum and three parts diluent; the result is multiplied by 4 to determine the serum concentration.

71. B Serum amylase usually peaks 2 to 12 hours following acute abdominal pain resulting from pancreatitis. Levels reach two to six times the URL and return to normal within 3 to 4 days.

72. Which of the following statements regarding the diagnosis of pancreatitis is correct?

A. Amylase and lipase are as predictive in chronic as in acute pancreatitis
B. Diagnostic sensitivity is increased by assaying both amylase and lipase
C. Measuring the urinary amylase:creatinine ratio is useful only when patients have renal failure
D. Serum lipase peaks several hours before amylase after an episode of acute pancreatitis

Chemistry/Enzymes/Disorders and disease/2

73. Which of the following conditions is associated with a high level of S-type amylase?

A. Mumps
B. Intestinal obstruction
C. Alcoholic liver disease
D. Peptic ulcers

Chemistry/Enzymes/Disorders and disease/Amylase/2

74. Which group of enzymes are considered drug-metabolizing enzymes, transforming xenobiotics into inactive, water-soluble compounds?

A. Aldolase
B. Cholinesterase
C. Cytochrome P-450
D. Glutamate dehydrogenase

Chemistry/Enzymes/1

75. Which of the following statements regarding amylase methods is true?

A. Dilution of serum may result in lower-than-expected activity
B. Methods generating NADH are preferred because they have higher sensitivity
C. Synthetic substrates can be conjugated to *p*-nitrophenol (PNP) for a kinetic assay
D. The reference range is consistent from method to method

Chemistry/Enzymes/Analytical methods/2

76. Which statement about the clinical utility of plasma or serum lipase is true?

A. Lipase is not increased in mumps, breast cancer, or ectopic pregnancy
B. Lipase is not increased as dramatically as amylase in acute pancreatitis
C. Increased plasma or serum lipase is specific for pancreatitis
D. Lipase levels are elevated in both acute and chronic pancreatitis

Chemistry/Enzymes/Lipase/2

Answers to Questions 72–76

72. B Amylase is not increased in all individuals with pancreatitis and can be increased in several non-pancreatic conditions. Lipase adds both sensitivity and specificity to the diagnosis of acute pancreatitis. Plasma or serum lipase becomes abnormal within 6 hours, peaks at approximately 24 hours, and remains abnormal for about 1 week following an episode of acute pancreatitis. In acute pancreatitis, the rate of urinary amylase excretion increases, and the amylase:creatinine clearance ratio is helpful in diagnosing some cases of pancreatitis.

73. A Both salivary and pancreatic amylases designated S-type and P-type, respectively, are present in normal serum. High amylase occurs in mumps, ectopic pregnancy, biliary obstruction, peptic ulcers, alcoholism, malignancies, and other nonpancreatic diseases.

74. C Cytochrome p-450 enzymes (CYP450) are involved in phase 1 reactions to transform drugs into inactive, water-soluble compounds for excretion through the kidneys. Aldolase plays a role in glycolysis, and cholinesterase hydrolyzes acetylcholine into choline and acetic acid. GDH catalyzes the conversion of glutamate to α-ketoglutarate and ammonia.

75. C Synthetic substrates such as maltotetraoseor 4-nitrophenyl maltoheptaoside can be used for kinetic assays. Many endogenous inhibitors of amylase, such as wheat germ, are found in serum. Diluted samples often show higher than expected activity caused by dilution of the inhibitor. Units of amylase activity vary widely depending upon the method of assay and calibration.

76. A Lipase is unaffected in mumps, breast cancer, or ectopic pregnancy. Lipase elevation is of greater magnitude and duration than amylase in acute pancreatitis. Lipase is also increased in peptic ulcers, renal insufficiency, and intestinal obstruction. Lipase levels are often low in chronic pancreatitis and cystic fibrosis.

77. In which condition would amylase but not lipase be elevated?
A. Pancreatic cancer
B. Peptic ulcer
C. Macroamylasemia
D. Renal failure

Chemistry/Enzymes/Disorders and disease/Lipase/2

78. The *most* commonly employed method of assay for plasma or serum lipase is based on:
A. Hydrolysis of olive oil
B. Rate turbidimetry
C. Immunoassay
D. Peroxidase coupling

Chemistry/Enzymes/Analytical methods/Lipase/1

79. Which of the following enzymes is usually depressed in liver disease?
A. Elastase-1
B. Glutamate dehydrogenase
C. Pseudocholinesterase
D. Aldolase

Chemistry/Enzymes/Disorders and disease/2

80. Which enzyme is measured in whole blood?
A. Chymotrypsin
B. Glucose-6-phosphate dehydrogenase
C. Glycogen phosphorylase
D. Lipase

Chemistry/Enzymes/1

Answers to Questions 77–80

77. C Macroamylasemia is an elevated blood amylase caused by formation of a complex between IgG and amylase.

78. D The most commonly used method for lipase assay is based upon the hydrolysis of a synthetic diglyceride substrate. This is hydrolyzed and forms glycerol, which is further oxidized by glycerophosphate oxidase, yielding H_2O_2. H_2O_2 is then further reduced in the presence of a dye precursor, N-Ethyl-N-(2-hydroxy-3sulfopropyl)-m-toluidine sodium salt (TOOS), producing a quinone dye product for colorimetric measurement.

$$\text{1,2 diglyceride} + H_2O \xrightarrow{\text{Lipase}}$$
$$\text{2} - \text{monoglyceride} + \text{fatty acid}$$
$$\text{2} - \text{monoglyceride} + H_2O \xrightarrow{\text{Monoglyceride esterase}}$$
$$\text{glycerol} + \text{fatty acid glycerol} + ATP \xrightarrow{\text{Glycerol kinase}}$$
$$\text{glycerol-3-phosphate} + ADP\ \text{glycerol-3-}PO_4 +$$
$$O_2 \xrightarrow{\text{Glycerophosphate oxidase}}$$
$$\text{dihydroxyacetone phosphate} + H_2O_2$$
$$H_2O_2 + \text{4-aminoantipyrene} + TOOS \xrightarrow{\text{Peroxidase}}$$
$$\text{quinoneimine dye} + H_2O$$

79. C Pseudocholinesterase is found mainly in the liver and functions to hydrolyze acetylcholine. Levels of pseudocholinesterase are decreased in patients with liver disease as a result of depressed synthesis. Elastase-1 is a pancreatic digestive enzyme and is reduced in persons with pancreatic insufficiency. Glutamate dehydrogenase is increased in necrotic jaundice, and aldolase is increased in necrotic jaundice and muscle disease.

80. B Glucose-6-phosphate dehydrogenase (G-6-PD) is measured on a whole blood hemolysate using glucose-6-PO_4 as the substrate, and forms 6-phosphogluconate as $NADP^+$ is converted to NADPH.

6.7

Clinical Endocrinology

1. Which of the following hormones is often decreased by approximately 25% in the serum of pregnant women who have a fetus with Down syndrome?

A. Estriol (E_3)
B. Human chorionic gonadotropin (hCG)
C. Progesterone
D. Estradiol (E_2)

Chemistry/Endocrine/Disorders and disease/Androgens/2

2. The syndrome of inappropriate antidiuretic hormone secretion (SIADH) causes:

A. Low serum vasopressin
B. Hypernatremia
C. Urine osmolality to be lower than plasma
D. Low serum electrolytes

Chemistry/Endocrine/Disorders and disease/ADH/2

3. Select the hormone which when elevated is associated with galactorrhea, pituitary adenoma, and amenorrhea.

A. Estradiol
B. Progesterone
C. Follicle-stimulating hormone (FSH)
D. Prolactin

Chemistry/Endocrine/Disorders and disease/Androgens/2

4. Zollinger-Ellison (Z-E) syndrome is characterized by significant (e.g., 20-fold) elevation of:

A. Gastrin
B. Cholecystokinin
C. Pepsin
D. Glucagon

Chemistry/Endocrine/Disorders and disease/Gastrin/2

5. Which statement *best* defines multiple endocrine neoplasia (MEN)?

A. It is associated with hyperplasia or neoplasia of at least two endocrine organs
B. Insulinoma is always present when the pituitary is involved
C. It is inherited as an autosomal recessive disorder
D. Plasma hormone levels from affected organs are elevated at least 10-fold

Chemistry/Endocrine/Disorders and disease/2

Answers to Questions 1–5

1. A Serum-free E_3 is often lower than expected for the gestational age in a pregnancy associated with Down syndrome. Unconjugated E_3 is produced in the placenta and fetal liver from dehydroepiandrosterone (DHEA), and levels rise throughout gestation.

2. D SIADH results in excessive secretion of vasopressin (or ADH) from the posterior pituitary, causing fluid retention and low plasma osmolality, sodium, potassium, and other electrolytes by hemodilution. It is suspected that urine osmolality is higher than plasma but urine sodium concentration is normal or increased.

3. D Serum prolactin may be increased from hypothalamic dysfunction or pituitary adenoma. When levels are greater than five times the URL, a pituitary tumor is suspected.

4. A Zollinger-Ellison (Z-E) syndrome is caused by a pancreatic or intestinal tumor secreting gastrin (gastrinoma) and results in greatly increased gastric acid production.

5. A Multiple endocrine neoplasia (MEN) syndrome is inherited as an autosomal dominant disease involving excess production of hormones from several endocrine glands. MEN I results from adenomas (usually benign) of at least two glands, including the pituitary, adrenal cortex, parathyroid, and pancreas.

6. Select the main estrogen produced by the ovaries and used to evaluate ovarian function.

A. Estril
B. Estradiol
C. Epiestriol
D. Hydroxyestrone

Chemistry/Endocrine/Androgens/1

7. Which statement *best* describes the relationship between luteinizing hormone (LH) and FSH in cases of dysmenorrhea?

A. Both are usually increased when there is pituitary adenoma
B. Increases in both hormones and a decrease in estrogen signal a pituitary cause of ovarian failure
C. Both hormones normally peak 1 to 2 days before ovulation
D. In menopause, the LH level at the midcycle peak is higher than the level of FSH

Chemistry/Endocrine/Androgens/2

8. When pituitary adenoma is the cause of decreased estrogen production, an increase of which hormone is *most* frequently responsible?

A. Prolactin
B. FSH
C. LH
D. TSH

Chemistry/Endocrine/2

9. Which set of results is *most* likely in an adult biological male with primary testicular failure?

A. Increased LH and FSH, and decreased testosterone
B. Decreased LH, FSH, and testosterone
C. Decreased testosterone, androstenedione, and FSH
D. Increased androstenedione, decreased testosterone, and normal FSH

Chemistry/Endocrine/Disorders and disease/Androgens/2

10. When should progesterone be measured when evaluating an adult biological female for anovulation?

A. At the onset of menses
B. During the first 7 days of the menstrual cycle
C. At the midcycle just after LH peaks
D. At the end of the menstrual cycle

Chemistry/Endocrine/Disorders and disease/Androgens/2

Answers to Questions 6–10

6. B Estradiol (E_2) is the major estrogen produced by the ovaries and is used to evaluate both ovarian function and menstrual cycle dysfunction.

7. C Both LH and FSH show a pronounced serum peak 1 to 2 days prior to ovulation and urine peak 20 to 44 hours before ovulation. In pituitary failure, levels of FSH and LH are reduced, and this reduction causes a deficiency of estrogen production by the ovaries. In patients with primary ovarian failure, LH and FSH are elevated because low estrogen levels stimulate release of luteinizing hormone–releasing hormone (LHRH) from the hypothalamus. Normally, the LH peak is sharper and greater than the FSH peak; however, in menopause, the FSH level usually becomes higher than that of LH.

8. A Prolactinoma can result in anovulation because high levels of prolactin suppress release of LHRH (gonadotropin-releasing hormone [GnRH]), causing suppression of GH, FSH, and estrogen.

9. A Primary testicular failure produces a picture of hypergonadotropism. LH and FSH are increased because the pituitary gland is normal and responds to decreased free testosterone. Androstenedione is an adrenal androgen that remains unaffected.

10. C Progesterone is often measured along with LH, FSH, estrogen, and prolactin to evaluate female infertility and dysmenorrhea. Low progesterone at midcycle indicates that ovulation did not occur.

11. A biological female showing signs of severe excessive pubic and facial hair growth (hirsutism) should be tested for which of the following hormones?

A. Estrogen and progesterone
B. HcG
C. GH
D. Testosterone and dehydroepiandrosterone sulfate

Chemistry/Endocrine/Disorders and disease/Androgens/2

12. The onset of menopause is usually associated with what hormonal changes?

A. Decreased estrogen, testosterone, and androgens
B. Decreased estrogen, FSH, LH, and progesterone
C. Decreased estrogen and progesterone, and increased LH and FSH
D. Decreased estrogen and progesterone, normal LH and FSH

Chemistry/Endocrine/Androgens/2

13. A quantitative sandwich enzyme immunoassay for intact serum hCG was performed on week 4 and the result was 40,000 mIU/mL (reference range 10,000–80,000 mIU/mL). The provider suspected a molar pregnancy and requested that the laboratory repeat the test checking for the hook effect. Which process would identify this problem?

A. Obtain a new plasma specimen and heat inactivate before testing
B. Obtain a urine specimen and perform the assay
C. Perform a qualitative pregnancy test
D. Perform a serial dilution of the sample and repeat the test

Chemistry/Endocrine/2

14. Which of the following statements is correct in assessing GH deficiency?

A. Pituitary failure may involve one, several, or all adenohypophyseal hormones, but GH deficiency is usually present
B. A normal random serum level of GH in a child under 6 years old rules out GH deficiency
C. Administration of arginine, insulin, or glucagon will suppress GH release
D. GH levels in the blood show little variation within a 24-hour period

Chemistry/Endocrine/GH/2

Answers to Questions 11–14

11. D Excessive hair growth in biological females results from excessive androgen production, which produces high levels of ovarian-derived testosterone. Dehydroepiandrosterone sulfate is produced only by the adrenals and would be useful in identifying those rare cases in which the cause is an androgen-secreting adrenal tumor.

12. C In menopause, estrogen production decreases to the point where the menstrual cycle and ovarian follicle maturation stop. The decreased estrogen causes the pituitary release of LH and FSH. In menopause, the FSH level at midcycle is higher than that of LH.

13. D The hook effect can cause results to be sufficiently low to cause misdiagnosis. It can be detected by diluting the sample (antigen) in which case the assay result will be greater than in the undiluted sample. The hook effect is the result of excessive antigen concentration and results in a dose-response (calibration) curve that reverses direction at very high antigen concentrations.

14. A Because GH is the most abundant pituitary hormone, it may be used as a screening test for pituitary failure in adults. In children, there is extensive overlap between normal and low GH levels, and a stimulation (provocative) test is usually needed to establish a diagnosis of deficiency. Certain drugs, such as arginine, insulin, propranolol, and glucagon, can be used to stimulate GH release. GH secretion peaks during sleep, and pulsed increases are seen after exercise and meals.

15. Which statement *best* describes the level of GH in patients with pituitary adenoma associated with acromegaly?

A. The fasting GH level is always elevated at least twofold

B. A glucose suppression test may be performed to establish a diagnosis

C. A normal fasting GH level rules out acromegaly

D. Patients produce a lower concentration of insulin-like growth factor 1 (IGF-1) than expected from their GH level

Chemistry/Endocrine/GH/2

16. Hyperparathyroidism is *most* consistently associated with:

A. Hypocalcemia

B. Hypocalciuria

C. Hypophosphatemia

D. Metabolic alkalosis

Chemistry/Endocrine/Parathyroid/2

17. The *best* method of analysis for serum PTH involves using antibodies that react with:

A. The amino (N)-terminal fragment of PTH

B. The carboxy (C)-terminal end of PTH

C. The N-terminal and either C-middle or C-terminal fragment

D. All fragments of PTH as well as intact hormone

Chemistry/Endocrine/Analytical methods/ Parathyroid/1

18. Which of the following is *most* often elevated in hypercalcemia associated with malignancy?

A. Parathyroid-derived PTH

B. Ectopic PTH

C. Parathyroid hormone–related protein (PTHrP)

D. Calcitonin

Chemistry/Endocrine/Disorders and disease/Parathyroid/1

19. Which is normally the most abundant corticosteroid hormone secreted by the adrenal cortex?

A. Cortisol

B. Dehydroepiandrosterone

C. Aldosterone

D. Corticosterone

Chemistry/Endocrine/Adrenal/1

20. Which of the following statements regarding adrenal cortical dysfunction is true?

A. Patients with Cushing syndrome usually have hyperkalemia

B. Cushing syndrome is associated with glucose intolerance

C. Addison disease is associated with hypernatremia

D. Addison disease is caused by elevated levels of cortisol

Chemistry/Endocrine/Disorders and disease/Adrenal/2

Answers to Questions 15–20

15. B Approximately 90% of patients with acromegaly have an elevated fasting GH level. The glucose suppression test is used to diagnose acromegaly. Patients with acromegaly also have high levels of IGF-1, which is overproduced by the liver in response to excess release of GH.

16. C Hyperparathyroidism causes increased resorption of calcium and decreased renal retention of phosphate. Increased serum calcium leads to increased urinary excretion. The distal collecting tubule of the nephron reabsorbs less bicarbonate as well as phosphate, resulting in acidosis.

17. C The biological activity of PTH resides in the N-terminal portion of the polypeptide, but the hormone is rapidly degraded and produces N-terminal, middle, and C-terminal fragments. The assay of choice for PTH is a two-site double-antibody sandwich method that measures intact PTH.

18. C Some malignancies (e.g., squamous, renal, bladder, and ovarian cancers) secrete PTHrP, causing hypercalcemia-associated malignancy. Because the region shared with PTH is small and poorly immunoreactive, the peptide does not cross-react in most assays for PTH. Calcitonin is a hormone produced in the medulla of the thyroid that opposes the action of PTH, and levels do not greatly influence serum calcium.

19. A Cortisol is the most abundant adrenal hormone. DHEA, an adrenal androgen, is the next most abundant adrenal hormone. Aldosterone is the principal mineral corticoid made by the adrenals, and corticosterone is the immediate precursor to aldosterone.

20. B Patients with Cushing syndrome have elevated levels of cortisol and other adrenal corticosteroids resulting in hypertension, hypernatremia, hypokalemia, and glycosuria. Addison disease results from adrenal hypoplasia and produces the opposite symptoms, including hypotension, hyponatremia, hyperkalemia, and hypoglycemia.

21. Which of the following statements about cortisol in Cushing syndrome is true?

A. 24-hour urinary free cortisol is a more sensitive test than plasma total cortisol
B. Patients with Cushing disease show pronounced diurnal variation in serum cortisol
C. Free cortisol is increased by a high-serum cortisol-binding protein concentration
D. An elevated serum total cortisol level is diagnostic of Cushing syndrome

Chemistry/Endocrine/Disorders and disease/Adrenal/2

22. Which of the following conditions is characterized by primary hyperaldosteronism caused by adrenal adenoma, carcinoma, or hyperplasia?

A. Cushing syndrome
B. Addison disease
C. Conn syndrome
D. Pheochromocytoma

Chemistry/Endocrine/Disorders and disease/Adrenal/2

23. Which of the following is the *most* common cause of Cushing syndrome?

A. Pituitary adenoma
B. Adrenal hyperplasia
C. Overuse of corticosteroids
D. Ectopic adrenocorticotropic hormone (ACTH) production by tumors

Chemistry/Endocrine/Disorders and disease/Adrenal/2

24. Which of the following is the mechanism causing Cushing disease?

A. Excess secretion of pituitary ACTH
B. Adrenal adenoma
C. Treatment with corticosteroids
D. Ectopic ACTH production by tumors

Chemistry/Endocrine/Disorders and disease/Adrenal/2

25. In which situation is the plasma or 24-hour urinary cortisol *not* consistent with the clinical picture?

A. In pregnant patients
B. In patients with a positive result on the overnight dexamethasone suppression test
C. In congenital adrenal hyperplasia
D. In Cushing syndrome caused by ectopic ACTH-producing tumors

Chemistry/Endocrine/Disorders and disease/Adrenal/2

26. Which test is used to distinguish Cushing *disease* from Cushing *syndrome* caused by adrenal tumors?

A. Low-dose overnight dexamethasone suppression
B. Inferior petrosal sinus sampling
C. Serum ACTH
D. 24-hour urine free cortisol

Chemistry/Endocrine/Disorders and disease/Adrenal/2

Answers to Questions 21–26

21. A When cortisol levels become elevated, free (unbound) cortisol is filtered by the glomeruli. Most of it is reabsorbed, but a significant amount reaches the urine as free cortisol. The 24-hour urinary free cortisol avoids the diurnal variation that may affect plasma free cortisol levels and is a more sensitive test than serum total or free cortisol.

22. C Conn syndrome is characterized by hypertension, hypokalemia, and hypernatremia, with increased plasma and urine aldosterone and decreased renin. Cushing syndrome results from excessive production of cortisol, and Addison disease results from deficient production of adrenal corticosteroids. Pheochromocytoma is a tumor of chromaffin cells that produces catecholamines.

23. C The most common cause of Cushing syndrome is the administration of medications with cortisol or glucocorticoid activity. Adrenal adenoma or carcinoma (non-ACTH–mediated Cushing syndrome) comprise about 20% of cases, and ectopic ACTH production accounts for 10% to 20%.

24. A Cushing disease refers to adrenal hyperplasia resulting from dysregulation of the hypothalamic–pituitary axis. Cushing syndrome may be caused by adrenal adenoma or carcinoma, ectopic ACTH-producing tumors, or excessive corticosteroid administration.

25. C Congenital adrenogenital syndrome (CAH) results from deficiency of an enzyme required for synthesis of cortisol, such as 21-hydroxylase or 11-hydroxylase.

26. C Serum ACTH assays are very helpful in distinguishing the cause of Cushing syndrome. Patients with adrenal tumors have ACTH values approaching zero while patients with ectopic ACTH tumors have values greater than 200 pg/dL. The high-dose dexamethasone suppression test is also used. Inferior petrosal sinus sampling is used to determine whether a high ACTH is from the pituitary glands or from an ectopic source.

27. Which is the *most* widely used screening test for Cushing syndrome?
A. Overnight low-dose dexamethasone suppression test
B. Corticotropin-releasing hormone (CRH) stimulation test
C. Inferior petrosal sinus sampling
D. Metyrapone stimulation test
Chemistry/Endocrine/Disorders and disease/Adrenal/2

28. Which test is the *most* specific for establishing a diagnosis of Cushing *disease*?
A. Low-dose dexamethasone suppression
B. High-dose dexamethasone suppression
C. 24-hour urine free cortisol
D. Petrosal sinus sampling after CRH stimulation
Chemistry/Endocrine/Disorders and disease/Adrenal/2

29. Which of the following statements about the diagnosis of Addison disease is true?
A. Patients with primary Addison disease show a normal response to ACTH stimulation
B. Primary and secondary Addison disease can often be differentiated by plasma ACTH
C. 24-hour urinary free cortisol is normal in Addison disease
D. Pituitary ACTH reserves are normal in secondary Addison disease
Chemistry/Endocrine/Adrenal/2

30. Which of the following statements regarding the catecholamines is true?
A. They are derived from tryptophan
B. They are produced by the zona glomerulosa of the adrenal cortex
C. Plasma levels show both diurnal and pulsed variation
D. They are excreted in urine primarily as free catecholamines
Chemistry/Endocrine/Catecholamines/2

31. Which assay is considered the *best* single screening test for pheochromocytoma?
A. Total urinary catecholamines
B. Vanillymandelic acid (VMA)
C. Homovanillic acid (HVA)
D. Plasma free metanephrines
Chemistry/Endocrine/Catecholamines/2

32. Which metabolite is *most* often increased in carcinoid tumors of the intestine?
A. 5-Hydroxyindolacetic acid (5-HIAA)
B. 3-Methoxy-4-hydroxyphenylglycol (MHPG)
C. 3-Methoxydopamine
D. HVA
Chemistry/Endocrine/Catecholamines/1

Answers to Questions 27–32

27. A Overnight low-dose dexamethasone suppression test is used to assess the negative feedback on the hypothalamus compared with cortisol. Corticotropin-releasing hormone (CRH) stimulation and petrosal sinus sampling are confirmatory tests for Cushing disease and are used when the high-dose dexamethasone suppression test is inconclusive. The metyrapone stimulation test measures the patient's ACTH reserve.

28. D Petrosal sinus sampling tests are confirmatory tests for Cushing disease. Although dexamethasone suppression tests have a high sensitivity, some individuals without Cushing syndrome have indeterminate results or abnormal results caused by medications or other conditions.

29. B ACTH (Cortrosyn) stimulation is used as a screening test for Addison disease. A subnormal response (low or no increase in serum cortisol) occurs in both primary and secondary Addison disease. Plasma ACTH is high in primary but is low in secondary Addison disease.

30. C Catecholamines—epinephrine, norepinephrine, and dopamine—are produced from the amino acid tyrosine by the chromaffin cells of the adrenal medulla and display both diurnal and pulsed variation. The zona glomerulosa is the outermost portion of the adrenal cortex, where aldosterone is mainly produced. Cortisol is made in the zona fasciculata.

31. D Catecholamines are metabolized as metanephrines and VMA. Measurement of plasma free metanephrine is about 96% sensitive for pheochromocytoma, and is the best single test followed by 24-hour urinary metanephrines, which is slightly less sensitive but more specific. Specificity and sensitivity for detecting pheochromocytoma approach 100% when both VMA and metanephrines are measured.

32. A 5-HIAA is a product of serotonin catabolism. Excess levels are found in the urine of patients with carcinoid tumors composed of argentaffin (enteroendrocrine) cells. Carcinoid tumors are usually found in the intestine or lung and produce serotonin and 5-hydroxytryptophan.

33. Which statement regarding the measurement of urinary catecholamines is true?

A. An increased excretion of total urinary catecholamines is specific for pheochromocytoma
B. 24-hour urinary catecholamine assay avoids pulse variations associated with measurement of plasma catecholamines
C. Total urinary catecholamine measurement provides greater specificity than measurement of urinary free fractionated catecholamines
D. Total urinary catecholamines are not affected by exercise

Chemistry/Endocrine/Catecholamines/2

34. Which method is *most* often used to measure fractionated catecholamines (epinephrine, norepinephrine, and dopamine)?

A. Measurement of fluorescence following oxidation by potassium ferricyanide
B. Measurement by HPLC with electrochemical detection
C. Measure of radioactivity after conversion by catechol-*O*-methyltransferase (COMT) to tritiated metanephrines
D. Measurement by immunoassay

Chemistry/Endocrine/Analytical methods/ Catecholamines/2

35. Which statement about sample collection for catecholamines and metabolites is true?

A. Blood for catecholamines is collected in the usual manner following a 12-hour fast
B. 24-hour urine sample for VMA, catecholamines, or metanephrines is collected in 1 mL of boric acid
C. 24-hour urine creatinine should be measured with VMA, HVA, or metanephrines
D. There is no need to discontinue medications if a 24-hour urine collection is used

Chemistry/Endocrine/Catecholamines/2

36. Which of the following statements applies to measurement of both VMA and metanephrines in urine?

A. Both can be oxidized to vanillin and measured at 360 nm without interference from dietary compounds
B. Both can be measured immunochemically after hydrolysis and derivatization
C. Both require acid hydrolysis prior to measurement
D. Both can be measured by specific HPLC and MS assays

Chemistry/Endocrine/Analytical methods/2

Answers to Questions 33–36

33. B Measurement of total urinary catecholamines is not a specific test for pheochromocytoma. Urine levels may be increased by exercise and in muscular diseases. Catecholamines in urine may also be derived from dietary sources rather than endogenous production. Most catecholamines are excreted as glucuronide, and the urinary free catecholamines increase only when there is increased secretion.

34. B HPLC–ECD (electrochemical detection) separates catecholamines by reverse-phase chromatography, then detects them by oxidizing the aromatic ring at +0.8 V. The method fractionates catecholamines into epinephrine, norepinephrine, and dopamine. Fluorescent methods show interference from several drugs. Immunoassays do not fractionate catecholamines.

35. C Renal clearance affects excretion of catecholamine metabolites; it is preferable to report VMA, HVA, and metanephrines, in micrograms per milligram of creatinine. A 4-hour fast is also recommended. Many drugs contain epinephrine, which may falsely elevate catecholamine levels; therefore, medications should be temporarily discontinued prior to testing, whenever possible. The 24-hour urine samples for catecholamines are usually preserved with 10 mL of 6 N HCl.

36. D Metanephrines, VMA, and HVA are most often measured by using HPLC-EDC. VMA and metanephrines can both be measured as vanillin after oxidation with periodate. However, these methods are affected by dietary sources of vanillin and must be excluded from the diet.

37. Urinary HVA is most often assayed to detect:
A. Pheochromocytoma
B. Neuroblastoma
C. Adrenal medullary carcinoma
D. Psychiatric disorders, such as manic depression
Chemistry/Endocrine/Catecholamines/1

38. Thyroid hormones are derived from the amino acid:
A. Phenylalanine
B. Methionine
C. Tyrosine
D. Histidine
Chemistry/Endocrine/Thyroid/1

39. Which statement regarding thyroid hormones is true?
A. Circulating levels of triiodothyronine (T_3) and thyroxine (T_4) are about equal
B. T_3 is about 10-fold more active than T_4
C. The rate of formation of monoiodotyrosine and diiodotyrosine is about equal
D. Most of the T_3 present in plasma is from its direct release from thyroid storage sites
Chemistry/Endocrine/Thyroid/2

40. Which of the following statements regarding thyroid hormones is true?
A. Both protein-bound and free T_3 and T_4 are physiologically active
B. Total T_3 and T_4 are influenced by the level of thyroxine-binding globulin (TBG)
C. Variation in thyroxine-binding protein levels affects both free T_3 and T_4
D. An elevated serum total T_4 and T_3 is diagnostic of hyperthyroidism
Chemistry/Endocrine/Thyroid/2

41. Which of the following conditions will increase total T_4 by increasing TBG?
A. Acute illness
B. Anabolic steroid use
C. Nephrotic syndrome
D. Pregnancy or estrogens
Chemistry/Endocrine/Disorders and disease/Thyroid/2

42. Select the *most* appropriate single screening test for thyroid disease.
A. Free T_4 index
B. Free T_3
C. Free T_4
D. TSH assay
Chemistry/Endocrine/Thyroid/2

Answers to Questions 37–42

37. B HVA is the major metabolite of dopamine, and urinary HVA is elevated in greater than 75% of patients with neuroblastoma.

38. C Thyroid hormones are derived from the enzymatic modification of tyrosine residues on thyroglobulin.

39. B T_3 is approximately 10 times more active physiologically than T_4, although levels of T_4 are about 50 times those of T_3. The rate of diiodotyrosine synthesis is twice that of monoiodotyrosine and the rate of coupling favors formation of T_4. Eighty percent of circulating T_3 is derived from enzymatic conversion of T_4 by iodothyronine-5′-deiodinase.

40. B Total serum T_4 and T_3 are dependent on both thyroid function and the amount of T_4-binding proteins, such as TBG. Total T_4 or T_3 may be abnormal in a patient with normal thyroid function if the TBG level is abnormal. For this reason, free T_3 and T_4 are more specific indicators of thyroid function than are measurements of total hormone. Only free hormone is physiologically active.

41. D Pregnancy and estrogens are the most common causes of increased TBG. Acute illness, anabolic steroids, and nephrotic syndrome decrease the level of TBG.

42. D TSH is produced by the anterior pituitary in response to low levels of free T_4 or T_3. A normal TSH rules out thyroid disease.

43. A patient previously diagnosed with primary hypothyroidism and started on T_4 replacement therapy is seen for follow-up testing after 2 weeks. The serum-free T_4 is normal, but the TSH is still elevated. What is the *most* likely explanation for these results?
- **A.** Laboratory error in measurement of free T_4
- **B.** Laboratory error in measurement of TSH
- **C.** *In vitro* drug interference with the free T_4 assay
- **D.** Results are consistent with a euthyroid patient in the early phase of therapy

Chemistry/Endocrine/Disorders and disease/Thyroid/3

44. The serum TSH level is almost absent in:
- **A.** Primary hyperthyroidism
- **B.** Primary hypothyroidism
- **C.** Secondary hyperthyroidism
- **D.** Euthyroid sick syndrome

Chemistry/Endocrine/Disorders and disease/Thyroid/1

45. Which assay is used to confirm difficult cases of hypothyroidism?
- **A.** Free T_3 assay
- **B.** Free T_4 index
- **C.** Thyrotropin-releasing hormone (TRH) stimulation test
- **D.** TBG assay

Chemistry/Endocrine/Disorders and disease/Thyroid/2

46. Which of the following statements is true regarding reverse T_3 (rT_3)?
- **A.** Formed in blood by degradation of T_4
- **B.** Physiologically active, but less than T_3
- **C.** Decreased in euthyroid sick syndrome
- **D.** Interferes with the measurement of serum T_3

Chemistry/Endocrine/Thyroid/2

47. A patient has an elevated serum free T_3 and free T_4 and undetectable TSH. What is the *most* likely cause of these results?
- **A.** Primary hyperthyroidism
- **B.** Secondary hyperthyroidism
- **C.** Euthyroid with increased TBG
- **D.** Euthyroid sick syndrome

Chemistry/Endocrine/Disorders and disease/Thyroid/3

48. A serum thyroid panel reveals an increase in total T_4, normal TSH, and normal free T_4. What is the *most* likely cause of these results?
- **A.** Primary hyperthyroidism
- **B.** Secondary hyperthyroidism
- **C.** Euthyroid with increased TBG
- **D.** Subclinical hypothyroidism

Chemistry/Endocrine/Thyroid/3

Answers to Questions 43–48

43. D Results of thyroid tests (especially in hospitalized patients) may sometimes appear discrepant because medications and nonthyroid illnesses can affect the test results. The pituitary is slow to respond to thyroxine replacement, and 6 to 8 weeks are usually required before TSH levels fall back to normal. In the early stage of therapy, the patient should be monitored by the free T_4 result. This patient's free T_4 is normal, indicating that replacement therapy is adequate. The high TSH sometimes seen in treated patients is called *pituitary lag*.

44. A Low TSH and a high T_3 occur in primary hyperthyroidism. High TSH and low T_4 levels occur in primary hypothyroidism but may also be seen in an acutely ill patient without thyroid disease (euthyroid sick syndrome). Secondary hyperthyroidism is caused by pituitary hyperfunction that increases TSH.

45. C The thyrotropin-releasing hormone (TRH) stimulation test is used to confirm borderline cases of abnormal thyroid function.

46. A Reverse T_3 (3,3´,5´-triiodothyronine) is formed from the deiodination of T_4 in blood. It is an inactive isomer of T_3. Reverse T_3 is increased in acute and chronic illnesses and is used to identify patients with euthyroid sick syndrome.

47. A An undetectable TSH with increased T_3 is caused by primary hyperthyroidism. In secondary hyperthyroidism, TSH will be elevated in addition to T_3. Patients with an increased TBG level will have an increase in total T_3 and T_4, but not free T_3, T_4, or TSH. Patients with euthyroid sick syndrome usually have a small decrease in free T_4 and a normal or slightly elevated TSH.

48. C Individuals with a normal TSH level are euthyroid, and an increase in total T_4 is caused by an increase in TBG. An increase in TBG causes an increase in total T_4 but not free T_4. Subclinical hypothyroidism is usually associated with high TSH but normal free T_3 and free T_4.

49. Which statement about TSH and T_4 in early pregnancy is correct?
A. TSH and thyroid hormones fall
B. TSH falls and thyroid hormones rise
C. TSH and thyroid hormones both rise
D. TSH rises and thyroid hormones fall
Chemistry/Endocrine/Thyroid/3

50. In which case might a very low plasma TSH result not correlate with thyroid status?
A. Euthyroid sick syndrome
B. Congenital hypothyroidism
C. When TBG is elevated
D. After high-dose corticosteroid treatment
Chemistry/Endocrine/Thyroid/3

Answers to Questions 49–50

49. B Estrogens released in pregnancy cause an increase in TBG, which causes an increase in total T_4 and T_3. In early pregnancy, hCG produced by the placenta stimulates the thyroid, causing an increase in free thyroid hormones. This suppresses TSH production.

50. D High doses of corticosteroids will suppress TSH production. Laboratory values in euthyroid sick syndrome may mimic mild hypothyroidism with normal thyroid function and TSH slightly increased because of lower levels of free T_3 or T_4.

6.8
Toxicology, Therapeutic Drug Monitoring, and Trace Metals

1. In which of the following cases is qualitative analysis of the drug usually adequate?
A. To determine whether the dose of a drug with a low therapeutic index is likely to be toxic
B. To determine whether a patient is complying with the physician's instructions
C. To adjust the dose if individual differences or disease alter the expected response
D. To determine whether the patient has been taking amphetamines

Chemistry/Therapeutic drug monitoring/1

2. The term *pharmacokinetics* refers to the:
A. Relationship between drug dose and the drug blood level
B. Concentration of drug at its sites of action
C. Relationship between blood concentration and therapeutic response
D. The relationship between blood and tissue drug levels

Chemistry/Therapeutic drug monitoring/1

3. The term *pharmacodynamics* is an expression of the relationship between:
A. Dose and physiological effect
B. Drug concentration at target sites and physiological effect
C. Time and serum drug concentration
D. Blood and tissue drug levels

Chemistry/Therapeutic drug monitoring/1

4. The study of pharmacogenomics involves which type of testing?
A. Familial studies to determine the inheritance of drug resistance
B. Testing drugs with cell cultures to determine the minimum toxic dosage
C. Testing for single nucleotide polymorphisms known to affect drug metabolism
D. Comparison of dose–response curves between family members

Chemistry/Therapeutic drug monitoring/1

5. Select the five pharmacological parameters that determine serum drug concentration.
A. Absorption, anabolism, perfusion, bioactivation, excretion
B. Liberation, equilibration, biotransformation, reabsorption, elimination
C. Liberation, absorption, distribution, metabolism, excretion
D. Ingestion, conjugation, integration, metabolism, elimination

Chemistry/Therapeutic drug monitoring/1

Answers to Questions 1–5

1. D Qualitative analysis is used when testing for abuse substances, when the goal is usually to determine whether the drug is present or absent, such as for amphetamines. Therapeutic drug monitoring is a quantitative procedure performed for drugs with a narrow therapeutic index.

2. A Pharmacokinetics is the mathematical expression of the relationship between drug dose and drug blood level.

3. B Pharmacodynamics is the relationship between the drug concentration at the receptor site (tissue concentration) and the response of the tissue to that drug.

4. C Pharmacogenomics refers to the study of genes that affect the concentration of a drug in an individual. One method is to test for single nucleotide polymorphisms (SNPs) by using DNA microarrays in genes. Genetic variations of one such enzyme may account for individual pharmacokinetic differences and can be used to predict the efficacy of the drug.

5. C Liberation is the release of the drug, and absorption is the transport of drug from the site of administration to blood. Distribution refers to the delivery of the drug to tissues. Metabolism is the process of chemical modification of the drug by cells. Excretion is the process by which the drug and its metabolites are removed from the body.

6. Which route of administration is associated with 100% bioavailability?
A. Sublingual
B. Intramuscular
C. Oral
D. IV

Chemistry/Therapeutic drug monitoring/2

7. The phrase "first-pass hepatic metabolism" means that:
A. 100% of a drug is excreted by the liver
B. All drug is inactivated by hepatic enzymes after one pass through the liver
C. Some drug is removed from the portal circulation, reducing bioavailability
D. The drug must be metabolized in the liver to an active form

Chemistry/Therapeutic drug monitoring/2

8. Which formula can be used to estimate dosage needed to give a desired steady-state blood level?
A. Dose per hour = clearance (milligrams per hour) × average concentration at steady state ÷ f
B. Dose per day = fraction absorbed – fraction excreted
C. Dose = fraction absorbed × (1/protein-bound fraction)
D. Dose per day = half-life × log V_d (volume distribution)

Chemistry/Therapeutic drug monitoring/1

9. For drugs with first-order elimination, which statement about drug clearance is true?
A. Clearance = elimination rate ÷ serum level
B. It is most often performed by the liver
C. It is directly related to half-life
D. Clearance rate is independent of dose

Chemistry/Therapeutic drug monitoring/2

10. Which statement about steady-state drug levels is true?
A. The absorbed drug must be greater than the amount excreted
B. Steady state can be measured after two elimination half-lives
C. Constant IV infusion will give the same minima and maxima as an oral dose
D. Oral dosing intervals give peaks and troughs in the dose–response curve

Chemistry/Therapeutic drug monitoring/2

Answers to Questions 6–10

6. D When a drug is administered intravenously, all of the drug enters the bloodstream. All other routes of administration require absorption through cells, and this process reduces the bioavailable fraction.

7. C Drugs given orally usually enter the blood via the portal circulation and are transported directly to the liver. Some drugs are excreted by the liver, and a fraction will be lost by hepatic excretion before the drug reaches the general circulation.

8. A After a patient receives a loading dose to rapidly bring the drug level up to the desired therapeutic range, a maintenance dose must be given at consistent intervals to maintain the blood drug level at the desired concentration. The dose per hour is determined by multiplying the clearance per hour by the desired average steady-state concentration, then dividing by *f* (bioavailable fraction).

9. A First-order elimination represents a linear relationship between the amount of drug eliminated per hour and the blood level of the drug. For drugs following linear kinetics, clearance equals the elimination rate divided by the drug concentration in blood. Clearance is inversely related to the drug's half-life and is accomplished mainly by the kidneys.

10. D The steady state is reached when the drug in the next dose is sufficient only to replace the drug eliminated since the last dose. Steady state can be measured after five drug half-lives. When drugs are infused through a steady IV drip, both the distribution and elimination rates are constant.

11. A peak blood level for gentamicin administered intramuscularly (therapeutic range 5–10 μg/mL) is 0.7 μg/mL. The preceding trough level was 0.5 μg/mL. What is the *most* likely explanation of these results?

A. Laboratory error made on peak measurement
B. Specimen for peak level was collected from wrong patient
C. Blood for peak level was drawn too soon
D. Elimination rate has reached maximum

Chemistry/Therapeutic drug monitoring/3

12. When should blood samples for trough drug levels be collected?

A. 30 minutes after peak levels
B. 45 minutes before the next dose
C. 1 to 2 hours after the last dose
D. Immediately before the next dose is given

Chemistry/Therapeutic drug monitoring/1

13. Of the following drugs, which is considered an antiseizure medication?

A. Phenytoin
B. Vancomycin
C. Gentamicin
D. Lithium

Chemistry/Therapeutic drug monitoring/1

14. Select the elimination model that *best* describes most oral drugs given at therapeutic doses.

A. One compartment, linear first-order elimination
B. Michaelis-Menton or nonlinear elimination
C. Two compartment with a biphasic elimination curve
D. Logarithmic elimination

Chemistry/Therapeutic drug monitoring/2

15. In the dose-response relationship, which is the *best* definition of the TD_{50} (toxic dose)?

A. The dose that would be predictive to result in death of 50% of the population
B. The dose that would produce an adverse effect in 50% of the population
C. The dose that would be ineffective in producing a therapeutic response in 50% of the population
D. A single, acute oral dose that has a lethal outcome in a 70-kg individual

Chemistry/Therapeutic drug monitoring/1

Answers to Questions 11–15

11. C Blood collection time for peak levels must not occur prior to complete absorption and distribution of drug. These results are most consistent with a peak sample having been drawn immediately after the intramuscular dose was given.

12. D The trough concentration of a drug is the lowest concentration obtained in the dosing interval. This occurs immediately before the absorption of the next dose given. Trough levels are usually collected just before the next dose is given.

13. A Phenytoin, also known as Dilantin, is used to treat seizures. Vancomycin and gentamicin are both classified as antibiotics, while lithium is a psychoactive drug.

14. A Most drugs given orally distribute uniformly through the tissues reaching rapid equilibrium, so both blood and tissues can be viewed as a single compartment. Elimination according to Michaelis-Menton kinetics is nonlinear because at high concentrations, the hepatic enzyme system becomes saturated, reducing the elimination efficiency. Therefore, at high serum concentrations, most first-order drugs transition to nonlinear elimination rates.

15. B The TD_{50} (toxic dose) is the dose that would produce an adverse, toxic response in 50% of the population. The LD_{50} is defined as the predicted dose that would result in death in 50% of the population, while the ED_{50} is the dose that would be beneficial or effective in 50% of the population.

16. Which fact must be considered when evaluating a patient who displays signs of drug toxicity?
A. Drug metabolites may need to be measured as well as parent drug
B. If the concentration of total drug is within therapeutic limits, the concentration of free drug cannot be toxic
C. If the drug has a wide therapeutic index, then it will not be toxic
D. A drug level cannot be toxic if the trough is within the published therapeutic range
Chemistry/Therapeutic drug monitoring/2

17. When a therapeutic drug is suspected of causing toxicity, which specimen is the *most* appropriate for an initial investigation?
A. Trough blood sample
B. Peak blood sample
C. Urine at the time of symptoms
D. Gastric fluid at the time of symptoms
Chemistry/Therapeutic drug monitoring/3

18. A chromatogram for blood alcohol (GC) gives broad trailing peaks and increased retention times for ethanol and internal standard. This is *most* likely caused by:
A. A contaminated injection syringe
B. Water contamination of the column packing
C. Carrier gas flow rate that is too fast
D. Oven temperature that is too high
Chemistry/Therapeutic drug monitoring/3

19. For which drug group are both peak and trough measurements usually required?
A. Antiarrhythmics
B. Analgesics
C. Tricyclic antidepressants
D. Aminoglycoside antibiotics
Chemistry/Therapeutic drug monitoring/2

20. A *stat* plasma lithium determined by using an ISE is measured at 14.0 mmol/L. Select the *most* appropriate course of action.
A. Immediately report this result
B. Check the sample for hemolysis
C. Call for a new specimen
D. Rerun the lithium calibrators
Chemistry/Therapeutic drug monitoring/3

21. Which of the following urine samples should be accepted for testing when processing samples for drugs of abuse (DAUs)?
A. Urine of abnormal color
B. Urine with an abnormal odor
C. Container with seal not applied across the lid
D. Sample with a volume of 50 mL
Chemistry/Toxicology/2

Answers to Questions 16–21

16. A Altered drug pharmacokinetics may result in toxicity even when the dose of drug is within the accepted therapeutic range. Two common causes of this are the presence of unmeasured metabolites that are physiologically active and the presence of a higher-than-expected concentration of free drug.

17. B When a drug is suspected of toxicity, the peak blood sample should be obtained because it is most likely to exceed the therapeutic limit.

18. B Water in a PEG column, such as Carbowax, used for measuring volatiles causes longer retention times and loss of resolution. Syringe contamination may cause the appearance of ghost peaks. Increased oven temperature or gas flow rate will shorten retention times and decrease peak widths.

19. D Aminoglycoside antibiotics cause damage to the eighth cranial nerve at toxic levels, resulting in hearing loss. When given at subtherapeutic doses, they fail to resolve infection. Most drugs falling in the other classes have a narrow peak–trough difference but are highly toxic when blood levels exceed the therapeutic range.

20. C A lithium level above 2.0 mmol/L is toxic. A level of 14 mmol/L would not occur unless the sample was contaminated with lithium. This would most likely result from collection in a green-top tube containing the lithium salt of heparin.

21. D Adulteration is a common problem with samples submitted for DAU testing. Urine with a volume under 30 mL, abnormal color, odor, or sign of adulteration should be rejected. The label should be placed across the entire lid so that the seal would be broken if the lid were removed after collection.

22. The enzyme-multiplied immunoassay technique (EMIT) for DAUs uses an:
A. Antibody conjugated to a drug
B. Enzyme conjugated to an antibody
C. Enzyme conjugated to a drug
D. Antibody bound to a solid phase
Chemistry/Toxicology/2

23. Which statement about EMIT is true?
A. Enzyme activity is inversely proportional to drug level
B. Formation of NADH is monitored at 340 nm
C. ALP is the commonly used conjugate
D. Assay use is restricted to serum
Chemistry/Toxicology/2

24. Which statement regarding cloned enzyme donor immunoassay (CEDIA) is true?
A. The enzyme used is G-6-PD
B. The enzyme donor and acceptor molecules are fragments of β-galactosidase
C. Drug concentration is inversely related to fluorescence
D. The antibody is covalently linked to the enzyme donor
Chemistry/Toxicology/2

25. Which statement is true regarding particle-enhanced turbidimetric inhibition immunoassay methods for therapeutic drugs?
A. Drug concentration is proportional to light scatter
B. Magnetic separation is needed to remove unbound conjugate
C. When particle-bound drug binds to antibody, light scattering is increased
D. Two antibodies to the drug are needed
Chemistry/Toxicology/2

26. Quantitation of a drug by GC-MS is usually performed in which mode?
A. Total ion chromatography
B. Selective ion monitoring
C. Ion subtraction
D. Selective reaction monitoring
Chemistry/Toxicology/1

27. A urine sample is received in the laboratory with the appropriate custody control form and a request for DAU screening. Which test result would be cause for rejecting the sample?
A. Post collection temperature is 95°F
B. pH is 5.0
C. Specific gravity is 5 mg/dL
D. Creatinine is 5 mg/dL
Chemistry/Toxicology/3

Answers to Questions 22–27

22. C In EMIT, the enzyme-labeled drug competes with drug in the sample for a limited amount of reagent the antibodies. When the antibody binds to the enzyme–drug conjugate, it blocks the catalytic site of the enzyme. Enzyme activity is directly proportional to the sample drug concentration because the quantity of unbound drug–enzyme conjugate will be highest when drug is present in the sample.

23. B Most EMIT assays use a two-reagent system. Reagent A contains substrate (usually glucose-6-PO_4), coenzyme (NAD^+), and antibody to the drug. Reagent B contains enzyme-labeled drug (usually G-6-PD-drug) and buffer. The rate of NADH production is proportional to the drug concentration. EMIT assays are commonly used to test for DAUs.

24. B Cloned enzyme donor immunoassay (CEDIA) is a homogeneous enzyme immunoassay that is commonly used to measure DAUs. Drug conjugated to a fragment of β-galactosidase that is catalytically inactive competes with the drug in the sample for a limited number of antibodies to the drug.

25. C Particle-enhanced turbidimetric inhibition immunoassays are homogeneous immunoassays frequently used to measure proteins and therapeutic drugs in serum or plasma. Polystyrene-modified latex particles conjugated to the drug (particle-bound drug) compete with the drug in the sample for a limited number of antibodies. If the drug concentration is low, more of the antibody binds to the particle-bound drug, increasing the turbidity of the reaction. Therefore, light scattering is inversely proportional to the drug concentration.

26. B Most GC-MS instruments use an electron beam to split the drug emerging from the column into its component ions. CG-MS instruments can be operated in two modes: total ion chromatography (TIC) and selective ion monitoring (SIM). SIM measures the abundance of one or more principal ions that provide sufficient specificity to eliminate potential interfering substances and greater quantitative sensitivity. TIC displays the retention time of all ions detected and their abundance. It is primarily used for identification of unknown compounds.

27. D The majority of DAU samples that have been adulterated can be detected by determining temperature (90°F–100°F), pH (4.5–8.0), specific gravity (1.003–1.019), and creatinine (20 mg/dL or greater). All the values listed are within the limits of an acceptable sample, with the exception of creatinine.

28. Which substance has the longest detection time in urine?
A. Amphetamines
B. Cocaine
C. Benzodiazepines
D. Marijuana
Chemistry/Toxicology/1

29. Which statement about the measurement of carboxyhemoglobin is true?
A. Treatment with alkaline dithionite is used to convert carboxyhemoglobin to oxyhemoglobin
B. Oxyhemoglobin has no absorbance at 540 nm, but carboxyhemoglobin does
C. Polychromic analysis is used to eliminate interference by oxyhemoglobin
D. Carboxyhemoglobin can be measured by potentiometry
Chemistry/Toxicology/2

30. Which of the following statements about blood alcohol measurement is correct?
A. Symptoms of intoxication usually begin when the level exceeds 0.05% w/v
B. The skin puncture site should be disinfected with isopropanol
C. The reference method is based upon enzymatic oxidation of ethanol by ADH
D. GC methods require extraction of ethanol from serum
Chemistry/Toxicology/2

31. Which specimen is the sample of choice for lead screening?
A. Whole blood
B. Hair
C. Serum
D. Urine
Chemistry/Toxicology/1

32. Which of the following enzymes can be used to measure plasma or serum salicylate?
A. Peroxidase
B. Salicylate esterase
C. Salicylate hydroxylase
D. *p*-Aminosalicylate oxidase
Chemistry/Toxicology/1

33. Which of the following tests is *least* essential to the operation of an ED at a general hospital?
A. Carboxyhemoglobin
B. Osmolality
C. Salicylate
D. Lead
Chemistry/Toxicology/2

Answers to Questions 28–33

28. D Marijuana is stored in fatty tissue and is metabolized slowly. In individuals who use marijuana several times per week, cannabinoids can be detected several weeks after last use. For chronic daily users, this extends to months after discontinuation.

29. C The absorbance spectra of oxy- and carboxyhemoglobin pigments overlap, and bichromatic or polychromatic analysis is required to accurately measure carboxyhemoglobin concentration.
In bichromatic analysis, oxyhemoglobin and methemoglobin are converted to deoxyhemoglobin by the addition of alkaline sodium dithionite. The ratio of absorbance at 541:555 nm is directly proportional to carboxyhemoglobin concentration.

30. A Symptoms of intoxication usually begin when the level exceeds 0.05% w/v. ADH is not specific for ethanol, and *in vitro* interference can occur with some ADH methods when skin is disinfected with other alcohols. For this reason, and to avoid interference with the interpretation of chromatograms for volatiles, blood samples are collected after disinfecting the skin site with benzalkonium chloride or other nonalcohol antiseptic. GLC is the legally accepted method of ethanol analysis. The low boiling point of ethanol permits direct analysis on blood or plasma diluted with water containing 1-propanol or another suitable internal standard.

31. A Lead accumulates in RBCs, bones, and neural tissues; whole blood, hair, and urine are suitable for demonstrating lead toxicity. The greatest sensitivity is obtained by using whole blood, which can detect exposure over time.

32. C The enzymatic assay of salicylate uses salicylate hydroxylase, which reduces salicylate with NADH and forms catechol and NAD^+.

33. D Toxicity from lead poisoning and most other trace metals is usually a chronic condition that does not often require immediate access to laboratory testing. The vast majority of acute toxicology situations seen in the ED involve poisoning with alcohol, acetaminophen, salicylate, abuse substances, or CO poisoning, and at a minimum, EDs should offer tests for these. Serum osmolality measured by freezing point depression is a sensitive surrogate test for drug and alcohol overdose.

34. A gastric fluid sample from a patient suspected of having taken an overdose of amphetamine is sent to the laboratory for analysis. The only test for amphetamines performed by the laboratory is EMIT. What is the *best* course of action?
A. Perform an EMIT assay for amphetamine
B. Refuse the sample and request urine
C. Dilute 1:10 with H_2O and filter; perform the test
D. Titrate to pH 7.0, then follow the procedure for measuring amphetamine in urine
Chemistry/Toxicology/3

35. A 6-year-old child being treated with phenytoin was recently placed on valproic acid for better control of seizures. After displaying signs of phenytoin toxicity, including ataxia, a *stat* phenytoin is determined to be 15.0 mg/L (reference range 10–20 mg/L). A peak blood level drawn 5 hours after the last dose is 18.0 mg/L. The valproic acid measured at the same time is within therapeutic limits. Quality control is within acceptable limits for all tests, but the provider questions the accuracy of the results. What is the *most* appropriate next course of action?
A. Repeat the valproic acid level using the last specimen
B. Repeat the phenytoin on both trough and peak samples using a different method
C. Recommend measurement of free phenytoin on the last specimen
D. Recommend a second trough level be measured
Chemistry/Toxicology/3

36. Which of the following trace elements is considered an essential micronutrient?
A. Thallium
B. Aluminum
C. Mercury
D. Selenium
Chemistry/Trace metals/1

37. When measuring trace metals other than lead in blood, what type of tube should be used?
A. Navy blue top
B. Green top
C. Purple top
D. Red top
Chemistry/Trace metals/Lead/1

38. Which whole blood level is suggestive of excessive exposure to lead in children but not adults?
A. 4 μg/dL
B. 14 μg/dL
C. 28 μg/dL
D. 32 μg/dL
Chemistry/Trace metals/Lead/2

Answers to Questions 34–38

34. B The gastric sample should not be used in place of serum or urine without documentation of acceptability by the reagent manufacturer or laboratory. EMIT is approved for measuring amphetamines in urine only.

35. C This patient's free phenytoin level should be measured, and the dose of phenytoin should be reduced to produce a free drug level that is within the therapeutic range. Phenytoin follows a nonlinear rate of elimination, which means that clearance decreases as blood levels increase. Valproic acid competes with phenytoin for binding sites on albumin.

36. D Trace elements can be divided into two categories: those that have no known biological purpose and those that do. The former includes thallium, mercury, lead, cadmium, and aluminum. All others can be considered essential trace elements, including selenium, which is a cofactor in enzymatic processes.

37. A To avoid trace contamination by metals present in the stopper lubricants, a tube with a navy blue top is used for measuring trace metals other than lead. These tubes are validated for most but not all trace metals.

38. B Because lead exposure in children leads to learning impairment, the cutoff for exposure recommended by the Centers for Disease Control and Prevention (CDC) is 5 μg/dL in venous whole blood.

39. What are the likely laboratory findings in a person suspected of having Wilson disease?

A. Blood copper and ceruloplasmin low, urinary copper excretion high
B. Blood and urine copper concentration high, ceruloplasmin low
C. Blood and urine copper concentration high, ceruloplasmin high
D. Blood and urine copper concentration low, ceruloplasmin low

Chemistry/Trace metals/Copper/2

40. Kashin-Beck disease, an osteoarthropathy seen in children, is associated with a low blood level of this trace metal.

A. Copper
B. Selenium
C. Cadmium
D. Arsenic

Chemistry/Trace metals/1

Answers to Questions 39–40

39. A Wilson disease is an autosomal recessive disease in which copper transport is abnormal. The gene causing the disease codes for an adenosine triphosphatase (ATPase, called *Wilson protein* or *ATP7B*) that is needed to excrete copper into bile and incorporate copper into ceruloplasmin. Absence of Wilson protein results in failure to load ceruloplasmin with copper. Therefore, blood levels of ceruloplasmin are low, and blood levels of copper are usually low because there is little ceruloplasmin to bind it.

40. B Kashin-Beck disease is a chronic joint disease in children and adolescents due to a selenium deficiency.

6.9
Tumor Markers

1. **Which of the following tumor markers is classified as a tumor suppressor gene?**
   A. *BRCA1*
   B. Carcinoembryonic antigen (CEA)
   C. hCG
   D. Nuclear matrix protein (NMP)
   Chemistry/Tumor markers/1

2. **In general, in which of the following situations is the analysis of a glycoprotein tumor marker, such as carbohydrate-associated antigen-125 (CA-125), *most* useful?**
   A. Testing for recurrence
   B. Prognosis
   C. Screening
   D. Diagnosis
   Chemistry/Tumor markers/1

3. **Which of the following enzymes increase in individuals with prostate and small cell lung cancer?**
   A. Creatine kinase-1 (CK-1)
   B. Gamma glutamyl transferase (GGT)
   C. Amylase
   D. LDH
   Chemistry/Tumor markers/2

4. **Which of the following is the *most* useful analyte to monitor for recurrence of ovarian cancer?**
   A. CA-15-3
   B. CA-19-9
   C. CA-125
   D. CEA
   Chemistry/Tumor markers/2

5. **Which tumor marker is associated with cancer of the urinary bladder?**
   A. CA-19-9
   B. CA-72-4
   C. Nuclear matrix protein 22 (NMP-22)
   D. Cathepsin D
   Chemistry/Tumor markers/2

Answers to Questions 1–5

1. A The *BRCA1* and *BRCA2* genes are tumor suppressor genes located on the long arm of chromosome 17 and mutation increases the risk of breast cancer.

2. A The major use of tumor markers is to monitor recurrence and therapy. Most tumor markers are often expressed at very low levels in normal cells so that the concentration in early malignancy overlaps that seen in normal individuals, making them ineffective for screening. Some tumor markers are useful predictors of disease progression and response to treatment.

3. A Creatine kinase-1 (CK-1 [CK-BB]) is not normally found in plasma or serum except in neonates. It may be present in persons with CNS damage and some other disorders, but its presence is often associated with various malignancies, especially prostate cancer and small cell carcinoma of the lung. GGT levels are very high in hepatoma, and amylase is elevated in pancreatic cancer. LDH is associated with various tumors.

4. C CA-125 is an oncofetal antigen, meaning that it is produced by genes that are active during fetal development but minimally active after birth except in malignant tissues. CA-15-3 is used mainly to monitor breast cancer treatment and recurrence. CA-19-9 is a glycoprotein shed from the surface of gastric, pancreatic, and colorectal cancer cells. CEA is most widely used as a tumor marker for colorectal cancer.

5. C Nuclear matrix protein 22 (NMP-22) is shed into urine in persons with bladder carcinoma.

6. A person presents with a cushingoid appearance and an elevated 24-hour urinary cortisol level. Plasma ACTH is very elevated, and the physician suspects that the cause is ectopic ACTH production. Which test would be *most* useful in substantiating this diagnosis?

A. Plasma cortisol
B. CA-50
C. ALP isoenzymes
D. AFP

Chemistry/Tumor markers/3

7. Which of the following tumor markers is used to monitor individuals with breast cancer for recurrence of disease?

A. Cathepsin D
B. CA-15-3
C. Retinoblastoma gene (*RB*)
D. Estrogen receptor (ER)

Chemistry/Tumor markers/2

8. Which of the following statements regarding Ph[1] is true?

A. It is seen exclusively in chronic myelogenous leukemia
B. It results from a translocation
C. It appears as a short-arm deletion of chromosome 21
D. It is associated with a poor prognosis

Chemistry/Tumor markers/1

9. What is the *primary* clinical utility of measuring CEA?

A. Diagnosis of liver cancer
B. Diagnosis of colorectal cancer
C. Screening for cancers of endodermal origin
D. Monitoring for recurrence of cancer

Chemistry/Tumor markers/1

10. Which tumor marker is used to determine the usefulness of trastuzumab (Herceptin) therapy for breast cancer?

A. Progesterone receptor (PR)
B. CEA
C. *HER-2/neu*
D. *Myc*

Chemistry/Tumor markers/1

11. A person is suspected of having testicular cancer. Which type of hCG test would be the *most* useful?

A. Plasma immunoassay for intact hCG only
B. Plasma immunoassay for intact hCG and the β-hCG subunit
C. Plasma immunoassay for the free α- and β-hCG subunits
D. Urine assay for hCG β-core

Chemistry/Tumor markers/2

Answers to Questions 6–11

6. C Most often, ectopic ACTH production occurs in lung cancer. Tumors of the lung are often associated with the production of placental-like ALP, and a positive finding would support the diagnosis of an ectopic (nonpituitary) source of ACTH. CA-50 is a marker for recurrence and treatment of GI and pancreatic cancers. AFP is the predominant protein produced by the fetus, and plasma levels are increased primarily in yolk sac, liver, and testicular tumors.

7. B CA-15-3 is used to monitor treatment and recurrence of breast cancer. However, abnormal plasma levels are seen in many nonmalignant conditions, and the test is not used for diagnostic purposes. Cathepsin D and estrogen receptor (ER) assays are performed to determine the prognosis of patients with breast cancer. The retinoblastoma gene (*RB*) is a tumor-suppressor gene found missing in persons with retinoblastoma.

8. B Ph[1] is formed by translocation of the long arms of chromosomes 9 and 22. The result is that part of the *ABL* gene of chromosome 9 becomes inserted into the *BCR* of chromosome 22. Approximately 95% of patients with chronic myelogenous leukemia have Ph[1]. It is also present in the lymphocytes of up to 25% of adults with acute lymphocytic leukemia (ALL).

9. D CEA is a glycoprotein that is secreted into plasma by various cancers of endodermal origin, including breast, lung, colorectal, and stomach cancers. Its clinical use is to detect recurrence and the need for second-look surgery in patients who have been treated and to evaluate the response to treatment.

10. C Trastuzumab is an antibody to the *HER-2/neu* gene product. *HER-2/neu* is an oncogene that is overexpressed in some breast cancers. The progesterone receptor (PR), like the estrogen receptor (ER), is used to identify patients with breast cancer who are more likely to respond to estrogen-suppression therapy. *Myc* is a group of oncogenes that are activated in various cancers, including lung, breast, colon, and stomach cancers; leukemia; and lymphoma.

11. B In addition to testicular cancer, hCG is produced by trophoblastic tumors and choriocarcinomas. Some of these tumors secrete the β-subunit without intact hCG. The use of an immunoassay that measures both the intact and free β-hCG will have greater sensitivity compared with an assay for intact hCG or an assay for only free subunits. Urinary β-core (urinary gonadotropin peptide) is a metabolic product of the β-subunit and has been used to monitor for persistence of trophoblastic disease and recurrence of some hCG-producing tumors.

12. A patient treated for a germ cell tumor has a total and free β-hCG assay performed prior to surgery. The result is 40,000 mIU/mL. One week after surgery, the hCG is 5,000 mIU/mL. Chemotherapy is started, and the hCG is measured 1 week later and found to be 10,000 mIU/mL. What does this indicate?

A. Recurrence of the tumor
B. Falsely increased hCG as a result of drug interference with the assay
C. Analytical error with the test reported as 5,000 mIU/mL
D. Transient hCG increase caused by chemotherapy

Chemistry/Tumor markers/3

13. An example of an oncofetal antigen that may also be utilized as a tumor marker would be:

A. PSA
B. 5-HIAA
C. AFP
D. ACTH

Chemistry/Tumor markers/1

14. Which type of cancer is associated with the highest level of AFP?

A. Hepatoma
B. Ovarian cancer
C. Testicular cancer
D. Breast cancer

Chemistry/Tumor markers/1

15. Which of the following assays is recommended as a screening test for colorectal cancer in individuals over 50 years of age?

A. CEA
B. AFP
C. Occult blood
D. Fecal trypsin

Chemistry/Tumor markers/2

16. Which of the following assays is used to determine the risk of cancer?

A. Epidermal growth factor receptor (EGFR)
B. Squamous cell carcinoma (SCC) antigen
C. *c-erbB-2* gene expression
D. *p53* gene mutation

Chemistry/Tumor markers/1

17. A person has elevated 24-hour urinary HVA and VMA levels. Urinary metanephrines, chromogranin A, and neuron-specific enolase levels are also elevated, but the 5-HIAA level is within the reference range. What is the *most* likely diagnosis?

A. Carcinoid tumors of the intestine
B. Pheochromocytoma
C. Neuroblastoma
D. Pancreatic cancer

Chemistry/Tumor markers/2

Answers to Questions 12–17

12. D Treatment of tumors with chemotherapy often causes a transient increase in the production of tumor markers as the drugs destroy tumor cells. Initiation of chemotherapy probably caused the hCG to double in the following week. The hCG assay should be monitored at regular intervals for several months because failure of hCG to decline or progressively increasing levels would suggest recurrence.

13. C AFP is considered an oncofetal antigen and is produced primarily during fetal development and is elevated in testicular cancer and hepatocarcinoma.

14. A AFP is increased in all patients with yolk sac tumors and greater than 80% of those with hepatoma. Ectopic AFP-secreting tumors are produced by ovarian, testicular, breast, GI, and bladder cancers, and these sources should be considered when 10-fold or higher elevations are seen in the absence of abnormal liver function.

15. C Bleeding in the GI tract occurs during the early stages of colorectal cancer, in which CEA is elevated in fewer than 60% of cases. AFP is elevated in only about 5% of colon cancers. Fecal trypsin is not a marker for colorectal cancer.

16. D The *p53* gene (tumor suppressor gene) produces a protein that downregulates the cell cycle. The *c-erbB-2* gene codes for a growth factor receptor with tyrosine kinase activity on the cell membrane. EGFR is a receptor for epidermal growth factor, and its overexpression in breast tissue is associated with a poorer prognosis. SCC antigen is found in the cytoplasm of tumors of squamous origin and is secreted in the plasma of patients with uterine cancer.

17. C Neuron-specific enolase is an isoenzyme specific to nervous tissue and found in neuroendocrine cells. Plasma levels are increased in neuroblastomas, carcinoid tumors, thyroid medullary carcinomas, and some lung cancers and seminomas. Urinary VMA, catecholamines, and metanephrines are increased in both pheochromocytoma (a tumor of chromaffin cells) and neuroblastoma (also a tumor of neuroectodermal cells derived from the neural crest neuroblasts of the sympathetic ganglia). Urinary HVA is increased in about 75% of patients with neuroblastoma but is not usually increased in pheochromocytoma. Chromogranin A is a protein that inhibits the release of catecholamines and is increased in pheochromocytoma, neuroblastoma, and carcinoid tumors. 5-HIAA is increased in carcinoid tumors (enterochromaffin tumors).

18. In which of the following situations is PSA *least* likely to be increased?
A. Precancerous lesions of the prostate
B. Post–prostate biopsy
C. Benign prostatic hypertrophy
D. Post–digital rectal examination
Chemistry/Tumor markers/1

19. Which of the following statements regarding PSA is true?
A. Complexed PSA in plasma is normally less than free PSA (fPSA)
B. fPSA less than 25% is a risk factor for malignant disease
C. A total PSA less than 4 ng/mL rules out malignant disease
D. A total PSA greater than 10 ng/mL is diagnostic of malignant disease
Chemistry/Tumor markers/2

20. A 55-year-old biological male with early-stage prostate cancer diagnosed through biopsy had their prostate gland removed (simple prostatectomy). Their PSA prior to surgery was 10.0 ng/mL. If the surgery was successful in completely removing the tumor cells, what would the PSA result be 1 month after surgery?
A. Undetectable
B. 1 to 3 ng/mL
C. Less than 4 ng/mL
D. Less than 10 ng/mL
Chemistry/Tumor markers/3

21. This glycoprotein is a Food and Drug Administration (FDA)–approved tumor marker for monitoring recurrence of ovarian cancer and evaluating the effectiveness of chemotherapy.
A. CA-15-3
B. CA-19-9
C. CA-125
D. CEA
Chemistry/Tumor markers/1

22. Which of the following is the *most* useful analyte to monitor for recurrence of colorectal cancer?
A. CA-15-3
B. CA-27-29
C. CA-125
D. CEA
Chemistry/Tumor markers/1

Answers to Questions 18–22

18. D Although digital rectal examination raises the prostatic acid phosphatase level, it does not increase the concentration of PSA in plasma. In addition to prostate cancer, PSA may be increased in acute or chronic prostate inflammation, benign prostate hypertrophy, and after transurethral prostate resection or prostate biopsy.

19. B In normal plasma, 55% to 95% of the PSA is bound to protease inhibitors and the remainder is fPSA. In individuals with a low ratio of fPSA:total PSA (less than 25% fPSA), this indicates a higher risk for prostate cancer.

20. A If the tumor were confined to the prostate, the PSA would be undetectable 1 month after successful surgery because there is no other tissue source of PSA. The half-life of PSA is 2.2 to 3.2 days, and the minimum detection limit of most assays is 0.2 ng/mL or lower. Therefore, it would require at least 2 weeks before the PSA level would be undetectable.

21. C CA-125 is a glycoprotein antigen shed by approximately 75% of ovarian cancers. It is an FDA-approved tumor marker for monitoring recurrence of ovarian cancer and evaluating the effectiveness of chemotherapy.

22. D CEA, an oncofetal antigen, is the most widely used tumor marker for colorectal cancer, though it is nonspecific. CA-15-3 and CA-27-29 are both used to monitor breast cancer treatment and recurrence. CA-125 is present in ovarian cancer and is monitored for a response to therapy.

23. If an individual is suspected of breast cancer associated with the *MUC1* gene, which combination of tumor markers provides the *best* evaluation of the protein expressed by the gene?

A. CA-19-9 and CEA
B. CA-27-29 and CA-15-3
C. β-hCG and CA-15-3
D. CA-125 and AFP

Chemistry/Tumor markers/2

24. As a tumor marker, elevation of this protein may indicate a poor prognosis in hematological cancers, such as multiple myeloma.

A. CA-125
B. β_2-Microglobulin
C. CA-19-9
D. CA-27-29

Chemistry/Tumor markers/2

25. Regarding the blood collection process for catecholamines, which statement is true?

A. The tube of choice is lithium heparin sample
B. The patient should avoid taking medications such as acetaminophen prior to collection
C. The patient should be seated in an upright position in the collection chair at least 30 minutes prior to collection
D. The patient should be fasting 8 to 12 hours prior to collecting the sample

Chemistry/Tumor markers/1

Answers to Questions 23–25

23. B CA-27-29 (also called BR-27-29) and CA-15-3 are useful in measuring different epitopes on the same antigen produced by the *MUC1* gene and both are elevated in an estimated 60% to 70% of individuals with advanced stage breast cancer.

24. B β_2-Microglobulin is found on the surface of nucleated cells and is a poor prognostic indicator for cancer recurrence in hematological malignancies, such as multiple myeloma or chronic lymphocytic leukemia.

25. B Prior to collection of a blood specimen for catecholamines, the patient should be instructed to avoid caffeine, over-the-counter medications such as acetaminophen, and certain foods. A 4-hour fast is recommended. The specimen of choice is nonhemolyzed EDTA plasma, separated and refrigerated within 30 minutes of collection. The patient should be in a supine position for 30 minutes prior to collection.

BIBLIOGRAPHY

1. *ASCP Quick Compendium of Medical Laboratory Sciences*. 2nd ed. ASCP Press; 2024.
2. Bishop ML, Fody EP, Van Siclen C, Mistler JM, Moy M. *Clinical Chemistry: Principles, Techniques, and Correlations*. 9th ed. Jones & Bartlett Learning; 2023.

CHAPTER 7

Hematology

7.1 *Blood Physiology*

7.2 *Normocytic Normochromic Anemia*

7.3 *Microcytic Hypochromic Anemia*

7.4 *Macrocytic Normochromic Anemia*

7.5 *Laboratory Evaluation of Anemia*

7.6 *Qualitative and Quantitative Nonmalignant Leukocyte Disorders*

7.7 *Myelodysplastic Syndromes*

7.8 *Lymphoproliferative and Myeloproliferative Neoplasms*

7.9 *Acute Leukemia*

7.10 *Laboratory Evaluation of Leukocyte Disorders*

7.1
Blood Physiology

1. **Which of the following is the preferred site for bone marrow aspiration and biopsy in an adult?**
   A. Iliac crest
   B. Sternum
   C. Tibia
   D. Spinous processes of a vertebra
   Hematology/Blood physiology/1

2. **What phagocytic cells produce lysozymes that are bactericidal?**
   A. Eosinophils
   B. Lymphocytes
   C. Platelets (PLTs)
   D. Neutrophils
   Hematology/Blood physiology/1

3. **The hematology analyzer results from a whole blood sample are 60% lymphocytes and an absolute count of 3,000. What do the findings indicate?**
   A. This is an expected finding for an infant
   B. This is suspicious for a lymphoblastic leukemia in a young child requiring further evaluation
   C. This is likely a viral infection in a symptomatic teenager
   D. This is an expected finding for an adult
   Hematology/Blood physiology/2

4. **An unknown nucleated erythrocyte has a pyknotic nucleus and pink cytoplasm. What is the likely identification?**
   A. Reticulocyte
   B. Polychromatophilic normoblast
   C. Basophilic normoblast
   D. Orthochromatophilic normoblast
   Hematology/Blood physiology/2

5. **The enzyme needed to incorporate iron into the protoporphyrin ring to complete the heme molecule is:**
   A. Deoxyhemoglobin
   B. Protoporphyrinogen oxidase
   C. Delta-amino levulinic acid
   D. Ferrochelatase
   Hematology/Blood physiology/1

Answers to Questions 1–5

1. A The iliac crest is the most frequently used site for bone marrow aspiration and biopsy. This site is the safest and most easily accessible, with the bone just beneath the skin, and neither blood vessels nor nerves are in the vicinity.

2. D Neutrophils are highly phagocytic and release lysozymes, peroxidase, and pyrogenic proteins. Eosinophils migrate to sites where there is an allergic reaction or parasitic infestation and release peroxidase, pyrogens, and other enzymes, including an oxidase that neutralizes histamine. Eosinophils are poorly phagocytic and do not release lysozyme.

3. A Adults and infants have an inverted differential mainly based on physiological need. Because of their naïve immune system, this is an expected finding for an infant. It would be considered an increased value in an adult patient. Using the relative and absolute counts as a guide, there is not enough information to determine the patient's age and a viral infection or a malignancy is not likely.

4. D In the stages of development for erythrocytes the stage that has a pyknotic nucleus and pink cytoplasm is the orthochromatophilic normoblast, which is the most common form of a nucleated RBC (NRBC). Younger stages, such as the basophilic normoblast, have more active RNA and have bluer cytoplasm. The middle stage that has purple cytoplasm is the polychromatophilic normoblast. Both basophilic normoblast and polychromatophilic normoblast are actively replicating DNA, so their nuclei will not be pyknotic.

5. D The heme molecule begins with the formation of delta-aminolevulinic acid (δ-ALA) from glycine and succinyl coenzyme A (CoA) with the help of ALA synthase. The final step after the protoporphyrin ring has been formed is to incorporate iron into the heme moiety, and the enzyme that does that is ferrochelatase. Protoporphyrinogen oxidase catalyzes the final step in the formation of the protoporphyrin ring.

6. Which of the following hemoglobin (Hgb) configurations represents the composition of Hgb F?
- **A.** 4 gamma chains
- **B.** 2 alpha and 2 gamma chains
- **C.** 4 beta chains
- **D.** 2 alpha and 2 beta chains

Hematology/Blood physiology/2

7. Which of the following organs is responsible for the "pitting process" in red blood cells (RBCs)?
- **A.** Liver
- **B.** Spleen
- **C.** Kidney
- **D.** Lymph nodes

Hematology/Blood physiology/1

8. Reticulocytosis usually indicates:
- **A.** Response to inflammation
- **B.** Neoplastic process
- **C.** Aplastic anemia
- **D.** RBC regeneration

Hematology/Blood physiology/2

Answers to Questions 6–8

6. B The structure of Hgb F is α_2-γ_2, which is the symbol for two alpha (α) and two gamma (γ) chains. Four beta chains (β_4) is the composition of Hgb H. Four gamma chains (γ_4) is Hgb Portland, and two alpha and two beta chains (α_2-β_2) is Hgb A.

7. B The spleen filters the blood, pitting imperfections from the erythrocyte without destroying the integrity of the membrane.

8. D Reticulocytes are polychromatophilic macrocytes, and the presence of reticulocytes indicates RBC regeneration. Bone marrow's appropriate response to anemia is to deliver RBCs prematurely to the peripheral circulation. In this way, reticulocytes and possibly NRBCs may be seen in the peripheral blood smear.

7.2
Normocytic Normochromic Anemia

1. The classification system of the erythrocytes in sickle cell disease (SCD) is:
A. Microcytic hypochromic
B. Macrocytic normochromic
C. Normocytic normochromic
D. Normocytic hypochromic
Hematology/Normocytic normochromic anemia/2

2. A patient's peripheral blood smear has 2+ spherocytes, 2+ schistocytes, and 3+ polychromasia. What does this indicate?
A. The patient likely has thalassemia major
B. The patient likely has extravascular hemolysis
C. The patient likely has iron-deficiency anemia
D. The patient likely has intravascular hemolysis
Hematology/Normocytic normochromic anemia/2

3. Which of the following is *not* associated with Hereditary Spherocytosis (HS)?
A. Increased osmotic fragility
B. Mean cell hemoglobin concentration (MCHC) greater than 36%
C. Intravascular hemolysis
D. Extravascular hemolysis
Hematology/Normocytic normochromic anemia/2

4. A lab report shows a mean cell volume (MCV) of 90 fL, and a mean cell hemoglobin concentration (MCHC) of 34%. Reticulocyte count is 5.5%. What can be concluded from these results?
A. The patient is healthy, and no further testing is required
B. The patient has a megaloblastic anemia, and a folate assay should be performed
C. The patient has iron-deficiency anemia that requires confirmation with iron studies
D. The patient has a hemolytic disorder, and additional testing is required
Hematology/Normocytic normochromic anemia/3

5. The classification of the erythrocytes seen in glucose-6-phosphate dehydrogenase (G-6-PD) deficiency is:
A. Microcytic normochromic
B. Microcytic hypochromic
C. Normocytic normochromic
D. Normocytic hypochromic
Hematology/Normocytic normochromic anemia/1

Answers to Questions 1–5

1. C Sickle cell disease (SCD) is a hemoglobinopathy caused by a qualitative defect in the hemoglobin molecule. Due to the qualitative defect, SCD patients produce Hgb S instead of Hgb A but in proportional quantities of erythrocytes and hemoglobin.
This indicates that the erythrocytes in SCD classify as normocytic normochromic.

2. D The presence of spherocytes indicates there is extravascular hemolysis present. The presence of schistocytes indicates that intravascular hemolysis is present. Physiologically, intravascular hemolysis eventually leads into extravascular hemolysis so the presence of schistocytes and spherocytes indicate intravascular hemolysis. Polychromasia indicates that there is a bone marrow response to the erythrocyte destruction and hypoxic need.

3. C Classic features of intravascular hemolysis, such as hemoglobinemia, hemoglobinuria, or hemosiderinuria, do not occur in HS. The hemolysis seen in HS is an extravascular process, rather than an intravascular process. Increased osmotic fragility and MCHC greater than 36% are common findings in HS.

4. D The lab report confirms a normocytic normochromic anemia. The increased reticulocyte count indicates a hemolytic process is occurring and rules out that the patient is healthy. Iron-deficiency anemia is a microcytic hypochromic anemia, which is confirmed with iron studies and has a low reticulocyte count. Megaloblastic anemia is a macrocytic normochromic anemia, which also presents with a low reticulocyte count.

5. C G-6-PD deficiency is a hemolytic disorder. Patients lack an enzyme that protects the erythrocytes against oxidative damage. As a result, there is accelerated erythrocyte destruction, which proportionally decreases the RBC count and the hemoglobin.
This indicates that the indices are normocytic normochromic.

6. Which is the major Hgb found in the RBCs of patients with hemoglobin C trait?
A. Hgb S
B. Hgb C
C. Hgb A_2
D. Hgb A
Hematology/Normocytic normochromic anemia/1

7. Select the amino acid substitution that is responsible for Hgb C disease.
A. Lysine is substituted for glutamic acid at the sixth position of the α-chain
B. Lysine is substituted for glutamic acid at the sixth position of the β-chain
C. Valine is substituted for glutamic acid at the sixth position of the α-chain
D. Glutamine is substituted for glutamic acid at the sixth position of the β-chain
Hematology/Normocytic normochromic anemia/1

8. Which of the following is *not* usually found in pyruvate kinase (PK) deficiency?
A. Echinocytes
B. Reticulocytosis
C. An increased indirect bilirubin
D. Decreased fluorescence in a qualitative PK assay
Hematology/Normocytic normochromic anemia/1

9. Which of the following electrophoretic results is consistent with sickle cell trait?

A. Hgb A: 40%	Hgb S: 35%	Hgb F: 5%
B. Hgb A: 60%	Hgb S: 40%	Hgb A_2: 2%
C. Hgb A: 0%	Hgb A_2: 5%	Hgb F: 95%
D. Hgb A: 80%	Hgb S: 10%	Hgb A_2: 10%

Hematology/Normocytic normochromic anemia/2

10. Autosplenectomy is associated with which of the following conditions?
A. Sickle cell trait
B. Hgb C disease
C. Hgb SC disease
D. Sickle cell disease
Hematology/Normocytic normochromic anemia/1

11. Which of the following is true of Paroxysmal nocturnal hemoglobinuria (PNH)?
A. It results from a somatic mutation in the *PIGA* gene that codes for GPI anchored proteins
B. It results from a biphasic antibody that binds and lyses at two different temperatures
C. It results from a mutant gene on the X chromosome
D. It is inherited as an autosomal recessive trait
Hematology/Normocytic normochromic anemia/1

12. Which of the following is *not* associated with hemolytic uremic syndrome (HUS)?
A. Renal failure
B. Thrombocytopenia
C. Hemoglobinuria
D. Reticulocytopenia
Hematology/Normocytic normochromic anemia/2

Answers to Questions 6–12

6. D The major Hgb in Hgb C trait is Hgb A, which constitutes 50% to 70% of the total. Hgb C makes up 20% to 40%, and Hgb A_2 and Hgb F are present in adequate amounts.

7. B The structural mutation for Hgb C is the substitution of lysine for glutamic acid at the sixth position of the β-chain. Because lysine is positively charged, the hemoglobin migrates toward the cathode at pH 8.6.

8. D Patients with a PK deficiency present with echinocytes, bilirubinemia, and reticulocytosis. When screening for a PK deficiency, adequate PK activity is confirmed by increased fluorescence on the qualitative PK assay, which represents the oxidation of NADH to NAD.

9. B Electrophoresis at alkaline pH usually shows 50% to 70% Hgb A, 20% to 40% Hgb S, and normal levels of Hgb A_2 in a patient with the sickle cell trait.

10. D Autosplenectomy occurs in sickle cell anemia as a result of repeated infarcts to the spleen caused by an overwhelming sickling phenomenon.

11. A PNH is a rare, acquired stem cell disorder that results from a somatic mutation in the phosphatidylinositol glycan A (*PIGA*) gene. The *PIGA* gene codes for the glycosylphosphatidylinositol (GPI) anchored proteins such as CD55 and CD59, which protect the blood cells against complement damage. As a result of the mutation, blood cells get destroyed through complement and patients become pancytopenic.

12. D Hemolytic anemia of HUS is associated with reticulocytosis. The anemia seen in HUS is multifactorial, with characteristic thrombocytopenia, schistocytes, and polychromasia commensurate with the anemia. There is also renal failure present as part of the triad of pathology in HUS.

13. The EMA (eosin-5-maleimide) binding test by flow cytometry is used in the identification of:
A. G-6-PD deficiency
B. HS
C. PK deficiency
D. PNH

Hematology/Normocytic normochromic anemia/2

14. Which antibody is associated with paroxysmal cold hemoglobinuria (PCH)?
A. Anti-I
B. Anti-i
C. Anti-M
D. Anti-P

Hematology/Normocytic normochromic anemia/1

15. Which of the following test results differentiates fragmentation and macrophage-mediated hemolysis?
A. Increased methemoglobin
B. Increased total bilirubin
C. Increased lactate dehydrogenase
D. Decreased hemopexin

Hematology/Normocytic normochromic anemia/2

16. Which of the following is a common finding in true forms of aplastic anemia?
A. A monoclonal disorder
B. Tumor infiltration
C. Peripheral blood pancytopenia
D. Defective DNA synthesis

Hematology/Normocytic normochromic anemia/1

17. In contrast with other congenital dyserythropoietic anemias (CDAs), CDA II is characterized by:
A. Bizarre multinucleated erythroblasts
B. Normocytic normochromic anemia
C. Megaloblastic erythropoiesis
D. An elevated myeloid:erythroid (M:E) ratio

Hematology/Normocytic normochromic anemia/2

18. Anemia can result from chronic kidney disease as a result of which of the following?
A. Ineffective erythropoiesis in the bone marrow
B. Insufficient hematopoiesis due to impaired stem cell signaling
C. Increased destruction due to uremia
D. Insufficient erythropoiesis due to a lack of erythropoietin production

Hematology/Normocytic normochromic anemia/2

Answers to Questions 13–18

13. B The EMA binding test is a more sensitive test for confirmation of HS. EMA is a fluorescent dye that binds to transmembrane proteins such as band 3, Rh, Rh Ag, and CD47 in the membrane of erythrocytes. When measured by a flow cytometer, spherocytes associated with HS show reduced mean fluorescent intensity (MFI) than standard erythrocytes and spherocytes caused by immune-mediated hemolysis.

14. D PCH is caused by the anti-P antibody, a cold autoantibody that binds to the patient's RBCs at low temperatures and fixes complement. In the classic Donath–Landsteiner test, hemolysis is demonstrated in a sample placed at 4°C then warmed to 37°C.

15. A Fragmentation hemolysis is also known as *intravascular hemolysis*, and macrophage-mediated hemolysis is also known as *extravascular hemolysis*. Commonalities between extravascular and intravascular hemolysis include increased total bilirubin and lactate dehydrogenase, and decreased hemopexin. Methemoglobin will be positive in intravascular hemolysis and negative in extravascular hemolysis.

16. C Aplastic anemia has many causes, such as chemical, drug, or radiation poisoning; congenital aplasia; and Fanconi syndrome. All result in depletion of hematopoietic precursors of all cell lines, leading to peripheral blood pancytopenia. There are conditions that produce a decreased amount of erythrocytes that are lumped into aplastic anemias but do not produce decreased amounts of all blood cells, but rather only red blood cells. These are not true aplastic anemias. They are hypoproliferative disorders that lead to anemias.

17. B There are four classifications of CDAs, each characterized by ineffective erythropoiesis, increased unconjugated bilirubin, and bizarre multinucleated erythroid precursors. Three of the four CDAs are classified as macrocytic normochromic, but CDA II is normocytic normochromic.

18. D Erythropoietin is produced in the renal tubule epithelial cells of the kidney. When there is damage to the kidney in chronic kidney disease, erythropoietin is reduced and consequently decreases erythrocyte production in the bone marrow, which causes anemia.

19. The severity of aplastic anemia is determined by which of the following?
- **A.** Bone marrow cellularity only
- **B.** Bone marrow cellularity and absolute neutrophil count
- **C.** Absolute neutrophil count, platelet count, and hemoglobin
- **D.** Bone marrow cellularity, absolute neutrophil count, and platelet count

Hematology/Normocytic normochromic anemia/1

20. Hemoglobinopathies are:
- **A.** Inherited qualitative defects in hemoglobin
- **B.** Inherited quantitative defects in hemoglobin
- **C.** Acquired qualitative defects in erythrocyte shape
- **D.** Acquired quantitative defects in erythrocyte biochemistry

Hematology/Normocytic normochromic anemia/2

21. Hereditary elliptocytosis (common HE) is an RBC membrane defect characterized by:
- **A.** Increased pencil-shaped cells
- **B.** Increased oval macrocytes
- **C.** Increased elongated erythrocytes with rounded ends
- **D.** Increased elliptocytes and spherocytes

Hematology/Normocytic normochromic anemia/2

Answers to Questions 19–21

19. D The severity of aplastic anemia can be differentiated by bone marrow cellularity, the degree of neutropenia as measured by the absolute neutrophil count, the degree of thrombocytopenia as measured by the platelet count, and the degree of anemia as measured by either a hemoglobin or reticulocyte count. At least two criteria plus the bone marrow cellularity are required to determine severity.

20. A Hemoglobinopathies are inherited qualitative defects in hemoglobin production. Single point mutations of an amino acid usually on the non-alpha globin chains cause aberrant qualitative hemoglobins to form, such as Hgb S or C.

21. C Common HE is a membrane defect characterized by defects in spectrin and protein 4.1. It is characterized by the presence of elliptocytes, which are elongated erythrocytes with a central pallor and rounded ends. Elliptocytes with spherocytes is characteristic of spherocytic HE. Ovalocytes may be seen in common HE, but the MCV is normocytic. Pencil-shaped cells are not elliptocytes.

7.3

Microcytic Hypochromic Anemia

1. Ferritin and UIBC can be used to differentiate between:
   A. Iron-deficiency anemia and β-thalassemia minor
   B. Iron-deficiency anemia and anemia of chronic inflammation
   C. Sideroblastic anemia and iron-deficiency anemia
   D. Alpha (α) thalassemia minor and β-thalassemia minor

   Hematology/Microcytic hypochromic anemia/1

2. Which of the following is *not* a characteristic finding in a patient with stage 3 iron-deficiency anemia?
   A. Microcytic, hypochromic RBC morphology
   B. Decreased serum iron levels
   C. Decreased total iron-binding capacity (TIBC)
   D. Decreased ferritin levels

   Hematology/Microcytic hypochromic anemia/2

3. Sideroblastic anemias are characterized by which of the following?
   A. Increased serum iron level
   B. Iron saturation over 60%
   C. Increased ferritin levels
   D. Increased ringed sideroblasts in the marrow

   Hematology/Microcytic hypochromic anemia/1

4. Which of the following conditions may be confused with iron-deficiency anemia on the peripheral blood smear?
   A. Sickle cell anemia
   B. β-Thalassemia minor
   C. α-Thalassemia major
   D. Hgb C disease

   Hematology/Microcytic hypochromic anemia/2

5. Which of the following sets of results is consistent with functional iron deficiency on the Thomas plot?
   A. Adequate sTfR/log ferritin and low reticulocyte hemoglobin content
   B. Decreased sTfR/log ferritin and low reticulocyte hemoglobin content
   C. Increased sTfR/log ferritin and low reticulocyte hemoglobin content
   D. Adequate sTfR/log ferritin and reticulocyte hemoglobin content

   Hematology/Microcytic hypochromic anemia/2

Answers to Questions 1–5

1. B Ferritin and unsaturated iron-binding capacity (UIBC) are used in the identification of iron disorders, such as iron-deficiency anemia and anemia of chronic inflammation. Both conditions present with different impairments in iron availability. Iron-deficiency anemia is characterized by iron insufficiency, whereas anemia of chronic inflammation is characterized by impaired ferrokinetics. Performing a ferritin and UIBC test can help differentiate between the two based on the disease pathology.

2. C In stage 3 iron-deficiency anemia, there is an increase in TIBC. Serum iron and ferritin levels are decreased. In stage 3, iron-deficiency anemia impaired hemoglobin production produces the microcytic hypochromic morphology associated with the condition.

3. D Sideroblastic anemias are a group of heterogeneous disorders that are defined by increased iron leading to toxicity risk in major organs. The hallmark feature for sideroblastic anemias is the presence of ringed sideroblasts in the marrow. Ringed sideroblasts are normoblasts with iron deposits forming a ring around the nucleus. Sideroblastic anemias produce increased serum iron, ferritin, and percent saturation studies, but those results can be present in other conditions.

4. B β-Thalassemia minor and iron-deficiency anemia are both classified as microcytic, hypochromic anemias with similar morphology on the peripheral blood smear. α-Thalassemia major is also microcytic hypochromic but is marked by significantly different peripheral blood findings than iron-deficiency anemia, such as NRBCs and marked polychromasia. Sickle cell disease and Hgb C are hemoglobinopathies that are normocytic normochromic.

5. A The Thomas plot tracks reticulated hemoglobin content against the ratio of the serum transferrin receptor and the log of ferritin (sTfR/log ferritin). Serum transferrin receptor increases, and ferritin decreases as iron deficiency progresses, so as the ratio increases, iron deficiency progresses. The hemoglobin content of reticulocytes precedes the hemoglobin content of mature erythrocytes, giving an early indicator of iron deficiency. These two parameters show higher sensitivity than traditional iron studies.

6. Subclinical anemia associated with iron deficiency can be verified by:
A. Serum transferrin levels
B. Hgb values
C. Myoglobin values
D. Serum ferritin levels

Hematology/Microcytic hypochromic anemia/3

7. Impaired globin chain production in β-thalassemia produces which of the following?
A. Increase in Hgb A, A2, and F
B. Decrease in Hgb A2
C. Increase in Hgb F and A2
D. Decrease in Hgb A and an increase in Hgb F and A2

Hematology/Microcytic hypochromic anemia/3

8. Impaired globin chain production in α-thalassemia produces which of the following?
A. Diminished production of all adult and fetal hemoglobin types
B. Increased production of Hgb A and decreased production of Hgb F and A2
C. Decreased production of all adult hemoglobin types and increased production of fused non-alpha hemoglobin types
D. Increased production of high-affinity hemoglobin types that compete with carbon dioxide to promote erythropoiesis

Hematology/Microcytic hypochromic anemia/2

9. What is the predominant Hgb found in patients with β-thalassemia major?
A. Hgb A2
B. Hgb A
C. Hgb C
D. Hgb F

Hematology/Microcytic hypochromic anemia/2

10. A lab report shows the following results on a 5-year-old female patient with pallor and fatigue: hematocrit (Hct) 32%, hemoglobin (Hgb) 10 g/dL, and RBC count of 5.0×10^{12}/L. What is the morphological classification of this anemia?
A. Normocytic, normochromic
B. Macrocytic, hypochromic
C. Microcytic, hypochromic
D. Normocytic, hyperchromic

Hematology/Microcytic hypochromic anemia/3

Answers to Questions 6–10

6. D The progression of iron deficiency ends with anemia, but there are two stages prior to the onset of the anemia that are defined as subclinical anemia. In these stages there is impaired iron bioavailability, but it has not caused anemia. In both subclinical stages (1 and 2), there is a decrease in ferritin levels. Stage 2 has additional impairments in circulating iron, marked by a decrease in serum iron and a subsequent increase in transferrin's binding capacity.

7. D When β-chains are impaired in β-thalassemia, this reduces Hgb A because it is composed of α- and β-chains. To compensate for the loss in β-chains, there is an increase in gamma (γ) and delta (δ) chains, which causes an increase in Hgb F and A2.

8. C In α-thalassemia, there is little or no production of the α-chains, resulting in severely depressed or no synthesis of all adult hemoglobin types. To compensate for the lack of Hgb A, A2, and F, the non-α chains (γ-, δ-, and β-chains) fuse together to produce aberrant hemoglobin types such as Hgb H, Portland, and Barts. These have high affinity for oxygen that results in impaired oxygen delivery.

9. D Patients with β-thalassemia major are unable to synthesize the β-chain; hence, little or no Hgb A is produced. However, γ-chains and δ-chains continue to be synthesized and lead to variable elevations of Hgb F in these patients. Owing to the delayed start of δ-chain production, the predominant hemoglobin present is Hgb F.

10. C The clinical presentation of fatigue and pallor suggests anemia. The results provided can be used to calculate the indices that will provide a morphological classification of this anemia. MCV is 64 fL (Hct/RBC × 10), MCH (mean corpuscular hemoglobin) is 20 pg (Hgb/RBC × 10), and MCHC is 31.3% (Hgb/Hct × 100). Therefore, the anemia is microcytic (MCV <80 fL) hypochromic (MCHC <32%).

11. Which of the following thalassemia disorders can be identified using polymerase chain reaction (PCR) followed by blotting with a single specific oligonucleotide probe?

A. α-Thalassemia
B. Hemoglobin S/β-thalassemia
C. β-Thalassemia
D. Hemoglobin C/β-thalassemia

Hematology/Microcytic hypochromic anemia/2

12. β-Thalassemia syndromes are stratified using:

A. The number of affected genes
B. Clinical presentation and transfusion dependence
C. Hemoglobin electrophoresis results
D. Complete blood count (CBC) results and the degree of anemia present

Hematology/Microcytic hypochromic anemia/2

Answers to Questions 11–12

11. A α-Thalassemia carriers have a full or partial deletion of one or two of their four globin genes. Genotyping can determine whether two deletions are *cis* or *trans* and is performed by using PCR with primers that are specific for the four most common deletions. β-Thalassemia may be caused by single base substitutions, deletions, or mutations in the flanking regions of the β-gene. Over 200 different mutations have been described, and 20 are relatively common. Approximately 90% of these can be detected by PCR coupled to electrophoresis. Multiplex ligation-dependent probe amplification (MLPA) and next-generation sequencing (NGS) are used to detect suspected cases that are negative.

12. A The number of affected genes is used to categorize α-thalassemia syndromes. β-Thalassemia syndromes have overlapping genetic and phenotypic results, making it difficult to clearly delineate the different subtypes. Instead, the thalassemia conditions must first be verified using the traditional testing with additional genetic or molecular testing to identify the clinical subtypes of the β-thalassemia.

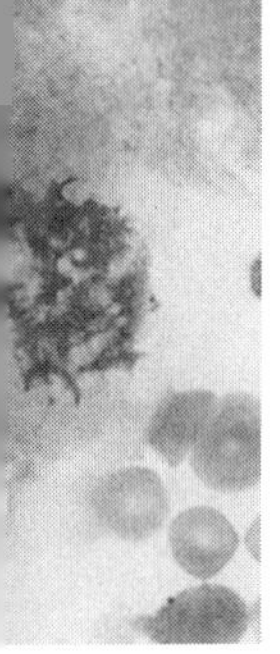

7.4

Macrocytic Normochromic Anemia

1. A peripheral blood smear shows dacryocytes, oval macrocytes, and hypersegmented neutrophils. Further testing revealed diminished folate levels. What condition is likely present?
A. Pernicious anemia
B. Iron-deficiency anemia
C. Bone marrow failure syndromes
D. Megaloblastic anemia
Hematology/Macrocytic normochromic anemia/3

2. Antibodies against parietal cells and/or intrinsic factors are present in which of the following conditions?
A. Celiac disease
B. Transcobalamin I deficiency
C. Gastrectomy
D. Pernicious anemia
Hematology/Macrocytic normochromic anemia/2

3. Which of the following are characteristics of congenital dyserythropoietic anemia?
A. Pancytopenia
B. Elevated reticulocyte count
C. Hypersegmented neutrophils
D. Macrocytic erythrocytes
Hematology/Macrocytic normochromic anemia/2

4. A patient with vitamin B_{12} anemia is prescribed a high dosage of folate. Which of the following is expected with this treatment?
A. An improvement in neurological problems
B. An improvement in hematological abnormalities
C. No expected improvement
D. Toxicity of the liver and kidneys
Hematology/Macrocytic normochromic anemia/3

5. The mechanism of anemia produced in patients with megaloblastic anemia is:
A. Insufficient erythropoiesis
B. Increased destruction of erythrocytes
C. Chronic blood loss
D. Ineffective erythropoiesis
Hematology/Macrocytic normochromic anemia/2

Answers to Questions 1–5

1. D Megaloblastic anemia results from a nutritional deficiency in either folic acid or vitamin B_{12}. These two vitamins are needed for thymine production. As a result of the deficiency, there is a lack of thymine, which is filled in with uracil in the DNA helix. As a result of this defect, erythrocytes become macrocytic, and neutrophils become hypersegmented. Additionally, there is bone marrow failure resulting in extramedullary hematopoiesis, which produce dacryocytes (teardrop cells).

2. D Pernicious anemia is caused by lack of intrinsic factor, which prevents vitamin B_{12} absorption. Intrinsic factor is produced by the parietal cells in the gastric mucosa. Antibodies to either parietal cells or intrinsic factor will impair vitamin B_{12} absorption and cause pernicious anemia. Gastrectomy impairs vitamin B_{12} absorption due to physical removal of parietal cells, but this is surgically mediated and not antibody mediated. Transcobalamin I deficiency causes a false decrease in vitamin B_{12} levels and is also not antibody mediated. Celiac disease or nontropical sprue is an autoimmune disorder that does affect vitamin B_{12} and folate absorption, but the antibodies mediating celiac disease target tissue transglutaminase or the endomysium of the gut.

3. D Congenital dyserythropoietic anemias (CDAs) are a group of disorders characterized by impaired division of normoblastic precursor producing bizarre morphology and decreased production in the bone marrow. White blood cells (WBCs) and platelets (PLTs) are not affected, so a pancytopenia is not produced in these disorders. Because of the impaired division, reticulocyte counts are decreased in these patients and the mature erythrocytes produced are large and macrocytic.

4. B Administration of folate to a patient with vitamin B_{12} deficiency will correct the hematological abnormalities, but the neurological problems will persist. This helps confirm vitamin B_{12} deficiency.

5. D Ineffective erythropoiesis is caused by destruction of erythroid precursor cells prior to their release from bone marrow. Megaloblastic anemia results from defective DNA synthesis; it is suggested that the asynchronous development of RBCs renders them more prone to intramedullary destruction, triggering hypoxic need and increased production of normoblastic precursors in the marrow.

6. A 60-year-old female patient is suffering from pernicious anemia due to chronic alcohol abuse. Which of the following laboratory data supports the likely condition for this patient?

A. RBC = 1.5×10^{12}/L; WBC =12,500/μL (12.5×10^9/L); PLT = 450,000/μL (450×10^9/L)
B. RBC = 5.5×10^{12}/L; WBC = 3,500/μL (3.5×10^9/L); PLT = 150,000/μL (150×10^9/L)
C. RBC = 3.0×10^{12}/L; WBC = 5,000/μL (5.0×10^9/L); PLT = 250,000/μL (250×10^9/L)
D. RBC = 2.5×10^{12}/L; WBC = 2,500/μL (2.5×10^9/L); PLT = 50,000/μL (50×10^9/L)

Hematology/Macrocytic normochromic anemia/3

7. A jaundiced patient is admitted with obstructive liver disease. Which of the following would be an *expected finding* in the peripheral blood smear from the patient?

A. Schistocytes
B. Macrocytes
C. Dacryocytes
D. Drepanocytes

Hematology/Macrocytic normochromic anemia/2

8. Which of the following is the correct order of the development of megaloblastic anemia? (Progression goes from left to right)

A. Anemia → Megaloblastic features in the BM → Oval macrocytes in the PB → Hypersegmentation of neutrophils → Decrease in vitamin levels
B. Decrease in vitamin levels → Anemia → Oval macrocytes in the PB → Hypersegmentation of neutrophils → Megaloblastic features in the BM
C. Decrease in vitamin levels → Hypersegmentation of neutrophils → Oval macrocytes in the PB → Megaloblastic features in the BM → Anemia
D. Megaloblastic features in the BM → Decrease in vitamin levels → Anemia → Hypersegmentation of neutrophils → Oval macrocytes in the PB

Hematology/Macrocytic normochromic anemia/2

9. Which of the following are *most* characteristic of the RBC indices associated with Fanconi anemia?

A. MCV 102 fL, MCHC 28%
B. MCV 62 fL, MCHC 30%
C. MCV 125 fL, MCHC 34%
D. MCV 88 fL, MCHC 33%

Hematology/Macrocytic normochromic anemia/2

10. Which of the following would be an *expected finding* in the bone marrow of patients with megaloblastic anemia?

A. Erythroid hyperplasia with increased reticulocytes
B. Giant metamyelocytes and nuclear-to-cytoplasmic asynchrony
C. Lymphocytic infiltration and fibrosis
D. Hypocellular marrow with increased fat content

Hematology/Macrocytic normochromic anemia/2

Answers to Questions 6–10

6. D Patients with pernicious anemia demonstrate pancytopenia with low WBC, PLT, and RBC counts. Because this is a megaloblastic process and a DNA maturation defect, all cell lines are affected. In the bone marrow, this results in abnormally large precursor cells, maturation asynchrony, hyperplasia of all cell lines, and a low M:E ratio.

7. B Patients with obstructive liver disease may have macrocytes on their peripheral blood smear because of an increased tendency toward deposition of lipid on the surface of RBCs. Consequently, the RBCs are larger or more macrocytic.

8. C Megaloblastic anemia begins with the deficiency in either vitamin B_{12} or folic acid. The vitamin deficiency leads to hypersegmentation of neutrophils, then oval macrocytes. After oval macrocytes are discovered in the peripheral blood (PB), there are changes in the bone marrow (BM) that produce nuclear-to-cytoplasmic asynchrony, which ultimately leads to the anemia signs and symptoms associated with the disease.

9. C The RBC indices in a patient with Fanconi anemia (FA) are macrocytic and normochromic. MCV values associated with macrocytosis are above 100 fL. MCHC values associated with normochromic erythrocytes are between 32% and 36%.

10. B The bone marrow of megaloblastic anemia patients show nuclear-to-cytoplasmic asynchrony (N:C asynchrony). The defect in DNA metabolism causes the nucleus to lag behind the cytoplasm, so the cytoplasm will be appropriate for the stage of development, but the nucleus will appear younger in comparison. The defect in DNA metabolism also affects leukocyte maturation, specifically neutrophils, making them appear larger than usual. This is most evident in the metamyelocyte stage of neutrophil development.

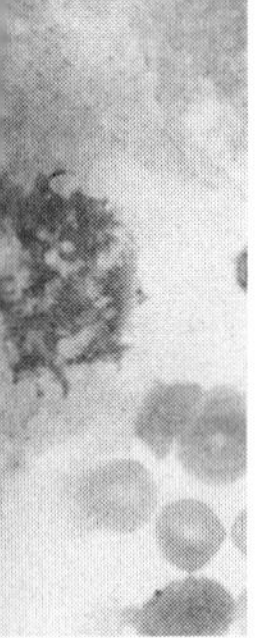

7.5

Laboratory Evaluation of Anemia

1. Variation in erythrocyte (RBC) size observed on the peripheral blood smear is described as:
A. Anisocytosis
B. Hypochromia
C. Poikilocytosis
D. Pleocytosis
Hematology/Laboratory evaluation of anemia/1

2. A lab report shows the following results:

RBC = $4.75 \times 10^6/\mu l$ ($4.75 \times 10^{12}/L$), Hgb = 13.5 g/dL, Hct = 40.5%

Calculate the MCV and MCHC results from these findings.
A. MCV = 88 fL, MCHC = 30%
B. MCV = 85 fL, MCHC = 33%
C. MCV = 100 fL, MCHC = 33%
D. MCV = 78 fL, MCHC = 28%
Hematology/Laboratory evaluation of anemia/2

3. A manual PLT count was performed on a patient with platelet clumping on their peripheral blood smear (PB smear) and a flagged PLT count on a CBC analyzer. An average of 36 PLTs were counted in the center square of an improved Neubauer hemacytometer. A 1:100 dilution with ammonium oxalate was used. What is the PLT count?
A. $3.6 \times 10^9/L$
B. $2.5 \times 10^9/L$
C. $4.0 \times 10^9/L$
D. $8.0 \times 10^9/L$
Hematology/Laboratory evaluation of anemia/2

4. An erythrocyte contains an aggregate of purple staining granules in one area of the cell. These are called:
A. Howell–Jolly bodies
B. Heinz bodies
C. Basophilic stippling
D. Pappenheimer bodies
Hematology/Laboratory evaluation of anemia/1

Answers to Questions 1–4

1. A A mature erythrocyte is approximately 7 to 8 µm in diameter. Variation in size is denoted by the term *anisocytosis* and reflected in the red cell distribution width (RDW). The higher RDW value, the greater the variation present. *Hypochromia* is a term that indicates increased central pallor in erythrocytes. The central pallor is the area of the erythrocyte devoid of hemoglobin, so the larger the central pallor, the lower the hemoglobin. *Poikilocytosis* denotes variation in RBC shape. *Pleocytosis* is used to describe the concentration of leukocytes present in body fluids and not in peripheral blood.

2. B MCV is calculated using the following formula = (Hct/RBC) × 10 and is expressed in femtoliters (fL). MCHC is calculated using the following formula = (Hgb/Hct) × 100 and is expressed in percentage (%) or grams per deciliter (g/dL). When the correct values are inserted into the formulas, the MCV is 85 fL and the MCHC is 33%, which is classified as normocytic normochromic.

3. A The formula used for calculating manual platelet counts by using a hemacytometer is (Number of cells counted × dilution factor) ÷ area counted. In this example, 36 × 100 = 3,600/0.1 = 36,000/mm^3 or $3.6 \times 10^9/L$.

4. D An aggregate of purple staining granules in one area of the erythrocyte consists of Pappenheimer bodies, which are composed of iron.

5. A patient is admitted in diabetic ketoacidosis. The patient's blood sugar on admission is 638 mg/dL. How will this affect the patient's CBC findings?
A. It will increase all cell counts due to the highly elevated plasma glucose
B. It will increase the patient's RBC, Hct, and Hgb, but decrease their WBC and PLT counts
C. It will increase their MCV and Hct, and lower their MCHC
D. It will decrease all cell counts plus Hct and Hgb and associated indices

Hematology/Laboratory evaluation of anemia/3

6. A patient has a reticulocyte count of 8% and Hct of 30%. What is the corrected reticulocyte count?
A. 1.4%
B. 5.3%
C. 3.5%
D. 14%

Hematology/Laboratory evaluation of anemia/2

7. A manual differential is performed on a 3-day-old premature infant. There are 55 NRBCs and the WBC count is 13,500/μL. What is the corrected WBC count?
A. 8,710/μL
B. 2,470/μL
C. 9,600/μL
D. 20,970/μL

Hematology/Laboratory evaluation of anemia/2

8. What effect would the buffer at pH 8.0 have on a Wright-stained smear?
A. RBCs would be stained too pink
B. WBC cytoplasm would be stained too blue
C. RBCs would be stained too blue
D. RBCs would lyse on the slide

Hematology/Laboratory evaluation of anemia/2

9. Which of the following erythrocyte inclusions can be visualized with new methylene blue but cannot be seen on a Wright-stained blood smear?
A. Basophilic stippling
B. Heinz bodies
C. Howell–Jolly bodies
D. Siderotic granules

Hematology/Laboratory evaluation of anemia/2

10. A lipemic sample is run on the Sysmex XN and has an MCHC of 44%. What other CBC parameters will be affected?
A. Hct and MCV
B. Hgb and MCH
C. RBC, Hct, and Hgb
D. Hgb and WBC count

Hematology/Laboratory evaluation of anemia/3

Answers to Questions 5–10

5. C The elevated glucose makes the plasma hypertonic. The hypertonic plasma causes the RBCs to swell and increase the MCV and Hct and falsely lowers the Hgb and consequently MCHC.

6. B In anemic states, the reticulocyte percentage is not a true measure of reticulocyte production. The following formula is used to correct the reticulocyte count for an anemia already present: Corrected reticulocyte count = reticulocytes (%) × (Hct ÷ 45), where 45 is the average Hct. In this case, 8 × (30 ÷ 45) = 5.3%.

7. A The NRBCs interfere with the counting of leukocytes due their proximity in morphology to small lymphocytes. The leukocyte count is falsely increased when NRBCs are present. When reviewed manually, NRBCs are counted alongside the manual differential and if the number exceeds 10 NRBCs the WBC count requires correction. In some children's hospitals, the number is reduced to 5 NRBCs to warrant a correction. The formula to correct the WBC count is (WBC × 100)/(NRBC+100), so in this example, (13,500 × 100)/(55 + 100) = 8,710/μL.

8. C The pH of the buffer is critical in Romanowsky staining. When the pH is too high (8.0 or above), the RBCs take up more alkaline dye (methylene blue), becoming too blue. Leukocytes also show poor cytoplasmic detail when the pH is increased.

9. B Heinz bodies are irregular, refractile, purple inclusions that are not visible with Wright staining but show up with supravital staining, such as new methylene blue or bromocresyl green. The other three inclusions can be seen with Wright or Wright-Giemsa staining.

10. B Lipemic plasma with an elevated MCHC will falsely increase the hemoglobin value. Hemoglobin is measured through spectrophotometry. Plasma and hemolysate is measured using a spectrophotometer and the signal strength is then converted to a hemoglobin concentration. Owing to the highly colored plasma, there is a higher signal strength and therefore a higher hemoglobin concentration. The hemoglobin concentration is also used to calculate the mean cell hemoglobin (MCH) which will also be falsely elevated. The formula for the MCH = (Hgb/RBC) × 10.
The MCHC is also falsely elevated due to the high hemoglobin concentration. The formula for the MCHC = (Hgb/Hct) × 100.

11. If RBC parameters follow the rule of three, the erythrocytes would be classified as:
A. Microcytic hypochromic
B. Normocytic normochromic
C. Macrocytic normochromic
D. Normocytic hypochromic
Hematology/Laboratory evaluation of anemia/1

12. A lab report shows the following results on a patient experiencing shortness of breath, hematuria, fatigue, and pallor: MCV 98 fL; MCH 30 pg; MCHC 34%, reticulocyte count 5.5% (uncorrected). What can be concluded from these findings?
A. The patient likely has a nutritional deficiency that requires confirmation with iron studies
B. The patient likely has a chronic inherited anemia that requires an altered treatment plan
C. The patient likely has a hemolytic disorder that requires confirmation to determine etiology
D. The patient may be suffering from bone marrow failure that requires immediate evaluation of their bone marrow
Hematology/Laboratory evaluation of anemia/3

13. You receive an EDTA (ethylenediaminetetraacetic acid) microtainer tube from a 2-day old infant with a Hgb of 16.5 g/dL. How should one proceed with making the blood smear?
A. Use a small drop of blood and lower the angle of the spreader slide
B. Use a large drop of blood and increase the angle of the spreader slide
C. Use a calibrated blood dropper with a variable angle for the spreader slide
D. Ask for a redraw to investigate the high hemoglobin
Hematology/Laboratory evaluation of anemia/2

14. What staining method is used most frequently to stain and manually count reticulocytes?
A. Immunofluorescence
B. Supravital staining
C. Romanowsky staining
D. Cytochemical staining
Hematology/Laboratory evaluation of anemia/1

15. The combination of low- voltage direct- current impedance with radiofrequency on a cell allows for:
A. Increased discrimination of cellular morphology
B. More sensitive detection of abnormal blood cells
C. Less interference from preanalytical variables when counting cells
D. Higher reproducibility of absolute blood cell counts
Hematology/Laboratory evaluation of anemia/2

Answers to Questions 11–15

11. B The rule of three indicates that the RBC count should be approximately one third of the hemoglobin value (MCH of 30 pg), and the hemoglobin should be one third of the hematocrit result (MCHC of 33%). Consequently, the hematocrit should be one ninth of the RBC count (MCV of 90 fL). These equate to normocytic normochromic erythrocytes.

12. C There are several supportive pieces of information to make conclusions. The clinical presentation suggests anemia, and the presence of hematuria is an indicator of a hemolytic process that is intravascular. The indices are supporting a normocytic normochromic anemia, which is consistent with the clinical presentation. Furthermore, the elevated reticulocyte count also supports a hemolytic picture. Hemolysis can be due to a variety of etiologies, so it is essential to investigate the probable cause of the hemolysis.

13. A Blood samples with high hemoglobin values should be extended on the slide to maximize the surface area of the monolayer for proper differential reading. To achieve this, the laboratory professional should lower the angle of the spreader slide. Because the blood is highly concentrated, as seen in many infant samples, a small drop of blood should be used.

14. B The reticulum within reticulocytes consists of ribonucleic acid (RNA), which cannot be stained with Wright stain. Supravital staining with new methylene blue is used to identify reticulocytes.

15. A Electronic cell counters use the principle of electrical impedance. Two electrodes are placed in a solution with blood cells. As a cell passes through the aperture of one of the electrodes, it interrupts the current and generates a voltage pulse, which is counted by the analyzer. Adding a radiofrequency (RF) signal allows for more detail of each blood cell to be collected, thereby facilitating better differentiation of each of the cells measured.

16. An increased RDW generated by a CBC analyzer should correlate with:
A. Marked spherocytes on the peripheral bloodsmear
B. A moderate or marked amount of anisocytosis
C. A moderate or marked amount of hypochromia
D. Presence of NRBCs or erythrocyte inclusions
Hematology/Laboratory evaluation of anemia/2

17. Which set of RBC indices suggests the presence of spherocytes on the peripheral blood smear?
A. MCV 76 μm^3 MCH 19.9 pg MCHC 28.5%
B. MCV 90 μm^3 MCH 30.5 pg MCHC 34.5%
C. MCV 79 μm^3 MCH 38.5 pg MCHC 39.0%
D. MCV 81 μm^3 MCH 27.0 pg MCHC 33.8%
Hematology/Laboratory evaluation of anemia/3

18. Which of the following hemoglobin types is produced with ferric iron and peaks at 630 nm on spectral absorption analysis?
A. Carboxyhemoglobin
B. Methemoglobin
C. Sulfhemoglobin
D. Deoxyhemoglobin
Hematology/Laboratory evaluation of anemia/1

19. Which condition will shift the oxyhemoglobin dissociation curve to the left?
A. Respiratory or metabolic acidosis
B. Respiratory or metabolic alkalosis
C. Increased 2,3-diphosphoglycerate (2,3-DPG) concentration
D. Increased quantities of aberrant hemoglobin types
Hematology/Laboratory evaluation of anemia/2

20. The pathophysiologic classification of anemias does *not* include which of the following?
A. Not producing enough RBCs s for oxygen needs
B. Producing inefficient RBCs s for oxygen needs
C. Acute blood loss
D. Premature destruction of RBCs
Hematology/Laboratory evaluation of anemia/1

21. A patient's peripheral blood smear reveals numerous NRBCs and pronounced polychromasia. In addition to decreased Hgb and decreased Hct values, what other CBC parameters may be evident?
A. Reduced PLTs
B. Increased MCHC
C. Increased MCV
D. Decreased RDW
Hematology/Laboratory evaluation of anemia/3

Answers to Questions 16–21

16. B The RDW parameter correlates with the degree of erythrocyte size variation (anisocytosis) seen on the morphological examination. It is expected to have less than 15% variation. Values above 15% RDW correlate to the degree (slight/few, moderate, or marked) of anisocytosis observed on the peripheral blood smear.

17. C Spherocytes have decreased cell diameter and volume, and this results in loss of central pallor and discoid shape. The loss of volume produces a microcytic MCV and elevated MCH and MCHC values. Typically, the MCHC is above 36% and would warrant review of the peripheral blood smear to rule out a problem with specimen integrity.

18. B Methemoglobin is produced when ferrous (divalent; Fe^{2+}) iron is reversibly oxidized to form ferric (trivalent; Fe^{3+}) iron in the heme molecule. Detection of methemoglobin requires spectral absorption analysis, which displays a peak at 630 nm.

19. B Respiratory or metabolic alkalosis will produce a shift to the left on the oxyhemoglobin dissociation curve and therefore increase O_2 affinity. Acidosis does the opposite. Shift to the left can also be produced with low concentration of 2,3-DPG. Aberrant hemoglobin types can either produce high affinity or low affinity. For example, Hgb Kansas causes a shift to the right, and Hgb Chesapeake causes a shift to the left.

20. C Anemias are classified morphologically by using laboratory data; pathophysiologically, based on the mechanism producing the anemia; and clinically, based on an assessment of symptoms. The pathophysiological mechanisms of anemia include insufficient erythropoiesis (not producing enough RBCs for the oxygen demands on the body), ineffective erythropoiesis (producing dysfunctional RBCs that are not effective for the oxygen demands), chronic blood loss (chronic bleeding that lessens the amount of erythrocytes needed for oxygen demands), and increased or premature destruction of functional erythrocytes. Acute blood loss is not considered a pathophysiological mechanism.

21. C The patient's abnormal peripheral blood smear indicates marked RBC regeneration, causing many reticulocytes to be released from the bone marrow. Because reticulocytes are larger than mature RBCs, MCV will be slightly elevated.

22. What RBC inclusion may be seen in the peripheral blood smear from a patient postsplenectomy?
A. Cabot rings
B. Howell–Jolly bodies
C. Basophilic stippling
D. Pappenheimer bodies
Hematology/Laboratory evaluation of anemia/1

23. A manual WBC count is performed, and 16 WBCs are counted in the four large corner squares of a Neubauer hemacytometer. The dilution is performed with ammonium oxalate at 1:100. What is the total WBC count?
A. 4.0×10^9/L
B. 8.0×10^9/L
C. 20.0×10^9/L
D. 200.0×10^9/L
Hematology/Laboratory evaluation of anemia/2

24. Review the following automated CBC values:

WBC = 22.5×10^9/L (flagged)	MCV = 87.2 fL
RBC = 2.89×10^{12}/L	MCH = 28.0 pg
Hgb = 8.1 g/dL	MCHC = 32.1%
Hct = 25.2%	PLT = 487×10^9/L

Many sickle cells are evident on review of the peripheral blood smear. Based on this finding and the results provided, what automated parameter of this patient is most likely inaccurate, and what follow-up test should be performed to accurately assess this parameter?
A. MCV/perform reticulocyte count
B. Hct/perform manual Hct
C. WBC/perform manual WBC count
D. Hgb/perform serum–saline replacement
Hematology/Laboratory evaluation of anemia/3

25. Review the following CBC results for a 2-day-old infant:

WBC = 15.2×10^9/L	MCV = 105 fL
RBC = 5.30×10^{12}/L	MCH = 34.0 pg
Hgb = 18.5 g/dL	MCHC = 33.5%
Hct = 57.9%	PLT = 213×10^9/L

These results indicate:
A. Macrocytic anemia
B. Microcytic anemia
C. Liver disease
D. Expected values for a 2-day-old infant
Hematology/Laboratory evaluation of anemia/2

Answers to Questions 22–25

22. B The spleen is responsible for removing (pitting) remnant DNA from erythrocytes without disrupting their membrane (culling). As a result of splenectomy, Howell–Jolly bodies, which are composed of residual DNA, may be seen in increased numbers.

23. A The formula for calculating manual cell counts using a hemacytometer is:

(Average number of cells counted × dilution factor) ÷ area counted.

or (16 x 100)/0.4 = 4,000

or 4.0 x 10^9*/L*

24. C When an automated WBC count is performed using a hematology analyzer, RBCs are lysed to allow enumeration of leukocytes. Sickle cells are often resistant to lysis within the limited time frame (less than 1 minute), during which the RBCs are exposed to the lysing reagent and the WBCs are subsequently counted. As a result, the nonlysed RBCs are counted along with WBCs, and this falsely increases the WBC count. When an automated cell counting analyzer indicates a review flag for the WBC count and sickle cells are noted on peripheral blood smear analysis, a manual WBC count must be performed. The manual method allows optimal time for sickle cell lysis and accurate enumeration of the leukocytes in the blood sample.

25. D During the first week of life, an infant has an average Hct of 55%. This value drops to a mean of 43% by the first month of life. The mean MCV of the first week is 108 fL; after 2 months, the average MCV is 96 fL. The mean WBC count during the first week is approximately 18×10^9/L, and this drops to an average of 10.8×10^9/L after the first month. The PLT count in newborns falls within the same normal range as in adults.

26. Refer to the following scatterplot, histograms, and automated values for a 45-year-old male patient. What follow-up verification procedure is indicated before the results can be released?

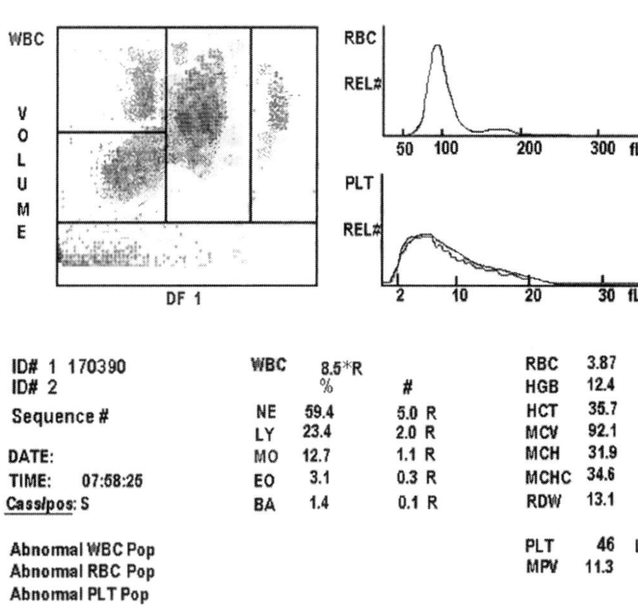

A. Redraw blood sample using a sodium citrate tube; multiply PLTs × 1.11
B. Dilute WBCs 1:10; multiply × 10
C. Perform plasma blank Hgb to correct for lipemia
D. Warm specimen at 37°C for 15 minutes; rerun specimen

Hematology/Laboratory evaluation of anemia/3

Answer to Question 26

26. A The image supports the presence of PLT clumps. On the WBC histogram, there are many particles being read below the threshold of leukocyte identification, indicating either the presence of abnormal RBC morphology or PLT clumps. Furthermore, the PLT histogram appears "bumpy," and the RBC histogram appears acceptable with no indications of abnormal size variation. This also supports the presence of PLT clumps in the sample. PLT clumping phenomenon is often induced *in vitro* by the anticoagulant EDTA. Redrawing a sample using a sodium citrate tube usually corrects this phenomenon and allows for accurate PLT enumeration. The PLT count must be multiplied by 1.1 to adjust for the amount of sodium citrate. PLT clumps cause a spurious decrease in the PLT count by automated methods. The WBC value has an "R" (review) flag because the PLT clumps have been falsely counted as WBCs, so a manual WBC count is needed.

27. Refer to the following scatterplot, histograms, and automated values for a 52-year-old female patient. What follow-up verification procedure is indicated before the results can be released?

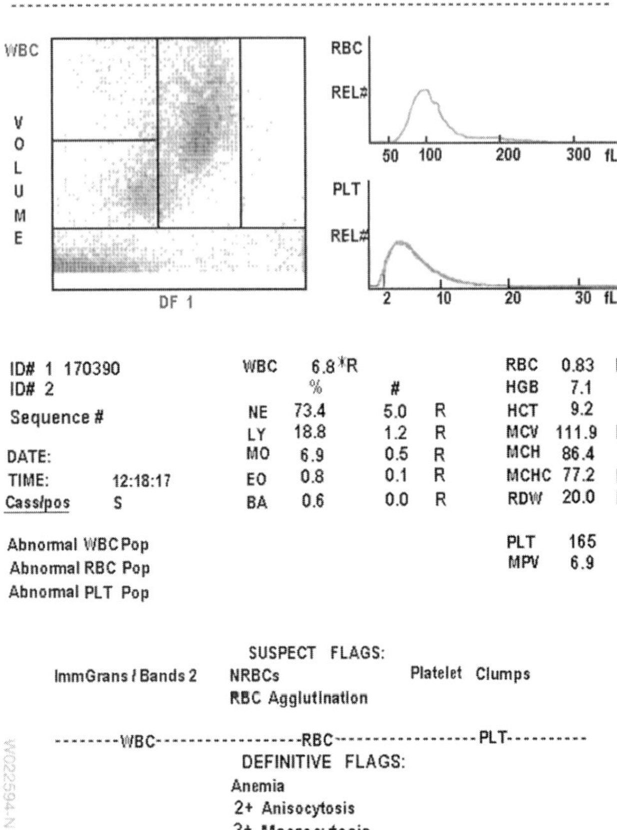

A. Redraw specimen using a sodium citrate tube; multiply PLTs × 1.11
B. Dilute WBCs 1:10; multiply × 10
C. Perform plasma blank Hgb to correct for lipemia
D. Warm the specimen at 37°C for 15 minutes; rerun the specimen

Hematology/Laboratory evaluation of anemia/3

Answer to Question 27

27. D The presence of high-titer cold agglutinin in a patient with cold autoimmune hemolytic anemia (AIHA) will interfere with automated cell counting. The most remarkable findings are falsely elevated MCV, MCH, and MCHC, as well as falsely decreased RBC count. The patient's RBCs will quickly agglutinate *in vitro* when exposed to ambient temperatures below body temperature. To correct for this phenomenon, the EDTA tube should be incubated at 37°C for 15 to 30 minutes, and then the specimen should be rerun.

28. **Refer to the following scatterplot, histograms, and automated values for a 33-year-old female patient. What follow-up verification procedure is indicated before the results can be released?**

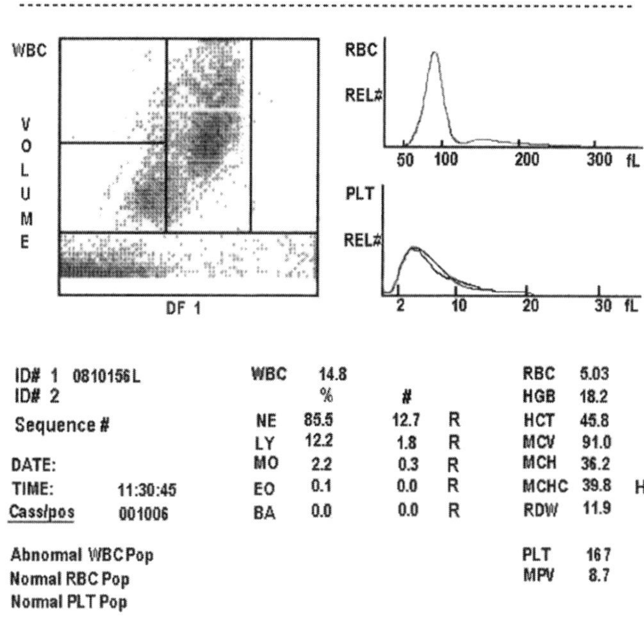

SUSPECT FLAGS:

Imm Grans / Bands 2

--------WBC------------------RBC-----------------PLT----------

DEFINITIVE FLAGS:

Leukocytosis
Neutrophilia %

W02594-N

A. Perform a manual Hct and redraw the sample using a sodium citrate tube; multiply PLTs × 1.11
B. Dilute WBCs 1:10; multiply × 10
C. Perform plasma blank Hgb to correct for lipemia
D. Warm the specimen at 37°C for 15 minutes; rerun the specimen

Hematology/Laboratory evaluation of anemia/3

Answer to Question 28

28. C The flag that warrants action to be taken is the elevated MCHC. This indicates either the presence of spherocytes or a problem with specimen integrity. The elevated MCHC warrants a correction in either the hemoglobin or hematocrit, which can be evaluated by spinning down a manual hematocrit and observing the plasma layer for any abnormality in the coloring of the plasma. Lipemia will appear as a milky white plasma, icteria (hyperbilirubinemia) will appear as a darker yellow or brown plasma, and hemolysis will appear as pink to red plasma. Additionally, the erythrocyte indices offer clues as well. The MCHC is calculated using the Hgb and Hct. If there is a problem with the hemoglobin, the MCH will be affected as well and the MCV will be unaffected (as indicated in the provided image). To address for the presence of highly colored plasma and correct the inaccurate hemoglobin, one of two procedures can be performed. First, a plasma (or saline) replacement can be performed in which the affected plasma is replaced with saline. It is crucial that there is a less than 10,000-cell difference between RBC counts before and after the saline replacement. A second procedure is to perform a plasma blank on the analyzer. A standard Hgb value (baseline Hgb) should be ascertained by using the patient's plasma and subsequently subtracted from the original falsely elevated Hgb value. The following formula can be used to correct for highly colored plasma:

Whole blood – [(Plasma Hgb) (1 – Hct/100)] = Corrected Hgb

29. Refer to the following scatterplot, histograms, and automated values for a 48-year-old male patient. What follow-up verification procedure is indicated before the five-part WBC differential results can be released?

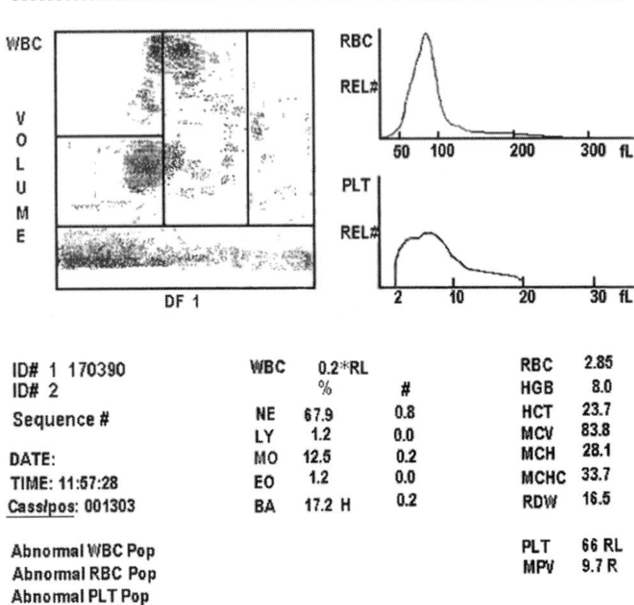

ID# 1 170390
ID# 2
Sequence #

DATE:
TIME: 11:57:28
Cass/pos: 001303

WBC	0.2*RL	
	%	#
NE	67.9	0.8
LY	1.2	0.0
MO	12.5	0.2
EO	1.2	0.0
BA	17.2 H	0.2

RBC	2.85
HGB	8.0
HCT	23.7
MCV	83.8
MCH	28.1
MCHC	33.7
RDW	16.5
PLT	66 RL
MPV	9.7 R

Abnormal WBC Pop
Abnormal RBC Pop
Abnormal PLT Pop

SUSPECT FLAGS:

WBC	RBC	PLT
Imm Grans/Bands2	NRBCs Micro RBCs RBC Fragments	Platelet Clumps Giant Platelets

--------WBC-----------------RBC-----------------PLT----------
DEFINITIVE FLAGS:

W02594-N

A. Dilute WBCs 1:10; multiply × 10
B. Redraw the sample using a sodium citrate tube; multiply WBCs × 1.11
C. Prepare buffy coat peripheral blood smears, and perform a manual differential
D. Warm specimen at 37°C for 15 minutes; rerun specimen

Hematology/Laboratory evaluation of anemia/3

Answer to Question 29

29. C The markedly decreased WBC count (0.2×10^9/L) indicates that a manual differential is necessary and that very few leukocytes will be available for differential cell counting. To increase the yield and thereby facilitate counting, differential smears should be prepared by using the buffy coat technique.

30. **Refer to the following scatterplot, histograms, and automated values for a 28-year-old female patient who has undergone preoperative laboratory testing. A manual WBC differential was requested by the provider. The WBC differential was not significantly different from the automated five-part differential; however, the medical laboratory scientist noted 3+ elliptocytes/ovalocytes while reviewing the RBC morphology. What is the *most* likely condition present in this patient?**

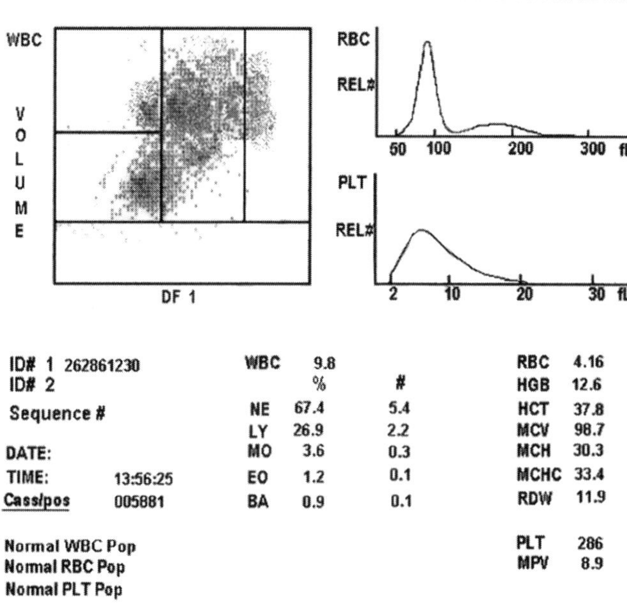

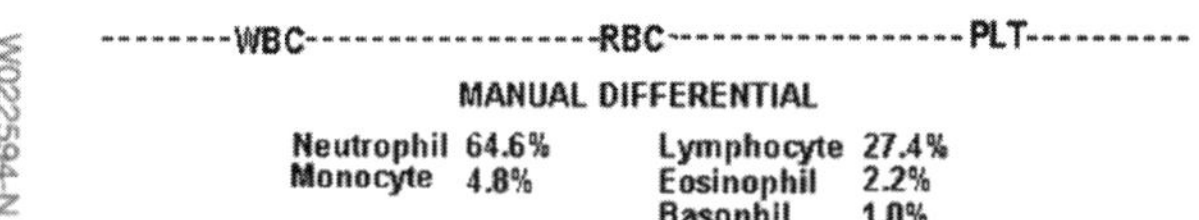

A. HS
B. HE
C. Cirrhosis
D. Hgb C disease

Hematology/Laboratory evaluation of anemia/2

Answer to Question 30

30. B The finding of ovalocytes as the predominant RBC morphology in peripheral blood is consistent with hereditary elliptocytosis or ovalocytosis (HE). This disorder is relatively common and can range in severity from an asymptomatic carrier state to homozygous HE with severe hemolysis. The most common clinical subtype is associated with no or minimal hemolysis. Therefore, HE is usually associated with a normal RBC histogram and cell indices and will go unnoticed without microscopic evaluation of the peripheral blood smear.

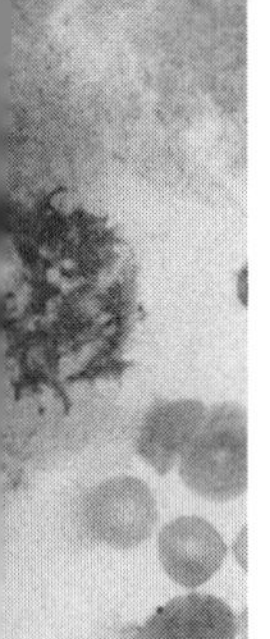

7.6

Qualitative and Quantitative Nonmalignant Leukocyte Disorders

1. Which of the following is a complication that may occur as a result of infectious mononucleosis infection?
A. Splenic infarctions
B. Dactylitis
C. Hemolytic anemia
D. Giant PLTs

Hematology/Qualitative and quantitative nonmalignant leukocyte disorders/2

2. Which of the following is an *expected* finding in patients with active HIV infection?
A. Regenerative shift to the left in WBCs
B. Target cells
C. Reactive lymphocytes
D. Pelgeroid neutrophils

Hematology/Qualitative and quantitative nonmalignant leukocyte disorders/1

3. This inclusion is seen as part of a stress response to infection and is composed of ribosomal RNA. What is the inclusion?
A. Döhle bodies
B. Basophilic stippling
C. Toxic granulation
D. Howell–Jolly bodies

Hematology/Qualitative and quantitative nonmalignant leukocyte disorders/1

4. Which of the following conditions is associated with the presence of metachromatic granules due to a buildup of mucopolysaccharides in granulocytes?
A. Chediak–Higashi anomaly
B. Alder–Reilly anomaly
C. May–Hegglin anomaly
D. Pelger–Huet anomaly

Hematology/Qualitative and quantitative nonmalignant leukocyte disorders/2

5. Which of the following conditions does *not* produce a lymphocyte count greater than 5.0×10^9/L?
A. Cytomegalovirus (CMV) infection
B. Syphilis infection
C. Hepatitis
D. Wiskott–Aldrich syndrome

Hematology/Qualitative and quantitative nonmalignant leukocyte disorders/2

Answers to Questions 1–5

1. C Patients with infectious mononucleosis may develop a potent cold agglutinin with anti-I specificity. This cold autoantibody can cause strong hemolysis and hemolytic anemia (cold autoimmune hemolytic anemia).

2. C HIV infection brings about several hematological abnormalities seen on peripheral blood smear examination. As in other viral infections, most patients display reactive lymphocytes and have granulocytopenia.

3. A Döhle bodies are RNA-rich areas within polymorphonuclear neutrophils (PMNs) that are oval and light blue. Although often associated with infectious states, they are seen in a wide range of conditions and toxic reactions, including hemolytic and pernicious anemias, chronic granulocytic leukemia, and therapy with antineoplastic drugs. Toxic granulation is also a stress response to infection but is composed of primary staining granules and not RNA. The other inclusions are found in erythrocytes and are not associated with infection.

4. B A buildup of mucopolysaccharides causes dark-staining metachromatic granules to form in the cytoplasm of neutrophils, eosinophils, and/or basophils. This is an inherited disorder that is called *Alder–Reilly anomaly (ARA)*. It should be noted that this inherited change to the granulocytes does not affect their function and will often go unnoticed unless a peripheral blood smear manual review is performed by the laboratory professional.

5. D The leukocyte count above 5.0×10^9/L indicates an absolute lymphocytosis, which can be seen in a variety of different infection types, such as CMV, syphilis, and hepatitis infections. In contrast, Wiskott–Aldrich syndrome produces a lymphocytopenia.

6. Which of the following is *not* a change associated with bacterial infections?
A. Neutrophilia
B. Hyposegmentation
C. Toxic granulation
D. Vacuolization

Hematology/Qualitative and quantitative nonmalignant leukocyte disorders/2

7. Which of the following is a risk associated with absolute neutrophil counts below 0.5 × 10^9/L?
A. Increased risk of opportunistic infections
B. Increased risk of leukemia relapse
C. Increased risk of bone marrow failure
D. Increased risk of disseminated intravascular coagulation (DIC)

Hematology/Qualitative and quantitative nonmalignant leukocyte disorders/2

8. The morphological characteristic(s) associated with Chédiak–Higashi syndrome is (are):
A. Pale blue cytoplasmic inclusions
B. Giant lysosomal granules
C. Small, dark-staining granules and condensed nuclei
D. Nuclear hyposegmentation

Hematology/Qualitative and quantitative nonmalignant leukocyte disorders/2

9. The familial condition of Pelger–Huët anomaly is important to recognize because this disorder must be differentiated from:
A. Infectious mononucleosis
B. May–Hegglin anomaly
C. Left shift
D. G-6-PD deficiency

Hematology/Qualitative and quantitative nonmalignant leukocyte disorders/2

10. A manual differential on a symptomatic patient shows marked reactive lymphocytes and lymphocytosis. The provider strongly suspects a viral infection and orders follow-up serological testing. The testing reveals negative heterophile antibody and EBV-IgM test results. Based on these findings, what is an *expected* laboratory result that confirms this clinical picture?
A. Heterophile antibody: positive
B. Epstein–Barr virus (EBV)–immunoglobulin M (IgM): positive
C. Direct antiglobulin test (DAT): positive
D. CMV–IgM: positive

Hematology/Qualitative and quantitative nonmalignant leukocyte disorders/3

Answers to Questions 6–10

6. B Neutrophil changes associated with infection may include neutrophilia, shift to the left, toxic granulation, Döhle bodies, and vacuolization. Pelgeroid hyposegmentation is noted in neutrophils from individuals with congenital Pelger–Huët anomaly and those with an acquired anomaly induced by drug ingestion or secondary to certain conditions, such as leukemia.

7. A An absolute neutrophil count (ANC) below 1.5 × 10^9/L is defined as neutropenia. Furthermore, an ANC below 0.5 × 10^9/L is defined as severe neutropenia. Neutropenia has a variety of etiologies ranging from blood malignancies to receiving marrow-suppressive therapies, but the primary risk of severe neutropenia is the increased risk of opportunistic infections.

8. B Chédiak–Higashi syndrome is a disorder of neutrophil phagocytic dysfunction caused by depressed chemotaxis and delayed degranulation. The degranulation disturbance is attributed to interference from the giant lysosomal granules characteristic of this disorder.

9. C Pelger–Huët anomaly is a benign familial condition reported in 1 out of 6,000 individuals. Care must be taken to differentiate Pelger–Huët cells from the numerous band neutrophils and metamyelocytes that may be observed during severe infection or a *shift-to-the-left* of immaturity in granulocyte stages. Morphology associated with pelgeroid neutrophils may resemble metamyelocytes and bands.

10. D If both the heterophile antibody test and the EBV-IgM tests yield negative results in a patient with reactive lymphocytosis and a suspected viral infection, serum should be analyzed for IgM antibodies to CMV. CMV belongs to the herpesvirus family and is endemic worldwide. CMV infection is the most common cause of heterophile-negative infectious mononucleosis.

11. Which of the following disorders results from a defective respiratory burst that leads to the onset of pyogenic infections in young children?

A. Chronic granulomatous disease of childhood
B. Bacterial sepsis
C. Gaucher disease
D. Niemann–Pick disease

Hematology/Qualitative and quantitative nonmalignant leukocyte disorders/2

12. A chronic myelogenous leukemia (CML) patient recovering from marrow suppressive therapy has an absolute monocyte count of 2.0 × 10^9/L. What should be the follow-up procedure to address this new finding?

A. A bone marrow biopsy and aspiration should be performed as this is a sign of relapsing CML
B. A cytogenetic karyotyping should be performed to rule out myelodysplasia
C. Flow cytometry should be conducted as this is an indicator of acute myelogenous leukemia (AML) transformation
D. This is likely a result of the recovery and nothing further is required

Hematology/Qualitative and quantitative nonmalignant leukocyte disorders/3

13. Which of the following results on an automated differential suggests that a peripheral blood smear should be reviewed manually?

A. Segmented neutrophils = 70%
B. Band neutrophils = 6%
C. Monocytes = 15%
D. Eosinophils = 2%

Hematology/Qualitative and quantitative nonmalignant leukocyte disorders/2

Answers to Questions 11–13

11. A Neutrophil phagocytosis and particle ingestion are associated with an increase in O_2 utilization called *respiratory burst*. The biochemical products of the respiratory burst involved in neutrophil particle ingestion during phagocytosis are H_2O_2 and O_2^-. The activated neutrophil discharges the enzyme NADPH oxidase into the phagolysosome, where it converts O_2 to O_2^-, which is then reduced to H_2O_2 to destroy the ingested bacterial antigen. When there is a defective respiratory burst, there is no effective killing mechanism, which leads to pus-forming (pyogenic) infections.

12. D It is a common occurrence after recovering from myelosuppressive therapy to observe a monocytosis. CML can progress into acute leukemia, but none of the other answer choices fit that progression.

13. C A relative monocyte count of 15% is abnormal, given that the baseline monocyte count in a normal differential is less than 10%. An increased monocyte count may signal a myeloproliferative process, such as chronic myelomonocytic leukemia, an inflammatory response, or abnormal lymphocytes that may have been counted as monocytes by an automated cell counter.

14. Review the scatterplot of WBCs provided. Which section of the scatterplot denotes the number of monocytes?

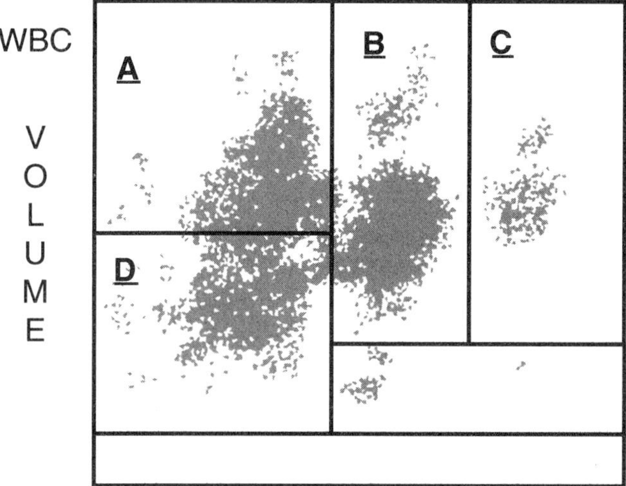

A. A
B. B
C. C
D. D

Hematology/Qualitative and quantitative nonmalignant leukocyte disorders/2

Answer to Question 14

14. A WBC identification is facilitated by analysis of the impedance, conductance, and light-scattering properties of WBCs. The scatterplot represents the relationship between volume (*x*-axis) and light scatter (*y*-axis). Monocytes account for the dots in section A, neutrophils are represented in section B, eosinophils are represented in section C, and lymphocytes are denoted in section D.

15. Review the following scatterplot, histograms, and automated values for a 21-year-old college student complaining of lassitude and a sore throat with enlarged cervical lymph nodes.

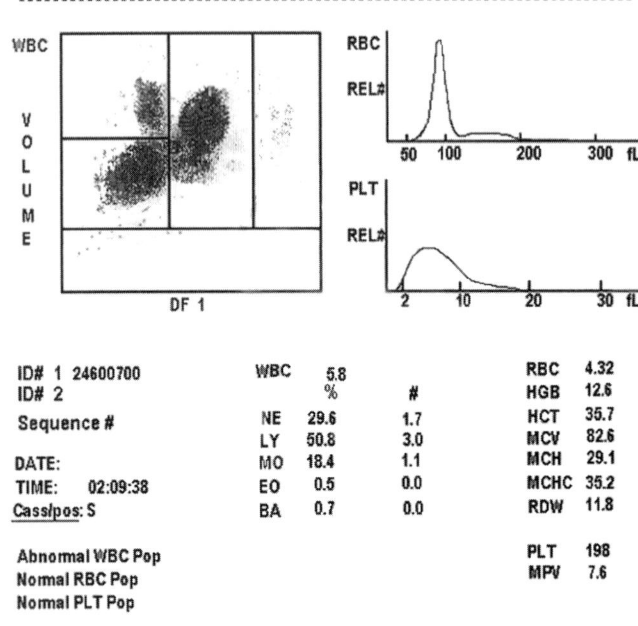

SUSPECT FLAGS:

--------WBC------------------RBC-----------------PLT---------

DEFINITIVE FLAGS:

Monocytosis %

W022594-N

WBC differential: 5 band neutrophils; 27 segmented neutrophils; 60 lymphocytes (55 atypical lymphocytes); 6 monocytes; 1 eosinophil; 1 basophil

What is the presumptive condition present in this patient?

A. Infectious mononucleosis
B. Monocytosis
C. Chronic lymphocytic leukemia (CLL)
D. β-Thalassemia

Hematology/Qualitative and quantitative nonmalignant leukocyte disorders/3

Answer to Question 15

15. A Lymphocytosis with numerous atypical lymphocytes is a hallmark consistent with infectious mononucleosis. The clinical presentation also supports this presumptive condition, specifically with the enlarged lymph nodes, sore throat, and extreme fatigue (lassitude). The automated results demonstrated abnormal WBC subpopulations, specifically lymphocytosis as well as monocytosis. However, on peripheral blood smear examination, 60 atypical lymphocytes and only 6 monocytes were noted. Atypical lymphocytes are often misclassified by automated cell counters as monocytes. Therefore, the automated analyzer differential must not be released, and the manual differential count must be relied on for diagnostic interpretation.

7.7
Myelodysplastic Syndromes

1. Which of the following *best* describes a myelodysplastic syndrome (MDS)?

A. A clonal proliferation of targeted myeloid or lymphoid cells causing systemic issues

B. A progressive group of disorders of hematopoiesis with qualitative abnormalities

C. A clonal proliferation of leukemic stem cells leading to a crowding out of resident hematopoietic cells

D. Uncontrolled proliferation of mutated cells to other organs

Hematology/Myelodysplastic syndromes/2

2. Intracytoplasmic bridging and oval macrocytes are markers associated with:

A. Dyserythropoiesis

B. Dysgranulopoiesis

C. Dysmegakaryopoiesis

D. Dysmyelopoiesis

Hematology/Myelodysplastic syndromes/2

3. Which of the following cytogenetic anomalies is seen in over 70% of MDS patients?

A. t(9,22)

B. t(8,21)

C. t(12,12)

D. del(5q)

Hematology/Myelodysplastic syndromes/1

4. A 70-year-old patient presents with fatigue and pancytopenia. A peripheral smear shows hypogranular neutrophils and oval macrocytes. Granulocytes and platelets do not appear abnormal. Iron studies and iron stores appear adequate. What is the *most* likely condition present?

A. MDS I

B. MDS II

C. MDS III

D. MDS IV

Hematology/Myelodysplastic syndromes/3

Answers to Questions 1–4

1. B A myelodysplastic syndrome is characterized by the presence of abnormal morphology and cytopenias that begin in the RBC line and eventually affect the other cell lines. MDS has the propensity to develop into acute leukemia with prominent dysplasia.

2. A Myelodysplastic syndromes are a group of progressive and heterogeneous disorders that display abnormal cellular division (dysplasia). Evidence of dyserythropoiesis includes intracytoplasmic bridging and oval macrocytes. Other evidence of dyserythropoiesis includes the presence of erythrocyte inclusions, microcytes with dimorphic RBC population, and ring sideroblasts.

3. D Myelodysplastic syndromes have a common cytogenetic anomaly that is seen in over 70% of patients. The anomaly is a deletion of the long arm of chromosome 5 labeled as del(5q).

4. A The presence of evidence supporting dyserythropoiesis without involvement of granulocytes and platelets indicates an earlier MDS, either MDS I or II. The adequate iron stores support MDS I more than MDS II.

5. A BM aspirate reveals 10% blasts, evidence of dyshematopoiesis across all three cell lines, and 20% ringed sideroblasts when stained with Prussian blue. What is the likely condition present?
A. MDS IV
B. MDS II
C. MDS III
D. MDS I

Hematology/Myelodysplastic syndromes/2

6. Atypical granulation and hyposegmentation of neutrophils are suggestive of:
A. Dyserythropoiesis
B. Dysmyelopoiesis
C. Dysmegakaryopoiesis
D. Transformation to AML

Hematology/Myelodysplastic syndromes/2

7. A CBC reveals the following results: WBC = 2.0 × 10^9/L, Hgb = 9.0 g/dL, PLT = 45 × 10^9/L. Bone marrow shows 8% blasts and dysplasia in erythroid precursors and megakaryocytes. Which World Health Organization (WHO) classification *best* fits?
A. MDS with isolated del(5q)
B. MDS with excess blasts-2 (MDS-EB2)
C. MDS with multilineage dysplasia
D. AML

Hematology/Myelodysplastic syndromes/3

8. A 70-year-old patient with MDS is being monitored for transformation. What change will be observed in the laboratory data that would support transformation?
A. Increase in ringed sideroblasts
B. Normalization of the platelet count
C. Blast count higher than 20%
D. Appearance of alternative RBC morphology or inclusions

Hematology/Myelodysplastic syndromes/3

9. The presence of giant platelets and hyperlobulation of megakaryocytes suggests:
A. Dyserythropoiesis
B. Dysmyelopoiesis
C. Dysmegakaryopoiesis
D. Transformation to AML

Hematology/Myelodysplastic syndromes/2

10. Early evidence of cytopenias suggests the pathology of MDS begins with:
A. Abnormal p53 housekeeping
B. Apoptosis of cellular precursors
C. Abnormal BM microenvironment
D. BM failure necessitating extramedullary hematopoiesis

Hematology/Myelodysplastic syndromes/2

Answers to Questions 5–10

5. C The presence of blasts below the 20% cutoff needed to identify the condition as an acute leukemia is suggestive of an MDS with excess blasts (MDS III). There are also ringed sideroblasts present, which carries over from MDS II, which also has increased ringed sideroblasts.

6. B Atypical granulation and pelgeroid hyposegmentation is considered evidence of dysmyelopoiesis. Other evidence includes hypogranulation or agranulation of neutrophils, nuclear-to-cytoplasmic asynchrony, hypersegmentation, and prominent nucleoli in nucleus.

7. C The abnormal production (dysplasia) in more than one cell line (erythroid and megakaryocytic) indicates it is multilineage. MDS-EB2 is identified as greater than 10% blasts, but under the 20% cutoff for AML, according to the WHO guidelines. The case shows under the 10% minimum that confirms this condition. The blast count is under the 20% that is needed to identify AML. The 5q- deletion is seen in over 70% of all MDS types so it cannot be tied to a specific MDS.

8. C According to the WHO guidelines, AML is identified as greater than 20% blasts in the bone marrow. If there is an MDS transformation into an AML, the results need to meet the 20% cutoff. Increase in ringed sideroblasts is seen in the earlier MDS stages and is not associated with transformation, which occurs in the later stages. Normalization of the platelet count and the presence of alternative RBC morphology or inclusions are associated with later stages of MDS, but CBC data, either quantitative or qualitative, are not used to identify transformation.

9. C Giant platelets and hyperlobulated megakaryocytes are evidence of abnormal megakaryocyte division. Additional findings include abnormal platelet granulation, circulating micromegakaryocytes, or megakaryocytes with small nuclei.

10. B Early-stage MDS begins with apoptosis, which prematurely destroys cellular precursors. Eventually there is abnormal housekeeping, which dysregulates cellular production, leading to the transformation to AML.

7.8 *Lymphoproliferative and Myeloproliferative Neoplasms*

1. **Which of the following driver mutations is found in over 95% of polycythemia vera (PV) patients?**
   A. *BCR::ABL*
   B. *CALR*
   C. *JAK2 V617F*
   D. *MPL*
   Hematology/Myeloproliferative neoplasms/2

2. **The PLTs produced in essential thrombocythemia (ET) are:**
   A. Increased in number and functionally abnormal
   B. Adequate in number and functionally abnormal
   C. Decreased in number and functional
   D. Decreased in number and functionally abnormal
   Hematology/Myeloproliferative neoplasms/2

3. **Which of the following cells is pathognomonic for Hodgkin lymphoma?**
   A. Niemann–Pick cells
   B. Reactive lymphocytes
   C. Flame cells
   D. Reed–Sternberg (RS) cells
   Hematology/Lymphoproliferative neoplasms/1

4. **In primary myelofibrosis (PMF), the characteristic RBC morphology is:**
   A. Codocytes
   B. Schistocytes
   C. Dacryocytes
   D. Ovalocytes
   Hematology/Lymphoproliferative neoplasms/1

5. **Which of the following is *not* included in the major diagnostic criteria for the identification of PV?**
   A. The presence of one of the driver mutations
   B. Elevated Hct and Hgb
   C. Trilineage hypercellularity in the bone marrow
   D. Low serum erythropoietin levels
   Hematology/Myeloproliferative neoplasms/2

Answers to Questions 1–5

1. C Over 95% of PV patients test positive for the *JAK2 V617F* mutation. This is a driver mutation that induces a gain of function in the Janus kinase 2 (JAK2) signal transduction pathway that is found in the hematopoietic stem cell (HSC). This is primarily responsible for the panmyelosis observed in PV patients. Activation of the JAK2 signal transduction pathway is capable of activating the erythropoietic signal pathway to induce erythropoiesis without erythropoietin (EPO) stimulation. The *V617F* indicates that the point mutation occurs at position 617 where valine replaces phenylalanine.

2. A In ET, the PLT count is extremely elevated. The PLTs are abnormal in function, leading to bleeding and thrombotic diathesis.

3. D The morphological common denominator in Hodgkin lymphoma is the RS cell. It is a large, binucleated cell with a dense nucleolus surrounded by clear space. These characteristics give the RS cell an "owl's eye" appearance. Niemann–Pick cells (foam cells) are histiocytes containing phagocytized sphingolipids that stain pale blue and impart a foamlike texture to the cytoplasm. Flame cells are plasma cells with a distinctive red cytoplasm. They are sometimes seen in the bone marrow of patients with multiple myeloma.

4. C The marked amount of fibrosis, both medullary and extramedullary, accounts for the irreversible change in RBC morphology to a teardrop shape or the formation of a dacryocyte. It is most associated with bone marrow failure, and the extramedullary hematopoiesis occurs in the vascular system of the liver and/or spleen.

5. D The diagnosis of PV requires confirmation between major and minor criteria. According to the 2022 WHO guidelines, the major criteria include confirmation of the following: (1) one of the driver mutations associated with the MPNs, (2) elevated Hgb (above 16.5 g/dL in males and 16.0 g/dL in females) or Hct (above 49% in males and 48% in females), (3) bone marrow showing trilineage hypercellularity (panmyelosis). A minor criterion is low serum EPO levels. The diagnosis may be made if all three major criteria are met or if two major criteria and one minor criterion are met.

6. LAP staining is performed from a lavender top tube on a patient with a regenerative left shift. Results are shown below:

Grading	Number of PMNs
0	90
1+	6
2+	4
3+	0
4+	0

What can be concluded from the findings?

A. The patient has CML
B. The patient has a leukemoid reaction
C. The test results are invalid due to EDTA and need to be repeated using a different anticoagulant
D. The test should be repeated after karyotyping is performed

Hematology/Myeloproliferative neoplasms/2

7. LAP staining performed on a patient gives the following results:

Grading	Number of PMNs
0	10
1+	48
2+	38
3+	3
4+	1

Calculate the LAP score.

A. 100
B. 117
C. 137
D. 252

Hematology/Myeloproliferative neoplasms/2

8. A manual differential is requested on a patient with hip pain and unexpected weight loss. Peripheral blood smear reveals moderate dacryocytes, polychromasia, and 4 NRBCs. CBC results show mild pancytopenia, a low hemoglobin, and normocytic normochromic erythrocytes. What test should be conducted next to confirm these findings?

A. Karyotyping for the Philadelphia chromosome
B. Flow cytometry for B-cell markers
C. Periodic acid–Schiff (PAS) staining to examine NRBCs
D. Bone marrow aspirate and biopsy with silver staining

Hematology/Myeloproliferative neoplasms/3

Answers to Questions 6–8

6. C The LAP score is used to evaluate the activity of leukocyte alkaline phosphatase (LAP) present in the tertiary granules of mature neutrophils and bands. Lower scores (below 20) are seen in CML, and higher scores (above 100) are seen in leukemoid reactions. EDTA diminishes LAP activity and causes a false positive interpretation for CML. Blood should be collected using either a heparinized capillary tube or a heparin tube.

7. C One hundred mature neutrophils are counted and scored. The LAP score is calculated as follows: (the number of 1+ cells × 1) + (2+ cells × 2) + (3+ cells × 3) + (4+ cells × 4). For this calculation, that is 48 + 76 + 9 + 4 = 137.

8. D The inconsistencies between what is evident on the peripheral blood smear and the CBC results supports a problem in the bone marrow. This is further supported by the presence of teardrop cells (dacryocytes), which is an indicator of hematopoiesis taking place outside the bone marrow (extramedullary). The logical next step is to evaluate the bone marrow for changes in hematopoiesis. Silver staining is used to evaluate collagen in the extracellular matrix (ECM), which is an indicator of myelofibrosis, which is consistent with what is present on the CBC and peripheral blood smear.

9. The following data are found in a 55-year-old patient with prominent joint pain in both hands. Platelet count = 650,000/μL, WBC count = 28,000/μL, RBC count = 4.50 x 10^6/μL. BM analysis revealed hyperlobulated dense megakaryocytes, granulopoiesis, and normoblastic maturation within expected reference limits. Cytogenetic karyotyping revealed *MPL* driver mutation present. What is the likely condition present in this patient?

A. CML
B. ET
C. Overt PMF
D. PV

Hematology/Myeloproliferative neoplasms/3

10. A characteristic finding in CML patients that differentiates it from other MPNs is:

A. Leukocytosis
B. Thrombocytosis
C. Erythrocytosis
D. A regenerative left shift

Hematology/Myeloproliferative neoplasms/2

11. Patients with Myeloproliferative neoplasms (MPNs) have an increased risk in developing:

A. Bone marrow failure
B. Splenomegaly
C. Myelodysplasia
D. Acute leukemia

Hematology/Myeloproliferative neoplasms/2

12. Which of the following may be used to differentiate between multiple myeloma and Waldenström macroglobulinemia?

A. Serum protein electrophoresis
B. Hyperviscosity of blood
C. Urine protein electrophoresis
D. Immunofixation electrophoresis

Hematology/Lymphoproliferative neoplasms/2

13. What is the characteristic finding evident in a peripheral blood smear from a patient with multiple myeloma?

A. Microcytic hypochromic cells
B. Intracellular inclusion bodies
C. Rouleaux
D. Hypersegmented neutrophils

Hematology/Lymphoproliferative neoplasms/1

Answers to Questions 9–13

9. B The findings are consistent with ET. The major diagnostic criteria established in the 2022 WHO guidelines indicate the following for the diagnosis of ET: (1) platelet count >450,000/μL, (2) BM exhibiting changes in the morphology of megakaryocytes including hyperlobularity and increased density, and (3) presence of one of the driver mutations associated with MPNs (*JAK2 V617F*, *MPL*, or *CALR*). These are all present in the patient in question, which supports the diagnosis of ET.

10. D CML is marked by an elevated WBC count demonstrating an increase in younger precursors in the blood (regenerative left shift). Elevated WBC count (leukocytosis), PLT count (thrombocytosis), or RBC count (erythrocytosis) is consistent with all myeloproliferative neoplasms and will not differentiate between the other MPNs and CML.

11. D MPNs have an increased risk of developing into acute leukemia. Many of the driver mutations can stimulate uncontrolled proliferation in the hematopoietic stem cells, which can transform into a clonal proliferation of leukemic stem cells. Splenomegaly is present in greater than 90% of MPN patients. Bone marrow failure is usually caused by increased apoptosis, and the opposite is true in MPNs. The driver mutations upregulate signal transduction leading to increased cellular proliferation rather than increased cellular destruction as seen in BM failure. Myelodysplasia is a qualitative defect in the structure and function of blood cells, and that is not consistent with the MPNs.

12. D Multiple myeloma and Waldenström macroglobulinemia are both lymphoproliferative disorders with different etiologies. Multiple myeloma results from an uncontrolled proliferation of malignant plasma cells that produces a monoclonal gammopathy on serum protein electrophoresis (SPE) and has specificity for either IgG or IgA on immunofixation electrophoresis (IFE). Waldenström macroglobulinemia results from a proliferation of plasma-like or prolymphocytes that also produces a monoclonal gammopathy on SPE but has specificity for IgM on IFE. Both conditions produce hyperviscosity and Bence Jones protein on urine protein electrophoresis (UPE) but have slight differences in the quantity of each.

13. C Multiple myeloma is a plasma cell dyscrasia that is characterized by overproduction of monoclonal immunoglobulin, which appears in the gamma fraction when proteins are separated on electrophoresis. Rouleaux are present in these patients as a result of increased viscosity and decreased albumin:globulin ratio.

14. The pathology of multiple myeloma does *not* include which of the following?

A. Expanding plasma cell mass
B. Overproduction of monoclonal immunoglobulins
C. Production of osteoclast activating factor (OAF) and other cytokines
D. Clonal proliferation of dysfunctional B-cell lymphoblasts

Hematology/Lymphoproliferative neoplasms/2

15. Waldenström macroglobulinemia is a malignancy of the:

A. Lymphoplasmacytoid cells
B. Adrenal cortex
C. Myeloblastic cell lines
D. Erythroid cell precursors

Hematology/Lymphoproliferative neoplasms/2

16. This condition is caused by a proliferation of cells that have an abundance of isoenzyme 5 that are characteristically resistant to tartaric acid. What condition is present and what is required to identify this condition?

A. Chronic lymphocytic leukemia (CLL) and a bone marrow aspirate
B. Multiple myeloma and an SPE with IFE
C. Hairy cell leukemia (HCL) and a TRAP stain
D. T-cell acute lymphoblastic leukemia (ALL) and flow cytometry

Hematology/Lymphoproliferative neoplasms/2

Answers to Questions 14–16

14. D Mutated plasmablasts in bone marrow undergo clonal replication and expand the plasma cell mass. Normal bone marrow is gradually replaced by malignant plasma cells, leading to pancytopenia. Most malignant plasma cells actively produce immunoglobulins. In multiple myeloma, the normally controlled and purposeful production of antibodies is replaced by inappropriate production of even larger amounts of useless immunoglobulin molecules. The normally equal production of light chains and heavy chains may be imbalanced. The result is the release of excess free light chains or free heavy chains. The immunoglobulins produced by a single clone of myeloma cells are identical. Any abnormal production of identical antibodies is referred to by the general term *monoclonal gammopathy*. Osteoclasts are bone cells active in locally resorbing bone and releasing calcium into blood. Nearby osteoblasts are equally active in utilizing the calcium in blood to form new bone. Multiple myeloma interrupts this balance by the secretion of at least two substances: interleukin 6 (IL-6) and OAF. As its name implies, OAF stimulates osteoclasts to increase bone resorption and release of calcium, which lead to lytic lesions of the bone.

15. A Waldenström macroglobulinemia is a malignancy of lymphoplasmacytoid cells, which manufacture IgM. Although the cells secrete immunoglobulin, they are not fully differentiated into plasma cells and lack the characteristic perinuclear halo, deep basophilia, and eccentric nucleus characteristic of classic plasma cells.

16. C Hairy cells are unique lymphoblasts that produce hair-like cytoplasmic projections that stain with high specificity with tartrate-resistant acid phosphatase (TRAP). What causes both of these findings is an abundance of isoenzyme 5. Nonerythroid blood cells have seven isoenzymes present, but isoenzyme 5 is the only one that is resistant to tartaric acid. Although this cytochemical reaction is fairly specific for HCL, TRAP activity has occasionally been reported in B-cell leukemia and, rarely, T-cell leukemia.

17. Review the following scatterplot, histograms, and automated values for a 61-year-old female experiencing fatigue and unexplained weight loss of 25 pounds.

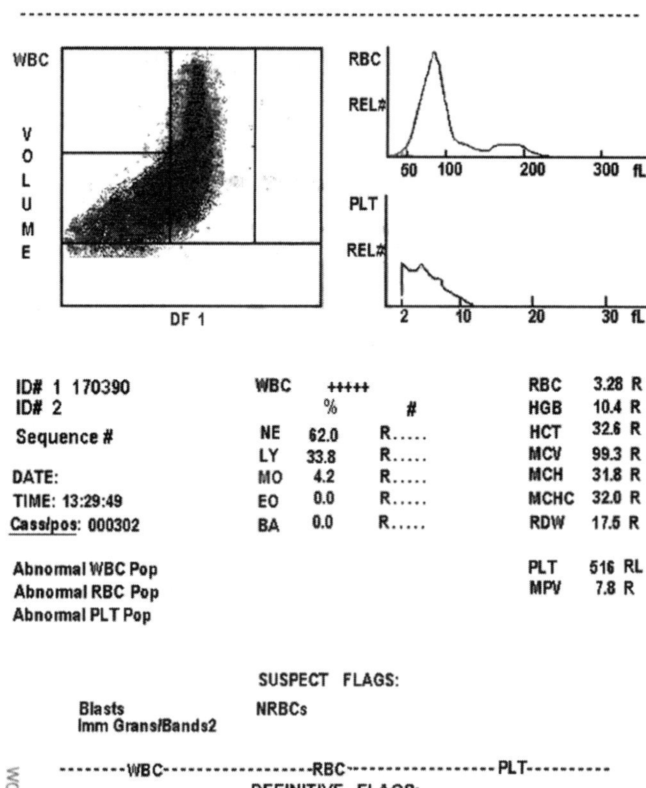

WBC differential: 14 band neutrophils; 50 segmented neutrophils; 7 lymphocytes; 4 monocytes; 10 metamyelocytes; 8 myelocytes; 1 promyelocyte; 3 eosinophils; 3 basophils; 2 NRBCs/100 WBCs

What is the presumptive condition present?

A. Leukemoid reaction
B. CML
C. AML
D. Megaloblastic leukemia

Hematology/Myeloproliferative neoplasms/3

18. Review the following CBC results for a 75-year-old male:

WBC = 158.2×10^9/L	MCV = 98 fL
RBC = 2.68×10^{12}/L	MCH = 31.7 pg
Hgb = 8.5 g/dL	MCHC = 32.6%
Hct = 26.5 %	PLT = 132×10^9/L

Differential: 96 lymphocytes; 2 band neutrophils; 2 segmented neutrophils; 25 smudge cells/100 WBCs

What is the *most* likely condition present?

A. ALL
B. CLL
C. Infectious mononucleosis
D. Myelodysplastic syndrome

Hematology/Lymphoproliferative neoplasms/2

Answers to Questions 17–18

17. B The "+++++" on the printout indicates that the WBC count exceeds the upper linearity of the analyzer. This markedly elevated WBC count, combined with the spectrum of immature granulocytic cells seen on peripheral blood smear examination, is highly presumptive of CML. It would still need to be confirmed with karyotyping and LAP staining.

18. B CLL is a disease of elderly individuals, classically associated with an elevated WBC count and relative and absolute lymphocytosis. Smudge cells are usually present in the peripheral blood smear due to the unstable fragility of the lymphocytes. CLL may occur with or without anemia or thrombocytopenia. The lack of immature blasts present on the differential rules out ALL. The lack of reactive (atypical) lymphocytes make infectious mononucleosis unlikely. Myelodysplastic syndromes may involve the erythroid, granulocytic, or megakaryocytic cell lines but not the lymphoid cells.

19. A 35-year-old patient presents to the primary care provider with a rash on the elbows that appears to be psoriasis. The patient's physical examination also reveals enlarged lymph nodes in the cervical and axillary areas. The provider biopsies the rash and orders a positron emission tomography (PET) scan to evaluate the enlarged lymph nodes. The skin biopsy reveals round lymphocytes with prominent nuclear clefts and cytoplasmic projections. What is the likely condition present based on these findings?

A. Hodgkin lymphoma
B. Non-Hodgkin lymphoma
C. Mycoses fungoides
D. Sézary syndrome

Hematology/Lymphoproliferative neoplasms/3

20. A complication of monoclonal gammopathies is:

A. Immunodeficiencies
B. Progression into acute leukemia
C. Adoption of additional driver mutations
D. Cold agglutinin disease

Hematology/Lymphoproliferative neoplasms/1

Answers to Questions 19–20

19. D These findings are consistent with Sézary syndrome. Sézary syndrome is a cutaneous T-cell lymphoma that begins as a skin rash and eventually progresses into a systemic lymphoproliferative neoplastic disorder. It typically begins with exposure to EBV that causes an uncontrolled proliferation of morphologically aberrant T cells. These T cells have a prominent nuclear cleft and are sometimes referred to as "butt cells." Mycosis fungoides is the same condition but has not progressed to the lymph nodes to cause pathology yet. Hodgkin lymphoma and non-Hodgkin lymphoma are both confirmed with a lymph node biopsy and the presence of RS cells that morphologically are different from Sézary cells.

20. D In the revised 2022 WHO classification, an associated complication that has been seen in monoclonal gammopathies is cold agglutinin disease. The excessive proliferation of immunoglobulins in these conditions can cause cold-reacting antibodies to bind to RBCs and cause agglutination.

7.9
Acute Leukemia

1. **The presence of which of the following inclusions indicates that leukemia is myeloid in origin?**
   A. Toxic granulation
   B. Vacuolization
   C. Auer rods
   D. Vacuolization with midnight blue cytoplasm
   Hematology/Acute leukemia/2

2. **The physical manifestations associated with leukemia are caused by:**
   A. Replacement of marrow precursors by leukemic stem cells causing impaired hematopoiesis
   B. Transformation of proliferating stem cells into dysfunctional stem cells and consequently impaired hematopoiesis
   C. Impaired bone marrow functionality leading to extramedullary hematopoiesis that is poorly
   D. Decreased erythropoietin production
   Hematology/Acute leukemia/2

3. **A peripheral blood smear is reviewed and there are predominant monoblasts and promonocytes. This is confirmed by biopsy. Additional testing revealed a *KMT2A* rearrangement and positive staining with ANAE. Based on these findings, which condition is likely?**
   A. AML, minimally differentiated
   B. AML, without maturation
   C. Acute myelomonocytic leukemia
   D. Acute monocytic leukemia
   Hematology/Acute leukemia/2

4. **ALL accounts for 75% of all cancers in which age group?**
   A. Infants
   B. Children <5 years of age
   C. Adolescents
   D. Adults in the ages of 20s and 30s
   Hematology/Acute leukemia/1

5. **Which acute leukemia has an increased risk of developing consumptive coagulopathy through the secretion of proteolytic enzymes?**
   A. AML, without maturation
   B. Acute promyelocytic leukemia (PML)
   C. Acute myelomonocytic leukemia
   D. Acute monocytic leukemia
   Hematology/Acute leukemia/2

Answers to Questions 1–5

1. C The presence of Auer rods is an indicator that the lineage of the malignant blasts are myeloid. Auer rods are primary granules that have been fused together to form needle-like structures. The primary granules are found only in stages of myeloid development and are not seen in lymphoid and monocytic lineages.

2. A The physical manifestations associated with leukemia present as a result of the pathology of the condition. Leukemia is an acquired condition with genomic instability. The unstable genetic or epigenetic change alters the function of the hematopoietic stem cell, which transforms into a leukemic stem cell. As a result, the hematopoietic stem cells are crowded out by the leukemic stem cell, which inhibits the function of all blood cells. For erythrocytes, there is impaired oxygen delivery, which produces fatigue, pallor, and shortness of breath. For leukocytes, there are impairments in host immune defenses, making the patient susceptible to infections. For platelets, there is impaired healing after injury, causing unplanned bleeding episodes to occur.

3. D Acute monocytic leukemia (AMoL) is responsible for less than 10% of all AML cases. It causes proliferation of monoblasts and promonocytes, which are considered blast equivalents according to the 2022 WHO guidelines. Additional results that support AMoL is the presence of the *KMT2A* rearrangement (most commonly with *MLLT3*) along with the positive staining with alpha naphthyl acetate esterase (ANAE).

4. B ALL accounts for 25% of all childhood cancers and up to 75% of all childhood leukemia. The largest stratified group of affected patients is children between ages 1 and 5 followed by adolescents. ALL has a bimodal occurrence, sometimes suffering a relapse when a patient is in their 40s or 50s.

5. B The increased risk of consumptive coagulopathy is associated with PML. This occurs through the release of proteolytic enzymes that activate thrombin. An example of a consumptive coagulopathy is DIC, in which concurrent hemorrhaging and thrombotic episodes occur.

6. Review the following laboratory results:

WBC = 6.0 × 10^9/L	Hgb = 6.0 g/dL
RBC = 1.90 × 10^{12}/L	Hct = 18.5%
PLT = 130 × 10^9/L	
Serum vitamin B_{12} and folic acid: within expected reference limits	

WBC Differential	Bone Marrow
6% PMNs	40% myeloblasts
40% lymphocytes	60% pronormoblasts
4% monocytes	40 orthochromatophilic NRBCs/100 WBCs
50% blasts	PAS: Positive with a coarse granular pattern

The results are *most* characteristic of:

A. Pernicious anemia
B. AML, without maturation
C. Acute erythroid leukemia
D. Acute myelomonocytic leukemia

Hematology/Acute leukemia/3

7. A 24-year-old male with Down syndrome presents with fever, pallor, lymphadenopathy, and hepatosplenomegaly. The CBC results are as follows:

WBCs = 10.8 × 10^9/L	RBCs = 1.56 × 10^{12}/L
8% PMNs	Hgb = 3.3 g/dL
25% lymphocytes	Hct = 11%
67% PAS-positive blasts exhibiting a coarse block pattern	PLTs = 2.5 × 10^9/L

These findings are suggestive of:

A. Hodgkin lymphoma
B. Myeloproliferative neoplasms
C. Leukemoid reaction
D. ALL

Hematology/Acute leukemia/3

8. A peripheral blood smear contains 75% blasts. Bone marrow revealed 90% myeloblasts with very few promyelocytes present. These stain positive for both Sudan Black B (SBB) and peroxidase. Given these values, which of the following disorders is *most* likely?

A. Acute myeloblastic leukemia, minimally differentiated
B. Acute myeloblastic leukemia with maturation
C. Acute undifferentiated leukemia (AUL)
D. ALL

Hematology/Acute leukemia/3

9. Leukemic lymphoblasts reacting with CD10 are characteristically seen in:

A. B-cell ALL
B. T-cell ALL
C. Null cell ALL
D. Common ALL

Hematology/Acute leukemia/2

10. A patient's peripheral blood smear and bone marrow both show 70% blasts. The cells are negative with myeloperoxidase (MPX/MPO) and SBB staining and positive for the Philadelphia chromosome. What is the likely condition present and the prognosis?

A. AML, poor prognosis
B. CLL, good prognosis
C. CML in blast crisis, good prognosis
D. ALL, poor prognosis

Hematology/Acute leukemia/3

Answers to Questions 6–10

6. C In acute erythroid leukemia, greater than 50% of nucleated bone marrow cells are erythroid and greater than 30% nonerythroid cells are blasts. The normoblasts stain positive with PAS with a coarse granular pattern.

7. D Common signs of ALL are hepatosplenomegaly , lymphadenopathy, and fever. Anemia and thrombocytopenia are usually present, and the WBC count is variable. The numerous lymphoblasts are generally PAS positive, producing a coarse block pattern.

8. A AML blasts stain positive for SBB and peroxidase, and the bone marrow is showing minimal progression to older stages of development. This is suggestive of AML without maturation.

9. D The majority of non-T-cell, non-B-cell ALL blast cells display the CALLA (CD10) marker. CALLA stands for common acute lymphoblastic leukemia antigen. Lymphoblasts of common ALL are TdT (terminal deoxynucleotidyl transferase) positive and CALLA positive but do not have surface membrane IgM or μ-chains and are pre-B-cell lymphoblasts.

10. D The negative staining with SBB and MPX is consistent with a nonmyeloid leukemia such as ALL. SBB stains phospholipids and other neutral fats present in the membrane of primary granules. Lymphoid cells rarely stain positive with MPX and SBB for this reason. The cytochemical stains used rule out CLL and CML as those stain blast cells, which are not seen in chronic leukemias. The presence of the Philadelphia chromosome is a good prognostic indicator for CML, but a poor prognosis in ALL patients.

11. A flow cytometry panel is evaluated for suspected ALL. The unknown cells stain positive for CD34, CD19, cCD22, and TdT. What condition is likely present?
A. Common B-cell ALL
B. Pre-B-cell ALL
C. Early precursor B-cell ALL
D. Mature T-cell ALL

Hematology/Acute leukemia/3

12. Acute promyelocytic leukemia has a defined karyotype present in over 95% of patients with this condition. What is the recurrent karyotype present?
A. t(15;17)
B. t(9,22)
C. t(8;21)
D. inv(16)

Hematology/Acute leukemia/2

13. Which of the following findings provides a favorable prognosis for AML patients?
A. *DEK:NUP214*
B. *BCR:ABL1*
C. Myelodysplasia-related findings
D. *CBFB:MYH11* fusion

Hematology/Acute leukemia/2

14. A 5-year-old patient is undergoing an AML laboratory evaluation. The following are identified: positive for CD41, CD42b, and CD61; strong expression with CD56; and negative for CD7, CD11b, CD13, CD36, CD45, CD38, and HLA-DR. What condition is *most* likely?
A. Acute myelomonocytic leukemia (AMML)
B. Acute monocytic leukemia (AMoL)
C. Acute megakaryoblastic leukemia (AMkL)
D. ALL

Hematology/Acute leukemia/3

Answers to Questions 11–14

11. C Positive staining for CD34, CD19, cCD22, and TdT are consistent with early staging of B-cell ALL. CD34 are found on all hematopoietic precursors. TdT is an early lymphoid marker seen in the early stages in both B- and T-cell development. CD22 begins their expression in the cytoplasm of B cells in the early stages of B-cell maturation and is then expressed on the surface of B cells in their mature stages.

12. A AML with t(15;17) is classified under the category "AML with Recurrent Genetic Abnormalities" by WHO. Acute PML is composed of abnormal promyelocytes with heavy granulation, sometimes obscuring the nucleus, and abundant cytoplasm. Acute PML contains a translocation that results in the fusion of a transcription factor called PML on chromosome 15 with the alpha (α)-retinoic acid receptor gene (*RAR*α) on chromosome 17.

13. D The focus of the 2022 WHO classification of leukemic disorders describes the prognosis for the different leukemia subtypes. These are tied to recurrent genetic abnormalities present along with other phenotypic findings.

14. C Acute megakaryoblastic leukemia (AMkL) affects platelet precursors or megakaryocytes. The platelet precursors exhibit positivity with traditional platelet markers such as CD41, CD42b, CD56, and CD61. They do not express CD markers associated with other cell types derived from the myeloid stem cell such as CD11b, CD13, HLA-DR, and CD45.

7.10

Laboratory Evaluation of Leukocyte Disorders

1. An M:E ratio of 10:1 indicates:

A. Erythroid hyperplasia
B. Granulocytic hyperplasia
C. Panmyelosis
D. Myelodysplasia

Hematology/Laboratory evaluation of leukocyte disorders/2

2. Which of the following is a characteristic of Auer rods?

A. They are composed of azurophilic granules
B. They stain positive on PAS staining
C. They are predominantly seen in CML
D. They are nonspecific esterase positive

Hematology/Laboratory evaluation of leukocyte disorders/1

3. The stain that selectively identifies phospholipids in the membranes of both primary and secondary granules is:

A. PAS
B. MPX
C. SBB
D. TdT

Hematology/Laboratory evaluation of leukocyte disorders/1

4. Sodium fluoride may be added to the naphthol ASD acetate (NASDA) esterase reaction. The fluoride is added to inhibit a positive reaction with:

A. Megakaryocytes
B. Monocytes
C. Erythrocytes
D. Granulocytes

Hematology/Laboratory evaluation of leukocyte disorders/1

5. Which of the following reactions are often positive in ALL but are negative in AML?

A. TdT and PAS
B. Chloroacetate esterase and nonspecific esterase
C. SBB and peroxidase
D. New methylene blue and acid phosphatase

Hematology/Laboratory evaluation of leukocyte disorders/2

Answers to Questions 1–5

1. B The M:E ratio reflects the relationship of RBC precursors to myeloid (granulocytic) precursors in the bone marrow. Because of their shortened life span in the marrow, there are two to three times more myeloid precursors than erythroid precursors. In this example, there are 10 times more granulocytic precursors, indicating an excessive proliferation of granulocytes in the marrow.

2. A Auer rods are needle-like inclusions composed of primary azurophilic granules and are present in the cytoplasm of myeloblasts and monoblasts in patients with acute leukemia.

3. C Phospholipids, neutral fats, and sterols are stained by SBB. The PAS reaction stains intracellular glycogen. Myeloperoxidase is an enzyme present in the primary granules of myeloid cells and, to a lesser degree, in monocytic cells. TdT is a DNA polymerase found in thymus-derived lymphocytes and some bone marrow–derived lymphocytes.

4. B NASDA stains monocytes (and monoblasts) and granulocytes (and myeloblasts). The addition of fluoride renders monocytic cells (and blasts) negative, thus allowing for differentiation from granulocytic cells, which remain positive.

5. A PAS is positive in about 50% of ALL with L1 and L2 morphology but is negative in ALL with L3 morphology (B-cell ALL). TdT is positive in all types of ALL except L3. Both TdT and PAS are negative in AML.

6. What is the benefit of having a defect in karyotyping in a leukemia patient?
- **A.** It allows for more expedient identification and treatment
- **B.** It is often correlated to a good prognosis
- **C.** It is used to establish staging of the leukemia
- **D.** It is often correlated to a targeted treatment plan

Hematology/Laboratory evaluation of leukocyte disorders/1

7. The WHO classification requires what percentage for the blast count in blood or bone marrow for the diagnosis of AML?
- **A.** At least 30%
- **B.** At least 20%
- **C.** At least 10%
- **D.** Any percentage

Hematology/Laboratory evaluation of leukocyte disorders/1

8. Which of the following tests are used to identify patterns of expression of antigens used in the identification of cellular lineages?
- **A.** Molecular diagnostics
- **B.** Immunophenotyping
- **C.** Whole genome sequencing
- **D.** Any percentage of blasts in the bone marrow

Hematology/Laboratory evaluation of leukocyte disorders/1

9. What is the primary benefit of using both molecular diagnostics and karyotyping in the laboratory evaluation of potential leukemia?
- **A.** Both test for genomic instability at two different levels, allowing for a broader determination of the leukemia present
- **B.** Both tests allow for expeditious identification and prompt planning for treatment
- **C.** Both tests are needed owing to their respective limitations in procedure
- **D.** Both are cost efficient and provide value in the diagnosis and treatment planning

Hematology/Laboratory evaluation of leukocyte disorders/2

10. Which of the following differentiates an immature T-cell and a mature T-cell phenotype?
- **A.** The expression of CD3 on the surface as opposed to the expression in the cytoplasm
- **B.** The expression of CD7 along with karyotyping
- **C.** The expression of both CD4 and CD8 in the early stages and choosing one of them in the later stages
- **D.** The amount of bone marrow cellularity present in the patient

Hematology/Laboratory evaluation of leukocyte disorders/2

Answers to Questions 6–10

6. D The primary benefit of finding an abnormal karyotype is that for many there is a targeted therapy addressing the genetic anomaly present. For example, all-trans retinoic acid (ATRA) used in PML targets the tyrosine kinase seen in the t(15,17) translocation.

7. B The WHO classification of AML requires that 20% or greater of nucleated bone marrow cells be blasts, whereas the French American–British (FAB) classification generally requires 30% or greater.

8. B Immunophenotyping is used to identify lineages through pattern recognition of antigens on the surface of the unknown cells, and it is performed by flow cytometry.

9. A Using molecular diagnostics and cytogenetic karyotyping adds value to the diagnosis. Molecular diagnostics focuses on the genetic abnormality at the nucleic acid level, whereas karyotyping focuses on the genetic abnormality at the chromosomal level.

10. C T-cells have the propensity to develop either into a T-helper cell or T-suppressor cell and that is directly tied to the CD markers they express on their surface. Younger cells will express both CD4 (T-helper) and CD8 (T-suppressor) on their surface, but as they mature, they only express either CD4 or CD8, not both.

BIBLIOGRAPHY

1. Kaushansky K, Lichtman MA, Prchal JT, Levi MM, Burns LJ, Lynch DC. *Williams Hematology.* 10th ed. McGraw-Hill; 2021.
2. Keohane EM, Butina MM, Mirza KM, Walenga JM. *Rodak's Hematology: Clinical Principles and Applications.* 7th ed. Elsevier; 2025.

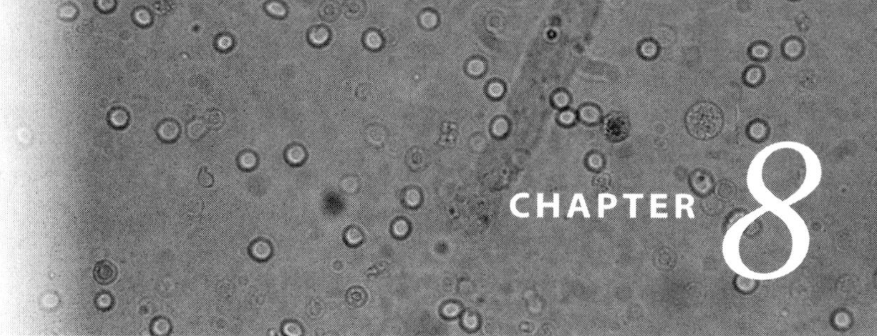

Hemostasis and Coagulation

8.1 *Coagulation Physiology*

8.2 *Primary Hemostasis Disorders: Platelet and Vascular Disorders*

8.3 *Secondary Hemostasis Disorders: Factor Deficiencies and Hemorrhagic Coagulation Disorders*

8.4 *Thrombosis Risk, Thrombotic Disorders, and Anticoagulant Therapies*

8.5 *Evaluation of Coagulopathies*

8.1

Coagulation Physiology

1. **Which of the following initiates *in vivo* coagulation by activation of factor VII?**
   A. Protein C
   B. Tissue factor (TF)
   C. Plasmin activator
   D. Thrombomodulin (TM)
   Hemostasis/Coagulation physiology/1

2. **Which of the following clotting factors plays a role in clot formation *in vitro*, but not *in vivo*?**
   A. Factor VIIa
   B. Factor IIa
   C. Factor XIIa
   D. Factor Xa
   Hemostasis/Coagulation physiology/1

3. **Vitamin K is responsible for:**
   A. Releasing von Willebrand factor (vWF) from the Weibel–Palade bodies when platelets activate
   B. Activating thrombin to initiate thrombin activable procoagulant processes *in vivo*
   C. Carboxylation of glutamate residues of some coagulation factors to initiate their activation
   D. Activating factors involved in the tenase and prothrombinase complexes
   Hemostasis/Coagulation physiology/2

4. **Which of the following is an endogenous activator of plasminogen secreted by endothelial cells?**
   A. Streptokinase
   B. Transglutaminase
   C. Tissue plasminogen activator (tPA)
   D. Urokinase
   Hemostasis/Coagulation physiology/1

Answers to Questions 1–4

1. B *In vivo*, activation of coagulation occurs on the surface of activated platelets (PLTs) or cells that have TF. The classical description of intrinsic, extrinsic, and common pathways does not take place *in vivo*. TF is found on the surface of many cells outside the vascular system (extrinsic). On vascular injury, TF is exposed to the vascular system. TF has high affinity for factors VII and VIIa. Protein C (choice A) is a natural inhibitor that is activated by the thrombin-thrombomodulin complex (choice D) with the help of protein S to neutralize factors V and VIII. Plasmin activator (choice C) is an agent that promotes fibrinolysis or clot dissolution.

2. C Factor XIIa does not play a role in coagulation *in vivo*; however, *in vitro*, the deficiency of this factor causes prolonged activated partial thromboplastin time (aPTT). *In vitro*, factor XII is activated by substances, such as glass, kaolin, and ellagic acid, and *in vivo* it may be activated by exposure to a negatively charged cell surface membrane, such as collagen, as well as to kallikrein and high-molecular-weight kininogen (HMWK). *In vivo*, factor XIIa plays an important role in the fibrinolytic system by activating plasminogen to plasmin. Plasmin degrades the fibrin clot at the site of injury. Deficiency of factor XII is associated with thrombosis and not with bleeding. Factors VIIa, Xa, and IIa play a role *in vivo* and *in vitro*.

3. C Vitamin K–dependent factors (II, VII, IX, and X) have a post-translational modification where they are missing a carboxyl group that facilitates calcium binding. Vitamin K donates the necessary carboxyl group on the glutamic acid residues of these factors to properly activate them.

4. C tPA is an endogenous (produced in the body) activator of plasminogen secreted by endothelial cells. It converts plasminogen to plasmin. Urokinase is another endogenous activator but is secreted by urinary epithelial cells, monocytes, and macrophages. Streptokinase is an exogenous (not made in the body) activator of plasminogen. An example of a transglutaminase is factor XIII, which is responsible for cross-linking the fibrin monomers.

5. Which of the following targets free plasmin to prevent binding to fibrin during fibrinolysis?
A. PAI-1
B. TAFI
C. α_2-Antiplasmin
D. α_2-Macroglobulin
Hemostasis/Coagulation physiology/2

6. A protein that plays a role in both primary and secondary hemostasis is:
A. Factor I
B. Factor VIII
C. Factor IX
D. Factor XI
Hemostasis/Coagulation physiology/2

7. PLT adhesion is dependent on:
A. Fibrinogen
B. Glycoprotein Ib
C. Glycoprotein IIb–IIIa complex
D. Calcium
Hemostasis/Coagulation physiology/1

8. Which of the following clotting factors are neutralized by proteins C and S?
A. Factors XII, XI
B. Factors XII, I
C. Factors I, II
D. Factors V, VIII
Hemostasis/Coagulation physiology/2

9. Which of the following inhibits PLT aggregation?
A. Thromboxane A_2
B. Thromboxane B_2
C. Prostacyclin
D. Antithrombin (AT)
Hemostasis/Coagulation physiology/1

10. Which platelet granule is responsible for fusing with the surface-connected canalicular system during their activation?
A. Dense granules
B. Alpha granules
C. Lysosomal granules
D. Azurophilic granules
Hemostasis/Coagulation physiology/1

11. What steps in the following coagulation cascade require platelet phospholipid or PF3?
1. Activation of factor X
2. Activation of factor II
3. Conversion of fibrinogen to fibrin
4. Conversion of prekallikrein to kallikrein
5. Activation of factor VII
A. Steps 1, 2, and 5
B. Steps 1, 2, and 3
C. Steps 1 and 4
D. Steps 2 and 4
Hemostasis/Coagulation physiology/2

Answers to Questions 5–11

5. C α_2-Antiplasmin is the main inhibitor of plasmin. It inhibits plasmin by forming a 1:1 stoichiometric complex with any free plasmin in plasma and, thus, prevents binding of plasmin to fibrin and fibrinogen. Plasminogen activator inhibitor-1 (PAI-1) regulates tPA release by targeting plasminogen, not plasmin. Thrombin activatable fibrinolysis inhibitor (TAFI) targets the carboxy residues on lysine present on fibrin to prevent binding of tPA to initiate fibrinolysis.

6. A Factor I (fibrinogen), along with the glycoprotein IIb–IIIa complex, is necessary for PLT aggregation, which is considered primary hemostasis. Factor I is also a substrate in the common pathway of coagulation, which is considered secondary hemostasis.

7. B Glycoprotein Ib is a PLT receptor for vWF. Glycoprotein Ib and vWF are both necessary for platelets to adhere to the exposed collagen. This is known as adhesion. Other proteins that play a role in PLT adhesion are glycoproteins V and IX.

8. D Factors V and VIII are clotting factors that are neutralized by proteins C and S. Protein C is activated by thrombin binding to thrombomodulin. Once activated, protein C complexes with protein S to neutralize factors V and VIII.

9. C Prostacyclin is released from the endothelium and is an inhibitor of PLT aggregation. Thromboxane A_2 (TXA2) promotes PLT aggregation. Thromboxane B_2 is an oxidized form of TXA2 and is excreted in urine. AT is a physiological anticoagulant that neutralizes thrombin-dependent clotting factors.

10. B There are approximately 50 to 80 alpha granules responsible for traveling from the organelle zone through the surface-connected canalicular system to the membrane to activate the platelet when the need arises.

11. A Platelet phospholipid or platelet factor 3 (PF3) is involved at several activation steps in the coagulation cascade. They are part of the tenase complex, which is responsible for activating factor X. They are also part of the prothrombinase complex, which is responsible for activating factor II (prothrombin). They are also involved in the activation of factor VII, which carries over to the tenase and subsequent prothrombinase complexes.

12. Megakaryocytes mature through a process called:
A. Mitosis
B. Meiosis
C. Endoreduplication
D. Translation

Hemostasis/Coagulation physiology/1

13. What are the primary procoagulant roles of the vascular system?
A. Prevent blood loss by initiating fibrinolysis
B. Secrete platelet growth factors and inhibit calcium production
C. Synthesize plasma inhibitors
D. Constrict and provide collagen for clotting activation

Hemostasis/Coagulation physiology/1

14. Patients who have a deficiency in AT have which type of problem?
A. Bleeding or hemorrhagic
B. Thrombotic
C. Bruising
D. Hypercalcemic

Hemostasis/Coagulation physiology/2

15. The activity of thrombin does *not* include:
A. Activation of protein C
B. Activation of factor XIII
C. Cross-linking of the fibrin monomers
D. Converting fibrinogen to fibrin

Hemostasis/Coagulation physiology/1

Answers to Questions 12–15

12. C Megakaryocytes mature differently than other blood cells. Megakaryocytes divide through the process of endoreduplication or endomitosis. Other blood cells divide through mitosis. Endoreduplication divides the nucleus without dividing the cytoplasm, causing the megakaryocyte to increase in size as it matures. Megakaryocytes are considered polyploidy, meaning that as the nucleus divides the number of chromosomes doubles and production capacity increases. The more nuclear lobes a megakaryocyte has, the more platelets it can produce.

13. D The vascular system is capable of procoagulant, anticoagulant, and fibrinolytic functions. The procoagulant functions of the vascular system involve vasoconstriction and initiate clotting factor activation. The trigger for clotting factor activation is exposure to subendothelial collagen.

14. B Antithrombin (AT) is a physiological anticoagulant that increases its activity in the presence of heparin. If a patient has a deficiency in AT, they will have problems with sufficiently anticoagulated their blood and predispose them to a thrombotic or hypercoagulable condition.

15. C Thrombin is the single factor that, once generated, has procoagulant, anticoagulant, and fibrinolytic functions. The anticoagulant properties of thrombin include activation of protein C. The procoagulant properties of thrombin include activation of factor XIII and converting fibrinogen to fibrin. Thrombin is not involved in the cross-linking of the fibrin monomers. This is the responsibility of factor XIII.

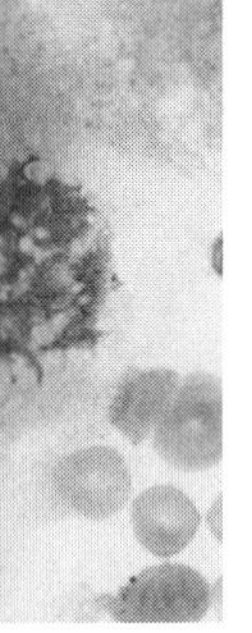

8.2

Primary Hemostasis Disorders: Platelet and Vascular Disorders

1. Thrombotic thrombocytopenic purpura (TTP) is characterized by:
A. Prolonged prothrombin time (PT)
B. Microangiopathic hemolytic anemia (MAHA)
C. Thrombocytosis
D. Decreased fibrinogen
Hemostasis/Primary hemostasis disorders/2

2. Chronic immune thrombocytopenia purpura (ITP) is characterized by:
A. Autoantibodies to platelets causing their destruction
B. Antibodies targeting viral antigen depositing on the surface of the platelets
C. Bacterial endotoxin damaging endothelial cells of the vasculature causing platelet deposition and aggregation
D. Increased production of megakaryocytes in the bone marrow causing thrombocytopenia
Hemostasis/Primary hemostasis disorders/2

3. Which of the following is an expected finding in a patient with classic von Willebrand disease?
A. Poor PLT aggregation with collagen agonist
B. aPTT within established reference intervals
C. Low PLT count
D. Low factor VIII:C levels
Hemostasis/Primary hemostasis disorders/2

4. Bernard–Soulier syndrome is associated with:
A. Decreased factor IX
B. Decreased factor VIII
C. Thrombocytopenia and giant PLTs
D. Primary and secondary waves of aggregation with PLT agonists
Hemostasis/Primary hemostasis disorders/2

5. Which of the following storage pool deficiencies is associated with increased susceptibility to opportunistic infections, eczema, and thrombocytopenia?
A. Chediak–Higashi syndrome
B. Wiskott–Aldrich syndrome
C. Hermansky–Pudlak syndrome
D. Thrombocytopenia absent radii syndrome
Hemostasis/Primary hemostasis disorders/2

Answers to Questions 1–5

1. B TTP is a quantitative PLT disorder associated with a triad of MAHA, thrombocytopenia, and renal failure and can also present as a pentad that includes fever and neurological abnormalities. The thrombocytopenia and MAHA are caused by uncleaved vWF that attracts and clumps platelets producing thrombocytopenia and hyaline microthrombi that shear erythrocytes to produce the schistocytes seen in MAHA. It does not involve clotting factors, so fibrinogen and PT will be within expected reference intervals.

2. A ITP can come in acute and chronic forms. Acute ITP is characterized by antiviral antibodies depositing on the PLT surface. Chronic ITP is characterized by autoantibodies to PLTs that bind and destroy them. Bacterial endotoxins damaging endothelial cells of the vascular system characterizes hemolytic uremic syndrome (HUS). Ineffective thrombopoiesis can be associated with a variety of vascular and PLT disorders, but they are not present in chronic ITP.

3. D von Willebrand disease (vWD) is an inherited, qualitative PLT disorder that results in increased bleeding, prolonged aPTT, and decreased factor VIII:C and vWF levels. PLT aggregation with collagen produce a monophasic primary wave of aggregation.

4. C Bernard–Soulier syndrome is associated with thrombocytopenia and giant PLTs. It is a qualitative PLT disorder caused by the deficiency of glycoprotein Ib. In Bernard–Soulier syndrome, PLT aggregation studies show an absence of aggregation with ristocetin and primary and secondary waves of aggregation with collagen, adenosine diphosphate (ADP), epinephrine, thrombin, and arachidonic acid. Factor VIII and IX assays are not indicated for this diagnosis.

5. B Storage pool deficiencies are initially differentiated based on the clinical presentation of albinism. Storage pool deficiencies associated with albinism are Chediak–Higashi syndrome and Hermansky–Pudlak syndrome. Wiskott–Aldrich syndrome is associated with increased susceptibility to opportunistic infections, eczema, and thrombocytopenia.

6. Which set of PLT responses would be *most* likely associated with Glanzmann thrombasthenia?
A. Strong PLT response to ADP and ristocetin; diminished aggregation to collagen
B. Strong PLT response to collagen; diminished aggregation to ADP and ristocetin
C. Strong PLT response to ristocetin; diminished aggregation to collagen, ADP, and epinephrine
D. Strong PLT response to ADP; diminished aggregation to collagen and ristocetin
Hemostasis/Primary hemostasis disorders/2

7. Which of the following is a characteristic of acute ITP?
A. Spontaneous remission within a few weeks
B. Predominantly seen in adults
C. Nonimmune PLT destruction
D. Insidious onset
Hemostasis/Primary hemostasis disorders/2

8. TTP differs from disseminated intravascular coagulation (DIC) in that:
A. aPTT is within expected reference intervals in TTP but prolonged in DIC
B. Schistocytes are not present in TTP but are present in DIC
C. PLT count is decreased in TTP but within expected reference intervals in DIC
D. PT is prolonged in TTP but decreased in DIC
Hemostasis/Primary hemostasis disorders/2

9. Several hours after birth, a baby boy develops petechiae and purpura and hemorrhagic diathesis. The PLT count is 18×10^9/L. The mom is PlA1 negative and does not have a diagnosis of ITP. What is the most likely explanation for the low PLT count?
A. Drug-induced thrombocytopenia
B. Secondary thrombocytopenia
C. Neonatal alloimmune thrombocytopenia
D. Neonatal autoimmune thrombocytopenia
Hemostasis/Primary hemostasis disorders/3

10. Which of the following is associated with post-transfusion purpura (PTP)?
A. Alloantibodies producing non–immune thrombocytopenia
B. Alloantibodies producing immune-mediated thrombocytopenia
C. Autoantibodies producing immune-mediated thrombocytopenia
D. Autoantibodies producing non–immune-mediated thrombocytopenia
Hemostasis/Primary hemostasis disorders/2

11. Hemolytic uremic syndrome (HUS) is produced by:
A. Uncleaved vWF attracting platelets to form circulating microthrombi
B. Antibodies targeting viral antigens depositing on platelet surface causing platelet destruction
C. Cytotoxins released by enteric pathogens damaging blood vessels causing platelet accumulation at injury site
D. Consumptive coagulopathy due to exacerbation of thrombin activation
Hemostasis/Primary hemostasis disorders/2

Answers to Questions 6–11

6. C Glanzmann thrombasthenia is a defect of glycoprotein IIb/IIIa that impairs PLT aggregation. As a result, response to endogenous platelet activators such as collagen, epinephrine, and ADP are impaired. Response to exogenous agonists such as ristocetin still produce a strong response.

7. A Acute ITP is an immune-mediated disorder found predominantly in children. It is commonly associated with viral infection. It is characterized by abrupt onset, and spontaneous remission usually occurs within several weeks.

8. A TTP is a PLT disorder in which PLT aggregation increases, resulting in thrombocytopenia. Schistocytes are present in TTP as a result of MAHA; however, the PT and aPTT are both normal. In DIC, the PT and aPTT are both prolonged, the PLT count is decreased, and schistocytes are seen in the peripheral blood smear.

9. C Neonatal alloimmune thrombocytopenia is similar to the hemolytic disease of the fetus and newborn. It results from immunization of the mother by fetal PLT antigens. The offending antibodies are commonly anti-PLT antigen A1 (PlA1), or human platelet antigen A1 (HPA-1a). Maternal antibodies cross the placenta, resulting in thrombocytopenia in the fetus.

10. B PTP is a rare form of alloimmune thrombocytopenia characterized by severe thrombocytopenia occurring after transfusion of blood or blood products. PTP is caused by antibody-related PLT destruction in previously immunized patients. In the majority of cases, the alloantibody produced is against PlA1 (HPA-1a).

11. C HUS is caused by enteric pathogens that produce cytotoxins, such as *E.coli O157: H7*. It is associated with ingestion of *E. coli*–contaminated foods and is commonly seen in children. The clinical manifestations in HUS are fever, diarrhea, thrombocytopenia, MAHA, and renal failure.

12. Hereditary hemorrhagic telangiectasia is a disorder of:

A. PLTs
B. Clotting proteins
C. Fibrinolysis
D. Connective tissue

Hemostasis/Primary hemostasis disorders/2

13. Which defect characterizes Gray syndrome?

A. PLT adhesion defect
B. Dense granule defect
C. Alpha granule defect
D. Coagulation defect

Hemostasis/Primary hemostasis disorders/2

14. Storage pool deficiencies are characterized by:

A. Monophasic curves with all endogenous agonists
B. Biphasic curves with all endogenous agonists
C. No or reduced response with endogenous agonists
D. Strong response with all agonists, endogenous and exogenous

Hemostasis/Primary hemostasis disorders/2

15. Iron-deficiency anemia and/or chronic inflammation cause which of the following?

A. Rebound thrombocytosis
B. Idiopathic thrombocytopenia
C. Postsplenectomy thrombocytosis
D. Thrombocytosis

Hemostasis/Primary hemostasis disorders/2

Answers to Questions 12–15

12. D Hereditary hemorrhagic telangiectasia (Osler–Weber–Rendu syndrome) is a connective tissue disorder associated with telangiectases (dilated capillaries) of the mucous membranes and skin. Lesions may develop on the tongue, lips, palate, face, hands, and nasal mucosa and throughout the gastrointestinal tract. This disorder is an autosomal dominant condition that usually manifests in adolescence or early adulthood.

13. C Gray syndrome is a PLT granule defect associated with a decrease in alpha granules resulting in decreased production of alpha granule proteins, such as platelet factor 4 (PF4) and beta thromboglobulin. Alpha granule deficiency results in the appearance of agranular PLTs when viewed in a Wright-stained blood smear.

14. C Storage pool deficiencies are defects in the granules, either dense or alpha. Dense granules contain ADP, epinephrine, calcium, and serotonin. ADP and epinephrine are endogenous agonists. As a result, there will be a diminished or minimal response with the endogenous agonists.

15. D Iron-deficiency anemia and chronic inflammation increase platelet production in a nonspecific way. Rebound thrombocytosis occurs specifically when marrow suppression therapy has stopped. Postsplenectomy thrombocytosis occurs after the spleen has been removed. The spleen holds approximately one third of the total circulating platelets and after the spleen has been removed, platelet production increases to compensate.

16. A 1-year-old infant was admitted with recurrent epistaxis for the past 5 days. Past medical history revealed easy bruising and a severe nosebleed that had occurred when he was 3 months of age, necessitating transfusion. The mother had a severe nosebleed 8 years ago. The father did not have a history of bleeding, but the infant's paternal grandfather passed away from a hemorrhagic stroke at a young age.

Admission Laboratory Results		
	Patient	**Reference Range**
Hgb	6.5 g/dL	13–15 g/dL
Platelet count	249×10^9/L	$150–450 \times 10^9$/L
PT	11.2 sec	11–13 sec
aPTT	34 sec	28–37 sec
ADDITIONAL LABORATORY TESTS		
Factor VIII activity	70%	50%–150%
Bleeding assessment tool (BAT)	Positive	
PLT aggregation:	Absent aggregation with ADP, epinephrine, and thrombin, adequate aggregation with ristocetin	

These clinical manifestations and laboratory results are consistent with which condition?

A. vWD
B. Bernard–Soulier syndrome
C. Glanzmann thrombasthenia
D. Factor VIII deficiency

Hemostasis/Primary hemostasis disorders/3

17. A 3-year-old was admitted with scattered petechiae and epistaxis. The patient had adequate growth and had no other medical problems except for viral gastroenteritis 3 weeks earlier. His family history was unremarkable.

Laboratory Results		
	Patient	**Reference Range**
PT	12 sec	10–13 sec
aPTT	35 sec	28–37 sec
PLT count	$18 \times 10^3/\mu L$	$150–450 \times 10^3/\mu L$
Peripheral blood smear: Normocytic normochromic with slight anisocytosis		

These clinical manifestations and laboratory results are consistent with which condition?

A. TTP
B. DIC
C. ITP
D. HUS

Hemostasis/Primary hemostasis disorders/3

Answers to Questions 16–17

16. C These clinical manifestations and laboratory results are consistent with Glanzmann thrombasthenia (GT). Epistaxis and easy bruising are characteristics of platelet disorders. The positive family history is indicative of an inherited bleeding disorder. Laboratory tests reveal a low hemoglobin (Hgb) level, likely due to the epistaxis episodes. The normal platelet count rules out any quantitative platelet disorder and Bernard–Soulier syndrome. Factor deficiencies and vWD are ruled out with the PT and aPTT values and factor VIII activity. The laboratory tests that confirm an inherited platelet disorder are PLT aggregation studies. Aggregation response to endogenous agonists is absent, but there is an adequate response to ristocetin. These results confirm GT.

17. C These clinical manifestations and laboratory results are consistent with ITP. In children, acute ITP occurs after a viral infection, in this case, viral gastroenteritis. The gastroenteritis can also be associated with HUS, but there would be signs of MAHA in HUS and that isn't present in this patient based on the peripheral blood smear. Another overlap between TTP, HUS, and ITP is found in the results of clotting factor assays PT and aPTT, which are within established reference intervals. Clinical manifestations are associated with petechiae, purpura, and mucous membrane bleeding, such as epistaxis and gingival bleeding. Abnormal laboratory tests include a very low PLT count, and other causes of thrombocytopenia should be ruled out in patients with suspected ITP.

18. A 12-year-old male has the following symptoms: visible bruising on arms and legs, bruising after sports activities, and excessive postoperative hemorrhage after tonsillectomy 3 months ago. His family history revealed that his mother suffers from heavy menstrual bleeding, and his maternal grandfather had recurrent nosebleeds and bruising.

Laboratory Results		
	Patient	**Reference Range**
BAT	Positive	Negative
PLT count:	350 × $10^3/\mu L$	200–450 × 10^3/×L
PT	11 sec	10–12 sec
aPTT	30 sec	28–37 sec
TT	13 sec	10–15 sec
PLT AGGREGATION		
Normal aggregation with all agonists		
Confirmatory Tests	**Patient**	**Reference Range**
vWF:Rco	25%	45%–140%
VIII:C	70%	50%–150%
vWF:antigen	30%	45%–185%
vWF multimers: Large and intermediate forms absent		

These clinical manifestations and laboratory results are consistent with which condition?

A. vWD type 1
B. vWD type 2A
C. vWD type 2B
D. vWD type 3

Hemostasis/Primary hemostasis disorders/3

Answer to Question 18

18. B These clinical manifestations and laboratory results are consistent with vWD type 2A. vWD results from either a qualitative or quantitative defect in vWF, which is responsible for platelet adhesion and for covalently binding to factor VIII. The clinical manifestations associated with vWD are easy bruising, epistaxis, and bleeding after surgery. Several tests are used in the identification of the subtypes of vWD. Screening tests include a bleeding assessment tool (BAT), PLT count, PT, aPTT, and thrombin time (TT). Confirmatory tests include vWF ristocetin cofactor activity (vWF:Rco; ristocetin-induced platelet aggregation [RIPA]), vWF antigen, vWF multimer analysis, and factor VIII activity. To rule out other qualitative or quantitative platelet disorders, platelet aggregation studies can also be performed. vWD types 1 and 3 are associated with diminished vWF antigen, vWF activity, and low factor VIII activity. Multimer analysis differentiates among subtypes. Type 1 shows adequate multimers with decreased vWF antigen concentration. Type 3 shows an absence of all multimers and decreased vWF antigen concentration. There are four subtypes of type 2 (2A, 2B, 2M, and 2N) that have distinct defects associated with them. Type 2A is similar to types 1 and 2 with diminished vWF activity and antigen but has normal factor VIII activity and aPTT. Multimer analysis shows a lack of intermediate and large multimers. Type 2B presents with a decreased platelet count and a lack of large multimers.

19. A 46-year-old female was admitted to the emergency department with complaints of headache, dizziness, lethargy, nausea, vomiting, and weakness. The patient had undergone a gastrectomy procedure 4 months earlier for removal of adenocarcinoma of the stomach and had been placed on mitomycin therapy. Diagnostic procedures indicated recurrence of the carcinoma.

Admission Results

Test	Patient	Reference Range
COMPLETE BLOOD COUNT (CBC)		
White blood cells (WBCs)	17.1×10^9/L	$4.8–10.8 \times 10^9$/L
RBCs	2.29×10^{12}/L	$3.80–5.50 \times 10^{12}$/L
Hgb	8.1 g/dL	12.0–15.2 g/dL
Hct	23%	37%–46%
MCV	95.7 fL	79–101 fL
MCH	35.4 pg	27–33 pg
MCHC	35.0%	31%–34 %
Red cell distribution width (RDW)	18.5	11.5–14.5
PLTs	48.0×10^9/L	$140–450 \times 10^9$/L
Mean PLT volume (MPV)	11.2	7.4–9.4
DIFFERENTIAL		
Segmented neutrophils	79	30%–70%
Band neutrophils	3	0%–10%
Lymphocytes	11%	20%–50%
Monocytes	6%	2%–12%
Basophils	1%	0%–2%
Nucleated RBCs (/100 WBCs)	3	0
Manual platelet count	18×10^9/L	$140–450 \times 10^9$/L
Peripheral blood smear	3+ anisocytosis, 3+ polychromasia, 3+ schistocytes	None
PT	12.2 sec	11–13 sec
aPTT	24 sec	22–38 sec
ADDITIONAL LABORATORY DATA		
Urinalysis	**Patient**	**Reference Range**
pH	5.0	5–7
Protein	30.0 mg/dL	0–15 mg/dL
RBCs	60–100/μL	0–5/μL
Casts	10/high-power field (hpf), granular/hyaline	Not detectable
Creatinine	3.9 mg/dL	0.7–1.3 mg/dL
BUN	39 mg/dL	8–22 mg/dL
Haptoglobin	5.0 mg/dL	50–150 mg/dL

These clinical manifestations and laboratory results are consistent with:

A. ITP
B. vWD
C. TTP
D. DIC

Hemostasis/Primary hemostasis disorders/3

20. Which of the following is correct regarding acquired TTP?

A. Autoimmune disease
B. Decreased PLT count
C. Decreased PLT aggregation
D. Decreased PLT adhesion

Hemostasis/Primary hemostasis disorders/2

Answers to Questions 19–20

19. C The clinical manifestations and laboratory results in this patient are consistent with TTP. The clinical manifestations of TTP include MAHA, thrombocytopenia, fever, renal failure, and neurological symptoms. The neurological symptoms in this patient are manifested by headache, dizziness, nausea, and vomiting. Weakness and lethargy are signs and symptoms of anemia. Low Hgb and hematocrit (Hct) with normal mean cell volume (MCV) and mean corpuscular hemoglobin concentration (MCHC) indicate a normocytic normochromic anemia. The presence of schistocytes in peripheral blood, with low platelet counts and low haptoglobin, are consistent with MAHA. The high blood urea nitrogen (BUN) and creatinine levels supported by high protein and cells found in the urinalysis are indicative of renal failure. The platelet count, performed on admission, was done on a hematology analyzer and was falsely elevated because of the presence of microcytes or fragmented red blood cells (RBCs). The manual platelet count was much lower. The coagulation tests are normal in TTP. In vWD, the platelet count is within expected reference intervals, and the aPTT is usually abnormal. ITP is characterized by thrombocytopenia but not hemolytic anemia (HA). DIC is associated with a low platelet count, HA, and abnormal coagulation studies. The acute onset of symptoms in this patient may be related to mitomycin used for the treatment of gastric carcinoma in this patient.

20. B TTP is a quantitative PLT disorder associated with increased intravascular PLT activation and aggregation resulting in thrombocytopenia. PT and aPTT results are normal in TTP.

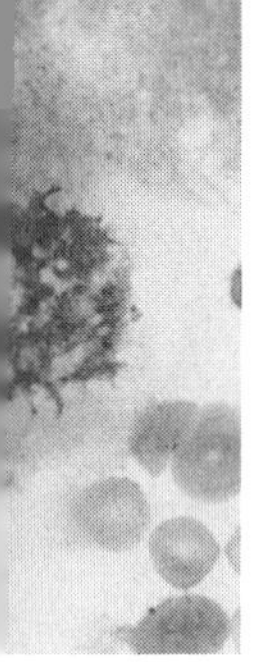

8.3

Secondary Hemostasis Disorders: Factor Deficiencies and Hemorrhagic Coagulation Disorders

1. Which test(s) would be prolonged in a patient with Stuart–Prower factor deficiency?
A. PT only
B. aPTT only
C. PT and aPTT
D. Thrombin time (TT)
Hemostasis/Secondary hemostasis disorders/2

2. A patient has a PT within the reference interval and a prolonged aPTT. Which coagulation factor is likely to be deficient?
A. Factor VII
B. Factor X
C. Factor IX
D. Calcium
Hemostasis/Secondary hemostasis disorders/2

3. Which test result would be within the reference interval in a patient with dysfibrinogenemia associated with liver disease?
A. TT
B. aPTT
C. Factor assays for II, V, VII, IX, and X
D. Fibrinogen level
Hemostasis/Secondary hemostasis disorders/2

4. A patient with a prolonged PT is given IV vitamin K. PT is corrected after 24 hours. Which clinical condition *most* likely caused these results?
A. Necrotic liver disease
B. Factor X deficiency
C. Fibrinogen deficiency
D. Obstructive jaundice
Hemostasis/Secondary hemostasis disorders/3

5. A patient has a prolonged PT and the aPTT is within the reference interval. Which factor is deficient?
A. Factor VII
B. Factor VIII
C. Factor IX
D. Factor X
Hemostasis/Secondary hemostasis disorders/2

Answers to Questions 1–5

1. C Stuart–Prower factor is also known as factor X, which is involved in the common pathway of the coagulation cascade; therefore, its deficiency prolongs both the PT and aPTT. Activated factor X along with activated factor V in the presence of calcium and PF3 form the tenase complex that converts prothrombin (factor II) to the activated thrombin (factor IIa).

2. C The aPTT is sensitive to the deficiency of coagulation factors in the intrinsic pathway (factors XII, XI, IX, and VIII) and the common pathway (factors X, V, II, and I). The PT is also sensitive to deficiencies of coagulation factors in the common pathway. If the PT is within the reference interval, and the aPTT is prolonged, this indicates a problem with the intrinsic pathway and not the common pathway since both tests can detect common pathway factor deficiencies.

3. D The level of plasma fibrinogen is within expected reference intervals. In a patient with dysfibrinogenemia, there are adequate quantities of fibrinogen, but they are not polymerized properly, causing abnormal results of the fibrinogen-dependent coagulation tests.

4. D Obstructive jaundice contributes to coagulation disorders by preventing vitamin K absorption. Vitamin K is fat soluble and requires bile salts for absorption. Parenteral administration of vitamin K bypasses the bowel, hence the need for bile salts.

5. A The PT is sensitive to the factors of the extrinsic (factor VII) and common pathways (factors X, V, II, and I). The aPTT is sensitive to the factors of the intrinsic and common pathways. With an aPTT within the reference interval and a prolonged PT, the factor deficiency is limited to the extrinsic pathway, which is factor VII.

6. Coagulation studies are performed on an infant suspected of having hemophilia. The provider orders a PT and aPTT and assays for factors VIII and IX. The results come back with the PT within reference interval and a prolonged aPTT. Factor VIII activity is 88% and factor IX activity is 5%. Which factor is deficient and what is the likely condition present?

A. Liver disease and factor V
B. Hemophilia A and factor VIII
C. Christmas disease and factor IX
D. Stuart–Prower deficiency and factor X

Hemostasis/Secondary hemostasis disorders/3

7. Which of the following is a characteristic of classic hemophilia?

A. Diminished PLT aggregation with endogenous and exogenous agonists
B. Autosomal recessive inheritance
C. Mild to severe anatomic bleeding depending on factor activity level
D. Multiple factor deficiencies

Hemostasis/Secondary hemostasis disorders/2

8. Refer to the following results:

PT = prolonged
aPTT = prolonged

Which disorder may be *ruled out* based on these findings?

A. Common pathway factor deficiency
B. vWD
C. DIC
D. Liver disease

Hemostasis/Secondary hemostasis disorders/3

9. The following results were obtained on a patient with menorrhagia: positive BAT, PLT count and PT within expected reference limits, and prolonged aPTT. Follow-up testing shows decreased vWF antigen, vWF activity, and factor VIII:C activity. Which of the following disorders is most consistent with these results?

A. Hemophilia A
B. vWD type 1
C. vWD type 2M
D. vWD type 3

Hemostasis/Secondary hemostasis disorders/3

10. The following laboratory results were obtained from a 40-year-old female: PT = 20 sec; aPTT = 50 sec; TT = 18 sec. What is the likely condition present?

A. Factor VII deficiency
B. Factor VIII deficiency
C. Factor X deficiency
D. Hypofibrinogenemia

Hemostasis/Secondary hemostasis disorders/3

Answers to Questions 6–10

6. C The PT evaluates the factor activity of the extrinsic and common pathways. The aPTT evaluates the factor activity of the intrinsic and common pathways. Thus, a common pathway factor deficiency is suspected when both the PT and aPTT are prolonged. In this situation, only the aPTT is prolonged, which supports the provider's suspicion of hemophilia and is limited to the factors of the intrinsic pathway: XI, IX, and VIII. Factor assays for VIII come back within reference limits, but factor IX is deficient. Factor deficiencies are defined as less than 50% activity on these factor assays. Factor IX is the Christmas factor and the disease produced is Christmas disease, or hemophilia B.

7. C Hemophilia A or classic hemophilia is characterized by mild to severe anatomical bleeding episodes, depending on the concentration of factor VIII:C. Patients will present with bleeding into joint or body cavities. Hemophilia A is inherited as a sex-linked disease that diminishes a single factor, in this case factor VIII:C. There is no dysfunction associated with PLT aggregation identified in hemophilia A.

8. B Prolonged PT and aPTT includes many different conditions, including liver disease due to procoagulant deficiencies in the intrinsic, extrinsic, and common pathways. Common pathway factor deficiencies also produce prolonged PT and aPTT. DIC is a consumptive coagulopathy in which all factors are consumed, thus producing a prolonged PT and aPTT. The only condition that can be ruled out is vWD, which produces dysfunction in the platelet as well as a prolonged aPTT due to an associated factor VIII deficiency.

9. B The results are consistent with vWD. These are confirmed by von Willebrand activity, antigen, and factor VIII assays. Hemophilia A is a sex-linked inherited deficiency of factor VIII, resulting in bleeding and abnormal aPTT, but it typically has no abnormalities of PLT function and/or number, as well as vWF antigen and antibody tests. There are six subtypes of vWD that are differentiated by specific vWF antigen, activity, multimer analysis, and factor VIII. Decreased vWF activity, antigen, and factor VIII assays are decreased, which is consistent with vWD type 1.

10. D Fibrinogen (factor I) is a clotting protein of the common pathway and is evaluated by the TT. In hypofibrinogenemia (fibrinogen concentration less than 100 mg/dL) PT, aPTT, and TT are prolonged. In factor VII deficiency, aPTT is within expected reference limits; in factor VIII deficiency, PT is within expected reference limits; and in factor X deficiency, TT is within expected reference limits.

11. The bleeding episodes in patients with afibrinogenemia are:

A. Anatomic
B. Systemic
C. From at least three orifices
D. Severe

Hemostasis/Secondary hemostasis disorders/2

12. Refer to the following results in a patient with mild systemic bleeding episodes:

PT = prolonged aPTT = prolonged PLT count = normal
PLT aggregation to endogenous agonists = absence of aggregation

Which of the following disorders may be indicated?

A. Factor VIII deficiency
B. Factor V deficiency
C. vWD disease
D. Factor IX deficiency

Hemostasis/Secondary hemostasis disorders/3

13. A newborn has large hematomas on their chest and legs at the time of delivery. There is some oozing from the umbilical stump that continues for several days after birth. Initial test screening results with PT, aPTT, platelet count, and BAT are within expected reference intervals. Select the best course of action to proceed with these findings.

A. Screen the infant's blood with 5 M urea
B. Repeat the test results at 6 months of age
C. Perform factor assays for VIII and IX
D. Nothing further is needed

Hemostasis/Secondary hemostasis disorders/3

14. Which of the following conditions is *not* associated with multiple factor deficiencies?

A. Hemophilia
B. Severe liver disease
C. DIC
D. Vitamin K deficiency

Hemostasis/Secondary hemostasis disorders/2

Answers to Questions 11–14

11. A The bleeding associated with afibrinogenemia (absence of fibrinogen) is considered anatomical, meaning bleeding into joints and other body cavities. Systemic or mucocutaneous bleeding is associated with primary hemostatic disorders affecting platelets and the vascular system. Bleeding from at least three orifices is a clinical indicator of DIC. Severity is determined by factor activity level and not qualified through the severity of symptoms.

12. B The prolonged PT and aPTT suggests a factor deficiency in the common pathway. The bleeding diathesis and the abnormal platelet aggregation studies are inconsistent with factor deficiencies. vWF is involved in both PLT adhesion and coagulation by complexing with factor VIII, but test results do not suggest vWD because the typical presentation involves PT results within expected reference limits and in this case it is prolonged. About 20% of factor V are housed in the alpha granules of platelets, so patients with factor V deficiency present with abnormal aggregation and systemic bleeding episodes.

13. A The presence of bleeding episodes and poor wound healing with unremarkable initial coagulation screening tests is strongly suggestive of a factor XIII deficiency. Factor XIII is a transglutaminase that is responsible for cross-linking the fibrin monomers once they have formed. The classic screening tests would not detect this deficiency because fibrin production is not altered. The initial screen for factor XIII deficiency is to mix patient plasma with 5 M urea and then confirm with a factor XIII assay.

14. A Most of the clotting factors are made in the liver. Therefore, severe liver disease results in multiple factor deficiencies. DIC is a consumptive coagulopathy secondary to another condition. The consumption of factors is due to the formation of microthrombi. Vitamin K deficiency affects the vitamin K–dependent factors (II, VII, IX, and X). Hemophilia is an inherited disorder of coagulation that is commonly associated with a single-factor deficiency in either factor VIII, which causes hemophilia A or classic hemophilia; factor IX, which causes hemophilia B or Christmas disease; or factor XI, which causes hemophilia C or Rosenthal syndrome.

15. The following laboratory results were obtained on a 22-year-old rickshaw driver with a history of ankle bleeds receiving factor replacement therapy.

PLT count within expected reference limits
PT within expected reference limits
aPTT prolonged
Mixing the patient's plasma with normal pooled plasma (NPP) corrected the prolonged aPTT on immediate testing. However, mixing followed by 2-hour incubation at 37°C caused prolonged aPTT.

What is the *most* probable cause of these laboratory results?

A. Lupus anticoagulant
B. Factor VIII deficiency
C. Factor IX deficiency
D. Factor VIII inhibitor

Hemostasis/Secondary hemostasis disorders/3

Answer to Question 15

15. D Factor VIII inhibitor is found in 20% to 25% of patients with hemophilia receiving replacement therapy. It may also develop in patients with immunologic problems, women after childbirth, and patients with lymphoproliferative and plasma cell disorders, or it may develop in response to medications. Factor VIII inhibitor is an IgG with an inhibitory effect that is time and temperature dependent. The presence of factor VIII inhibitor causes elevated aPTT in the face of a normal PT. Mixing studies in factors VIII and IX deficiencies will correct the prolonged aPTT both at the immediate mixing stage and after incubation for 2 hours. aPTT would not be corrected by mixing studies in the presence of factor VIII inhibitor. In addition, factor VIII inhibitor is associated with bleeding. Lupus anticoagulant is associated with thrombosis and not bleeding unless it coexists with thrombocytopenia, which is not the case in this patient.

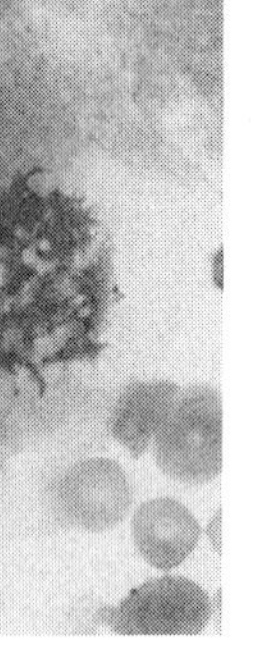

8.4

Thrombosis Risk, Thrombotic Disorders, and Anticoagulant Therapies

1. Prolonged aPTT caused by a pathological circulating anticoagulant is:
A. Corrected with factor VIII–deficient plasma
B. Corrected with factor IX–deficient plasma
C. Corrected with NPP
D. Not corrected with NPP
Hemostasis/Thrombosis risk/2

2. How does kidney disease, such as nephrotic syndrome, contribute to thrombosis risk?
A. It does not contribute to thrombosis risk
B. It decreases the risk of thrombosis by reabsorbing essential proteins needed for proper hemostasis
C. It increases the risk of thrombosis by increasing the circulation of naturally occurring inhibitors
D. It increases the risk of thrombosis through protein loss of essential anticoagulants
Hemostasis/Thrombosis risk/2

3. Choose the correct statement about warfarin (Coumadin) from the following choices.
A. It is a vitamin B recycling antagonist
B. Piggyback therapy is required at the start of the therapeutic regimen
C. It needs AT as a cofactor to increase its effectiveness *in vivo*
D. The aPTT is used to make adjustments to its dosage
Hemostasis/Thrombosis risk/2

4. Which statement regarding protein C is correct?
A. It is activated by thrombin
B. It is activated by fibrinogen
C. It activates cofactors V and VIII
D. Free protein S is its cofactor
Hemostasis/Thrombosis risk/1

Answers to Questions 1–4

1. D In the presence of a pathological circulating anticoagulant (also known as an *antiphospholipid antibody*), a mixing study using normal pooled plasma does not correct the prolonged aPTT. These anticoagulants are IgM or IgG, which target the anionic surfaces of the different phospholipids in the body. They also interfere with phospholipid-dependent clotting assays such as the aPTT. A prolonged aPTT caused by a factor deficiency is ruled out with a corrected result in the mixing study with normal pooled plasma (NPP). NPP contains 100% of the factors needed to complete clot formation, so when this occurs in a patient with a missing factor, the NPP replaces the missing factor and corrects the clotting time.

2. D Nephrotic syndrome creates protein imbalances that lead to protein loss. The proteins lost are essential naturally occurring inhibitors (anticoagulants) such as AT. The loss of AT disrupts the regulation of procoagulant activation, leading to thrombus formation.

3. B Warfarin (Coumadin) is a vitamin K antagonist drug that inhibits the recycling of vitamin K essential to the synthesis and activation of the vitamin K–dependent factors (II, VII, IX, and X) but also disrupts the activation of vitamin K–dependent inhibitors (protein C, protein S, and protein Z). Diminished activation of naturally occurring inhibitors interferes with the regulation of procoagulant activation, thus increasing the risk of thrombosis. The half-life of the inhibitors is 6 to 8 hours, indicating that the risk is highest at the start of therapy, necessitating piggyback therapy with another anticoagulant, usually a form of heparin. AT is a heparin (not warfarin) cofactor. The international normalized ratio (INR) is used to monitor warfarin dosage.

4. D Free protein S in the plasma functions as a cofactor of protein C and, as such, enhances its activity. Activated protein C (APC) inactivates factors Va and VIIIa. Protein C binds to the endothelial cell protein C receptor on thrombomodulin, which is complexed with thrombin, so thrombin alone is not responsible for protein C activation.

5. Which of the following mutations is associated with activated protein C resistance (APCR)?
A. Prothrombin G20210
B. Factor V Leiden
C. Methylenetetrahydrofolate reductase
D. Philadelphia chromosome
Hemostasis/Thrombosis risk/2

6. An admitted patient who had a total knee replacement has been on unfractionated heparin for the past 7 days. Which combination of tests is expected to be abnormal?
A. PT and aPTT only
B. PT, aPTT, TT
C. aPTT, TT, fibrinogen assay
D. PT, aPTT, TT, and PLT count
Hemostasis/Thrombosis risk/3

7. Which of the following drugs inhibits ADP-mediated PLT aggregation?
A. Heparin
B. Warfarin
C. Aspirin
D. Prasugrel
Hemostasis/Thrombosis risk/2

8. A patient is given Lovenox in the hospital. Which test can be used to monitor his therapy?
A. PT-INR
B. Chromogenic anti-Xa
C. TT
D. aPTT
Hemostasis/Thrombosis risk/2

9. Which test is commonly used to monitor warfarin therapy?
A. INR
B. aPTT
C. Chromogenic anti-Xa
D. Ecarin clotting time
Hemostasis/Thrombosis risk/2

10. Which of the following markers evaluates thrombosis risk as an antifibrinolytic agent?
A. Homocysteine
B. High-sensitivity C-reactive protein (CRP)
C. Lipoprotein A
D. Anticardiolipin antibodies
Hemostasis/Thrombosis risk/1

Answers to Questions 5–10

5. B APCR is tied to the single most common cause of inherited thrombosis, factor V Leiden. Affected individuals are predisposed to thrombosis, mainly after age 40 years. Physiologically, protein C neutralizes activated factor V, but in patients with factor V Leiden, factor V is resistant to the neutralization of protein C, thus causing APCR. Heterozygous individuals may not manifest thrombosis unless other clinical conditions coexist.

6. D Heparin is a therapeutic anticoagulant with an AT activity. Heparin also inhibits factors XIIa, XIa, Xa, and IXa. In patients receiving heparin therapy, PT, aPTT, and TT are all prolonged. Being on unfractionated heparin for more than 5 days increases the risk for heparin-induced thrombocytopenia (HIT), which produces a low platelet count. Quantitative fibrinogen assay, however, is not affected by heparin therapy.

7. D Prasugrel (Effient) is an antiplatelet drug that reduces PLT aggregation by irreversibly blocking P2Y12 receptors on the PLT surface membrane, thereby inhibiting PLT aggregation to ADP. Aspirin is another antiplatelet drug that inhibits PLT aggregation by blocking the action of the enzyme cyclooxygenase. Warfarin and heparin are anticoagulant drugs that act against clotting factors.

8. B Lovenox (enoxaparin) is a low-molecular-weight heparin (LMWH). It is derived from unfractionated heparin and is nine sugars long. It is administered subcutaneously and targets factors Xa and IIa. It is the preferred form of heparin to use because of its lower risk of HIT. In contrast to unfractionated heparin, which uses the aPTT to monitor, Lovenox uses the chromogenic anti-Xa assay because that is its target.

9. A Warfarin is a vitamin K recycling antagonist. It inhibits vitamin K–dependent factors (II, VII, IX, and X) and vitamin K–dependent inhibitors, such as proteins C, S, and Z. Warfarin therapy is monitored with the INR. An INR of 2.0 to 3.0 is used as the target when monitoring warfarin therapy for prophylaxis and treatment of deep vein thrombosis (DVT). A higher dose of warfarin (giving an INR of 2.5–3.5) is required for patients with mechanical heart valves.

10. C Thrombosis risk markers are valuable to evaluate a person's risk for developing thrombosis prior to its occurrence. Lipoprotein (a) is an antifibrinolytic agent that inhibits fibrinolysis two different ways. It acts as a competitive inhibitor of plasminogen binding sites on fibrin and also binds to tPA to stimulate the release of PAI-1 from endothelial cells. Homocysteine and high-sensitivity CRP are also thrombosis risk markers but are not antifibrinolytic agents. Anticardiolipin antibodies are a form of antiphospholipid antibodies that also increases thrombosis risk.

11. The presence of lupus anticoagulants is *confirmed* by which of the following criteria?
A. Increased aPTT
B. Failure to correct aPTT in mixing studies
C. Neutralization of the antibody by high concentration of phospholipids
D. Confirmation that abnormal coagulation tests are due to factor deficiencies

Hemostasis/Thrombosis risk/3

12. Which of the following is a characteristic of Pentasaccharide?
A. Requires regular and consistent monitoring
B. Specifically acts on factors Xa and IIa
C. Has a longer half-life compared to unfractionated heparin (UFH) and LMWH
D. Is the largest in size of all the heparin anticoagulants

Hemostasis/Thrombosis risk/1

13. Which of the following tests is *most* likely to be abnormal in patients taking aspirin?
A. PLT morphology
B. PLT count
C. PLT aggregation with collagen as an agonist
D. PLT aggregation with thrombin as an agonist

Hemostasis/Thrombosis risk/2

14. Which of the following is used to treat HIT/HITTS?
A. Enoxaparin
B. Argatroban
C. Coumadin
D. Prasugrel

Hemostasis/Thrombosis risk/2

15. Interpret the following data:
aPTT with the addition of calcium chloride = 30 sec
aPTT with the addition of calcium chloride and excess APC = 54 sec
What is the next step to confirm these findings?
A. Nothing further is needed
B. The test results should be repeated with a 2-hour incubation
C. Test the patient for factor V Leiden
D. The patient should be started on Warfarin immediately

Hemostasis/Thrombosis risk/3

Answers to Questions 11–15

11. C The 2020 International Society of Hemostasis and Thrombosis standards recommend the following criteria for the identification of lupus anticoagulants: (1) positive screen resulting from the prolongation of one or more of the phospholipid-dependent clotting tests, such as aPTT or diluted Russell viper venom test (DRVVT); (2) presence of an inhibitor confirmed by mixing studies on DRVVT and aPTT (not corrected without preincubation); (3) confirmatory test on DRVVT and aPTT, which is evidence that the inhibitor is directed against phospholipids, irrespective of the results of the mixing studies by neutralizing the antibodies with a high concentration of phospholipids mixed with equal parts (1:1) patient plasma and pooled normal plasma (PNP).

12. C Pentasaccharide (PS; fondaparinux) is a small glycosaminoglycan that is five sugars long and derived from UFH. PS is a stable chemical anticoagulant that is 1,728 daltons in molecular weight, making it the smallest of all the heparins used for anticoagulant therapies. It targets factor Xa and not IIa as LMWH does. It can be monitored using the chromogenic Xa. It has 100% bioavailability and does not bind to platelet factor 4 (PF4), so the risk for HIT is very low. It has the longest half-life of all the heparins as a result of its bioavailability and can remain stable for 17 hours (compared to 4 hours for LMWH and 30 minutes for UFH).

13. C Aspirin is an antiplatelet drug. It prevents PLT aggregation by inhibition of cyclooxygenase. Aspirin has no effect on the PLT count, PLT morphology, or PT.

14. B Heparin-induced thrombocytopenia and thrombosis syndrome (HIT/HITTS) is a consequence of prolonged use of UFH. UFH acts as a hapten that allows IgG molecules to bind to PF4 molecules on PLTs. LMWH (enoxaparin) also cross-reacts with the PF4 molecule so it shouldn't be used to treat HIT/HITTS. Warfarin (Coumadin) is too slow and is not recommended either. Prasugrel (Effient) is a antiplatelet agent that competitively inhibits the ADP response by binding to the ADP receptor PGY12. Direct thrombin inhibitors such as argatroban are the treatment of choice for HIT/HITTS.

15. C This is the APCR screening test. The baseline tube has a time of 30 sec and the experimental tube has a time of 54 sec. The ratio between the baseline and experimental tube times is less than 2 (30 sec/54 sec), indicating there is APCR. The next step to confirm this is to isolate the factor V Leiden mutation through reverse transcription polymerase chain reaction (RT-PCR) assay.

16. Which of the following mutations causes an increase in factor II levels as a result of a substitution of guanine for adenine at the 3′ untranslated region?

A. Factor V Leiden
B. Prothrombin G20210A
C. Methylenetetrahydrofolate reductase
D. *PML::RARA*

Hemostasis/Thrombosis risk/2

17. Which therapy is appropriate for the treatment of a patient with a high titer of factor VIII inhibitors?

A. Porcine complex concentrate
B. Bypassing agents such as recombinant factor VIIa (rVIIa)
C. Cryoprecipitate containing factor X concentrate
D. Fresh frozen plasma (FFP) containing concentrated factor VIII

Hemostasis/Thrombosis risk/2

18. Hyperhomocysteinemia may be a risk factor for:

A. Bleeding
B. Thrombocythemia
C. Thrombosis
D. Thrombocytopenia

Hemostasis/Thrombosis risk/2

19. A 30-year-old female was referred to the hospital for evaluation for multiple spontaneous abortions and current complaint of pain and swelling in her right leg. Her family history is unremarkable.

Laboratory Tests	Patient	Reference Range
PT	14.5 sec	11–13 sec
aPTT	63.0 sec	28–37 sec
TT	12.0 sec	10–15 sec
DRVVT	62.0 sec	
aPTT mixing study 1:1	60.0 sec	
1:2	58.0 sec	
1:4	55.0 sec	
1:8	54.0 sec	
1:16	53.0 sec	
1:32	50.0 sec	
Mixing study with excess phospholipid	24.0 sec	

These clinical manifestations and laboratory results are consistent with:

A. Factor VIII inhibitor
B. Factor VIII deficiency
C. Anticardiolipin antibodies
D. Lupus anticoagulant

Hemostasis/Thrombosis risk/3

Answers to Questions 16–19

16. B Prothrombin G20210A is defined as a single-point mutation where guanine is replaced with adenine at the 3′ untranslated region of the prothrombin gene, resulting in increased concentration of plasma prothrombin above 130% activity level and, thus, is a risk factor for thrombosis.

17. B In the case of developed inhibitors, rVIIa is effective for the treatment. Factor VIIa can directly activate factor X to factor Xa in the absence of factors VIII and IX. rVIIa does not stimulate anamnestic responses in patients with factor VIII inhibitor. The antibodies produced are against factor VIII concentrate, so it cannot be used. Porcine complex concentrate, cryoprecipitate, and FFP contain multiple factors that decrease the effectiveness of the factor VIII and cannot be used.

18. C Elevated plasma homocysteine is a risk factor for the development of DVT, coronary heart disease, and stroke. Homocysteinemia may be inherited or acquired. Acquired homocysteinemia is caused by dietary deficiencies of vitamins B_6, B_{12}, and folic acid.

19. D These clinical manifestations and laboratory results are consistent with lupus anticoagulant. Pain and swelling in the patient's right leg may be indicative of thrombosis. Women with repeated spontaneous abortions have lupus anticoagulant or another antibody to phospholipid. Normal TT rules out fibrinogen disorders. The aPTT test performed on serial mixtures of patient plasma and normal plasma did not correct the prolonged aPTT. This result is indicative of an inhibitor. A mixing study with excess phospholipid should be performed and a correction will confirm the presence of a lupus anticoagulant.

20. A patient was put on subcutaneous LMWH postoperatively after being involved in a car crash necessitating surgery and immobilization. The patient had the following laboratory results on admission: PLT count = 350 × 10^9/L; PT = 12 sec (reference 10–13 sec); aPTT = 35 sec (reference 28–37). After 6 days of Lovenox, the patient complained of pain and swelling in her left leg. Her PLT count dropped to 85 = 10^9/L, and her aPTT result was 36 sec. The physician suspected HIT and ordered the PLT aggregation test to be performed immediately. The heparin-induced PLT aggregation test result was negative. Heparin therapy was continued. Several days later, the patient developed a massive clot in her left leg that necessitated amputation.
Which of the following should have been recognized or initiated?

A. The patient should have been placed on UFH
B. The heparin dose should have been increased
C. The negative PLT aggregation does not rule out HIT
D. The patient should have been placed on warfarin therapy

Hemostasis/Thrombosis risk/3

Answer to Question 20

20. C LMWH therapy should be stopped immediately when clinical symptoms indicate HIT. The blood sample should be tested at least 4 hours after heparin therapy is discontinued. Early sampling for HIT testing may give a false-negative result because of the neutralization of antibody by heparin. UFH should not be used in patients who develop HIT because UFH has a higher risk of developing HIT. Warfarin therapy can be started in patients who respond to heparin therapy, but the challenge is that it must be piggybacked with UFH until the INR reaches a stable therapeutic range (2.0–3.0), which takes several days. In this case, warfarin therapy cannot be used in this patient. The first step in the treatment of HIT is discontinuation of heparin.

8.5

Evaluation of Coagulopathies

1. **The specimen of choice for assessment of factor activity is:**
   A. Platelet-poor plasma in 3.2% sodium oxalate
   B. Platelet-poor plasma in 3.2% sodium citrate
   C. Platelet-rich plasma in 2% lithium heparin
   D. Platelet-rich plasma in 2.5 mL EDTA
   Hemostasis/Evaluation of coagulopathies/1

2. **Which blood:anticoagulant ratio is correct for coagulation testing?**
   A. 4:1
   B. 5:1
   C. 9:1
   D. 10:1
   Hemostasis/Evaluation of coagulopathies/1

3. **A patient has a Hct of 62% and has coagulation studies collected in a 3.2% sodium citrate tube with a 9:1 ratio of blood to anticoagulant. What would be the expected PT and aPTT results given this information?**
   A. Both will be prolonged as compared to the reference interval
   B. Both will be shortened as compared to the reference interval
   C. The PT will be within the reference interval and the aPTT will be prolonged
   D. Both will be within the reference interval
   Hemostasis/Evaluation of coagulopathies/2

4. **Which reagents are used in the PT test?**
   A. Thromboplastin and sodium chloride
   B. Thromboplastin and potassium chloride
   C. Thromboplastin and calcium
   D. Actin and calcium chloride
   Hemostasis/Evaluation of coagulopathies/1

5. **Which clotting factor is *not* measured by the PT and aPTT?**
   A. Factor VIII
   B. Factor IX
   C. Factor V
   D. Factor XIII
   Hemostasis/Evaluation of coagulopathies/2

Answers to Questions 1–5

1. B To conduct an evaluation of factor activity, platelets must be in low concentration in the plasma, which is platelet-poor plasma. This is because platelets activate the clotting cascade. Using platelet-rich plasma will mask deficiencies in factor activity, making them more difficult to detect. The anticoagulant of choice is 3.2% sodium citrate, which is sufficient to chelate the calcium in the blood sample that also activates certain coagulation factors. Heparin, sodium oxalate, and EDTA all inhibit factor activity and consequently are not used for routine evaluation of factor activity. .

2. C The optimal blood-to-anticoagulant ratio is 9:1. The anticoagulant supplied in this amount is sufficient to bind all the available calcium in the blood sample, thereby preventing clotting.

3. A The increased Hct reduces the volume of plasma and the concentration of factors for the amount of anticoagulant present in a standard 3.2% sodium citrate with a 9:1 ratio of blood to anticoagulant. Therefore, there is excess anticoagulant available to bind to reagent calcium, resulting in a prolongation of PT and aPTT. For more accurate results, the plasma: anticoagulant ratio can be modified by decreasing the amount of anticoagulant in the collection tube by using the following formula:

$$(0.00185)\ (V)\ (100 - H) = C$$

where V = blood volume in milliliters (mL); H = patient's hematocrit (Hct); and C = volume (mL) of anticoagulant. A new sample should be drawn with a corrected anticoagulant volume to obtain accurate PT and aPTT results.

4. C Thromboplastin and calcium (combined into a single reagent) replace tissue thromboplastin and calcium necessary, *in vivo*, to activate factor VII to factor VIIa. This ultimately generates thrombin from prothrombin via the coagulation cascade.

5. D Factor XIII is not measured by PT or aPTT. Factor XIII (fibrin stabilizing factor) is a transglutaminase responsible for creating covalent bonds between fibrin monomers. The PT and aPTT measure the clotting factor activity until fibrin monomers are formed. In the absence of factor XIII, hydrogen bonds link the fibrin monomers, rendering them less stable.

6. A modification of which procedure can be used to measure fibrinogen?
A. PT
B. aPTT
C. TT
D. Fibrin degradation products
Hemostasis/Evaluation of coagulopathies/1

7. Which fragments of fibrin clot degradation are measured by the D-dimer test?
A. Fragments X and Y
B. Fibrinopeptide A and B
C. Fragments D and E
D. The D-D domains
Hemostasis/Evaluation of coagulopathies/1

8. Which of the following clotting factors are measured by the aPTT test?
A. Factors II, VII, IX, X
B. Factors VII, X, V, II, I
C. Factors XII, XI, IX, VIII, X, V, II, I
D. Factors XII, VII, X, V, II, I
Hemostasis/Evaluation of coagulopathies/2

9. Which of the following is correct regarding the INR?
A. It uses the international sensitivity ratio (ISR)
B. It standardizes PT results
C. It standardizes aPTT results
D. It is used to monitor heparin therapy
Hemostasis/Evaluation of coagulopathies/2

10. Which of the following test results can help confirm dysfibrinogenemia?
A. Prolonged TT and reptilase time
B. Prolonged TT and reptilase time within expected reference interval
C. Prolonged reptilase time and TT within expected reference interval
D. TT and reptilase time within expected reference interval
Hemostasis/Evaluation of coagulopathies/2

11. Which statement is correct regarding sample storage for the PT test?
A. Stable for 24 hours if the sample is capped
B. Stable for 24 hours if the sample is refrigerated at 4°C
C. Stable for 4 hours if the sample is stored at 4°C
D. Should be run within 8 hours
Hemostasis/Evaluation of coagulopathies/2

Answers to Questions 6–11

6. C Fibrinogen can be quantitatively measured by modification of the TT using the Clauss method. The modifications that allow for quantitation of fibrinogen are dilution of patient's platelet poor plasma and incorporation of a fibrinogen calibration curve. There is an inverse relationship between the clotting time and fibrinogen concentration.

7. D D-dimer is a specific product resulting from digestion of cross-linked fibrin only. It consists of two D domains called *D-D fragment*. In the D-dimer test, monoclonal antibody is directed against D-dimer antigen and quantified based on instrument cutoffs. The D-dimer test is used to rule in consumptive coagulopathies and can help differentiate between systemic fibrinolysis and thromboembolic disorders. Fragments X, Y, D, and E are produced by the action of plasmin on fibrinogen and fibrin.

8. C The aPTT test evaluates the clotting factors in the intrinsic pathway (XII, XI, IX, and VIII) as well as those in the common pathway (X, V, II, and I).

9. B INR is used to standardize PT results to adjust for the differences in thromboplastin reagents made by different manufacturers and used by various institutions. The INR calculation uses the international sensitivity index (ISI) value and is used to monitor an oral anticoagulant, such as warfarin. INR is not used to standardize aPTT testing.

10. A TT and reptilase time (RT) both detect fibrinogen activation to fibrin. The thrombin time uses thrombin, whereas the RT uses batroxobin isolated from the venom of the *Bothrops atrox* that catalyzes fibrinogen to become fibrin. In the case of dysfibrinogenemia, there is an adequate amount of fibrinogen but it is dysfunctional. Consequently, both the TT and RT will be prolonged.

11. A According to Clinical Laboratory Standards Institute (CLSI) guidelines, plasma samples for PT testing, if capped, are stable for 24 hours at room temperature. Refrigerating the sample causes cold activation of factor VII and, therefore, shortened PT results. aPTT samples are stable for 4 hours if stored at 4°C.

12. Which substrate is used in a chromogenic factor assay?
A. *p*-Nitroaniline (pNa)
B. Chlorophenol red
C. Prussian blue
D. Ferricyanide
Hemostasis/Evaluation of coagulopathies/1

13. vWF activity is measured by:
A. Patient's platelets mixed with ristocetin
B. Reagent platelets mixed with collagen
C. Patient's platelets mixed with thrombin
D. Reagent platelets mixed with ristocetin
Hemostasis/Evaluation of coagulopathies/2

14. The NBA and the Bethesda titer are used to:
A. Quantify the amount of factor VIII activity in a patient's PPP
B. Quantify the amount of factor VIII inhibitor in a patient's PPP
C. Quantify the amount of vWF in a patient's PPP
D. Quantify the amount of fibrinogen in a patient's PPP
Hemostasis/Evaluation of coagulopathies/2

15. Which of the following is an appropriate screening test for the detection of a lupus anticoagulant?
A. TT
B. DRVVT
C. Reptilase time (RT)
D. Fibrinogen assay
Hemostasis/Evaluation of coagulopathies/2

16. A fresh blood sample was sent to the laboratory at 8:00 a.m. for the PT test. At 4:00 p.m., the doctor requested for the aPTT test to be done on the same sample. What should the scientist do to address this situation?
A. Rerun the aPTT on the 8:00 a.m. sample and report the result
B. Request a new sample for aPTT
C. Run the aPTT in duplicate and report the average
D. Mix patient plasma with normal plasma and run the aPTT
Hemostasis/Evaluation of coagulopathies/3

Answers to Questions 12–16

12. A The chromogenic, or amidolytic, assays use a color-producing substance, known as *chromophore.* The chromophore used for the coagulation laboratory is *p*-nitroaniline (pNa). pNa is bound to a synthetic oligopeptide substrate. The protease cleaves the chromogenic substrate at the site binding the oligopeptide to the pNa, which results in release of pNa. Free pNa has a yellow color; the color intensity of the solution is proportional to protease activity and is measured by a photodetector at 405 nm.

13. D vWF activity is also called *ristocetin-induced platelet aggregation* (RIPA). In the RIPA assay, reagent platelets are mixed with ristocetin and their aggregation activity is measured. Patient platelets are not used because there are subtypes of vWD that produce dysfunctional platelets in addition to the impaired vWF activity. This differentiates between those subtypes.

14. B The NBA is the Nijmegen-Bethesda assay. Both the NBA and the Bethesda titer measure the amount of factor VIII inhibitor present in the patient's platelet-poor plasma (PPP). In order to measure this, a factor VIII assay is performed on incubated plasma with pooled normal plasma (PNP) and then corrections from a baseline level are used to extrapolate the amount of factor VIII inhibitor present.

15. B Russell viper venom (RVV) reagent contains factors X and V, activating enzymes that are strongly phospholipid dependent. The reagent also contains RVV, Ca^{2+}, and phospholipid. In the presence of phospholipid autoantibodies, such as lupus anticoagulant, the reagent phospholipid is partially neutralized, causing prolongation of clotting time. TT evaluates fibrinogen. RT also uses snake venom but it measures factor X activation and it uses the venom from *Bothrops atrox*. Fibrinogen assay and TT are not indicated for the diagnosis of lupus anticoagulant.

16. B The medical laboratory scientist should request a new sample for the aPTT test. According to the CLSI guidelines, samples for aPTT should be centrifuged and tested within 2 hours after collection. However, the sample is stable for 4 hours if stored at 4°C. aPTT evaluates the clotting factors in the intrinsic and common coagulation pathways, including factor VIII (intrinsic) and factor V (common). Factors VIII and V are cofactors necessary for fibrin formation. However, they are both labile. Storage beyond 4 hours causes falsely elevated aPTT results.

17. The P2Y12 ADP receptor agonist assay may be used to monitor PLT aggregation inhibition to which of the following drugs?
A. Warfarin
B. Heparin
C. LMWH
D. Clopidogrel (Plavix)
Hemostasis/Evaluation of coagulopathies/2

18. When performing a factor VIII activity assay, a patient's platelet-poor plasma is mixed with:
A. Normal pooled plasma
B. Factor VIII–deficient plasma
C. Plasma with a high concentration of factor VIII
D. Normal control plasma
Hemostasis/Evaluation of coagulopathies/1

19. A standard 4.5-mL blue-top tube filled with 3.0 mL of blood was submitted to the laboratory for PT and aPTT tests. The sample is from a patient undergoing surgery the following morning for a tonsillectomy. Which of the following is the necessary course of action by the medical laboratory scientist?
A. Run both tests in duplicate and report the average result
B. Reject the sample and request a new sample
C. Report the PT result
D. Report the aPTT result
Hemostasis/Evaluation of coagulopathies/3

20. Which of the following PLT aggregating agents demonstrates a monophasic aggregation curve when used in the optimal concentration?
A. Thrombin
B. Collagen
C. ADP
D. Epinephrine
Hemostasis/Evaluation of coagulopathies/1

Answers to Questions 17–20

17. D The VerifyNow P2Y12 test is used to assess a patient's response to antiplatelet drugs, such as clopidogrel (Plavix) and prasugrel (Effient). These drugs are given orally along with aspirin for prevention of thrombosis or as alternative antiplatelet drugs for patients who cannot tolerate or are not sensitive to aspirin. Clopidogrel and prasugrel prevent PLT aggregation by irreversibly binding to P2Y12, which is a PLT membrane receptor for ADP. The VerifyNow P2Y12 test is a whole blood test and uses ADP as an aggregating agent to measure the level of PLT aggregation impaired by these medications. The baseline value for PLT aggregation is established. The percent (%) change from baseline aggregation is calculated and reported as % P2Y12 inhibition.

18. B Coagulation factor assays are based on the ability of the patient's plasma to correct any specific factor-deficient plasma. To measure for factor VIII activity in a patient's plasma, diluted patient plasma is mixed with factor VIII–deficient plasma. The aPTT test is performed on the mixture. Each laboratory should calculate its own normal ranges, which are based on the patient population, reagents, and instrument used. A range of 50% to 150% is considered normal.

19. B A 4.5-mL blue-top tube contains 4.5 mL blood + 0.5 mL sodium citrate. The tube should be 90% full. A tube with 3.0 mL blood should be rejected because the quantity is not sufficient (QNS). QNS samples alter the necessary blood: anticoagulant ratio (9:1). The excess anticoagulant in a QNS sample binds to the reagent calcium, resulting in prolongation of PT and aPTT.

20. B Collagen is the only commonly used agent that demonstrates a single-wave (monophasic) response preceded by a lag time.

BIBLIOGRAPHY

1. Keohane EM, Butina MM, Mirza KM, Walenga JM. *Rodak's Hematology: Clinical Principles and Applications.* 7th ed. Elsevier; 2025.
2. Kaushansky K, Lichtman MA, Prchal JT, Levi MM, Burns LJ, Lynch DC. *Williams Hematology.* 10th ed. McGraw-Hill; 2021.

CHAPTER 9

Microbiology

9.1 *Basic Concepts and Microscopy*

9.2 *Preanalytical Procedures*

9.3 *Antimicrobials and Susceptibility Methods*

9.4 *Enterobacterales*

9.5 *Nonfermentative Bacilli*

9.6 *Miscellaneous and Fastidious Gram-Negative Rods*

9.7 *Gram-Positive and Gram-Negative Cocci*

9.8 *Aerobic Gram-Positive Rods, Spirochetes, Mycoplasmas, Ureaplasmas, and Chlamydia*

9.9 *Anaerobic Bacteria*

9.10 *Mycobacteria*

9.11 *Mycology*

9.12 *Virology*

9.13 *Parasitology*

9.1

Basic Concepts and Microscopy

1. Bacteria can be identified in the laboratory using these two major criteria for classification:

A. Colonial morphology and cellular morphology
B. Phenotypic and genotypic characteristics
C. Nucleotide sequencing and epigenetic traits
D. Biochemical and colonial morphology

Microbiology/Basic concepts/Classification/2

2. All the following characteristics listed are considered genotypic, *except:*

A. The ratio of pyrimidines to purines
B. Cellular structures including antigens and flagella
C. Genome-to-genome distance
D. Nucleic acid–base composition

Microbiology/Basic concepts/2

3. A genome-to-genome distance between bacteria is defined as:

A. The order of bases along a strand of DNA or RNA
B. The extent to which two organisms contain G+C and A+T content in the genome
C. A computerized calculation that uses inference from simulations
D. Evaluation of multiple coding sequences in an organism and determining the average nucleotide identity

Microbiology/Basic concepts/2

4. An organism that includes species of the same genetic makeup with differential physiological characteristics that can be identified using biochemical methods is termed:

A. Genotype
B. Serotype
C. Subspecies
D. Biotype

Microbiology/Basic concepts/2

5. The process by which two bacteria contact each other via a pilus and transfer genetic material is referred to as:

A. Replication
B. Transformation
C. Generalized transduction
D. Conjugation

Microbiology/Basic concepts/1

Answers to Questions 1–5

1. B All the items listed in the responses listed are criteria that can be used to identify and classify bacteria; however, the two major types of criteria used for classification are those that are physically visible or phenotypic and those that are based on the genetic sequence.

2. B The only response that is not part of the genetic makeup or composition of the nucleic acids is the cellular structures that include antigens and flagella. Antigens can be detected using antibodies conjugated to an enzyme or other indicator for visualization. Flagella, pili, or fimbriae may be visualized using special staining characteristics. or nucleic acids present in the bacteria, termed *genotypic*.

3. C Genome-to-genome distance is based on simulated computerized algorithms that compare and eliminate errors from wet-lab experiments or genetic sequencing to calculate similarities. Organisms are considered related with a genome-to-genome distance (GGD) of 70%.

4. D A biotype is an organism that demonstrates two forms of the same species with the same genetic makeup that express different physiological characteristics that are identifiable using biochemical methods. A serotype is based on antigenic differences; a genotype indicates differences in sequence or gene variants in the nucleic acids; and subspecies do not demonstrate enough variation to be a new species or a new biotype.

5. D Some genera of microorganisms produce a protein structure or pilus. The primary function of this protein is to serve as a tube or connection for bacteria to transfer mobile genetic elements from one cell to another. This process is known as *conjugation*. Conjugative plasmids that carry accessory physiological functions for survival, such as antibiotic resistance, can transfer between cells, propagating the genetic resistance markers to multiple cells protecting the population.

6. Bacteria that are capable of growth in the presence or absence of oxygen are considered:
A. Obligately aerobic
B. Facultatively anaerobic
C. Microaerophilic
D. Capnophilic
Microbiology/Basic concepts/1

7. A bacterial cell appendage that is external to the peptidoglycan layer in gram-positive organisms and the outer membrane in gram-negative bacteria can be termed as all the following *except:*
A. Capsule
B. Slime layer
C. Biofilm
D. Protein coat
Microbiology/Basic concepts/1

8. Microscopy continues to play a pivotal role in the clinical laboratory. This type of microscopy has the widest use and application within the clinical laboratory.
A. Darkfield microscopy
B. Phase contrast microscopy
C. Electron microscopy
D. Brightfield microscopy
Microbiology/Microscopy/1

9. A technologist was viewing an organism using binocular standard brightfield microscope using the 40× objective lens. Calculate the total magnification used to view the specimen.
A. 10× magnification
B. 40× magnification
C. 400× magnification
D. 4,000× magnification
Microbiology/Microscopy/2

10. When reviewing a direct smear of a sputum specimen in the clinical laboratory, all the following items should be included in the final Gram stain report *except:*
A. Gram stain reactions of the organisms
B. Cellular shape of the organisms
C. Cellular structure including appendages of the organisms
D. Cellular arrangements of the organisms
Microbiology/Basic concepts/2

Answers to Questions 6–10

6. B Bacteria that can grow in the presence of oxygen or the absence of oxygen are considered facultative anaerobes. Anaerobic atmospheric conditions typically consist of three gases: 80% to 90% nitrogen, 5% to 10% hydrogen, and 5% to 10% CO_2.

7. D Bacteria that can produce a layer of extracellular polysaccharide includes both gram-positive and gram-negative microorganisms. Organisms that produce a capsule of polysaccharide produce the material in response to specific environments and mediate attachment as well as prevent recognition by the immune system. The capsule is typically found external to the peptidoglycan layer in gram-positive bacteria. Biofilm or slime layers also contain polysaccharides but have variation in chemical makeup and can be produced by a monomicrobic or polymicrobic population of bacteria.

8. D Brightfield or light microscopy is the most widely used type of microscopy used in the clinical laboratory. It permits the visualization of most clinically significant agents of infections except viruses.

9. C The total magnification is calculated by multiplying the ocular magnification, which is typically 10× on most standard brightfield microscopes, by the magnification of the objective lens. In this case, 40× multiplied by 10× = a total magnification of 400×.

10. C When observing a sputum specimen on a Gram stain using a direct smear, the specific Gram stain reactions of the organisms must be reported. Organisms that stain purple are considered gram positive; those that appear red to pink are gram negative. The shape of the cells and the arrangements are also of clinical significance. Examples include gram-positive cocci in clusters, gram-positive rods, gram-negative diplococci, etc. The structure of the cells is implied based on the Gram stain characteristics but is not considered a separate reportable characteristic.

11. A Gram stain of a sputum specimen appeared dark purple and contained gram-positive rods, gram-positive cocci, and gram-positive diplococci. The white blood cells (WBCs) also appeared purple upon review. What is the likely cause of this discrepancy?
A. There is no discrepancy, and the Gram stain should be reported
B. The gram-positive diplococci are most likely gram-negative
C. The specimen may be too thick and did not properly decolorize
D. The specimen was over-decolorized
Microbiology/Microscopy/2

12. Some organisms are difficult to visualize on Gram stain because of their physiology and structure, such as the causative agent of syphilis, *Treponema pallidum*. What microscopic method is used to visualize these organisms?
A. Phase contrast microscopy
B. Darkfield microscopy
C. Brightfield microscopy
D. Fluorescent microscopy
Microbiology/Microscopy/1

Answers to Questions 11–12

11. C Sputum samples are often viscous. The sample should be spread thin prior to Gram staining. The WBCs should not stain purple. This sample may be too thick and was under-decolorized. The sample can be treated with more alcohol:acetone decolorizer and restained with the secondary stain, or the microbiologist can make a new smear if there is additional sample.

12. B Although rarely used in a clinical laboratory, spirochetes such as *Treponema pallidum* can be visualized using a darkfield microscope. The organisms will appear light in a dark background. Darkfield microscopy has been replaced in most laboratories with serological techniques for the diagnosis of syphilis.

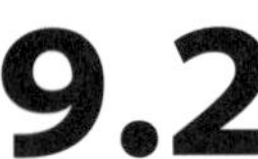

9.2

Preanalytical Procedures

1. The aseptic collection of blood cultures requires that the skin be cleansed with:
A. 2% iodine and then 70% alcohol solution
B. 70% alcohol and then 2% iodine or an iodophor
C. 70% alcohol and then 95% alcohol
D. 95% alcohol only
Microbiology/Preanalytical/1

2. When cleansing the skin with alcohol and then iodine for the collection of blood cultures, the iodine (or iodophor) should remain intact on the skin for at least:
A. 10 seconds
B. 30 seconds
C. 60 seconds
D. 5 minutes
Microbiology/Preanalytical/1

3. Manufacturers add 0.006% to 0.083% sodium polyanethol sulfonate (SPS) to nutrient broth medium for the collection of blood cultures to improve recovery of pathogens. What is the purpose of SPS in the medium?
A. It inhibits complement and blocks phagocytosis
B. It promotes formation of blood clots
C. It enhances growth of anaerobes
D. It functions as a preservative
Microbiology/Preanalytical/2

4. A flexible cotton or polyester nasopharyngeal swab is the collection device of choice for recovery of which organism from the nasopharynx?
A. *Staphylococcus aureus*
B. *Streptococcus pneumoniae*
C. *Corynebacterium diphtheriae*
D. *Bacteroides fragilis*
Microbiology/Preanalytical/1

5. Semisolid transport media, such as Amies, Stuart, or Cary-Blair, are suitable for the transport of swabs for culture of most pathogens *except*:
A. *Neisseria gonorrhoeae*
B. *Escherichia coli*
C. *Campylobacter fetus*
D. *Streptococcus pneumoniae*
Microbiology/Preanalytical/1

Answers to Questions 1–5

1. B To attain asepsis of the skin, 70% alcohol followed by 2% iodine or chlorhexidine gluconate is used for obtaining blood cultures. Chlorhexidine is not recommended for children <2 months of age. Povidone-iodine is recommended but requires much longer contact time with the patient's skin and is then followed by 70% isopropyl alcohol.

2. B The iodine or other iodophor solution should remain on the skin for 30 seconds in adults and children >2 months of age. If povidone-iodine is used, it must remain on the skin for 1.5 to 2.0 minutes to achieve similar antisepsis when cleansing the skin for a blood culture.

3. A SPS is used in most commercial blood culture products because it functions as an anticoagulant and prevents phagocytosis and inhbitis complement activation. In addition, SPS neutralizes some aminoglycoside antibiotics. Addition of SPS may inhibit some *Neisseria* spp., *Gardnerella vaginalis, Streptobacillus moniliformis,* and *Peptostreptococcus.* Inhibition of microorganism growth may be overcome in continuous monitoring blood culture systems by ensuring adequate sample volume is inoculated to the blood culture bottles or the addition of 1.2% gelatin to the media.

4. C *C. diphtheriae* must be recovered from the deep layers of the pseudomembrane that forms in the nasopharyngeal area. A flexible cotton- or polyester-tipped nasopharyngeal swab is the best choice for collecting a specimen for culture from the posterior nares and pharynx.

5. A Specimens for culture of *N. gonorrhoeae* are best if plated immediately or transported in a medium containing activated charcoal to absorb inhibitory substances that hinder their recovery from the specimens.

6. Select the method of choice for recovery of anaerobic bacteria from a deep wound abscess.
A. Cotton fiber swab of the abscess area
B. Skin snip of the surface tissue
C. Needle aspirate after surface decontamination
D. Swab of the scalpel used for débridement
Microbiology/Preanalytical/2

7. In general, specimens for the collection and identification of microorganisms should be completed:
A. During the initial exposure period, when the patient has no symptoms
B. During the convalescent state, when the patient is recovering
C. During the clinical state, when all characteristic signs or symptoms are present
D. During the prodromal or acute state, during the first sign of symptoms
Microbiology/Preanalytical/2

8. Following the collection of a specimen for culture or identification of a microorganism, the sample should be transported to the laboratory:
A. Immediately, and within 15 minutes to preserve the viability of the organism
B. Generally within 2 hours of collection for most microorganisms
C. Generally within 4 hours is acceptable for most samples
D. Within 24 hours, as the microorganisms can remain viable within the specimen for long periods
Microbiology/Preanalytical/2

9. Specimens for viral culture should be transported in media containing:
A. Antibiotics and 5% sheep blood
B. Saline and 5% sheep blood
C. 22% bovine albumin
D. Antibiotics and protein nutrient
Microbiology/Preanalytical/1

10. Cerebrospinal fluid (CSF) should be cultured immediately, but if delayed, the specimen should be:
A. Refrigerated at 4°C to 6°C
B. Frozen at –20°C
C. Stored at room temperature for no longer than 24 hours
D. Incubated at 37°C and cultured as soon as possible
Microbiology/Preanalytical/1

Answers to Questions 6–10

6. C Anaerobic specimens are easily contaminated with organisms present on the skin or mucosal surfaces. Needle aspiration of an abscess following surface decontamination prevents contamination with nonpathogenic organisms and provides the least exposure to ambient oxygen that would decrease the viability and recovery of anaerobic bacteria from the specimen.

7. D Specimens for the recovery of microorganisms should be collected during the time when a patient is experiencing signs and symptoms of illness. This is generally within the first 2 to 3 days and before the patient has received any antimicrobial, antiviral, or antifungal medication.

8. B Following the collection of a sample, transport should be to the laboratory within 2 hours. This ensures viability and recovery for most pathogenic organisms. However, there are several pathogens that require specialized media or may be placed in transport media that would support the viability of the organisms when a longer transport time is inevitable, such as to a reference laboratory.

9. D Media for transporting specimens for virus culture include Hanks' balanced salt solution with bovine albumin, Amies media, Stuart medium, Eagle's tissue culture medium, Leibovitz-Emory medium, or commercially available M4, M5, or universal transport media. Media used for transporting specimens for viral culture require the addition of a nutrient source, such as fetal calf serum, gelatin, or albumin. Antibiotics are also included to prevent bacterial contamination. Specimens should be refrigerated (not frozen) after being placed in the transport media until the culture media can be inoculated or processed for additional diagnostic tests.

10. D Fastidious organisms, such as *Neisseria* and *Haemophilus,* frequently isolated from the CSF of patients with bacterial meningitis are preserved by placing the fluid in 3% to 7% CO_2 at 35°C to 37°C (or at room temperature for no longer than 30 minutes), if the specimen cannot be cultured immediately.

11. Which specimen collection and processing procedure is (are) appropriate for the diagnosis of *Chlamydia* spp. genital infection?

A. Obtain urethral, cervical swabs and urine specimens placed in transport media
B. Plate onto blood and chocolate agar
C. Inoculate into thioglycollate (THIO) broth
D. Plate to modified Thayer-Martin (MTM) agar within 24 hours

Microbiology/Preanalytical/2

12. Select the primary and differential culture media of choice for recovery of most fecal pathogens.

A. MacConkey, blood, bird seed, and *Campylobacter* (Campy) agars
B. Hektoen, MacConkey, MacConkey-sorbitol, Campy blood, colistin–nalidixic acid (CNA) agars; Selenite broth (SEL)
C. CNA and Christensen urea agars and thioglycollate media
D. Blood, Campy, Mueller-Hinton agars, and thioglycollate media

Microbiology/Preanalytical/1

13. Select the culture media of choice for recovery of *Vibrio cholerae* from a stool specimen.

A. MacConkey agar and thioglycollate media
B. Thiosulfate–citrate–bile–sucrose (TCBS) agar and alkaline peptone water (APW) broth
C. Blood agar and SEL broth
D. CNA agar

Microbiology/Preanalytical/1

14. Columbia CNA agar is used primarily for the selective isolation of:

A. *Neisseria* species
B. *Enterobacteriaceae*
C. *Pseudomonas aeruginosa*
D. *Staphylococcus aureus*

Microbiology/Preanalytical/1

15. In the United States, most blood agar plates are prepared with 5% or 10% red blood cells (RBCs) obtained from:

A. Sheep
B. Horses
C. Humans
D. Dogs

Microbiology/Preanalytical/1

Answers to Questions 11–15

11. A Chlamydiae are strict intracellular organisms and must be cultured using living cells (e.g., cyclohexamide-treated McCoy cells). Direct smears can also be made at the time of culture. Fluorescein-conjugated monoclonal antibodies may be used to identify the organisms in infected cells. Cell cultures present limitations but are used if legal situations (e.g., sexual abuse) are implied. Commercially available kits for antigen detection and nucleic acid amplification and hybridization techniques, which have been approved by the Food and Drug Administration (FDA), are not culture methods and are more sensitive and specific than culture methods.

12. B Hektoen agar selectively isolates pathogenic gram-negative microorganisms, especially *Salmonella* and *Shigella*. MacConkey agar differentiates lactose fermenters from nonfermenters. MacConkey with sorbitol isolates *Escherichia coli* O157:H7. CNA agar contains antibiotics that prohibit growth of gram-negative coliforms but not gram-positive cocci. Campy blood agar contains the antibiotics cephalothin, trimethoprim, vancomycin, polymyxin B, and amphotericin B to prevent growth of *Enterobacterales*, *Pseudomonas* spp., and fungi. Selenite broth selectively inhibits many gram-positive and gram-negative microorganisms.

13. B TCBS agar is used to grow *V. cholerae*, which appear as yellow or blue colonies because of the use of both citrate and sucrose. APW is used as an enrichment broth and should be subcultured to TCBS agar at 24 hours for further evaluation of *Vibrio* colonies.

14. D CNA agar inhibits the growth of gram-negative bacteria and is used to isolate gram-positive cocci from specimens. This medium is especially useful for stool and wound cultures because these may contain large numbers of gram-negative rods.

15. A Sheep RBCs are used in blood agar plates because they are readily available and less inhibitory than cells of other species. Sheep blood agar provides the nutrients for the growth of most bacteria (nutritional media) and can be considered differential based on the organism's ability to lyse or hemolyze the RBCs.

16. All the following are appropriate when attempting to isolate *N. gonorrhoeae* from a genital specimen *except*:
- **A.** Transport the genital swab in charcoal transport medium
- **B.** Plate the specimen directly on MTM medium
- **C.** Plate the specimen directly on New York City or Martin-Lewis agar
- **D.** Culture specimens in ambient oxygen at 37°C

Microbiology/Preanalytical/1

17. Chocolate agar and MTM agar are used for the recovery of:
- **A.** *Haemophilus* spp. and *Neisseria* spp., respectively
- **B.** *Haemophilus* spp. and *N. gonorrhoeae*, respectively
- **C.** *Neisseria* spp. and *Streptococcus* spp., respectively
- **D.** *Streptococcus* spp. and *Staphylococcus* spp., respectively

Microbiology/Preanalytical/1

18. Cycloserine–cefoxitin–fructose agar (CCFA) is used for the recovery of:
- **A.** *Yersinia enterocolitica*
- **B.** *Yersinia intermedia*
- **C.** *Clostridium perfringens*
- **D.** *Clostridioides difficile*

Microbiology/Preanalytical/1

19. Xylose lysine deoxycholate (XLD) agar is a highly selective medium used for the recovery of which bacteria?
- **A.** *Staphylococcus* spp. from normal flora
- **B.** *Yersinia* spp. that do not grow on Hektoen agar
- **C.** *Enterobacteriaceae* from gastrointestinal specimens
- **D.** *Streptococcus* spp. from stool cultures

Microbiology/Stool culture/Media/1

20. A sheep blood agar plate is used as a primary isolation medium for the recovery of the following potential pathogens from a wound specimen *except*:
- **A.** β-Hemolytic streptococci and coagulase-positive staphylococci
- **B.** *Haemophilus influenzae* and *Haemophilus parainfluenzae*
- **C.** *Proteus* spp. and *Escherichia coli*
- **D.** *Pseudomonas* spp. and *Acinetobacter* spp.

Microbiology/Preanalytical/2

Answers to Questions 16–20

16. D MTM, New York City, and Martin-Lewis agars contain blood components needed to support the growth of *N. gonorrhoeae* as well as antibiotics that prevent growth of normal genital microbiota. Some strains may be inhibited by vancomycin in the selective media. A chocolate agar plate, without antimicrobials, should be inoculated simultaneously. The culture must be incubated in 3% to 7% carbon dioxide (CO_2) at 35°C. Cultures should be held a minimum of 72 hours before being considered negative.

17. B Chocolate agar provides X factor (hemin) and V factor (nicotinamide adenine dinucleotide [NAD]) required for the growth of *Haemophilus* spp. Thayer-Martin medium is a chocolate agar containing the antibiotics colistin, nystatin, vancomycin, and trimethoprim that permit isolation of *N. gonorrhoeae* in specimens containing large numbers of contaminating bacteria.

18. D CCFA is used for recovery of *C. difficile* from stool cultures. Cycloserine and cefoxitin inhibit growth of gram-negative bacteria in the stool specimen. *C. difficile* ferments fructose, forming acid that, in the presence of neutral red, causes the colonies to become yellow.

19. C XLD agar is selective for gram-negative bacteria because of a high concentration (0.25%) of deoxycholate, which inhibits gram-positive bacteria and some gram-negative rods. In addition, XLD is differential for *Shigella* and *Salmonella* spp. The medium contains xylose, lactose, and sucrose, which are fermented by many gram-negative bacteria producing yellow colonies. *Shigella* does not ferment the sugars and produces red (or clear) colonies. Xylose is present in lower quantity than lactose and sucrose. *Salmonella* spp. rapidly uses up the small amount of xylose and switches to decarboxylate lysine in the medium, causing production of ammonia changing the media back to red. Some *Salmonella* produce hydrogen sulfide (H_2S) from sodium thiosulfate and therefore appear as red colonies with black centers.

20. B Both gram-positive cocci and gram-negative bacilli will grow on blood agar plates, but the medium is used in conjunction with a selective medium, such as CNA agar, for gram-positive cocci and MacConkey agar for gram-negative bacilli. *H. influenzae* requires X and V factors, and *H. parainfluenzae* requires V factor. The primary isolation medium for *Haemophilus* is chocolate agar.

21. Prereduced and vitamin K_1-supplemented blood agar plates are recommended for the culture and isolation of:

A. *Mycobacterium marinum* and *Mycobacterium avium intracellulare*
B. *Bacteroides, Peptostreptococcus,* and *Clostridium* spp.
C. *Proteus* spp.
D. *Enterococcus* spp.

Microbiology/Preanalytical/2

22. Select the medium best suited for the recovery of *Y. enterocolitica* from a patient with gastroenteritis.

A. Hektoen agar
B. Cefsulodin–irgasan–novobiocin (CIN) agar
C. Blood agar
D. Eosin methylene blue agar

Microbiology/Preanalytical/1

23. Cold enrichment of feces (incubation at 4°C) in phosphate-buffered saline prior to subculture onto enteric media enhances the recovery of:

A. Enterotoxigenic *Escherichia coli*
B. *Salmonella paratyphi*
C. *Hafnia alvei*
D. *Yersinia enterocolitica*

Microbiology/Preanalytical/1

24. A typical routine stool culture should include media for the isolation of *E. coli* O157:H7 as well as:

A. *Salmonella, Shigella, Yersinia, Campylobacter,* and *Staphylococcus aureus*
B. *Vibrio cholerae, Brucella,* and *Yersinia* spp.
C. *Staphylococcus aureus*, group B streptococci, and group D streptococci
D. *Clostridioides difficile, Clostridium perfringens,* and *Yersinia* spp.

Microbiology/Preanalytical/2

25. Which agar that is used for routine stool cultures is the medium of choice for the isolation of *Yersinia* strains from stool specimens?

A. *Salmonella–Shigella* agar
B. Hektoen enteric agar
C. MacConkey agar
D. CNA agar

Microbiology/Preanalytical/2

Answers to Questions 21–25

21. B Anaerobic culture media can be prereduced before sterilization by boiling, saturation with oxygen-free gas, and addition of cysteine or other thiol compounds. The final oxidation reduction potential (Eh) of the medium should be approximately −150 mV to minimize the effects of exposure of organisms to oxygen during inoculation.

22. B CIN agar inhibits the growth of many *Enterobacterales* and gram-positive organisms. *Yersinia* spp. may also be cultured using MacConkey and *Salmonella-Shigella* agars. *Y. enterocolitica* are seen as "bull's eye" colonies on CIN agar after 48 hours at room temperature.

23. D Cold enrichment is especially useful when specimens contain large numbers of normal microbiota. In addition to *Yersinia*, the technique has been used to enhance recovery of *Listeria monocytogenes* from specimens containing other bacteria.

24. A *V. cholerae* and *C. difficile* are usually not included in a routine stool culture. If *Vibrio* spp. are suspected, a special request should be included. Although MacConkey agar will support the growth of *Vibrio* spp., normal enteric microbiota overgrows these organisms. *C. difficile* culture requires special media (e.g., CCFA) that inhibit other anaerobic and facultative anaerobic organisms, and culture should be requested specifically if symptoms warrant. MacConkey agar with sorbitol will allow the *E. coli* O157:H7 to be recovered. *Yersinia* spp. can be detected on a regular MacConkey agar plate.

25. C CIN medium is the best agar for the isolation of *Yersinia* strains because it inhibits growth of other coliforms, but it is not used routinely in clinical laboratories. *Yersinia* spp. grow well on MacConkey agar incubated at 37°C, but the colonies are much smaller than the other *Enterobacterales* species. Therefore, 25°C is the temperature recommended for isolation. Some serotypes of *Yersinia* may be inhibited on more selective media, such as *Salmonella–Shigella* or Hektoen enteric agar. CNA agar inhibits the growth of gram-negative bacteria.

26. A 12-month-old child presented to the emergency department with a fever of 103°F and appeared listless. The child had been diagnosed with an ear infection 3 days earlier. A lumbar puncture was performed, but only one tube of CSF was obtained. The single tube of CSF should be submitted first to which department?

A. Chemistry
B. Microbiology
C. Hematology
D. Cytology/Histology

Microbiology/Preanalytical/2

27. A 65-year-old outpatient submitted a 24-hour urine specimen for protein and creatinine tests. When the sample arrived at the laboratory, the requisition also included an order for mycobacteria culture from the same sample. Should the microbiology laboratory accept this 24-hour specimen for culture?

A. Yes, if the specimen is kept on ice
B. Yes, if the specimen is for aerobic culture only
C. No, the specimen must be kept at room temperature
D. No, the specimen is unsuitable for the recovery of mycobacteria

Microbiology/Preanalytical/3

28. A lymph node biopsy specimen obtained from a 30-year-old patient was submitted to the microbiology laboratory for culture and acid-fast bacilli (AFB) smear for mycobacteria. The specimen was fixed in formalin. This specimen should be:

A. Accepted for AFB smear preparation and cultured
B. Rejected
C. Held at room temperature for 24 hours and then cultured
D. Cultured for anaerobes only

Microbiology/Preanalytical/3

Answers to Questions 26–28

26. B Typically when collecting CSF, it is aliquoted into sterile collection tubes that are numbered sequentially in the order of collection. Tube 1 is used for chemistry and immunology studies because these tests are less affected by the presence of blood cells or bacteria that may be introduced during the procedure. Tube 2 is used for culture. Tube 3 may be used for microbiology if larger sample volumes are needed, and if there is a fourth tube, that is generally used for cell counts, differentials, and flow cytometry because it is the least likely to be contaminated from cells introduced during the procedure. If there is only one tube, microbiology should receive the sample first to avoid contamination with external microorganisms to ensure the accuracy of the results.

27. D In general, a 24-hour urine specimen is unsuitable for culture; a first morning specimen is best for the recovery of mycobacteria in the urine.

28. B Specimens submitted for culture and recovery of any bacteria should be submitted without fixatives.

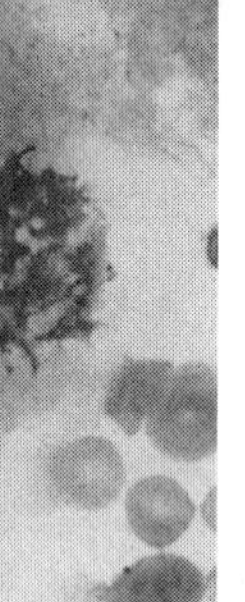

9.3
Antimicrobials and Susceptibility Methods

1. **The *most* used rapid disk detection method for the presence of β-lactamase–producing bacteria is:**
   A. Chromogenic cephalosporin
   B. Penicillin
   C. Oxidase
   D. Chloramphenicol acetyltransferase
   Microbiology/Susceptibility methods/2

2. **The *breakpoint* of an antimicrobial drug refers to:**
   A. The amount needed to cause bacteriostasis
   B. An MIC of 16 µg/mL or greater
   C. An MIC of 64 µg/mL or greater
   D. The optimal therapeutic level of drug that is achievable in serum
   Microbiology/Susceptibility methods/2

3. **Which of the following variables may change the results of an MIC?**
   A. Inoculum size
   B. Incubation time
   C. Purity of the bacterial isolate
   D. Incubation temperature
   Microbiology/Susceptibility methods/2

4. **According to the Kirby-Bauer standard antimicrobial susceptibility testing method, what is the proper way to interpret the zone size of a motile, swarming organism, such as a *Proteus* species?**
   A. The swarming area should be ignored
   B. The results of the disk diffusion method are invalid
   C. The swarming area should be measured as the growth boundary
   D. The isolate should be retested after diluting to a 0.05 McFarland standard
   Microbiology/Susceptibility methods/2

5. **An isolate of *S. aureus* was cultured from an ulcer obtained from the leg of a 79-year-old patient with diabetes. The organism showed resistance to methicillin. This isolate should be additionally tested for resistance or susceptibility to:**
   A. Erythromycin
   B. Gentamicin
   C. Vancomycin
   D. Kanamycin
   Microbiology/Susceptibility methods/3

Answers to Questions 1–5

1. A β-Lactamase production by bacteria that are resistant to penicillin, cephalosporins, and other β-lactams is detected using various methods. The most common method used is a chromogenic cephalosporin (e.g., nitrocefin) disk. The nitrocefin is hydrolyzed by β-lactamase into acidic products that can be detected as a color change by a pH indicator. However, the disk detection method lacks sensitivity for the detection of β-lactamase production in some organisms such as strains of *Staphylcoccus aureus*. Any isolate that tests negative should be confirmed using a microdilution minimal inhibitory concentration (MIC) method.

2. D The term *breakpoint* refers to an antimicrobial concentration in the serum or body fluid associated with optimal therapy using the customary dosing schedule. An organism is susceptible if inhibited if the MIC is at or below the breakpoint.

3. D *In vitro* testing of antimicrobials is reliable if the method is standardized including the inoculum size, incubation time, and temperature. In addition, failure to achieve proper pure culture isolation may result in inaccurate results associated with the identification of a specific organism. Different microorganisms have different sensitivity patterns.

4. A A thin film of growth appearing in the zone area of inhibition around the susceptibility disk should be ignored when swarming *Proteus* or other motile organisms are encountered.

5. C MRSA (methicillin-resistant *Staphylococcus aureus*) isolates are usually tested for susceptibility or resistance to vancomycin, a glycopeptide.

6. In breakpoint antimicrobial drug testing, interpretation of susceptible (S), intermediate (I), and resistant (R) refers to testing antibiotics by using:

A. The amount needed to cause bacteriostasis
B. Only the specific concentrations necessary to report S, I, or R
C. An MIC of 64 µg/mL
D. A dilution of drug that is one tube less than the toxic level

Microbiology/Susceptibility methods/1

7. Antimicrobials exhibit different specificity related to their bacterial targets; this is used to categorize the agents and is referred to as:

A. Selective toxicity
B. Mode of action
C. Spectrum of activity
D. Pharmacokinetics

Microbiology/Antimicrobials/1

8. This antimicrobial binds to DNA gyrase and topoisomerase IV enzyme, inhibiting DNA synthesis in both gram-positive and gram-negative microorganisms.

A. β-Lactams
B. Lipopeptides
C. Fluoroquinolones
D. Aminoglycosides

Microbiology/Antimicrobials/1

9. This antimicrobial disrupts the cell membrane of gram-negative bacteria and is also used in selective culture media to inhibit their growth.

A. Vancomycin
B. Penicillin
C. Colistin
D. Tetracycline

Microbiology/Antimicrobials/2

10. Antimicrobial resistance that is due to the normal structure, physiology, and genetics of an organism is called:

A. Extrinsic resistance
B. Natural resistance
C. High resistance
D. Intrinsic resistance

Microbiology/Antimicrobials/1

Answers to Questions 6–10

6. B Breakpoint susceptibility testing is performed by selecting only two appropriate drug concentrations for testing. If the results show growth at both concentrations, then resistance (R) is indicated; growth only at the lower concentration signifies an intermediate (I) result; no growth at either concentration is interpreted as susceptible (S).

7. B The various targets for antimicrobials are used to classify them based on specificity, which is termed *mode of action*.

8. C Fluoroquinolones inhibit DNA synthesis by binding DNA gyrase and topoisomerase IV in both gram-positive and gram-negative organisms. Common fluoroquinolines include ciprofloxacin and levofloxacin.

9. C Colistin is a polymyxin and disrupts the cell membrane of gram-negative bacteria. It is also used in selective media such as CNA to support the growth of gram-positive organisms and prevent overgrowth by gram-negative bacteria.

10. D Bacteria have several natural mechanisms that provide resistance to antimicrobials. These mechanisms are a result of the presence of specific genetic determinants and structural and physiological properties of the bacteria. These methods are considered intrinsic antimicrobial resistance because they are part of the normal biology of the microorganism.

9.4

Enterobacterales

1. **Biochemically, the *Enterobacterales* are gram-negative rods that:**
   A. Ferment glucose and are oxidase negative
   B. Ferment glucose, produce indophenol oxidase, and form gas
   C. Ferment lactose and reduce nitrite to nitrogen gas
   D. Ferment lactose and produce indophenol oxidase
   Microbiology/Biochemical/Enterobacterales/1

2. **The ortho-nitrophenyl-β-galactopyranoside (ONPG) test is most useful when differentiating:**
   A. *Salmonella* spp. from *Pseudomonas* spp.
   B. *Escherichia coli* from most species of *Shigella*
   C. *Klebsiella* spp. from *Enterobacter* spp.
   D. *Proteus vulgaris* from *Salmonella* spp.
   Microbiology/Biochemical/Enterobacterales/2

3. **The Voges-Proskauer (VP) test detects which product of glucose fermentation?**
   A. Acetoin
   B. Nitrite
   C. Acetic acid
   D. Hydrogen sulfide (H_2S)
   Microbiology/Biochemical/Enterobacterales/1

4. **At which pH does the methyl red (MR) test become positive?**
   A. 7.0
   B. 6.5
   C. 6.0
   D. 4.5
   Microbiology/Biochemical/Enterobacterales/1

5. **A positive Simmons citrate test is seen as a:**
   A. Blue color in the medium after incubation at 35°C
   B. Red color in the medium after incubation at 35°C
   C. Yellow color in the medium after incubation at 35°C
   D. Green color in the medium after incubation at 35°C
   Microbiology/Biochemical/Enterobacterales/1

Answers to Questions 1–5

1. A The Order *Enterobacterales* consists of seven families and more than 250 species and represents the most encountered isolates in clinical specimens. All *Enterobacterales* ferment glucose, are nonsporulating, and are oxidase negative (except for *Plesiomonas shigelloides*, which is oxidase positive).

2. B The ONPG test detects β-galactosidase activity and is most useful in distinguishing late lactose fermenters from lactose nonfermenters. Some strains of *E. coli* are slow lactose fermenters and may be confused with *Shigella* spp., which do not ferment lactose. *E. coli* are ONPG positive, whereas *Shigella* spp. are typically ONPG negative (except *Shigella sonnei*).

3. A Acetoin, an end product of glucose fermentation, is converted to diacetyl after the addition of the VP reagents (β-naphthol and 40% potassium hydroxide [KOH]). Diacetyl is seen as a red- to pink-colored complex.

4. D Both MR and VP tests detect acid production from the fermentation of glucose. The MR test specifically detects mixed acid fermentation, which lowers the pH in the broth. MR is read at a pH around 4.5, which indicates a positive result; yellow is a negative result; any shade of orange is considered inconclusive.

5. A The Simmons citrate test determines whether an organism can utilize citrate as the sole source of carbon. The medium turns blue, indicating the presence of alkaline products, such as carbonate. Tubes are incubated a minimum of 24 hours at 35°C with a loose cap before reading. Some organisms are capable of growth on citrate and will not produce a color change. Heavy growth without a color change may be a positive test; if the agar does not turn blue, incubate up to 4 days and repeat with a smaller inoculum.

6. In the test for urease production, ammonia reacts to form which product?
A. Ammonium citrate
B. Ammonium carbonate
C. Ammonium oxalate
D. Ammonium nitrate
Microbiology/Biochemical/Enterobacterales/1

7. Which of the following reagents is added to detect the production of indole in the tube method?
A. *p*-Dimethylaminobenzaldehyde and hydrochloride
B. Bromcresol purple
C. Methyl red
D. Cytochrome oxidase
Microbiology/Biochemical/Enterobacterales/1

8. Decarboxylation of the amino acids lysine, ornithine, and arginine results in the formation of:
A. Ammonia
B. Urea
C. Carbonate
D. Amines
Microbiology/Biochemical/Enterobacterales/1

9. Lysine iron agar (LIA) showing a purple slant and a blackened butt indicates:
A. *Escherichia coli*
B. *Citrobacter* spp.
C. *Salmonella* spp.
D. *Proteus* spp.
Microbiology/Biochemical/Enterobacterales/2

10. Putrescine is an alkaline amine product of which bacterial enzyme?
A. Arginine decarboxylase
B. Phenylalanine deaminase
C. Ornithine decarboxylase
D. Lysine decarboxylase
Microbiology/Biochemical/Enterobacterales/1

11. Which genera are positive for phenylalanine deaminase?
A. *Enterobacter, Escherichia,* and *Salmonella*
B. *Morganella, Providencia,* and *Proteus*
C. *Klebsiella* and *Enterobacter*
D. *Proteus, Escherichia,* and *Shigella*
Microbiology/Biochemical/Enterobacterales/1

12. Kliger iron agar (KIA) differs from triple-sugar iron agar (TSI) in the:
A. Ratio of lactose to glucose
B. Ability to detect H_2S production
C. Use of sucrose in the medium
D. Color reaction denoting production of acid
Microbiology/Biochemical/Enterobacterales/2

Answers to Questions 6–12

6. B The test for urease production is based on the ability of the colonies to hydrolyze urea in Stuart broth or Christensen agar to form CO_2 and ammonia. These products form ammonium carbonate, resulting in alkalinization. This turns the pH indicator (phenol red) pink at pH 8.1.

7. A The indole tube test detects the conversion of tryptophan (present in the media) to indole by the enzyme tryptophanase. Indole is detected by the reaction with the aldehyde group of *p*-dimethylaminobenzaldehyde (the active reagent in Kovac and Ehrlich reagents) in acid, forming a red complex.

8. D Specific decarboxylases split dibasic amino acids (lysine, arginine, and ornithine), forming alkaline amines. These products turn the pH indicators in the medium (cresol red and bromcresol purple) from yellow to purple.

9. C LIA is used as an aid for the identification of *Salmonella* species. It contains phenylalanine, lysine, glucose, thiosulfate, ferric ammonium citrate, and bromcresol purple. *Salmonella* spp. produce H_2S from thiosulfate. This reduces ferric ammonium citrate, forming ferrous sulfate and causing the butt to blacken. *Salmonella* also decarboxylate lysine to produce alkaline amines, giving the slant its purple color and differentiating it from *Citrobacter* spp., which are lysine decarboxylase negative.

10. C Putrescine is the amine product of the decarboxylation of ornithine.

11. B Phenylalanine deaminase oxidatively deaminates phenylalanine, forming phenylpyruvic acid. When a solution of ferric chloride is added, the iron reacts with phenylpyruvic acid, forming a green-colored complex. Phenylalanine deaminase is found in the genera *Morganella, Providencia,* and *Proteus* and is an excellent test to determine whether an organism belongs to this group. Rarely, isolates of *Enterobacter* may be phenylalanine deaminase positive as well.

12. C Both KIA and TSI contain 10-fold more lactose than glucose, peptone, and phenol red to detect acid production (turns yellow) and sodium thiosulfate and ferrous ammonium sulfate to detect H_2S production. However, TSI contains sucrose, and KIA does not. Organisms fermenting either sucrose or lactose will turn the slant of the agar tube yellow. Therefore, some organisms (e.g., many species of *Cedecea, Citrobacter, Edwardsiella,* and *Serratia*) will produce a yellow slant on TSI but a red slant on KIA.

13. The malonate test is *most* useful in differentiating which members in the Order *Enterobacterales*?
A. *Shigella*
B. *Proteus*
C. *Salmonella enterica* subgroups 2, 3
D. *Serratia*
Microbiology/Biochemical/Enterobacterales/2

14. Which genera in the Order *Enterobacterales* are known to cause diarrhea and are considered enteric pathogens?
A. *Enterobacter*, *Klebsiella*, *Providencia*, and *Proteus*
B. *Escherichia*, *Salmonella*, *Shigella*, and *Yersinia*
C. *Pseudomonas*, *Moraxella*, *Acinetobacter*, and *Aeromonas*
D. *Enterobacter*, *Citrobacter*, and *Morganella*
Microbiology/Pathogenicity/Enterobacterales/1

15. An isolate of *E. coli* O157-H7 recovered from the stool of a patient with severe bloody diarrhea typically can be biochemically identified by the inability to metabolize which carbohydrate?
A. Sorbitol (fermentation)
B. Mannitol (oxidation)
C. Raffinose (fermentation)
D. Sucrose (fermentation)
Microbiology/Biochemical/Enterobacterales/1

16. The taxonomy and identification of isolates of *Shigella* have been traditionally determined by serotypes; however, care must be taken when utilizing this method because serological cross reactions occur with:
A. *Escherichia coli*
B. *Salmonella* spp.
C. *Pseudomonas* spp.
D. *Proteus* spp.
Microbiology/Serotype/Enterobacterales/2

17. Which species of *Shigella* is *most* associated with diarrheal disease in the United States?
A. *S. dysenteriae*
B. *S. flexneri*
C. *S. boydii*
D. *S. sonnei*
Microbiology/Pathogenicity/Enterobacterales/1

18. Which of the following phenotypic tests *best* differentiates *Shigella* species from *E. coli*?
A. H_2S, VP, citrate, and urease
B. Lactose, indole, ONPG, and motility
C. H_2S, MR, citrate, and urease
D. Gas, citrate, and VP
Microbiology/Biochemical/Enterobacterales/2

Answers to Questions 13–18

13. C The malonate test determines whether an organism can utilize sodium malonate as the sole source of carbon. Malonate is broken down, forming alkaline metabolites that raise the pH of the broth above 7.6. This causes bromthymol blue to turn from green to deep blue (Prussian blue). *E. coli, Shigella,* and most *Salmonella* are malonate negative, whereas *Enterobacter* and *Salmonella enterica* subgroups 2, 3a, and 3b are positive. *Proteus, Providencia, Serratia,* and *Yersinia* are also malonate negative.

14. B *Escherichia, Salmonella, Shigella,* and *Yersinia* are responsible for most enteric diarrhea cases attributable to the *Enterobacteriaceae* family.

15. A An isolate of *E. coli* (shiga-like producing toxin of *E. coli* [STEC]) recovered from a stool culture in hemorrhagic colitis can be definitely identified by serotyping. The isolate is identified as *E. coli* by the usual biochemical reactions. The strain of *E. coli* responsible for hemorrhagic colitis is O157:H7 and is usually negative for sorbitol fermentation. Colonies of this strain of *E. coli* appear colorless on MacConkey agar with sorbitol added.

16. A Historically, *Shigella* spp. were taxonomically defined by serotypes, which were also used along with biochemical tests to differentiate the organism from other *Enterobacteriaceae* such as *Escherichia coli*. However, some of the serotypes are very closely related to specific enteroinvasive *E. coli* serotypes that complicate the identification of a clinical isolate. Molecular characterization has replaced classic serotyping, organizing *Shigella* spp. into three genetic clusters. Serological classification may not reflect accurate results for some isolates.

17. D The *Shigella* spp. are lactose nonfermenters that, for the most part, are biochemically inert and are classified into serogroups A, B, C, and D because of their biochemical similarity. *S. sonnei* (serogroup D) is the species most often isolated from diarrhea cases in the United States.

18. B *E. coli*, when positive for lactose, indole, and ONPG, are usually motile. *Shigella* species do not ferment lactose or produce indole, lack β-galactosidase, and are nonmotile.

19. Which genera in the Order *Enterobacterales* are usually nonmotile at 36°C?
A. *Shigella, Klebsiella,* and *Yersinia*
B. *Escherichia, Edwardsiella,* and *Enterobacter*
C. *Proteus, Providencia,* and *Salmonella*
D. *Serratia, Morganella,* and *Hafnia*
Microbiology/Phenotypic characteristics/ Enterobacterales/1

20. Fever, abdominal cramping, watery stools, and fluid and electrolyte loss preceded by bloody stools 2 to 3 days before is characteristic of shigellosis but may also result from infection with:
A. *Campylobacter* spp.
B. *Salmonella* spp.
C. *Proteus* spp.
D. *Yersinia* spp.
Microbiology/Pathogenicity/Enterobacterales/2

21. Which group of biochemical tests, along with colony morphology on primary media, aids *most* in the phenotypic and biochemical identification of *Enterobacterales*?
A. MR and VP, urease, and blood agar plate
B. Phenylalanine deaminase, urease, and CDC agar plate
C. Bacitracin, β-lactamase, and MacConkey agar plate
D. Indole, oxidase, MacConkey, and blood agar plates
Microbiology/Biochemical/Enterobacterales/2

22. Which group of phenotypic and biochemical tests *best* identifies the *Morganella* and *Proteus* genera?
A. Motility, urease, and phenylalanine deaminase
B. Malonate, glucose fermentation, and deoxyribonuclease (DNase)
C. Indole, oxidase, MR, and VP
D. Indole, citrate, and urease
Microbiology/Biochemical/Enterobacterales/2

23. Which group of phenotypic and biochemical tests *best* differentiates *Klebsiella aerogenes* from *Edwardsiella tarda*?
A. Motility, citrate, and urease
B. H_2S production, sucrose fermentation, indole, and VP
C. Lysine decarboxylase, urease, and arginine dihydrolase
D. Motility, H_2S production, and DNase
Microbiology/Biochemical/Enterobacterales/2

Answers to Questions 19–23

19. A *Shigella* spp. and *Klebsiella* spp. are, for the most part, nonmotile. *Yersinia* can be motile at 22°C but is nonmotile at 36°C. Other members of the Order *Enterobacterales* that have been isolated from human specimens and are usually nonmotile include *Leminorella, Rahnella*, and *Tatumella* (considered unusual enteric pathogens).

20. A *Shigella* spp. and *Campylobacter* spp. are both causes of diarrhea, abdominal pain, fever, and sometimes vomiting. Blood is present in the stools of patients infected with *Shigella* because of invasion and penetration of the bowel by the organisms. Young children may also exhibit bloody stools when infected with *Campylobacter*.

21. D All *Enterobacterales* species are oxidase negative (except *Plesiomonas shigelloides*). *E. coli* and *Proteus* spp. comprise most of the organisms recovered from clinical specimens and can be initially identified through rapid phenotypic testing without additional overnight testing. *E. coli* displays a positive indole test, and the colonial morphology on MacConkey agar is distinctive, showing flat, pink (lactose-positive) colonies with a ring of bile precipitation. *Proteus* spp. swarm on blood agar and are indole negative.

22. A *Morganella* and *Proteus* spp. are motile, produce urease, and deaminate phenylalanine.

23. B

Test	*K. aerogenes* (% positive)	*E. tarda* (% positive)
H_2S	0	100
Sucrose	>90	0
Indole	<20	100
VP	100	0
Citrate	95	0

24. *Cronobacter sakazakii* can *best* be differentiated from *Enterobacter cloacae* by which of the following characteristics?
A. Yellow pigmentation and negative sorbitol fermentation
B. Pink pigmentation and positive arginine dihydrolase
C. Yellow pigmentation and positive urease
D. H_2S production on TSI

Microbiology/Biochemical/Enterobacterales/2

25. Members of the genus *Cedecea* are *best* differentiated from *Serratia* spp. by which phenotypic or biochemical test result?
A. Positive motility
B. Positive urease
C. Positive phenylalanine deaminase
D. Negative DNase

Microbiology/Biochemical/Enterobacterales/2

26. Which of the following organisms is biochemically confused with the *Salmonella* species and on plated media?
A. *Escherichia coli*
B. *Citrobacter freundii*
C. *Enterobacter cloacae*
D. *Shigella dysenteriae*

Microbiology/Biochemical/Emterobacterales/2

27. A gram-negative rod is recovered from a catheterized urine sample from a nursing home patient. The lactose-negative isolate tested positive for indole, urease, ornithine decarboxylase, and phenylalanine deaminase and negative for H_2S. The most probable identification is:
A. *Edwardsiella* spp.
B. *Morganella* spp.
C. *Ewingella* spp.
D. *Shigella* spp.

Microbiology/Biochemical/Enterobacterales/3

28. Which single biochemical test *best* separates *Klebsiella oxytoca* from *K. pneumoniae*?
A. Urease
B. Sucrose
C. Citrate
D. Indole

Microbiology/Biochemical/Enterobacterales/1

29. Which of the following organisms, found in normal fecal flora, may be mistaken phenotypically and/or biochemically for the genus *Yersinia*?
A. *Klebsiella* spp.
B. *Proteus* spp.
C. *Escherichia coli*
D. *Enterobacter* spp.

Microbiology/Biochemical/Enterobacterales/2

Answers to Questions 24–29

24. A *C. sakazakii* is best differentiated from *E. cloacae* by sorbitol fermentation (95% positive for *E. cloacae* and 0% for *C. sakazakii*). In addition, *E. cloacae* is usually positive for urease and malonate (65% and 75%, respectively) and *C. sakazakii* is usually negative (1% and less than 20%, respectively). Both are usually motile and arginine dihydrolase positive.

25. D DNase is not produced by *Cedecea* spp. but is produced (along with proteinases) by *Serratia* spp. Other key phenotypic biochemical differential tests include lipase (positive for *Cedecea*, negative for *Serratia*) and gelatin hydrolysis (negative for *Cedecea*, positive for *Serratia*).

26. B *C. freundii* strains, such as *Salmonella* spp., are usually H_2S producers and may be confused with *Salmonella* spp. unless the proper biochemical tests are utilized. *C. freundii* and *Salmonella* spp. are adonitol, indole, and malonate negative. However, *C. freundii* is potassium cyanide (KCN) positive, whereas *Salmonella* spp. are KCN negative. (*C. freundii* are late lactose fermenters and appear colorless at 24 hours on MacConkey agar.)

27. B *Morganella* spp. are biochemically similar to *Proteus* spp., both being lactose negative, motile, and positive for phenylalanine deaminase and urease. However, *Morganella* spp. can be differentiated from *Proteus* spp. based on H_2S, indole, ornithine decarboxylase, and xylose fermentation. *Ewingella* spp. are usually positive (70%) for lactose fermentation, whereas the other three genera are lactose negative.

28. D *K. oxytoca* and *K. pneumoniae* are almost identical biochemically except for the ability to produce indole. Both organisms are nonmotile and usually test positive for urease, sucrose, and citrate. However, *K. oxytoca* is indole positive, and *K. pneumoniae* is indole negative.

29. B *Proteus* spp. are urease positive, as are approximately 70% of *Y. enterocolitica* isolates. Both organisms are lactose negative and motile. However, *Yersinia* is motile at 22°C and not at 35°C (demonstrated by using motility media).

30. When utilizing traditional stool culture methods for the identification of enteric pathogens, when is it necessary to subculture both pink (lactose-positive) and colorless (lactose-negative) colonies from an initial stool culture on MacConkey agar and test further for possible pathogens?

A. Most *Shigella* strains are lactose positive
B. Most *Salmonella* strains are maltose negative
C. Most *Proteus* spp. are lactose negative
D. Pathogenic *Escherichia coli* can be lactose positive or lactose negative

Microbiology/Biochemical/Enterobacterales/2

31. A suspected case of plague requires which of the following procedures to confirm *Yersinia pestis*?

A. Collection of multiple sets of blood culture specimens
B. Slow-growing, lactose-negative colonies should be identified using an automated platform
C. All samples should be sent directly to a Laboratory Response Network (LRN) member laboratory
D. Slow-growing, lactose-negative colonies should be processed in a biosafety level 3 (BSL-3) laboratory and identified using a nucleic acid amplification test (NAAT)

Microbiology/Enterobacterales/2

32. A group of elementary students became ill after eating undercooked ground beef prepared in the school cafeteria. The suspected pathogen, *E. coli* serotype O157:H7, is usually recovered using which of the following media?

A. Xylose lysine deoxycholate agar
B. MacConkey agar
C. MacConkey agar with sorbitol
D. Hektoen agar

Microbiology/Enterobacterales/2

33. Which organism is sometimes mistaken for *Salmonella* using traditional biochemical methods for identification?

A. *Citrobacter freundii* strains
B. *Proteus mirabilis* strains
C. *Shigella sonnei* strains
D. *Escherichia coli*

Microbiology/Biochemical/Enterobacterales/2

Answers to Questions 30–33

30. D Most *E. coli* ferment lactose and appear pink to red on MacConkey agar; however, some strains are slow fermenters and may appear colorless. The *E. coli* strain O157:H7 causes the enteric disease hemorrhagic colitis and can be differentiated from nonpathogenic *E. coli* by the inability to ferment D-sorbitol. O157:H7 *E. coli* ferments D-sorbitol slowly or not at all and appears as colorless colonies on MacConkey–sorbitol agar.

31. D *Y. pestis* is on the list of agents of bioterrorism. Isolation and identification should be performed in a facility with a level 3 biosafety rating. Recovery of *Y. pestis* is highest if the specimen is cultured within 2 hours of collection. Slow-growing, lactose-negative colonies from a suspected case of plague must never be placed on an automated platform, due to the risk of aerosolization. Isolates should be transferred to a LRN laboratory using LRN protocols in a BSL-3 facility. A variety of molecular assays are available for rapid identification.

32. C *E. coli* O157:H7 ferments lactose and, therefore, appears as dark pink colonies on MacConkey agar. To differentiate *E. coli* O157:H7 from normal fecal flora, MacConkey agar with sorbitol is used. *E. coli* O157:H7 does not ferment sorbitol, and usually are colorless colonies.

33. A *C. freundii* and *Salmonella* spp. are H_2S positive and indole, VP, and phenylalanine deaminase negative. Biochemical characteristics that help to differentiate *C. freundii* from *Salmonella* include lactose fermentation (50% of *C. freundii* are lactose positive, whereas 100% of *Salmonella* are lactose negative) and urease production (70% of *Citrobacter* are positive and greater than 99% of *Salmonella* are negative).

34. A bloody stool cultured from a 26-year-old patient after 3 days of severe diarrhea showed the following results at 48 hours after being cultured on the following media:

MacConkey agar: Scant normal microbiota present with many non–lactose-fermenting colonies. Non–lactose-fermenting colonies are nonmotile, and oxidase, indole, urease, and H_2S negative.
Hektoen enteric agar: Many blue-green colonies
Campylobacter blood agar and *C. difficile* agar: No growth

The *most* likely identification is:
A. *Shigella* spp.
B. *Salmonella* spp.
C. *Proteus* spp.
D. *Escherichia coli*

Microbiology/Enterobacterales/3

35. Which of the following organisms is generally positive for β-galactosidase (utilizes lactose)?
A. *Salmonella* spp.
B. *Shigella* spp.
C. *Proteus* spp.
D. *Escherichia coli*

Microbiology/Biochemical/Enterobacterales/1

36. In the Kauffmann-White schema, the combined antigens used for serological identification and classification of the *Salmonella* spp. are:
A. O antigens
B. H antigens
C. Vi and H antigens
D. O, Vi, and H antigens

Microbiology/Serotype/Enterobacterales/1

37. The Shiga-like toxin (verotoxin) is produced mainly by which *Enterobacterales* species?
A. *Klebsiella pneumoniae*
B. *Escherichia coli*
C. *Salmonella typhimurium*
D. *Enterobacter cloacae*

Microbiology/Pathogenicity/Enterobacterales/1

Answers to Questions 34–37

34. A *Shigella* is the most likely organism. *E. coli* are usually indole and motility positive, and *Proteus* are motility and urease positive. Most *Salmonella* are H_2S positive. *Shigella* and *Campylobacter* cause bloody diarrhea because they invade the epithelial cells of the large bowel; however, *Campylobacter* spp. do not grow on MacConkey agar, and they are oxidase positive.

35. D *Salmonella, Shigella, Proteus, Providencia,* and *Morganella* are usually lactose nonfermenters. Others—including certain strains of *E. coli, S. sonnei, Hafnia alvei, Serratia marcescens*, and some *Yersinia*—appear to be lactose nonfermenters because they lack the permease enzyme that actively transports lactose across the cell membrane. However, true lactose nonfermenters do not possess β-galactosidase. The test for β-galactosidase uses the substrate *o*-nitrophenyl-β-galactopyranoside. At an alkaline pH, β-galactosidase hydrolyses the substrate, forming *o*-nitrophenol, which turns the medium yellow.

36. D The Kaufmann-White schema groups *Salmonella* spp. using the somatic O (heat-stable) antigens and subdivides them into serotypes based on the flagellar H (heat-labile) antigens. The Vi (or K) antigen is a capsular polysaccharide that may be removed by heating. In the United States, commercially available slide agglutination tests utilize polyvalent antisera (A, B, C-1, C-2, D, E, and Vi) to group the *Salmonella* spp. because 95% of isolated organisms belong to groups A through E with the Vi antiserum identifying the capsular or "K" antigen of *Salmonella* serotype Typhi. Antiserum is also used against the flagella ("H") antigens. If the Vi antigen is positive and the O antigen is negative, the isolate must be heated in boiling water for 15 minutes to remove the capsule and retested with the antisera. Serodiagnostic techniques are used for only two members of the *Enterobacterales: Salmonella* Typhi and *Yersinia pestis.*

37. B Strains of *E. coli* that produce one or both Shiga-like toxins (SLT I and SLT II) can cause bloody diarrhea (hemorrhagic colitis). In the United States, *E. coli* strain O157:H7 is the serotype most often associated with hemorrhagic colitis.

38. A leg culture from a patient in a long-term care facility grew gram-negative rods on MacConkey agar as pink to dark pink oxidase-negative colonies. Given the following results, which is the *most* likely organism?

TSI = A/A	Indole = Neg	MR = Neg
VP = +	Citrate = +	H_2S = Neg
Urease = +	Motility = Neg	

A. *Klebsiella pneumoniae* subsp. *ozaenae*
B. *Proteus vulgaris*
C. *Enterobacter cloacae*
D. *Klebsiella pneumoniae* subsp. *pneumoniae*

Microbiology/Enterobacterales/3

39. Four blood cultures were taken over a 24-hour period from a 20-year-old patient with severe diarrhea. The cultures grew motile (room temperature), gram-negative rods. A urine specimen obtained via catheterization also showed gram-negative rods (100,000 colonies/mL). Given the following results, which is the *most* likely organism?

TSI = A/A gas	Indole = +
VP = Neg	MR = +
H_2S = Neg	Citrate = Neg
Urease = Neg	Lysine decarboxylase = +
Phenylalanine deaminase (PD) = Neg	

A. *Proteus vulgaris*
B. *Salmonella typhi*
C. *Yersinia enterocolitica*
D. *Escherichia coli*

Microbiology/Enterobacterales/3

40. A stool culture from a 30-year-old patient suffering from bloody mucoid diarrhea demonstrated the following results on differential enteric media:

MacConkey agar = Clear colonies
XLD agar = Clear colonies
Hektoen agar = Green colonies
Salmonella–Shigella agar = Small, clear colonies

Which phenotypic tests are *most* appropriate for identification of this enteric pathogen?

A. TSI, motility, indole, urease, *Shigella* typing with polyvalent sera
B. TSI, motility, indole, lysine, *Salmonella* typing with polyvalent sera
C. TSI, indole, MR, VP, citrate
D. TSI, indole, MR, and urease

Microbiology/Enterobacterales/3

Answers to Questions 38–40

38. D *K. pneumoniae* subsp. *pneumoniae* and *E. cloacae* display similar IMViC (indole, MR, VP, and citrate) reactions and TSI results. However, approximately 65% of *E. cloacae* strains are urease positive compared with 98% of *K. pneumoniae* subsp. *pneumoniae*. *Enterobacter* spp. are motile, and *Klebsiella* are nonmotile. *K. pneumoniae* subsp. *ozaenae* is typically VP negative and 10% are urease positive.

39. D Typically, the IMViC reactions for the organisms listed are:

E. coli:	(++00) (PD = Neg)
S. typhi:	(0+00)
Y. enterocolitica:	(V+00)
P. vulgaris:	(++00) (PD = +)

Note: Indole reaction is variable (V) for Y. enterocolitica.

40. A The most likely organism is a species of *Shigella*. Typically, *Salmonella* spp. produce H_2S-positive colonies that display black centers on the differential media (except on MacConkey agar). The biochemical tests listed are necessary to differentiate *Shigella* from *E. coli* because some *E. coli* strains cross-react with *Shigella*-typing sera. *Shigella* spp. are one of the most common causes of bacterial diarrhea; group D (*S. sonnei*) and group B (*S. flexneri*) are the most often isolated species.

41. A leg wound culture from a hospitalized 70-year-old individual with diabetes grew motile, lactose-negative colonies on MacConkey agar. Given the following biochemical reactions at 24 hours, what is the *most* probable organism?

H_2S (TSI) = Neg	Indole = Neg
MR = Neg	VP = +
DNase = +	Citrate = +
Urease = Neg	
PD = Neg	
Ornithine and lysine decarboxylase = +	
Arginine decarboxylase = Neg	
Gelatin hydrolysis = +	

A. *Proteus vulgaris*
B. *Serratia marcescens*
C. *Proteus mirabilis*
D. *Enterobacter cloacae*

Microbiology/Enterobacterales/3

42. Three blood culture specimens taken from a 30-year-old patient with cancer receiving chemotherapy and admitted with a urinary tract infection (UTI) grew lactose-negative, motile, gram-negative rods prior to antibiotic therapy. Given the following biochemical reactions, which is the *most* likely organism?

H_2S (TSI) = +	Indole = +	MR = +
VP = Neg	Citrate = Neg	Urease = +
DNase = +	PD = +	
Gelatin hydrolysis = +		
Ornithine decarboxylase = Neg		

A. *Proteus vulgaris*
B. *Proteus mirabilis*
C. *Proteus penneri*
D. *Klebsiella pneumoniae*

Microbiology/Enterobacterales/3

43. Three consecutive stool cultures from a 25-year-old patient produced scant normal fecal flora on MacConkey and Hektoen agars. However, colonies on CIN agar displayed "bull's eye" colonies after 48 hours of incubation. The patient had been suffering from enterocolitis with fever, diarrhea, and abdominal pain for 2 days. What is the *most* likely identification of this gram-negative rod?

A. *Escherichia coli*
B. *Proteus mirabilis*
C. *Yersinia enterocolitica*
D. *Klebsiella pneumoniae*

Microbiology/Enterobacterales/3

44. A 6-year-old patient was admitted to the hospital following 2 days of severe diarrhea. Cultures from three consecutive stool samples contained blood and mucus. Patient history revealed that the child had eaten a hamburger at a fast-food restaurant 3 days earlier. Which pathogen is *most* likely responsible for the following results?

Growth on:
XLD agar = Yellow colonies
Hektoen enteric agar = Yellow colonies
MacConkey agar = Light pink and dark pink colonies
MacConkey with sorbitol agar = Few dark pink and many colorless colonies

A. *Salmonella* spp.
B. *Shigella* spp.
C. *Escherichia coli* O157:H7
D. *Yersinia enterocolitica*

Microbiology/Enterobacterales/3

Answers to Questions 41–44

41. B *S. marcescens* has been implicated in numerous nosocomial infections and is recognized as an important pathogen with invasive properties. Gelatin hydrolysis and DNase are positive for *Proteus* spp. and *Serratia*, but the negative urease and phenylalanine deaminase are differential. *E. cloacae* do not produce DNase, gelatinase, or lysine decarboxylase but will display red-pigmented colonies on MacConkey agar similar to *S. marcescens*.

42. A Although *P. mirabilis* is more frequently recovered from patients with UTIs, *P. vulgaris* is commonly recovered from immunosuppressed patients. *P. mirabilis* is indole negative and ornithine decarboxylase (ODC) positive but otherwise it is very similar to *P. vulgaris*. *P. penneri* is indole and ODC negative, which differentiates it from both species.

43. C Most members of the *Enterobacterales* produce detectable growth on MacConkey agar within 24 hours. *Y. enterocolitica* produces non–lactose-fermenting colonies on MacConkey agar, salmon-colored colonies on Hektoen agar, and yellow or colorless colonies on XLD agar. If *Y. enterocolitica* is suspected, specialized agar (CIN) is employed. The typical "bull's eye" colonies, dark red with a translucent border, can be confused with *Aeromonas* spp. that appear similarly on CIN agar. To differentiate, an oxidase test must be performed because *Yersinia* spp. are oxidase negative and *Aeromonas* spp. are oxidase positive.

44. C Inflammation with bleeding of the mucosa of the large intestine (hemorrhagic colitis) is a result of an enterohemorrhagic *E. coli* (EHEC) infection associated with certain serotypes, such as *E. coli* O157:H7. The source of the *E. coli* infection is from ingestion of undercooked ground beef contaminated with fecal matter or drinking raw milk.

45. Following a 2-week camping trip to the southwest United States, a 65-year-old patient was hospitalized with a high fever and an inflammatory swelling of the axilla and groin lymph nodes. Several blood cultures were obtained, and cultures showed growth of gram-negative rods resembling "closed safety pins." The organism growth demonstrated non–lactose-fermenting colonies on MacConkey agar. Phenotypic testing demonstrated a nonmotile rod that was biochemically inert. What is the *most* likely pathogen identified?

A. *Yersinia pestis*
B. *Klebsiella pneumoniae*
C. *Proteus vulgaris*
D. *Morganella morganii*

Microbiology/Enterobacterales/3

46. Direct spread of pneumonic plague disease occurs by which route?

A. Fecal–oral route
B. Rat bite
C. Ingestion of contaminated tissue
D. Inhalation of contaminated aerosolized droplets

Microbiology/Pathogenicity/Enterobacterales/2

47. Which isolates of the Order *Enterobacterales* most commonly produce extended-spectrum β-lactamase (ESBL)?

A. *Escherichia coli* and *Klebsiella pneumoniae*
B. *Yersinia enterocolitica* and *Yersinia pestis*
C. *Morganella morganii* and *Proteus vulgaris*
D. *Salmonella typhi* and *Shigella sonnei*

Microbiology/Enterobacterales/1

48. Which of the following *Shigella* spp. serotypes is the *most* often isolated in the United States?

A. Serotype A (*S. dysenteriae*)
B. Serotype B (*S. flexneri*)
C. Serotype C (*S. boydii*)
D. Serotype D (*S. sonnei*)

Microbiology/Serotype/Enterobacterales/1

49. Which organism is transmitted by ingesting undercooked ground beef or raw milk resulting in inflammation and bleeding of the mucosa in the large intestine (i.e., hemorrhagic colitis), which can also lead to hemolytic uremic syndrome (HUS)?

A. *Escherichia coli* (STEC/EHEC/VTEC)—Shiga toxin
B. *Escherichia coli* (ETEC)—enterotoxigenic
C. *Escherichia coli* (EAEC)—enteroaggregative
D. *Proteus mirabilis*

Microbiology/Pathogenicity/Enterobacterales/2

Answers to Questions 45–49

45. A *Y. pestis* is the cause of bubonic and pneumonic plague. Bubonic plague causes swelling of the groin lymph nodes (bubos), whereas pneumonic plague involves the lungs. The infection caused by bubonic plague may result in fulminant bacteremia that is usually fatal. The transmission is from rodents (rats, ground squirrels, or prairie dogs) to humans by the bite of fleas (vectors) or by ingestion of contaminated animal tissues. Pneumonic plague is acquired via droplet transmission of aerosolized particles when there is close contact with other pneumonic plague victims. Human-to-human transmission is possible with the pneumonic plague.

46. D Bubonic plague involves an inflammatory swelling of the lymph nodes of the axilla and groin, whereas pneumonic plague is associated with aerosolized droplets that are inhaled (respiratory route of infection). Both infections are caused by the same member of the Order *Enterobacterales*, family Yersiniaceae—*Y. pestis*.

47. A Point mutation occurs in most members of the *Enterobacterales* that result in production of a β-lactamase that hydrolyzes broad-spectrum antibiotics, such as the cephalosporins, as well as penicillin and monobactam antibiotics. These are known as *ESBL producers*. The most common ESBL organisms are *K. pneumoniae* and *E. coli*. ESBL strains are detected by demonstrating resistance to β-lactam antibiotics.

48. D *S. sonnei* (serotype D) is the most isolated species of *Shigella* in the United States and Europe. Humans are the only reservoirs, and of the estimated 500,000 cases of shigellosis in the United States per year, *S. sonnei* is responsible for 85% of the infections.

49. A *E. coli* (STEC) is the organism referred to as enterohemorrhagic *E. coli* (EHEC) and is also known as verocytotoxin-producing *E. coli* (VTEC), which produces a toxin similar to the Shiga toxin produced by *S. dysenteriae*. STEC strains encode Shiga toxin 1 (Stx1) and/or Shiga toxin 2 (Stx2). Inflammation and bleeding of the mucosa of the large intestine can lead to kidney failure and HUS. HUS is characterized by low platelet counts and hemolytic anemia, leading to transfusions and dialysis and death. The two most common serotypes are O157:H7 and O157:NM (nonmotile). Unlike dysentery, the wet preps of the stools usually lack WBCs.

50. This organism is transmitted by ingesting contaminated fresh water and/or shellfish, resulting in watery, dysentery-like stools and chronic diarrhea. Culture on stool media and initial testing show the following results:

MacConkey agar = Both lactose-fermenting and non–lactose-fermenting colonies
Sheep blood agar = Nonhemolytic, shiny, opaque, smooth, nonspreading
Oxidase = + DNase = Neg String test = Neg

What is the *most* likely preliminary identification?

A. *Proteus vulgaris*
B. *Escherichia coli*
C. *Salmonella* spp.
D. *Plesiomonas shigelloides*

Microbiology/Enterobacterales/3

51. Which reagent(s) is (are) used to develop the red color indicative of a positive reaction in the nitrate reduction test?

A. Sulfanilic acid and α-naphthylamine
B. Ehrlich and Kovac reagents
C. *o*-Nitrophenyl-β-D-galactopyranoside
D. Kovac reagent

Microbiology/Biochemical/Enterobacterales/1

52. Which is the *best* rapid test to differentiate *P. shigelloides* from a *Shigella* species on selective enteric agar?

A. Oxidase
B. Indole
C. TSI agar
D. Urease

Microbiology/Biochemical/Enterobacterales/2

53. A 49-year-old individual who traveled to Mexico City returned with severe dysentery. The patients' symptoms are fever; abdominal cramping; and bloody, mucoidal, frequent stools. In addition to this, many WBCs are present in the Gram-stained smear. Stool culture gave the following results:

Gram staining = gram-negative rods	Lactose = +
Indole = +	Lysine decarboxylase = Neg
Urease = Neg	Motility = Neg

What is the *most* likely organism?

A. *Salmonella* spp.
B. *Proteus mirabilis*
C. *Escherichia coli*
D. Enteroinvasive *E. coli* (EIEC)

Microbiology/Enterobacterales/3

Answers to Questions 50–53

50. D *P. shigelloides* is the only oxidase-positive member of the *Enterobacterales* and causes gastroenteritis from consuming uncooked shellfish. Although rare, extraintestinal infections include wounds, bacteremia, and meningitis.

51. A In the nitrate test, nitrites formed by bacterial reduction of nitrates will diazotize sulfanilic acid. The diazonium compound complexes with α-naphthylamine, forming a red product. Media containing nitrates are used for the identification of nonfermenters. When testing nonfermenters, it is wise to confirm a negative reaction using zinc dust. The diazonium compound detects nitrites only, and the organism may have reduced nitrates to nitrogen, ammonia, nitrous oxide, or hydroxylamine. Zinc ions reduce residual nitrates in the media to nitrites. A red color produced after the addition of zinc indicates the presence of residual nitrates, confirming a true negative reaction. If a red or pink color does not occur after adding zinc, then the organism reduces the nitrate to a product other than nitrite, and the result is considered positive.

52. A *P. shigelloides* is a non–lactose-fermenter (NLF) that will resemble *Shigella* spp. on MacConkey agar. Both are TSI Alk/Acid and urease negative. *Plesiomonas* produces indole and *Shigella* usually demonstrates delayed production of indole. However, *Plesiomonas* is oxidase positive, whereas *Shigella* spp. are oxidase negative.

53. D EIEC produces dysentery like that by *Shigella*, with invasion and destruction of the intestinal mucosal epithelium. Leukocytes are seen on the Gram-stained smear. Adults who travel to foreign countries with inadequate sanitation or food processing are at greatest risk.

54. An 80-year-old patient was admitted to the hospital with a fever of 102°F. A sputum Gram stain revealed many gram-negative rods. Following overnight incubation, the organism grew on MacConkey agar and blood agar. The patient was diagnosed with pneumonia. The following biochemical results were obtained from the pure colonies isolated on the blood agar:

H_2S = Neg	Lactose = +	Urease = +
Citrate = +	Indole = +	VP = +
Motility = Neg	Resistance to ampicillin and carbenicillin	

What is the *most* likely identification?

A. *Klebsiella oxytoca*
B. *Proteus mirabilis*
C. *Escherichia coli*
D. *Klebsiella pneumoniae*

Microbiology/Enterobacterales/3

55. An immunocompromised 58-year-old patient on chemotherapy received 2 units of packed RBCs. The patient died 3 days later, and the report from the autopsy revealed that the patient's death resulted from septic shock. The blood bags were submitted for culture, and the following results were noted:

GROWTH OF AEROBIC GRAM-NEGATIVE RODS ON BOTH MACCONKEY AND BLOOD AGARS

Lactose = Neg	Sucrose = +	Citrate = Neg
Indole = Neg	VP = Neg	H_2S = Neg
Urease = +	Motility 22°C = +	Motility 37°C = Neg

What is the *most* likely identification?

A. *Escherichia coli*
B. *Yersinia enterocolitica*
C. *Enterobacter cloacae*
D. *Citrobacter freundii*

Microbiology/Enterobacterales/3

56. A pediatric patient who had had been camping with family was admitted to the hospital with severe bloody diarrhea and complications of HUS. Several stool specimens were submitted for culture and the following results noted:

Gram staining = Many gram-negative rods, with no WBCs seen
Blood agar = Normal flora MacConkey agar = Normal flora
MacConkey agar with sorbitol = Many clear colonies (sorbitol negative)
Hektoen agar = Normal flora Campy agar = No growth

What is the *most* likely identification?

A. *Yersinia* spp.
B. *E. coli* O157:H7
C. *Salmonella* spp.
D. *Shigella* spp.

Microbiology/Enterobacterales/3

Answers to Questions 54–56

54. A *K. oxytoca* is like *K. pneumoniae* except that the indole test is positive for *K. oxytoca*.

55. B *Y. enterocolitica* has been associated with fatal bacteremia and septic shock from contaminated blood transfusion products. The motility at room temperature is a clue to this identification.

56. B *E. coli* O157:H7 is usually the most common isolate from bloody stools of the EHEC group; illness results from consuming contaminated undercooked beef. These strains are waterborne and foodborne, and the infections from *E. coli* O157:H7 are greatest during the summer months in temperate climates.

57. **A 14-year-old patient presented to the emergency department; the patient had been to the doctor's office 2 days ago with abdominal pain, diarrhea, and a low-grade fever. The patient was diagnosed at the emergency department with pseudoappendicular syndrome. The stool sample contained blood and WBCs. Culture and biochemical tests showed the following results:**

AEROBIC GRAM-NEGATIVE RODS ON MACCONKEY AGAR (CLEAR COLONIES)		
Campy agar = No growth		
Lactose = Neg	Sucrose = +	Citrate = Neg
Indole = Neg	VP = Neg	H_2S = Neg
Motility 37°C = Neg	Motility 22°C = +	Hektoen agar = NF

What is the *most* likely identification?

A. *Yersinia enterocolitica*
B. *Salmonella* spp.
C. *Shigella* spp.
D. *Escherichia coli*

Microbiology/Enterobacterales/3

58. **A patient exhibits fever, chills, abdominal cramps, diarrhea, vomiting, and bloody stools 10 to 12 hours after eating. Which organisms will *most* likely grow from this patient's stool culture?**

A. *Salmonella* or *Yersinia* spp.
B. *Escherichia coli* O157:H7 or *Shigella* spp.
C. *Staphylococcus aureus* or *Clostridium perfringens*
D. *Salmonella* or *Staphylococcus* spp.

Microbiology/Enterobacterales/3

59. **Which biochemical tests should be performed to identify colorless colonies growing on MacConkey agar (swarming colonies on blood agar) from a catheterized urine specimen?**

A. Indole, phenylalanine deaminase, and urease
B. Glucose, oxidase, and lactose utilization
C. Phenylalanine deaminase and bile solubility
D. H_2S and catalase

Microbiology/Enterobacterales/3

60. **Matrix-assisted laser desorption/ionization time-of-flight mass spectrometry (MALDI-TOF MS) cannot clearly differentiate which of the following two organisms?**

A. *Escherichia coli* and *Salmonella* spp.
B. *Yersina pestis* and *Yersina enterocolitica*
C. *Klebsiella oxytoca* and *Pseudomonas aeruginosa*
D. *Plesiomonas shigelloides* and *Escherichia coli*

Microbiology/Enterobacterales/2

61. **A patient presented with severe diarrhea. Stool culture did not identify any unusual pathogenic bacteria and was reported to the primary care provider following 48 hours of incubation as normal flora. However, the patient continued to experience severe symptoms. A syndromic nucleic acid panel was ordered by the provider and returned a positive result for *E. coli* O157-H7. What is the reason for the discrepancy between the culture and the molecular test?**

A. The technologist erroneously reported normal flora
B. Stool cultures can be negative whereas NAAT has a lower limit of detection
C. The patient likely acquired a new infection after the stool specimen was collected
D. The NAAT may have been contaminated from another sample

Microbiology/Enterobacterales/3

Answers to Questions 57–61

57. A Blood and leukocytes can be present in stools. Patients exhibiting appendicitis-like symptoms with lactose-negative colonies growing on MacConkey agar (small colonies at 24 hours, but larger colonies at 48 hours if incubated at room temperature) should be tested for the growth of *Y. enterocolitica*.

58. B Both *E. coli* O157:H7 and *Shigella* spp. are invasive and cause bloody stools.

59. A A swarmer on blood agar would most likely be a *Proteus* spp. A lactose nonfermenter and swarmer that is often isolated from UTIs is *P. mirabilis*.

60. B MALDI-TOF MS is relatively accurate when identifying the *Enterobacterales* to the genus level. However, at the time of this writing, new species may not be included, and it is limited in the ability to differentiate *Y. pestis* from *Y. enterocolitica*.

61. B Traditional stool cultures and enzyme immunoassays may produce false-negative results for the identification of *E. coli* O157-H7. NAAT has a much a lower limit of detection than the other methods, resulting in the identification of approximately 58% more infections caused by this pathogenic bacterium.

9.5
Nonfermentative Bacilli

1. **What are the *most* appropriate biochemical screening tests to presumptively differentiate and identify the gram-negative nonfermentative bacilli (NFB) from the *Enterobacterales*?**
   A. Catalase, decarboxylation of arginine, growth on blood agar
   B. Motility, urease, morphology on blood agar
   C. Oxidase, TSI, nitrate reduction, growth on MacConkey agar
   D. Oxidase, indole, and growth on blood agar
   Microbiology/Biochemical/NFB/2

2. **Presumptive biochemical tests used for identification of the *Pseudomonas* spp. are:**
   A. Oxidase, oxidation–fermentation (OF) glucose (open), OF glucose (sealed), motility, pigment production
   B. Growth on blood agar plate (BAP) and eosin–methylene blue (EMB) agars, lysine decarboxylation, catalase
   C. Growth on MacConkey, EMB, and XLD agars and motility
   D. Growth on mannitol salt agar and flagellar stain
   Microbiology/Biochemicasl/NFB/2

3. **Which tests are *most* appropriate to differentiate *Pseudomonas aeruginosa* from *Pseudomonas putida*?**
   A. Oxidase, motility, pyoverdin
   B. Oxidase, motility, lactose
   C. Oxidase, ONPG, DNase
   D. Mannitol, nitrate reduction, growth at 42°C
   Microbiology/Biochemical/NFB/2

4. **Which test group *best* differentiates *Acinetobacter* spp. from *P. aeruginosa*?**
   A. Oxidase, motility, nitrate reduction
   B. MacConkey growth, 37°C growth, catalase
   C. Blood agar growth, oxidase, catalase
   D. Oxidase, TSI, MacConkey growth
   Microbiology/Biochemical/NFB/2

Answers to Questions 1–4

1. C NFB will grow on the slant of TSI or KIA, but they do not acidify the butt (glucose fermentation), as do the *Enterobacterales*. NFB can be cytochrome oxidase positive or negative, but all the *Enterobacterales*, except *Plesiomonas shigelloides,* are oxidase negative. *Enterobacterales* grow well on MacConkey agar and reduce nitrate to nitrite, but NFB grow poorly or not at all on MacConkey agar, and most do not reduce nitrate. Nearly 70% of NFB recovered from clinical specimens are strains of *P. aeruginosa, Acinetobacter* spp., or *Stenotrophomonas maltophilia.*

2. A OF tubes are used to determine fermentation and oxidation of glucose or other carbohydrates in bacillus species (glucose oxidation positive and glucose fermentation negative). The positive cytochrome oxidase test and pigment production indicate a possible *Pseudomonas* species. Several NFB produce pigments that aid in species identification: *P. aeruginosa* produces pyoverdins (green), pyocyanin (blue aqua pigment), pyrorubrin (red), or pyomelanin (brown) diffusible pigments on MacConkey agar. The characteristic grapelike odor of aminoacetophenone and growth at 42°C are characteristic of *P. aeruginosa.*

3. D Both organisms are oxidase positive, are motile, and produce pyoverdin. Both are negative for ONPG and DNase. The differentiating tests are:

Test	*P. aeruginosa*	*P. putida*
Mannitol	+	Variable (25% Pos)
Reduction of nitrate to nitrite	+	Neg
42°C growth	+	Neg

4. A *Acinetobacter* spp. are nonmotile rods, which appear as coccobacillary forms in clinical specimens. All are oxidase negative and catalase positive. *P. aeruginosa* reduces nitrate to nitrite, whereas *Acinetobacter* spp. do not. The genus *Acinetobacter* is divided into two groups: saccharolytic or glucose-oxidizing species and asaccharolytic or nonglucose species.

5. In addition to motility, which biochemical test *best* differentiates *Acinetobacter* spp. and *Alcaligenes faecalis*?
A. TSI agar
B. Oxidase
C. Urease
D. Flagellar stain
Microbiology/Biochemical/NFB/2

6. The *most* noted phenotypic and biochemical differences between *P. aeruginosa* and *Stenotrophomonas maltophilia* are:
A. Oxidase, catalase, and TSI
B. Oxidase, catalase, and ONPG
C. Oxidase, 42°C growth, and polar tuft of flagella
D. Catalase, TSI, and pigment
Microbiology/Biochemical/NFB/2

7. Which NFB is usually associated with a lung infection related to cystic fibrosis (CF)?
A. *Pseudomonas fluorescens*
B. *Pseudomonas aeruginosa*
C. *Pseudomonas putida*
D. *Burkholderia pseudomallei*
Microbiology/Pathogenicity/NFB/2

8. A nonfermenter recovered from an eye wound is oxidase positive, motile with polar monotrichous flagella, and grows at 42°C. Colonies on blood agar are nonhemolytic, dry, wrinkled or smooth, buff to light brown, and difficult to remove from the agar. In which DNA homology group should this organism be placed?
A. *Pseudomonas stutzeri*
B. *Pseudomonas fluorescens*
C. *Pseudomonas putida*
D. *Burkholderia pseudomallei*
Microbiology/NFB/3

9. Which organism is associated with immunodeficiency syndromes and melioidosis (a glanders-like disease)?
A. *Pseudomonas aeruginosa*
B. *Pseudomonas stutzeri*
C. *Pseudomonas putida*
D. *Burkholderia pseudomallei*
Microbiology/Pathogenicity/NFB/2

10. Which phenotypic characteristics and biochemical tests are used to differentiate *Burkholderia cepacia* from *S. maltophilia*?
A. Pigment on blood agar, oxidase, DNase
B. Pigment on MacConkey agar, motility
C. Glucose, maltose, lysine decarboxylase
D. TSI agar, motility, oxidase
Microbiology/Biochemical/NFB/2

Answers to Questions 5–10

5. B The two genera, *Acinetobacter* and *Alcaligenes*, are very similar. Both use oxidation for the metabolism of carbohydrates, with some strains being asaccharolytic. Both grow well on MacConkey agar. However, *Acinetobacter* is nonmotile and oxidase negative. *Alcaligenes* is motile by peritrichous flagella and oxidase positive.

6. C The two genera, *Pseudomonas* and *Stenotrophomonas*, are motile and grow well on MacConkey agar. However, *P. aeruginosa* is oxidase positive and grows at 42°C but is motile by polar monotrichous flagella. *S. maltophilia* is oxidase negative, does not grow at 42°C, and is motile by a polar tuft of flagella.

7. B *P. aeruginosa* is often recovered from the respiratory secretions of patients with CF. If the patient is chronically infected with the mucoid strain of *P. aeruginosa*, the biochemical identification is very difficult. The mucoid strain results from the production of large amounts of alginate, a polysaccharide that surrounds the cell forming a biofilm.

8. A *P. stutzeri* produces buff to brown, dry, wrinkled nonhemolytic colonies that are tough and adhere to the media as well as smooth colonies. *B. pseudomallei* produces similar colony types but is distinguished by biochemical tests and susceptibility to the polymyxins.

9. D *B. pseudomallei* produces wrinkled colonies resembling *P. stutzeri*. Infections may be asymptomatic to severe, causing skin abscesses, internal abscesses in several organs, acute pulmonary disease, and sepsis. The organism has become geographically widespread in Australia, Southeast Asia, Africa, the Americas, and China as well as throughout other areas in Asia and India.

10. A Both organisms produce yellowish pigment, but the oxidase and DNase tests are differential.

Test	*B. cepacia*	*S. maltophilia*
Pigment on BAP	Green-yellow	Lavender-green
Oxidase	+	Neg
DNase	Neg	+
Motility	+	+
Glucose OF (oxidation)	+	+
Maltose OF (oxidation)	+	+
Lysine decarboxylase	+	+

11. The following phenotypic characteristics biochemical results were obtained from a pure culture of gram-negative rods recovered from the pulmonary secretions of a 10-year-old CF patient with pneumonia:

Oxidase = +	Motility = +
Glucose OF (oxidation) = +	Gelatin hydrolysis = +
Pigment = Red, nonflurorescent	Arginine dihydrolase = +
Growth at 42°C = +	

Which is the *most* likely organism?
A. *Burkholderia pseudomallei*
B. *Pseudomonas stutzeri*
C. *Burkholderia cepacia*
D. *Pseudomonas aeruginosa*
Microbiology/Biochemical/NFB/3

12. *Alcaligenes faecalis* is biochemically distinguished from *Bordetella bronchiseptica* with which test?
A. Urease (rapid)
B. Oxidase
C. Growth on MacConkey agar
D. Motility
Microbiology/Biochemical/NFB/1

13. *Chryseobacterium* spp. are biochemically distinguished from *Acinetobacter* spp. by which of the following two tests?
A. Oxidase, growth on MacConkey agar
B. Oxidase and OF (glucose)
C. TSI and urea hydrolysis
D. TSI and VP
Microbiology/Biochemical/NFB/2

14. A gram-negative coccobacillus was recovered on chocolate agar from the CSF of an immunosuppressed patient. The organism was nonmotile and positive for indophenol oxidase but failed to grow on MacConkey agar. The organism was highly susceptible to penicillin. The *most* probable identification is:
A. *Acinetobacter* spp.
B. *Pseudomonas aeruginosa*
C. *Pseudomonas stutzeri*
D. *Moraxella lacunata*
Microbiology/Biochemical/NFB/2

15. Cetrimide is used as a selective isolation agar for which organism?
A. *Acinetobacter* spp.
B. *Pseudomonas aeruginosa*
C. *Moraxella* spp.
D. *Stenotrophomonas maltophilia*
Microbiology/Biochemical/NFB/2

Answers to Questions 11–15

11. D The oxidase test and red pigment (pyorubin), as well as growth at 42°C, distinguish *P. aeruginosa* from the other nonfermenters listed, particularly *B. cepacia*, which is also associated with CF.

12. A *Alcaligenes* spp. and *Bordetella* spp. (nonpertussis) are two organisms that are very similar biochemically, but *B. bronchiseptica* is urease positive. Both organisms are oxidase positive, grow on MacConkey agar, and are motile by peritrichous flagella. *B. bronchiseptica* grows well on MacConkey agar, but other species of *Bordetella* are fastidious gram-negative rods. *B. bronchiseptica* is the cause of mild respiratory infections, whereas *B. pertussis* is the cause of whooping cough.

13. A *Chryseobacterium* spp. and *Acinetobacter* spp. often produce a yellow pigment on blood or chocolate agar and are nonmotile. *Acinetobacter* spp. are oxidase negative, grow on MacConkey agar, and are coccobacillary on the Gram-stained smear. In contrast, *Chryseobacterium* spp. are oxidase positive, do not typically grow on MacConkey agar or demonstrate delayed, poor growth, and are typically rod shaped.

14. D *Moraxella* spp. are oxidase positive and nonmotile, and this distinguishes them from *Acinetobacter* spp. and most *Pseudomonas* spp. *Moraxella* spp. are highly sensitive to penicillin, but *Acinetobacter* spp. and *Pseudomonas* spp. are penicillin resistant. *M. lacunata* is implicated in infections involving immunosuppressed patients. *M. lacunata* is usually associated with eye infections but can also be the cause of bacteremia and respiratory infections in the immunosuppressed patient.

15. B Growth on Cetrimide (acetyltrimethylammonium bromide) agar is used for the isolation and presumptive identification of *P. aeruginosa*. Except for *P. fluorescens*, the other pseudomonads are inhibited along with related nonfermentative bacteria. Colonies of *P. aeruginosa* appear as yellow-green to blue-green colonies on Cetrimide agar. Cetrimide is toxic to many bacteria by releasing nitrogen and phosphorus.

16. A specimen from a 15-year-old burn patient was cultured after débridement, and the following results were obtained:

Oxidase = +	Lysine decarboxylase = Neg
Catalase = +	Motility = +
Ornithine decarboxylase Neg	Glucose = + for = oxidation
Arginine dihydrolase = +	Maltose = Neg for oxidation
Penicillin = Resistant	Aminoglycosides = Susceptible
Colistin (polymixin B) = Susceptible	

These results indicate which of the following organisms?

A. *Acinetobacter* spp.
B. *Moraxella lacunata*
C. *Pseudomonas aeruginosa*
D. *Alcaligenes* spp.

Microbiology/NFB/3

17. A yellow pigment–producing organism on chocolate agar was recovered from the blood of a neonate. The isolate is nonmotile, oxidase positive, and demonstrates no growth on MacConkey agar. What is the *most* likely organism?

A. *Acinetobacter* spp.
B. *Pseudomonas aeruginosa*
C. *Burkholderia cepacia*
D. *Elizabethkingia meningoseptica*

Microbiology/NFB/3

18. A culture from an intra-abdominal abscess produced orange-tan colonies on blood agar producing the following results:

Oxidase = +	Nitrate reduction = +
KIA = Alk/Alk (H_2S)+	Motility = + (single polar flagellum)
DNase = +	Ornithine decarboxylase = +
Growth at 42°C = Neg	MacConkey agar = colorless colonies (non–lactose fermenter)

The *most* likely identification is:

A. *Shewanella putrefaciens*
B. *Acinetobacter* spp.
C. *Pseudomonas aeruginosa*
D. *Chryseobacterium* spp.

Microbiology/NFB/3

19. *Chryseobacterium* spp. and *B. cepacia* are easily differentiated by which biochemical test?

A. Motility
B. OF glucose
C. Oxidase
D. Cetrimide agar

Microbiology/Biochemical/NFB/1

20. A 15-year-old patient complained of severe eye irritation after removing soft contact lenses. A swab specimen of the infected right eye was obtained by an ophthalmologist, who ordered culture and sensitivity testing. The sample was inoculated on blood agar and MacConkey agar. Following 24 hours of incubation, the isolate was identified as an oxidase-positive, gram-negative rod. The organism appeared as round, flat, and colorless colonies on MacConkey agar that autofluoresced under ultraviolet light. What is the *most* likely identification?

A. *Burkholderia cepacia*
B. *Pseudomonas aeruginosa*
C. *Stenotrophomonas maltophilia*
D. *Acinetobacter* spp.

Microbiology/NFB/3

Answers to Questions 16–20

16. C *P. aeruginosa* is a cause of a significant number of burn wound infections; these organisms can exist in distilled water and underchlorinated water. *Acinetobacter* spp. are oxidase negative and *Moraxella* spp. are highly susceptible to penicillin.

17. D All species of *Acinetobacter* are oxidase negative, are nonmotile, and grow on MacConkey agar. *Elizabethkingia* spp. produce yellow pigment (like some *Acinetobacter*) but are oxidase positive and do not grow well on MacConkey agar. *B. cepacia* also produces a yellow pigment but is motile. *P. aeruginosa* is motile and grows on MacConkey agar.

18. A *S. putrefaciens* produces abundant H_2S on KIA or TSI. *Shewanella* spp. are the only nonfermenters that produce H_2S on these media.

19. A *B. cepacia* (93%) are weakly oxidase positive and motile. *Chryseobacterium* spp. are oxidase positive but are nonmotile.

20. B *P. aeruginosa* is an opportunistic organism that is not part of the human normal microbiota. Contact lens solution contamination, eye injury, or contact lens eye trauma are factors that contribute to *P. aeruginosa* eye infections. The characteristic blue-green pigment (pyocyanin) fluoresces and is produced by *P. aeruginosa*.

21. Which of the listed *Pseudomonas* spp. is associated with the following virulence factors: exotoxin A, endotoxins, proteolytic enzymes, antimicrobial resistance, and production of alginate?
A. *Pseudomonas fluorescens*
B. *Pseudomonas putida*
C. *Pseudomonas stutzeri*
D. *Pseudomonas aeruginosa*
Microbiology/Pathogenicity/NFB/3

22. A 20-year-old horse groomer exhibited a "glanders-like" infection. The patient has a history of several open wounds on the hands 2 weeks before presenting with swelling of the lymph nodes. A gram-negative rod was recovered from a blood culture that grew well on blood and MacConkey agars. Most of the biochemical tests were negative, including the cytochrome oxidase test. What is the *most* likely identification?
A. *Burkholderia mallei*
B. *Pseudomonas aeruginosa*
C. *Pseudomonas stutzeri*
D. *Burkholderia pseudomallei*
Microbiology/NFB/3

23. A Vietnam War veteran presented with a "glanders-like" infection (melioidosis). Several blood cultures produced gram-negative rods that were positive for cytochrome oxidase, oxidized glucose and xylose, and grew at 42°C. What is the *most* likely organism?
A. *Stenotrophomonas maltophilia*
B. *Burkholderia pseudomallei*
C. *Pseudomonas aeruginosa*
D. *Acinetobacter* spp.
Microbiology/NFB/3

24. Cytochrome oxidase-positive, gram-negative NFB were recovered from a stool sample of a patient with CF. The isolates produced wet (mucoid) light blue colonies on tryptic soy agar. Which identification is *most* likely?
A. *Acinetobacter* spp.
B. *Pseudomonas putida*
C. *Pseudomonas stutzeri*
D. *Pseudomonas aeruginosa*
Microbiology/NFB/2

25. Several postoperative hospitalized patients were colonized with gram-negative coccobacilli capable of growth on MacConkey agar. Specimens were obtained from blood, urine, and wound sites. Biochemical testing revealed oxidase-negative, nonmotile organisms. Which of the following is the *most* likely cause of the nosocomial infection?
A. *Acinetobacter* spp.
B. *Pseudomonas aeruginosa*
C. *Burkholderia cepacia*
D. *Pseudomonas putida*
Microbiology/NFB/3

Answers to Questions 21–25

21. D *P. aeruginosa* is highly resistant to many antimicrobial drugs as well as being one of the most often cultured opportunistic organisms. This virulence factor allows for many nosocomial infections, such as UTI, wounds (in burn patients), bacteremia, respiratory tract infection, and central nervous system infection.

22. A *B. mallei* is rarely transmitted to humans. It is the causative agent of glanders in mules, donkeys, and horses. It is not part of the human skin microbiota, and the most likely transmission to humans is through broken skin.

23. B *B. pseudomallei* infections often produce abscesses in organs (liver, spleen, lungs) as well as on the skin, in soft tissue, and in joints and bones. Vietnam War veterans especially may harbor these organisms, which were historically limited to tropical and subtropical environments (Southeast Asia and Australia) but have become more geographically widespread. The organism may surface years later after surviving in a latent state within phagocytes.

24. D Patients with CF are often colonized with *P. aeruginosa*. *P. aeruginosa* produces alginate that accounts for the "wet, mucoid" appearance. The overproduction of alginate (biofilm) inhibits phagocytosis and increases the antibiotic resistance of the organism. The light blue color results from lower production of polyamine. The result is chronic infections in patients with CF with the "wet" form of *P. aeruginosa*.

25. A *Acinetobacter* spp. often colonize immunocompromised patients through IV or urinary catheters. *Acinetobacter* spp. are nonmotile, oxidase-negative coccobacilli that grow well on MacConkey agar.

26. A nosocomial infection involving an 80-year-old patient, recovering from pneumonia, produced many oxidase-negative colonies on MacConkey agar. Further testing results are:

Motility = +	Maltose = +	Resistant to most β-lactams
Glucose = +	Resistant to most aminoglycosides	

The *most* likely identification is:

A. *Acinetobacter* spp.
B. *Stenotrophomonas maltophilia*
C. *Pseudomonas aeruginosa*
D. *Burkholderia gladioli*

Microbiology/NFB/3

27. A non–lactose-fermenting gram-negative bacterium was isolated from a burn wound specimen. Which of the following is the *best* choice of tests to differentiate *P. aeruginosa* from *Acinetobacter* spp.?

A. Growth on MacConkey agar, catalase, growth at 37°C
B. Oxidase, motility, growth at 42°C
C. Growth on blood agar, oxidase, growth at 35°C
D. String test and coagulase test

Microbiology/NFB/3

28. MALDI-TOF MS is limited in the ability to differentiate some of the uncommon species of *Pseudomonas* as well as other gram-negative NFB. What is the *most* likely limitation associated with using this method to identify these organisms?

A. Difficulty spotting sufficient organisms on the test card
B. Lack of clinical isolates for an accurate identification
C. There is no limitation to identify NFB using this method
D. Failure to lyse and release the proteins in the matrix

Microbiology/NFB/3

Answers to Questions 26–28

26. B *S. maltophilia* are oxidase negative, whereas all the other choices are oxidase positive. (*B. gladioli* are weakly oxidase positive and rarely recovered from human infections.)

27. B *P. aeruginosa* has a distinctive grape odor. The *best* tests to differentiate it from *Acinetobacter* spp. are growth at 42°C, oxidase, and motility, which give the following results:

	42°C Growth	Oxidase	Motility
P. aeruginosa	+	+	+
Acinetobacter spp.	+/Neg	Neg	Neg

28. B The major limitation to identifying many of the species in the genera included in the gram-negative NFB is the lack of data that is available in the commercial databases. This is simply due to the infrequent isolation of many of the organisms in clinical infections.

9.6

Miscellaneous and Fastidious Gram-Negative Rods

1. A visitor to South America who returned with diarrhea is suspected of being infected with *Vibrio cholerae.* Select the *best* isolation medium for recovery and identification of this organism.

A. MacConkey agar
B. Blood agar
C. TCBS agar
D. XLD agar

Microbiology/Biochemical/Media/2

2. A curved gram-negative, oxidase-positive organism was recovered from a stool culture of a patient experiencing watery diarrhea demonstrating green colonies on TCBS agar and smooth, convex, nonhemolytic colonies on blood agar. Given the following results, what is the *most* likely identification?

Lysine decarboxylase = +	Arginine decarboxylase = Neg
Indole = +	KIA = Alk/Acid
VP = Neg	Lactose = Neg
Urease = ± (variable)	String test = Neg
Arabinose = +	Sucrose = Neg

A. *Vibrio cholerae*
B. *Vibrio parahaemolyticus*
C. *Shigella* spp.
D. *Salmonella* spp.

Microbiology/GNR/3

3. A gram-negative S-shaped rod recovered from CAMP-CVA (cefoperzaone, vancomycin, amphotericin B) selective media incubated in a microaerobic atmosphere (5% O_2, 10% CO_2, and 85% N) for *Campylobacter* species demonstrated the following biochemical results:

Catalase = +	Oxidase = +	Nitrate reduction = +
Motility = +	Hippurate hydrolysis = +	
Growth at 42°C = + nonpigmented		

The *most* likely identification is:

A. *Pseudomonas aeruginosa*
B. *Campylobacter jejuni*
C. *Campylobacter fetus*
D. *Pseudomonas putida*

Microbiology/GNR/3

Answers to Questions 1–3

1. C The growth of yellow or green colonies on the selective TCBS agar is dependent on whether the organism ferments sucrose (producing yellow colonies). *Vibrio* spp. also grow well on 5% sheep blood, chocolate, and MacConkey agars. Enrichment with alkaline peptone broth, pH 8.4, helps recover *Vibrio* spp. from stool specimens.

2. B *V. parahaemolyticus* appear as green colonies on TCBS agar, whereas *V. cholerae* appear as yellow colonies on TCBS. *V. parahaemolyticus* is positive for arabinose and negative for sucrose, whereas *V. cholerae* is negative for arabinose and positive for sucrose. *V. cholerae* is the only *Vibrio* species that causes a positive string test result. In the test, a loopful of bacterial colonies is suspended in sodium deoxycholate, 0.5%, on a glass slide. After 60 seconds, the inoculating loop is lifted out of the suspension. *V. cholerae* forms a long string resembling a string of pearls. *Salmonella* spp. and *Shigella* spp. are oxidase negative.

3. B The only *Campylobacter* spp. that hydrolyze hippurate are *C. jejuni* subsp. *jejuni, C. jejuni* subsp. *doylei,* and *C. curvus. C. curvus,* which is infrequently isolated from human samples, requires H_2 for growth. Some strains of *P. aeruginosa* grow on agar selective for *Campylobacter* at 42°C. *C. fetus* usually will not grow at 42°C but will grow at 25°C and 37°C.

4. Which atmospheric condition is needed to recover the commonly encountered *Campylobacter* spp. from clinical specimens inoculated onto a Campy-selective agar at 35°C to 37°C and 42°C?

A. 5% O_2, 10% CO_2, and 85% N_2
B. 20% O_2, 10% CO_2, and 70% N_2
C. 20% O_2, 20% CO_2, and 60% N_2
D. 20% O_2, 5% CO_2, and 75% N_2

Microbiology/GNR/2

5. Which group of tests *best* differentiates *Arcobacter* spp. from *C. jejuni*?

A. Catalase, oxidase, and Gram stain
B. Catalase, oxidase, and nalidixic acid sensitivity
C. Catalase, oxidase, and cephalothin sensitivity
D. Urease, nitrate, aryl sulfatase, and hippurate hydrolysis

Microbiology/Biochemical/GNR/2

6. Which of the following biochemical tests should be done *first* to differentiate *Aeromonas* spp. from the *Enterobacterales*?

A. Urease
B. OF glucose
C. Oxidase
D. Catalase

Microbiology/Biochemical/GNR/2

7. Which are the *most* reliable biochemical tests that can be performed to differentiate *Aeromonas hydrophila* from *Plesiomonas shigelloides*?

A. Oxidase and motility
B. DNase and Voges-Proskauer test
C. Indole and lysine decarboxylase
D. Growth on MacConkey and blood agar

Microbiology/Biochemical/GNR/2

8. Which genus of small gram-negative oxidase- and catalase-positive coccobacilli is associated mainly with animals but may cause endocarditis and bacteremia as well as wound and dental infections in humans?

A. *Aggregatibacter*
B. *Pseudomonas*
C. *Campylobacter*
D. *Vibrio*

Microbiology/Pathogenicity/GNR/2

Answers to Questions 4–8

4. A *Campylobacter* spp. are best recovered in a microaerobic atmosphere (reduced O_2). The use of a CO_2 incubator is not recommended because the amount of O_2 and CO_2 do not permit any but the most aerotolerant *Campylobacter* to survive. Cultures for *Campylobacter* should be incubated for 48 to 72 hours before reporting no growth.

5. D *Arcobacter* spp. are *Campylobacter*-like bacteria. *A. butzleri* has been isolated from patients with diarrhea, bacteremia, endocarditis, and peritonitis. Both *A. butzleri* and *C. jejuni* are catalase and oxidase positive. However, *Arcobacter* spp. are aryl sulfatase and hippurate negative, which differentiates them from *Campylobacter jejuni*.

6. C *Aeromonas hydrophilia* and other *Aeromonas* spp. have been implicated in acute diarrhea as well as cellulitis and wound infections. Infections usually follow exposure to contaminated soil, water, or food. *Aeromonas* growing on enteric media are differentiated from the *Enterobacterales* species by demonstrating oxidase-positive colonies. The *Aeromonas* are sometimes overlooked as pathogens because most strains grow on selective enteric agar as lactose fermenters.

7. B Both of these bacteria cause diarrhea, grow well on enteric agar, and may be confused with other pathogenic gram-negative rods. Both organisms are positive for oxidase, motility, indole, and lysine decarboxylase. The following reactions are differential:

Test	*A. hydrophilia*	*P. shigelloides*
β-Hemolysis on sheep blood agar	+	Neg
DNase	+	Neg
Voges-Proskauer	+	Neg

8. A *Aggregatibacter* spp. share many biochemical characteristics of the *Haemophilus* spp. Infections most often associated with this gram-negative coccobacillus are subacute bacterial endocarditis and periodontal disease (its main habitat is the mouth). The most common human isolate is *Aggregatibacter actinomycetemcomitans*, which grows slowly on chocolate agar. It is positive for catalase, nitrate reduction, and glucose fermentation. It does not grow on MacConkey agar and is negative for oxidase, urease, indole, X, and V requirements.

9. Which of the following tests may be used to differentiate *Cardiobacterium hominis* from *Aggregatibacter* spp.?

A. Gram stain
B. Indole
C. Anaerobic incubation
D. Oxidase

Microbiology/Biochemical/GNR/1

10. A mixture of slender gram-negative rods and coccobacilli with rounded ends was recovered from blood cultures after a patient's root canal surgery. Given the following biochemical results after 48 hours of incubation, what is the *most* likely organism?

Catalase = Neg	Ornithine decarboxylase = +
Urease = Neg	Lysine decarboxylase = +
Oxidase = +	X and V requirement = Neg
Indole = Neg	Carbohydrates = Neg (no acid produced)
Growth on blood and chocolate agar = + (with pitting of agar)	
Growth on MacConkey agar = Neg	

A. *Eikenella corrodens*
B. *Aggregatibacter* spp.
C. *Cardiobacterium hominis*
D. *Proteus* spp.

Microbiology/GNR/3

11. *Kingella kingae* can *best* be differentiated from *Eikenella corrodens* on which primary culture medium?

A. Sheep blood agar
B. Chocolate agar
C. MacConkey agar
D. Xylose lysine deoxycholate agar

Microbiology/GNR/2

12. *K. kingae* is usually associated with which type of infection?

A. Middle ear infection
B. Endocarditis
C. Meningitis
D. Urogenital infection

Microbiology/Pathogenicity/GNR/1

Answers to Questions 9–12

9. B *C. hominis* (indole positive) is a gram-negative coccobacillus biochemically similar to *Aggregatibacter* spp. (indole negative). Like *Aggregatibacter* spp., it is a cause of endocarditis. However, *Cardiobacterium* spp. are positive for cytochrome oxidase and negative for nitrate reduction and catalase, whereas most *Aggregatibacter* spp. are variable for oxidase and positive for nitrate reduction and catalase. *C. hominis* will grow on blood agar after 48 to 72 hours in 5% CO_2 at 35°C, but *Aggregatibacter* requires chocolate agar.

10. A *E. corrodens* is a part of the normal microbiota of the upper respiratory tract and the mouth. It is often seen after trauma to the head and neck, dental infections, and human bite wounds. It requires blood for growth. The organism causes pits in the agar where colonies are located. The smell of bleach may be apparent when the plates are uncovered for examination. *Aggregatibacter* spp. and *C. hominis* both utilize several carbohydrates, and *Proteus* spp. are oxidase negative.

11. A Both *K. kingae* and *E. corrodens* are gram-negative rods that are oxidase positive and catalase negative. Both grow well on blood and chocolate agars and cause pitting of the media, and neither grows on MacConkey or XLD agar. However, *K. kingae* strains produce a narrow zone of β-hemolysis on sheep blood agar like that of group B streptococci.

12. B *Kingella* spp. are gram-negative coccobacilli or plump-looking rods. They are part of the normal flora of the upper respiratory and urogenital tracts of humans. Infection is seen primarily in patients having underlying heart disease, poor oral hygiene, or iatrogenic mucosal ulcerations (e.g., radiation therapy), in whom the organism is recovered from blood cultures.

13. Cultures obtained from a dog bite wound produced yellow, tan, and slightly pink colonies on blood and chocolate agar, with a margin of finger-like projections appearing as a film around the colonies. Given the following results following 24 hours of incubation, which is the *most* likely organism?

Oxidase = +	Catalase = +
No growth on MacConkey agar	Motility = Neg

A. *Aggregatibacter* spp.
B. *Eikenella* spp.
C. *Capnocytophaga* spp.
D. *Pseudomonas* spp.

Microbiology/GNR/3

14. Smooth gray colonies showing no hemolytic activity were recovered from an infected cat scratch wound culture; the colonies grew on blood and chocolate agar (a musty odor was noted) but failed to grow on MacConkey agar. The organism is a gram-negative pleomorphic rod that is catalase and oxidase positive and strongly indole positive. The *most* likely organism is:

A. *Haemophilus* spp.
B. *Pasteurella* spp.
C. *Proteus* spp.
D. *Pseudomonas* spp.

Microbiology/GNR/3

15. Which culture medium should be used to recover *B. pertussis* from a nasopharyngeal specimen?

A. Chocolate agar
B. Blood agar
C. MacConkey agar
D. Bordet-Gengou agar

Microbiology/Coccobacillus/2

16. Which medium is recommended for the recovery of *Brucella* spp. from blood and bone marrow specimens?

A. Blood culture broth media, blood and chocolate agar
B. Blood culture bottles with *Brucella* broth
C. Bordet-Gengou agar plates and THIO broth
D. Blood culture bottles with THIO broth

Microbiology/Coccobacillus/2

17. In addition to CO_2 requirements and biochemical characteristics, *B. melitensis* and *B. abortus* are differentiated by growth on media containing which two dyes?

A. Basic fuchsin and thionine
B. Methylene blue and crystal violet
C. Carbol fuchsin and iodine
D. Safranin and methylene blue

Microbiology/Biochemical/Coccobacilli/2

Answers to Questions 13–17

13. C The *Capnocytophaga* species *C. gingivalis*, *C. granulosa*, *C. haemolytica*, *C. leadbetteri*, *C. periodontitidis*, *C. sputigena*, and *C. ochracea* are part of the normal oropharyngeal flora of humans; however, *C. canimorsus* and *C. cynodegmi* are associated with infections resulting from dog bite wounds and cat bites as well as scratch wounds.

14. B *Pasteurella multocida* is part of the normal oral flora of cats and dogs and is frequently recovered from infected bite wounds. It produces large amounts of indole and therefore an odor resembling that of colonies of *E. coli*. *Pseudomonas* spp. are also catalase and oxidase positive but grow on MacConkey agar and do not produce indole.

15. D *B. pertussis* is an oxidase-positive, nonmotile, gram-negative coccobacillus and appears as small, round colonies resembling droplets of mercury on Bordet-Gengou media with sheep blood agar. It is fastidious and does not grow on chocolate or MacConkey agar. Cultures should be incubated at 35°C to 37° for up to 1 week in an ambient atmosphere before calling a negative culture. This organism is the cause of whooping cough, which can be prevented by immunization with the diphtheria, tetanus, pertussis vaccine.

16. A Recovery of *Brucella* spp. is typically very sensitive using traditional blood culture media along with blood and chocolate agar. Solid media can be incubated in ambient air or 5% to 10% CO_2. Colonies are typically visible on solid media within 24 to 48 hours. *Brucella* is the cause of undulant fever (acquired by ingesting infected, unpasteurized milk products) and is responsible for many cases of fever of unknown origin. *Brucella melitensis* is the most frequently recovered species.

17. A *B. abortus* can be differentiated from *B. melitensis* by the following reactions:

	H_2S	Urease	CO_2 Requirement	Basic Fuchsin	Thionin (20 mg)
B. melitensis	Neg	V	Neg	+ growth	+ growth
B. abortus	+	+	+/V	+ growth	Neg (no growth)

18. Enriched culture medium containing which amino acids is required for growth of *Francisella tularensis*?
A. Leucine and ornithine
B. Arginine and lysine
C. Cysteine and cystine
D. Histidine and tryptophan
Microbiology/Biochemical/GNR/1

19. Which culture medium is recommended for the recovery of *Legionella pneumophila* from clinical specimens?
A. Chocolate agar
B. Bordet-Gengou agar
C. New yeast extract agar
D. Buffered charcoal–yeast extract (BCYE) agar
Microbiology/Media/GNR/1

20. *Haemophilus aegyptius* causes ocular infections ("pink eye") and requires X and V factors in the primary culture medium for growth. *H. aegyptius* and *H. influenzae* can be identified and differentiated by which two biochemical tests?
A. Indole and xylose
B. Glucose and urease
C. Oxidase and catalase
D. Aminolevulinic acid (ALA) test and oxidase
Microbiology/Biochemical/Coccobacilli/1

21. *Haemophilus* species that require the V factor (NAD) are easily recovered on which primary culture medium?
A. Blood agar made with sheep RBCs
B. Blood agar made with horse RBCs
C. Chocolate agar
D. Xylose agar
Microbiology/Coccobacillus/2

22. Which of the following growth factors are responsible for satellite growth of *Haemophilus* spp. around colonies of *Staphylococcus aureus* growing on sheep blood agar?
A. NAD and hemin
B. Lactose
C. Indole
D. Oxidase
Microbiology/Biochemical/Coccobacilli/1

23. Which of the following primary culture media and biochemical tests can be used to identify *H. haemolyticus* and *H. parahaemolyticus?*
A. Sheep blood agar and chocolate agar
B. Horse blood agar and Mueller-Hinton agar with X and V strips
C. Brain–heart infusion (BHI) agar with sheep RBCs added
D. Chocolate agar and Mueller-Hinton agar with X factor added
Microbiology/Coccobacillus/2

Answers to Questions 18–23

18. C *F. tularensis* (the causative agent of tularemia) is a fastidious gram-negative rod that is best recovered from lymph node aspirates and tissue biopsies. It is oxidase negative, nonmotile, and inert biochemically. Cysteine blood agar is the medium of choice or any enriched media that contains sulfhydryl compounds (cysteine, cystine, thiosulfate, or IsoVitaleX). *F. tularensis* will grow on commercially prepared chocolate agar because it contains X factor and is supplemented with IsoVitaleX. *F. tularensis* may not grow well on MacConkey agar.

19. D *L. pneumophila* should be recovered on BCYE agar. This agar is nonselective but can be made more selective for *Legionella* spp. with the addition of the antibiotics cefamandole, polymixin B, and anisomycin. Any small, glistening, convex colonies on BCYE agar after 2 to 3 days of incubation that do not grow on l-cysteine–deficient BCYE agar or routine nonselective media should be further tested for confirmation of *L. pneumophila*.

20. A Both *H. influenzae* and *H. aegyptius* are glucose, urease, oxidase, and catalase positive. *H. influenzae* (biotype II) is positive for both indole and xylose, whereas *H. aegyptius* is negative for both tests. *H. aegyptius* is responsible for epidemics of conjunctivitis in children.

21. C The V factor, NAD, must first be released from RBCs before it can be assimilated by *Haemophilus* spp. Chocolate agar is made by heating blood agar to lyse RBCs. The released NAD is directly available to the *Haemophilus* species. Chocolate agar also contains the X factor (hemin). All *Haemophilus* spp. except *H. ducreyi* require V factor, whereas X factor is required by *H. influenzae*, *H. aegyptius*, *H. haemolyticus*, and *H. ducreyi*.

22. A *Staphylococcus aureus* growing on sheep blood agar produces NAD (V factor) as a metabolic by-product and β-hemolysins which lyse sheep RBCs, releasing hemin (X factor). This feature allows pinpoint-sized colonies of *Haemophilus* spp. to grow around *Staphylococcus aureus* as satellite colonies.

23. B Production of β-hemolysis is used to distinguish these two species from other *Haemophilus* with the same X and V requirements. Horse blood agar furnishes X factor and, when supplemented with yeast extract, supports the growth of *Haemophilus* spp. Sheep blood agar is not used because it contains growth inhibitors for some *Haemophilus* spp.
H. haemolyticus requires both X and V factor, whereas *H. parahaemolyticus* only requires V factor.

24. The majority of *H. influenzae* invasive infections are caused by which of the following capsular serotypes?

A. a and c
B. a and b
C. b and c
D. c and d

Microbiology/Serotype/Coccobacilli/2

25. Which of the following, usually recovered from blood cultures, is generally associated with subacute bacterial endocarditis?

A. *Haemophilus influenzae*
B. *Haemophilus ducreyi*
C. *Aggregatibacter aphrophilus*
D. *Haemophilus haemolyticus*

Microbiology/Pathogenicity/GNR/1

26. Which *Haemophilus* species is difficult to isolate and recover from genital ulcers and swollen lymph nodes?

A. *Haemophilus aegyptius*
B. *Haemophilus ducreyi*
C. *Haemophilus haemolyticus*
D. *Haemophilus parahaemolyticus*

Microbiology/Pathogenicity/Coccobacilli/1

27. Which of the following is a characteristic of strains of *H. influenzae* that are resistant to ampicillin?

A. Production of β-lactamase enzymes
B. Hydrolysis of chloramphenicol
C. Hydrolysis of urea
D. All these options

Microbiology/Antibiotic sensitivity/Coccobacilli/1

28. A small, gram-negative coccobacillus recovered from the CSF of a 2-year-old unvaccinated child demonstrated the following characteristics:

Indole = +	Glucose = + (acid)
X requirement = +	V requirement = +
Urease = +	Lactose = Neg
Sucrose = Neg	Nonhemolytic

Which is the *most* likely infectious agent?

A. *Haemophilus parainfluenzae*
B. *Haemophilus influenzae*
C. *Haemophilus ducreyi*
D. *Aggregatibacter aphrophilus*

Microbiology/GNR/3

Answers to Questions 24–28

24. B The majority of *H. influenzae* invasive infections are caused by capsular serotypes a and b. The non-typable (NTHi) strains do not have a capsule and are part of the normal respiratory flora. As a result of the widespread use of the *H. influenzae* type b (Hib) vaccine, an increase in infections with NTHi has been noted. Life-threatening infections with *H. influenzae* are rarely reported in the United States. Serotyping of *Haemophilus* is performed by mixing colonies with agglutinating antibodies available as commercial agglutination kits.

25. C *A. aphrophilus* is primarily associated with subacute bacterial endocarditis and does not require either X or V factor for growth and is differentiated from the *Haemophilus* species by its ability to produce acid from lactose and a positive ALA test. *H. influenzae* and *H. haemolyticus* are incapable of synthesizing protoporphyrin from Δ-ALA and are negative for this test.

26. B *H. ducreyi* requires exogenous X factor and causes genital lesions referred to as "soft chancres." It is difficult to grow and requires commercial chocolate agar or gonococcus base medium containing 1% to 2% hemoglobin, 5% fetal bovine serum, and 1% IsoVitaleX enrichment with and without 3 µg/mL vancomycin. Some strains are sensitive to vancomycin. The primary culture media must be incubated at 30°C to 33°C in a 3% to 5% CO_2 moist environment for 2 to 3 days. Recovery of *H. ducreyi* from specimens constitutes a reportable sexually transmitted disease (chancroid).

27. A Most *H. influenzae* strains produce β-lactamase, which hydrolyses and inactivates the β-lactam ring of ampicillin (and penicillin). However, cephalosporins, and carbapenems along with agents that contain a β-lactamase inhibitor combined with a β-lactam may be effective for treatment of an *H. influenzae* infection.

28. B *H. influenzae* can cause meningitis in young, unvaccinated children. Although several biotypes of *H. parainfluenzae* produce indole and urease, *H. parainfluenzae* does not require X factor for growth. *H. influenzae* is sucrose negative and *H. parainfluenzae* is sucrose positive. *H. ducreyi* requires X factor, but not V factor. *A. aphrophilus* does not require either X factor or V factor for growth.

29. The ALA test (porphyrins) is a confirmatory procedure for which conventional biochemical test used for identification of *Haemophilus influenzae* from non-*influenzae* species?
A. X factor requirement
B. V factor requirement
C. Urease production
D. Indole production
Microbiology/Biochemical/Coccobacilli/1

30. An elderly patient who cared for several domestic cats was hospitalized with suspected cat scratch disease (CSD). Blood cultures appeared negative, but after several days, a small, slightly curved pleomorphic gram-negative bacillus grew on BHI agar supplemented with 5% horse blood. Other traditional biochemical methods demonstrated negative results. What is the *most* likely identification?
A. *Bartonella* spp.
B. *Brucella* spp.
C. *Kingella* spp.
D. *Haemophilus* spp.
Microbiology/GNR/3

31. A 5-year-old nonimmunized patient with a persistent cough, fever, and flu-like symptoms was admitted to the hospital. Nasopharyngeal swabs were cultured on 15% blood, chocolate, Bordet-Gengou, and Regan-Lowe (with 10% charcoal) agars. All media grew a gram-negative coccobacillus after 3 days of incubation. Carbohydrate and biochemical tests demonstrated negative results. What is the *most* likely identification?
A. *Haemophilus influenzae*
B. *Bordetella pertussis*
C. *Haemophilus parainfluenzae*
D. *Bordetella bronchiseptica*
Microbiology/GNR/3

32. A 29-year-old individual who often hunted rabbits and spent a lot of time in the woods was admitted to the hospital with skin ulcers on the upper extremities. At 48 hours, a small coccobacillus was recovered from the aerobic blood culture bottle. The organism stained poorly with Gram stain. Samples collected from the ulcers did not grow on primary culture media. What is the *most* likely identification?
A. *Pseudomonas aeruginosa*
B. *Pseudomonas fluorescens*
C. *Chryseobacterium* spp.
D. *Francisella tularensis*
Microbiology/GNR/3

Answers to Questions 29–32

29. A The X factor requirement for growth is the cause of many inaccuracies when identifying *Haemophilus* spp. False-negative results have been attributed to the presence of small amounts of hemin in the basal media, or X factor carryover from colonies transferred from primary culture media containing blood. The ALA test determines the ability of an organism to synthesize protoporphyrin intermediates in the biosynthetic pathway to hemin from the precursor compound Δ-ALA. *Haemophilus* species that need exogenous X factor to grow are unable to synthesize protoporphyrin from Δ-ALA and are negative for the ALA test. These species include *H. influenzae*, *H. haemolyticus*, *H. aegyptius*, and *H. ducreyi*.

30. A *Bartonella* spp., frequently the cause of zoonoses infections, are difficult to grow on primary culture media because they are facultative intracellular organisms. *Bartonella henselae is* the organism found in domestic cats, the main reservoir. When CSD is suspected from the patient's history, a peripheral thin blood smear stained with Giemsa should be performed. *Bartonella* bacteremia can be cyclic and may result in negative blood cultures and negative blood smears. *Bartonella* spp. are biochemically inert—that is, they are negative for oxidase, catalase, indole, and urease tests. Serological assays, including enzyme immunoassay (EIA) and immunofluorescent antibody tests (indirect fluorescent antibody [IFA]) remain the diagnostic test of choice for *Bartonella* infection.

31. B *B. pertussis,* the cause of whooping cough, is highly contagious during the 5- to 10-day period after acquisition. The incidence of whooping cough is greater in nonimmunized individuals and therefore is higher in children younger than 1 year. *B. bronchiseptica* is only rarely found in humans but may cause respiratory disease in animals. Unlike *B. pertussis,* it is positive for nitrite, urease, and motility.

32. D *F. tularensis* requires cysteine and cystine to grow. It may grow on chocolate agar supplemented with IsoVitaleX and also on charcoal yeast extract agar used to isolate *Legionella*.

33. A neonate was readmitted to the hospital with a diagnosis of meningitis. CSF revealed gram-negative straight rods. Following 24 hours of incubation, the organism grew on 5% sheep blood and chocolate agars displaying a yellow pigment. On MacConkey agar, it appeared as a non–lactose fermenter (NLF). Colonies were oxidase, DNase, and gelatinase positive, and oxidized glucose and mannitol. What is the *most* likely identification?

A. *Haemophilus influenza*
B. *Elizabethkingia meningoseptica*
C. *Stenotrophomonas maltophilia*
D. *Acinetobacter* spp.

Microbiology/GNR/3

34. A 46-year-old dog warden was admitted to the hospital with several puncture wounds encountered while wrangling a stray dog. Following 48 hours of incubation in 10% CO_2 the isolate demonstrated small yellow colonies on 5% sheep blood and chocolate agars and no growth on MacConkey agar. Gram stain showed gram-negative curved fusiform rods. Isolated colonies were oxidase and catalase positive. What is the *most* likely identification?

A. *Capnocytophaga canimorsus*
B. *Francisella tularensis*
C. *Legionella pneumophila*
D. *Pseudomonas aeruginosa*

Microbiology/GNR/3

35. The AACEK (formerly HACEK) group of organisms consisting of *Aggregatibacter (Haemophilus) aphrophilus*, *Actinobacillus actinomycetemcomitans*, *Cardiobacterium hominis*, *Eikenella corrodens*, and *Kingella* spp. are known by this acronym to denote which type of infection?

A. Urinary tract infection
B. Subacute bacterial endocarditis
C. Pharyngitis
D. Tonsillitis

Microbiology/Pathogenicity/2

36. Gastric biopsy material was obtained from a 35-year-old patient. A suspected case of *H. pylori* could presumptively be identified and then ultimately confirmed by which of the following methods?

A. Urea broth test and polymerase chain reaction (PCR)
B. Gram staining and culture
C. Acid-fast staining and culture
D. Giemsa staining and culture

Microbiology/GNR/2

37. Which acronym is used in reference to the slow-growing group of gram-negative bacteria indicated in subacute bacterial endocarditis?

A. HLACK
B. AACEK
C. ANBBC
D. NBCCBS

Microbiology/GNR/1

Answers to Questions 33–37

33. B *Elizabethkingia meningoseptica* can cause septicemia and meningitis in neonates and immunocompromised adults. The ability to encapsulate, produce proteases, and survive in chlorinated tap water are factors that contribute to hospital-acquired infections with this bacterium.

34. A *C. canimorsus* are part of the oral flora of dogs. The organisms require at least 5% CO_2 for growth and grow slowly on blood and chocolate agars. Colonies can grow in 48 hours if cultured in high CO_2 on BHI agar with 5% sheep blood.

35. B Blood cultures growing small, gram-negative rods should alert the microbiologist to the possibility of infection with one of the five AACEK (formerly HACEK) organisms.

36. A Tissue specimens are immersed in urea broth or placed in urea agar. A positive test indicates the presence of urease produced by *H. pylori*. Another method is the urea breath test, which is less invasive. PCR amplification or *in situ* hybridization are useful approaches for the detection of *H. pylori* in gastric biopsy specimens.

37. B AACEK (formerly HACEK) denotes the following slow-growing gram-negative bacilli causing subacute bacterial endocarditis: *Aggregatibacter aphrophilus; Aggregatibacter actinomycetemcomitans; Cardiobacterium hominis; Eikenella corrodens;* and *Kingella kingae.*

38. A 20-year-old patient presented with soft chancres in the genital area and swollen lymph nodes. A culture specimen was taken but failed to grow after 4 days on chocolate agar, sheep blood agar, and MTM agar. A Gram stain demonstrated small, pleomorphic gram-negative rods. What is the *most* likely presumptive identification?

A. *Neisseria gonorrhoeae*
B. *Haemophilus ducreyi*
C. *Haemophilus influenzae*
D. *Moraxella* spp.

Microbiology/Coccobacilli/3

39. A 7-year-old child became ill after eating a chicken sandwich from a fast-food restaurant. After 24 hours of gastroenteritis, a stool swab was obtained for culture, with normal fecal microbiota identified on MacConkey and XLD agars following 18 hours of incubation. Furthermore, growth was observed on Campy blood agar at 42°C and 37°C. Which traditional biochemical test(s) differentiates *C. jejuni* subsp. *doylei* from *C. jejuni* subsp. *jejuni*?

A. Urease
B. Hippurate hydrolysis
C. Cephalothin and nalidixic acid antibiotic disks
D. Growth at 25°C

Microbiology/Biochemical/GNR/3

40. Culture of the sputum specimen from a 13-year-old patient with CF grew a predominance of short, gram-negative rods that tested oxidase negative. On MacConkey, chocolate, and blood agar plates, the organism appeared to have lavender-green pigmentation. Further testing showed the following:

Motility = +	DNase = +
Glucose = + (oxidative)	Maltose = + (oxidative)
Lysine decarboxylase = +	Esculin hydrolysis = +

What is the *most* likely identification?

A. *Stenotrophomonas maltophilia*
B. *Acinetobacter* spp.
C. *Pseudomonas aeruginosa*
D. *Burkholderia cepacia*

Microbiology/GNR/3

41. A patient with a human bite wound on the right forearm arrived at the clinic for treatment. The wound was inflicted 36 hours earlier. A swab of the wound exudate was submitted for culture. After 48 hours of incubation, the laboratory results were as follows:

Gram-staining = Gram-negative straight, slender rods
Chocolate agar plate = "Pitting" of the agar by small, yellow, opaque colonies
Oxidase = + Motility = Neg Catalase = Neg
Glucose = +
Growth in increased CO_2 = + Growth at 42°C = Neg

What is the *most* likely identification of this facultative anaerobe?

A. *Pseudomonas aeruginosa*
B. *Acinetobacter* spp.
C. *Kingella kingae*
D. *Eikenella corrodens*

Microbiology/GNR/3

Answers to Questions 38–41

38. B *H. ducreyi* may take up to 7 days to grow on chocolate agar (requiring X factor for growth) and preferably at 30°C to 33°C with high humidity. Testing for chancroid disease requires specialized media.

39. C To separate *C. jejuni* subsp. *jejuni* from *C. jejuni* subsp. *doylei* (both are positive for hippurate hydrolysis and grow at 37°C and 42°C), it is best to use cephalothin (30-µg disk) and nalidixic acid (30-µg disk) antibiotic sensitivity testing. *C. jejuni* subsp. *jejuni* are resistant to cephalothin and susceptible to nalidixic acid. *C. jejuni* subsp. *doylei* are susceptible to both disks.

40. A *S. maltophilia* is the third most frequently isolated nonfermentative gram-negative rod in the clinical laboratory. Patients with CF are at greater risk for infections because of previous antimicrobial treatment and recurrent pneumonia and because some strains may be colonizers.

41. D *E. corrodens* is part of the normal microbiota of the human mouth and typically "pits" the agar. This organism is capnophilic (needing increased CO_2).

42. A dog bite wound to the thumb of a 20-year-old patient became infected. Culture grew a gram-negative, slender rod, which was a facultative anaerobe. The following results were noted:

Oxidase = +	Motility = Neg
Catalase = +	Capnophilic = +
"Gliding" on the agar was noted.	

What is the *most* likely identification?

A. *Pseudomonas aeruginosa*
B. *Capnocytophaga canimorsus*
C. *Acinetobacter* spp.
D. *Proteus mirabilis*

Microbiology/GNR/3

43. A *Haemophilus* species recovered from a throat culture specimen obtained from a 59-year-old patient undergoing chemotherapy required hemin (X factor) and NAD (V factor) for growth. The isolate also hemolyzed horse erythrocytes on blood agar. What is the *most* likely species?

A. *H. ducreyi*
B. *H. parahaemolyticus*
C. *H. haemolyticus*
D. *H. aegyptius*

Microbiology/Coccobacilli/3

44. The majority of syndromic molecular encephalitis panels are able to detect which capsule types of *Haemophilus influenzae*?

A. Type b
B. Types a and f and nontypeable strains
C. Type a and f
D. Type f

Microbiology/Molecular/Coccobacilli/2

45. A CSF sample obtained from a 2-week-old infant with suspected bacterial meningitis grew gram-negative rods on blood and chocolate agars. The following results were noted:

MacConkey agar = No growth	ONPG = +
Glucose (open) OF = +	Urease = Neg
Glucose (closed) OF = Neg	Catalase = +
Indole = +	Oxidase = +
Motility = Neg	Pigment = Yellow
42°C growth = Neg	

What is the correct identification?

A. *Pseudomonas aeruginosa*
B. *Elizabethkingia meningoseptica*
C. *Acinetobacter* spp.
D. *Escherichia coli*

Microbiology/GNR/3

Answers to Questions 42–45

42. B *C. canimorsus* is associated with septicemia or meningitis following dog bites. All *Capnocytophaga* strains are capnophilic, facultative anaerobic, gram-negative, slender or filamentous rods with tapered ends.

43. C *H. haemolyticus* requires both X and V factors for growth and lyses horse erythrocytes.

44. B NAATs have been developed that are capable of detecting *H. influenzae* types a and f and nontypeable species. *H. influenzae* type b is no longer commonly isolated in serious infections as a result of the use of the Hib vaccine.

45. B *Elizabethkingia meningoseptica* is a well-known cause of neonatal meningitis. It grows well on chocolate agar, producing yellow-pigmented colonies.

46. During the summer break, several elementary school teachers, all middle-aged, from the same school district attended a 3-day seminar in Chicago. Upon returning home, three female teachers from the group were hospitalized with pneumonia, flu-like symptoms, and a nonproductive cough. Routine testing of sputum samples revealed normal flora. Further testing with BCYE agar with L-cysteine and α-ketoglutarate in 5% CO_2 produced growth of opaque colonies that stained faintly, showing thin gram-negative rods. What is the *most* likely identification?

A. *Legionella pneumophila*
B. *Haemophilus influenzae*
C. *Eikenella corrodens*
D. *Streptococcus pneumoniae*

Microbiology/GNR/3

47. A tissue biopsy specimen of the stomach was obtained from a 38-year-old patient diagnosed with gastric ulcers. The specimen was transported immediately and processed for culture and histology. At 5 days, the culture produced colonies of gram-negative (curved) bacilli on chocolate and *Brucella* agar with 5% sheep blood. The cultures were held at 35°C to 37°C in a microaerophilic atmosphere. The colonies tested positive for urease. The *most* likely identification is:

A. *Escherichia coli*
B. *Helicobacter pylori*
C. *Enterococcus faecalis*
D. *Streptococcus gallolyticus*

Microbiology/Bacteria/3

Answers to Questions 46–47

46. A *L. pneumophila* is the cause of pneumonia and can occur as part of an epidemic sporadically or as a nosocomial infection or may be community acquired. The appearance of mottled, cut-glass colonies on BCYE agar under low power and the use of a direct immunofluorescent technique on sputum samples determine the presence of *L. pneumophila*. The most common environmental sites for recovery are shower heads, faucets, water tanks, and air-conditioning systems.

47. B *H. pylori* is not easily cultured for growth and identification. Tissue samples should be transported in appropriate media and tested immediately. Other means of successful identification are rapid urease test on biopsy material; urea breath test; and serological tests for the detection of antibodies to *H. pylori* by enzyme-linked immunosorbent assay (ELISA) and IFA procedures.

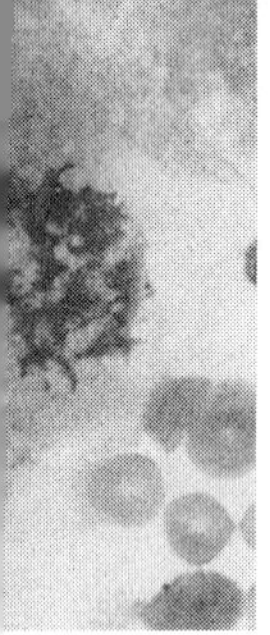

9.7

Gram-Positive and Gram-Negative Cocci

1. **The quick biochemical test used to separate *Staphylococcus* and *Micrococcus* spp. from *Streptococcus* spp. is:**
   A. Bacitracin
   B. Catalase
   C. Hemolysis pattern
   D. Microdase
   Microbiology/Biochemical/GPC/1

2. ***Micrococcus* and *Staphylococcus* spp. are differentiated by which quick biochemical test?**
   A. Fermentation of glucose (OF tube)
   B. Catalase test
   C. Gram stain
   D. Microdase
   Microbiology/Biochemical/GPC/1

3. **Lysostaphin can be used to differentiate *Staphylococcus* from which other gram-positive, catalase-positive organisms?**
   A. *Streptococcus*
   B. *Aerococcus*
   C. *Micrococcus*
   D. *Enterococcus*
   Microbiology/Biochemical/GPC/1

4. **Which of the following traditional quick tests can be used to preliminarily identify *S. aureus*?**
   A. Slide coagulase test
   B. Microdase
   C. Lysostaphin
   D. Catalase test
   Microbiology/Biochemical/GPC/1

5. **Which of the following enzymes contribute to the virulence of *S. aureus*?**
   A. Urease and lecithinase
   B. Hyaluronidase and β-lactamase
   C. Lecithinase and catalase
   D. Cytochrome oxidase
   Microbiology/Pathogenicity/GPC/1

Answers to Questions 1–5

1. B The catalase test (utilizing a 3% hydrogen peroxide [H_2O_2] solution stored in a brown bottle under refrigeration) is positive for the *Staphylococcus* and *Micrococcus* spp. However, some strains of catalase-negative staphylococci have been identified. Members of the *Streptococcaceae* family are negative.

2. D The Microdase disk, or modified oxidase test, is used to differentiate *Micrococcus, Macrococcus,* and *Mammaliicoccus* (all positive) from *Staphylococcus* spp. (negative).

3. C Lysostaphin is an endopeptidase that cleaves the glycine-rich pentapeptide cross-bridges in the staphylococcal cell wall peptidoglycan, causing lysis of the organism or cell death The susceptibility of staphylococci to lysostaphin (less than 200 μg/mL) is used to differentiate them from the micrococci. Staphylococci are susceptible and show a 10- to 16-mm zone of inhibition, whereas micrococci are not inhibited and will grow up to the disk.

4. A The slide coagulase test is a quick test that uses rabbit plasma with ethylenediaminetetraacetic acid (EDTA) to detect bound coagulase or "clumping factor" on the surface of the cell wall, which reacts with the fibrinogen in the plasma. This test is not positive for all strains of *S. aureus,* and a negative result must be confirmed by the tube method for detecting "free coagulase" or extracellular coagulase. The tube test is usually positive within 4 hours at 35°C; however, a negative result must then be incubated at room temperature for the remainder of 18 to 24 hours. Some strains produce coagulase slowly or produce fibrinolysin, which dissolves the clot at 35°C. Latex agglutination procedures may also be used that utilize fibrinogen and immunoglobulin G (IgG)-coated latex beads that detect protein A on the staphylococcal cell wall.

5. B In addition to coagulase, the virulence of *S. aureus* is attributed to hyaluronidase, which damages the intercellular matrix (basement membrane) of tissues. β-Lactamase–producing strains are able to inactivate penicillin and ampicillin, making the organism resistant to the antibiotics. Lecithinase is not produced by *S. aureus,* and urease is not a virulence factor.

6. Toxic shock syndrome is attributed to infection with:
A. *Staphylococcus epidermidis*
B. *Staphylococcus hominis*
C. *Staphylococcus aureus*
D. *Staphylococcus saprophyticus*
Microbiology/Pathogenicity/GPC/1

7. Which *Staphylococcus* species, in addition to *S. aureus*, also produces extracellular free coagulase that is detectable using the tube coagulase test?
A. *S. intermedius*
B. *S. saprophyticus*
C. *S. hominis*
D. *S. haemolyticus*
Microbiology/Biochemical/GPC/2

8. *S. aureus, S. epidermidis, S. haemolyticus,* and *S. hominis* can produce a substance that inhibits phagocytosis and penetration of antibiotics. What is this virulence factor?
A. Alginate
B. Biofilm or polysaccharide capsule
C. Panton-Valentine leukocidin (PVL)
D. Delta toxin
Microbiology/Pathogenicity/GPC/1

9. *S. saprophyticus* can be differentiated from *S. epidermidis* by its resistance to:
A. 5 μg of lysostaphin
B. 5 μg of novobiocin
C. 10 units of penicillin
D. 0.04 unit of bacitracin
Microbiology/Antibiotic sensitivity/GPC/Staphylococcus/1

10. The following results were observed by using a tube coagulase test:

Coagulase at 4 hours = +	Coagulase at 18 hours = Neg
DNase = +	Novobiocin = Sensitive (16-mm zone)
β-Hemolysis on blood agar	Mannitol salt agar plate = + (acid production)

What is the *most* probable identification?
A. *Staphylococcus saprophyticus*
B. *Staphylococcus epidermidis*
C. *Staphylococcus aureus*
D. *Staphylococcus hominis*
Microbiology/GPC/3

Answers to Questions 6–10

6. C *S. aureus* is the organism most often recovered from female patients. These strains produce toxic shock syndrome toxin 1 (TSST-1). Toxic shock syndrome is attributed to the use of certain highly absorbent tampons by menstruating females. The toxin is also recovered from sites other than the genital area and produces fever and life-threatening systemic damage as well as shock.

7. A Several clinically significant staphylococci will test positive for extracellular free coagulase using the tube testing method. These include *S.* biovar *anaerobius, S. hyicus, S. intermedius, S. dephini, S. pseudintermedius,* and *S. coagulans. S. intermedius* is often associated with dog bite wounds and can be misidentified as *S. aureus* if only coagulase testing is performed. A clinical isolate from a wound that is catalase-positive, gram-positive cocci in clusters that is β-hemolytic, white-to-yellow, creamy, and opaque on blood agar may be presumptively identified as *S. aureus.* When using traditional biochemical testing methods, additional confirmatory testing is required for definitive identification. *S. intermedius* may give a positive latex agglutination coagulase test.

8. B *Staphylococcus* spp. are capable of producing an extracellular slime (exopolysaccharide or biofilm) that enhances the adhesion of these organisms to indwelling plastic catheters. The extracellular slime or biofilm inhibits phagocytosis, allows the organism to adhere to surfaces, and also inhibits the action or penetration of antibiotics. The slime production is considered a virulence factor.

9. B *S. saprophyticus* is coagulase negative and resistant to 5 μg of novobiocin. When using the standardized Kirby-Bauer sensitivity procedure, a 6- to 12-mm zone of growth inhibition is considered resistant. Susceptible strains measure 16 to 27 mm (inhibition) zones.

10. C *S. aureus* can produce fibrinolysins that dissolve the clot formed by the coagulase enzyme. The tube method calls for an incubation of 4 hours at 35°C to 37°C and 18 to 24 hours at room temperature. Both must be negative to interpret the result as coagulase negative. This organism is coagulase positive and, therefore, is identified as *S. aureus.*

11. *S. aureus* recovered from a wound culture gave the following antibiotic sensitivity pattern by the standardized Kirby-Bauer method (S = sensitive; R = resistant):

Penicillin = R	Ampicillin = S
Cephalothin = R	Cefoxitin = R
Vancomycin = S	Methicillin = R

Which is the drug of choice for treating this infection?
A. Penicillin
B. Ampicillin
C. Cephalothin
D. Vancomycin
Microbiology/Antibiotic sensitivity/GPC/2

12. Which of the following traditional biochemical tests can be used to separate *S. aureus* from *S. intermedius*?
A. Acetoin
B. Catalase
C. Slide coagulase
D. Urease
Microbiology/Biochemical/GPC/2

13. A gram-positive coccus recovered from a wound ulcer from a 31-year-old patient with diabetes showed pale yellow, creamy, β-hemolytic colonies on blood agar. Given the following biochemical test results, what is the *most* likely identification?

Catalase = +
Glucose OF: Positive (oxidation) open tube, negative (fermentation) sealed tube
Mannitol salt = Neg
Slide coagulase = Neg
Microdase = +

A. *Staphylococcus aureus*
B. *Staphylococcus epidermidis*
C. *Micrococcus* spp.
D. *Streptococcus* spp.
Microbiology/Biochemical/GPC/3

14. Urine cultured from the catheter of an 18-year-old female patient produced more than 100,000 col/mL on CNA agar. Colonies are catalase positive, coagulase negative by the latex agglutination slide method as well as the tube coagulase test. What is the *most* reliable follow-up test for a preliminary identification of the isolate?
A. Lactose fermentation
B. Urease
C. Catalase
D. Novobiocin susceptibility
Microbiology/Biochemical/GPC/3

Answers to Questions 11–14

11. D Vancomycin is used for strains of *S. aureus* that are resistant to the β-lactams. However, strains of *S. aureus* have been identified with high-level resistance to vancomycin (MIC >8 μg/mL) and reduced or intermediate susceptible (MIC 4–8 μg/mL). Two additional agents can be used against resistance strains: linezolid and daptomycin.

12. A The production of acetoin by *S. aureus* from glucose or pyruvate differentiates it from *S. intermedius*, which is also coagulase positive (positive for clumping factor and free coagulase or tube test). This test is the Voges-Proskauer (VP) test. Acetoin production is detected by addition of 40% KOH and 1% α-naphthol to the VP test broth after 48 hours of incubation. A distinct pink color within 10 minutes denotes a positive test result.

13. C *Micrococcus* spp. utilize glucose oxidatively but not under anaerobic conditions (sealed tube). *Staphylococcus* spp. utilize glucose oxidatively and anaerobically. The catalase differentiates the Micrococcaceae family (positive) from the Streptococcaceae family (negative). The microdase test differentiates the *Staphylococcus, Macrococcus,* and *Mammaliicoccus* (all negative) from the *Micrococcus* spp. (positive).

14. D *S. epidermidis* and *S. saprophyticus* are the two possibilities because they are both catalase positive, coagulase negative, urease positive, and ferment lactose. Novobiocin susceptibility can be used to differentiate these two species. *S. epidermidis* is sensitive, but *S. saprophyticus* is resistant to 5 μg of novobiocin. UTIs caused by *S. saprophyticus* are often seen in cultures from sexually active young females.

15. A *Staphylococcus* spp. recovered from a wound (cellulitis) demonstrated β-hemolysis on blood agar and is negative for the slide coagulase test (clumping factor) and sensitive to novobiocin. Utilizing traditional biochemical methods, what would be the *next* test to assist with preliminary identification of the isolate?
A. Tube coagulase test
B. β-Hemolysis on blood agar
C. Mannitol salt agar plate
D. Penicillin-binding protein 2 (PBP2) latex agglutination
Microbiology/Biochemical/GPC/3

16. Furazolidone (Furoxone) susceptibility is a test used to differentiate:
A. *Staphylococcus* spp. from *Micrococcus* spp.
B. *Streptococcus* spp. from *Staphylococcus* spp.
C. *Staphylococcus* spp. from *Pseudomonas* spp.
D. Gram-positive, catalase-positive cocci
Microbiology/Antimicrobial sensitivity/GPC/2

17. Which of the following rapid biochemical tests can be performed to differentiate micrococci from staphylococci?
A. Catalase
B. Coagulase
C. Modified oxidase
D. Novobiocin susceptibility
Microbiology/Biochemical/GPC/2

18. *Streptococcus* species exhibit which of the following properties?
A. Aerobic, oxidase positive, and catalase positive
B. Facultative anaerobic, oxidase negative, catalase negative
C. Facultative anaerobic, β-hemolytic, catalase positive
D. May be α-, β-, or γ-hemolytic, catalase positive
Microbiology/Biochemical/GPC/2

19. Which group of β-hemolytic streptococci is associated with erythrogenic toxin production?
A. Group A
B. Group B
C. Group C
D. Group G
Microbiology/Pathogenicity/GPC/1

20. A fourfold rise in titer of which antibody would indicate a recent infection with group A β-hemolytic streptococci?
A. Anti-streptolysin O
B. Anti-streptolysin S
C. Anti-A
D. Anti-B
Microbiology/Pathogenicity/GPC/1

Answers to Questions 15–20

15. D *S. aureus* is novobiocin sensitive and cannot be ruled out by a negative clumping factor test. Most *S. aureus* produce β-hemolysis on sheep blood agar plates and are mannitol salt positive (produce acid and are not inhibited by the high salt concentration). The tube test (to detect free coagulase) should be performed because the slide test was negative.

16. D *Staphylococcus, Macrococcus, Mammaliicoccus, Kocuria,* and some species of *Rothia* are susceptible to furazolidone, giving zones of inhibition that are 15 mm or greater. *Micrococcus, Planococcus*, and some *Rothia* spp. are resistant to furazolidone, giving zones of 6 to 9 mm. The test may be used in conjunction with other traditional biochemical tests but is not reliable independently as a means for definitive identification. The test is performed as a disk susceptibility procedure using a blood agar plate.

17. C The modified oxidase test (Microdase) is used to rapidly identify catalase-positive gram-positive cocci as *Micrococcus* spp. (positive) or *Staphylococcus* spp. (negative). Filter paper disks that are saturated with oxidase reagent (tetramethyl-*p*-phenylenediamine in dimethylsulfoxide) are used. A colony of the isolate is rubbed onto the paper. Oxidase-positive organisms produce a purple color within 30 seconds or a blue color within 2 minutes if using the commercial product Microdase.

18. B *Streptococcus* spp. are facultative anaerobes that also grow aerobically and are oxidase and catalase negative.

19. A Group A β-hemolytic streptococci are the cause of scarlet fever, and some strains produce toxins (pyrogenic exotoxins A, B, and C). *Streptococcus pyogenes* can cause of puerperal fever, streptococcal toxic shock, rheumatic fever, and a severe necrotizing fasciitis bacterial infection.

20. A The anti-streptolysin O (ASO) titer is used to indicate a recent infection with group A β-hemolytic streptococci. Streptolysin O may also be produced by some strains of groups C and G streptococci.

21. The L-pyrrolidonyl-β-napthylamide (PYR), hippurate, and CAMP tests can be used for the presumptive identification of which group of β-hemolytic streptococci?
A. Groups A and B
B. Groups C and D
C. Group C
D. Group F
Microbiology/Biochemical/GPC/1

22. To diagnose streptococcal pharyngitis, primary culture plates of blood agar and blood agar with sulfamethoxazole-trimethoprim (SXT) can be used to differentiate which streptococci?
A. α-Hemolytic streptococci
B. β-Hemolytic streptococci
C. *Streptococcus pneumoniae*
D. *Enterococcus faecalis*
Microbiology/Biochemical/GPC/1

23. β-Hemolytic streptococci, not of group A or B, usually exhibit which of the following reactions?

	Bacitracin	SXT
A.	Susceptible	Resistant
B.	Resistant	Resistant
C.	Resistant	Susceptible
D.	Susceptible or resistant	Susceptible

Microbiology/Antibiotic sensitivity/GPC/2

24. A false-positive CAMP test result for the presumptive identification of group B streptococci may occur if the plate is incubated in a(n):
A. Anaerobically or CO_2 incubator
B. Ambient air incubator
C. 35°C incubator
D. 37°C incubator
Microbiology/Biochemical/GPC/3

25. Which biochemical test can be used to differentiate α-hemolytic streptococci from the *Enterococcus* spp. and *S. gallolyticus* growing on blood agar?
A. Bacitracin disk test
B. CAMP test
C. Hippurate hydrolysis test
D. Bile esculin test
Microbiology/Biochemical/GPC/1

Answers to Questions 21–25

21. A The bacitracin A disk test is no longer used, but the PYR, hippurate hydrolysis, and CAMP tests can be used for the presumptive identification of the β-hemolytic streptococci. The CAMP test (first described by Christie, Atkins, and Munch-Petersen in 1944; CAMP is an acronym of the authors' names) refers to a hemolytic interaction (flaming arrowhead) that is seen on a blood agar plate between the β-hemolysins produced by most strains of *S. aureus* and an extracellular protein produced by both hemolytic and nonhemolytic isolates of group B streptococci. In addition to group A, groups C, F, and G are also β-hemolytic and give a positive test result for bacitracin (a zone of inhibition of any size). Therefore, a positive bacitracin A disk test does not confirm the presence of group A β-hemolytic streptococci. Group A streptococci test positive for PYR but negative for hippurate and the CAMP test. Group B streptococci test negative in the PYR test but positive in the hippurate and CAMP tests. Groups C, G, and F test negative in all three tests.

22. B SXT is inhibitory to most streptococci except *S. pyogenes* and *Streptococcus agalactiae*. For this reason, SXT is used in a commercially available streptococcal selective agar (SSA) for the detection of group A streptococci. Latex agglutination test kits are used for the rapid detection of β-hemolytic streptococci Lancefield groups A, B, C, F, and G.

23. D Streptococci that are not group A or B may be either resistant or susceptible to bacitracin but are usually susceptible to SXT.

β-Hemolytic Streptococci	Bacitracin	Sulfamethoxazole-Trimethoprim
Group A	Susceptible	Resistant
Group B	Resistant	Resistant
Non-A, non-B	Susceptible or resistant	Susceptible

24. A In a CAMP test, the plate must be placed in an ambient air incubator at 35°C to 37°C. Group A streptococci may be CAMP positive if the plate is incubated in a candle jar, in high CO_2 atmosphere, or anaerobically.

25. D The bile esculin test differentiates bacteria that can hydrolyze esculin and also grow in the presence of 4% bile salts or 40% bile. The bile esculin slant or agar plate is inoculated on the surface and incubated for 24 to 48 hours in a non-CO_2 incubator. Group D streptococci (enterococci and nonenterococci) are positive, causing blackening of half or more of the slant within 48 hours. Viridans streptococci are negative (do not grow or hydrolyze esculin).

26. The bile solubility test causes the lysis of:
A. *Streptococcus gallolyticus* colonies on a blood agar plate
B. *Streptococcus pneumoniae* colonies on a blood agar plate
C. Group A streptococci in broth culture
D. Group B streptococci in broth culture
Microbiology/Boiochemical/GPC/1

27. ***S. pneumoniae*** **and the α-hemolytic viridans streptococci can be differentiated by which test?**
A. Optochin P disk test, 5 μg/mL or less
B. Bacitracin A disk test, 0.04 unit
C. CAMP test
D. Bile esculin test
Microbiology/Biochemical/GPC/2

28. The salt tolerance test (6.5% salt broth) can be used to presumptively identify:
A. *Streptococcus pneumoniae*
B. *Streptococcus gallolyticus*
C. Viridans streptococci
D. *Enterococcus faecalis*
Microbiology/Biochemical/GPC/1

29. In addition to ***E. faecalis*****, which other streptococci will grow in 6.5% salt broth?**
A. Group A streptococci
B. Group B streptococci
C. *Streptococcus pneumoniae*
D. *Streptococcus gallolyticus*
Microbiology/Biochemical/GPC/2

30. The PYR hydrolysis test is a presumptive test for which group of β-hemolytic streptococci?
A. Group A and *Enterococcus*
B. Group A and B β-hemolytic streptococci
C. Non–group A or non–group B β-hemolytic streptococci
D. *Streptococcus pneumoniae* and *Streptococcus gallolyticus*
Microbiology/Biochemical/GPC/1

31. A pure culture of β-hemolytic streptococci recovered from a leg wound ulcer gave the following reactions:

CAMP test = Neg	Hippurate hydrolysis = Neg
Bile esculin = Neg	6.5% salt = Neg
PYR = Neg	Bacitracin = Resistant
Optochin = Resistant	SXT = Sensitive

The *most* likely identification is:
A. Group A streptococci
B. Group B streptococci
C. *Enterococcus* spp.
D. Non–group A, non–group B streptococci
Microbiology/GPC/3

Answers to Questions 26–31

26. B The bile solubility test can be performed directly by dropping 2% sodium deoxycholate onto a few well-isolated colonies of *S. pneumoniae*. The bile salts speed up the autolysis observed in pneumococcal cultures. The colonies lyse and disappear when incubated at 35°C for 30 minutes, leaving a partially hemolyzed area on the plate. The same phenomenon can be seen using a broth culture; addition of 10% deoxycholate to broth containing *S. pneumoniae* results in visible clearing of the suspension after incubation at 35°C for 3 hours.

27. A Optochin (P disk) at a concentration of 5 μg/mL or less inhibits the growth of *S. pneumoniae* but not viridans streptococci. However, optochin at a concentration more than 5 μg/mL inhibits viridans streptococci as well if incubated under 5% CO_2 at 35ºC for 18 to 24 hours. A zone of inhibition of 14 mm or more around the 6-mm disk is considered a presumptive identification of *S. pneumoniae*. A questionable zone size should be confirmed by performing a bile solubility test.

28. D *E. faecalis* will grow in 6.5% salt, and the nonenterococci (*S. gallolyticus* and *S. equinus*) will not. This test distinguishes the enterococci group from *S. gallolyticus* and *S. equinus* (nonenterococci group). Both groups grow on bile esculin agar. Viridans streptococci are negative for 6.5% salt growth and will not grow on bile esculin agar.

29. B Approximately 80% of group B streptococci can grow in 6.5% salt broth; however, they do not hydrolyze esculin or grow in media containing 4% bile salts.

30. A The PYR hydrolysis test is highly specific for group A streptococci and *Enterococcus* spp. The test detects the pyrrolidonyl arylamidase enzyme, which hydrolyzes PYR.

31. D The β-hemolytic streptococci—not of groups A or B—are sensitive to SXT and may be either sensitive or resistant to bacitracin. Groups A and B are both resistant to SXT. Group A and *E. faecalis* are PYR positive. *E. faecalis* is also positive for bile esculin and 6.5% salt broth. Latex agglutination tests identify β-hemolytic groups A, B, C, F, and G.

32. β-Hemolytic streptococci, greater than 50,000 col/mL, were isolated from a urinary tract catheter specimen. Given the following reactions, what is the *most* likely identification?

CAMP test = Neg	Hippurate hydrolysis = Neg
Bile solubility = Neg	6.5% salt = +
PYR = +	Bile esculin = +
SXT = Resistant	Bacitracin = Resistant
Optochin = Resistant	Vancomycin = Resistant

A. Group A streptococci
B. Group B streptococci
C. *Enterococcus faecalis, Enterococcus faecium*
D. Non–group A, non–group B streptococci
Microbiology/GPC/3

33. *Abiotrophia* spp., previously known as nutritionally variant streptococci (NVS), require specific thiol compounds, cysteine, or the active form (pyridoxal) of vitamin B_6. Which of the following tests supplies these requirements for growth?
A. CAMP test
B. Bacitracin susceptibility test
C. Bile solubility test
D. Staphylococcal cross-streak test
Microbiology/Biochemical/GPC/1

34. Many β-hemolytic streptococci recovered from a wound were found to be penicillin resistant. Given the following biochemical results, what is the *most* likely identification?

Bile esculin = +	PYR = +	6.5% salt = +
Hippurate hydrolysis = +	Bile solubility = Neg	
SXT = Resistant		

A. *Enterococcus faecalis*
B. *Streptococcus pneumoniae*
C. *Streptococcus gallolyticus*
D. Group B streptococci
Microbiology/GPC/3

35. Which two biochemical tests can be used to differentiate α-hemolytic *S. gallolyticus (S. equinus* group) from *Streptococcus salivarius (S. salivarius* group), which is also α-hemolytic?
A. Bile esculin and 6.5% salt broth
B. Starch hydrolysis and acid production from mannitol
C. Bacitracin and PYR
D. SXT susceptibility and PYR
Microbiology/Biochemical/GPC/2

Answers to Questions 32–35

32. C VRE (vancomycin-resistant *Enterococcus*) denotes *E. faecalis* and *Enterococcus facium*, which have shown resistance to most antimicrobials used to treat infections caused by gram-positive cocci (ampicillin, methicillin, and other β-lactams) and many are resistant to vancomycin. Group A streptococci are sensitive to bacitracin and negative for bile esculin and 6.5% salt broth. Group B streptococci will grow in 6.5% salt broth but are negative for bile esculin and PYR. The non–group A, non–group B streptococci will not grow in 6.5% salt broth and are sensitive to SXT. *E. faecalis* is positive for bile esculin, 6.5% salt broth, and PYR.

33. D The staphylococcal streak, across the *Abiotrophia* inoculum, provides the nutrients needed. Very small colonies of *Abiotrophia* spp. can be seen growing adjacent to the staphylococcal streak on the blood agar plate in a manner like the satellite phenomenon of *Haemophilus* spp. around *S. aureus*. *Abiotrophia* spp. are normal microbiota of the oral cavity but may cause life-threatening infections when introduced into sterile areas (cause of endocarditis). Blood culture media will supply the necessary nutrients for their recovery.

34. A *E. faecalis* is resistant to penicillin and ampicillin as well as some of the aminoglycoside antibiotics. Pneumococci, group B streptococci, and *S. gallolyticus* are PYR negative.

35. B *S. equinus* group and *S. salivarius* group are physiologically and biochemically similar. They are both PYR and 6.5% salt broth negative and bile esculin positive, but only *S. equinus* group organisms are typically positive for mannitol. *S. salivarius* group organisms are also typically positive for urea hydrolysis. See the following chart:

	Bacitracin	PYR	Bile Esculin	6.5% Salt	Mannitol	Urease
S. equinus Group	R	Neg	+	Neg	Variable	Neg
S. salivarius Group	R	Neg	+	Neg	Neg	Variable

36. Two blood cultures obtained from a neonate grew β-hemolytic streptococci with the following reactions:

CAMP test = +	Hippurate hydrolysis = +
Bile solubility = Neg	6.5% salt = +
Bacitracin = Resistant	Bile esculin = Neg
PYR = Neg	
SXT = Resistant	

Which is the *most* likely identification?
A. Group A streptococci
B. Group B streptococci
C. *Enterococcus faecalis*
D. Non–group A, non–group B streptococci
Microbiology/GPC/3

37. MTM medium is used primarily for the selective recovery of which pathogenic *Neisseria* spp. organism from genital specimens?
A. *N. gonorrhoeae*
B. *N. lactamica*
C. *N. sicca*
D. *N. flavescens*
Microbiology/Culture/GNC/1

38. A female was experience painful or burning urination and a yellow vaginal discharge. A gram-negative, oxidase-positive diplococcus is recovered from a urogenital specimen on MTM agar. The organism can be presumptively identified as:
A. *Neisseria gonorrhoeae*
B. *Neisseria meningitidis*
C. *Neisseria lactamica*
D. *Neisseria sicca*
Microbiology/GNC/3

39. Colonies growing on MTM agar and showing a 4+ reaction with the Superoxol test may be considered as a rapid preliminary test for:
A. *Neisseria gonorrhoeae*
B. *Neisseria meningitidis*
C. *Neisseria lactamica*
D. *Moraxella catarrhalis*
Microbiology/Biochemical/GNC/1

40. Nonpathogenic *Moraxella* spp. capable of growing on selective media for *Neisseria* can be differentiated from pathogenic *Neisseria* spp. by which phenotypic test?
A. Catalase test
B. 10-unit penicillin disk on blood agar
C. Oxidase test
D. Superoxol test
Microbiology/Biochemical/GNC/1

Answers to Questions 36–40

36. B Group B streptococci (*S. agalactiae*) are resistant to both bacitracin and SXT. Unlike group A and *E. faecalis*, the group B streptococci are negative for PYR. With some exceptions, group B streptococci will grow in 6.5% salt broth. Group B strep infections in newborns are the result of premature rupture of the mother's membranes. The infection in a newborn happens within the first 5 days after birth and results in fever, sepsis, meningitis, and respiratory distress.

37. A Both *N. gonorrhoeae* and *N. meningitidis* grow selectively on MTM agar as a result of the addition of vancomycin and colistin, which inhibit gram-positive and gram-negative bacteria, respectively. Trimethoprim is added to inhibit swarming of *Proteus* spp. because a rectal swab may be used for culture. Nystatin and amphotericin B are used to prevent growth of yeasts and molds from vaginal specimens. *N. lactamica* will grow on MTM agar but is rarely involved in human infection.

38. D All the *Neisseria* spp. listed grow on MTM agar except *Neisseria sicca* and all are oxidase positive. *N. lactamica* is a nonpathogenic component of normal throat microbiota resembling *N. meningitidis*, but it grows well on selective MTM agar. Presumptive identification of *N. gonorrhoeae* is stated only if the individual patient is female and experiencing symptoms of urogenital infection. However, the identification must be confirmed by further testing, such as carbohydrate utilization tests, DNA tests, or rapid latex slide agglutination tests because avirulent strains and normal vaginal and rectal microbiota resemble *Neisseria* spp.

39. A *N. gonorrhoeae* recovered from selective MTM media give an immediate 4+ positive reaction (bubbling) when 30% H_2O_2 is added. The catalase test uses 3% H_2O_2. This is not a presumptive test for *N. gonorrhoeae*; further testing is required. *N. meningitidis* and *N. lactamica* give a weak or delayed bubbling reaction. *M. catarrhalis* is catalase positive, whereas the Superoxol reactions are negative, weak, or delayed and it shows a variable growth pattern on MTM agar.

40. B *Moraxella* spp. are oxidase and catalase positive, as are the gonococci. *Neisseria* spp. and *M. catarrhalis* will keep their typical cocci morphology after overnight incubation on blood agar with a 10-unit penicillin disk (CO_2 incubation). Other *Moraxella* spp. form long filaments or long spindle-shaped cells when grown near a 10-unit penicillin disk.

41. A Gram stain of a urethral discharge from a male patient showing extracellular and intracellular gram-negative diplococci within segmented neutrophils is a presumptive identification for:

A. *Neisseria gonorrhoeae*
B. *Neisseria meningitidis*
C. *Moraxella catarrhalis*
D. *Neisseria lactamica*

Microbiology/GNC/3

42. The β-galactosidase test aids in the identification of which *Neisseria* species?

A. *N. lactamica*
B. *N. meningitidis*
C. *N. gonorrhoeae*
D. *N. flavescens*

Microbiology/Biochemical/GNC/1

43. Cystine tryptic digest (CTA) media used for identification of *Neisseria* spp. should be incubated in:

A. A CO_2 incubator at 35°C for 24 hours
B. A CO_2 incubator at 42°C for up to 72 hours
C. A non-CO_2 incubator at 35°C for up to 72 hours
D. An anaerobic incubator at 35°C for up to 72 hours

Microbiology/Biochemical/GNC/2

44. Culture on MTM media of a vaginal swab produced several colonies of gram-negative diplococci that were catalase and oxidase positive and Superoxol negative. Given the following carbohydrate reactions, select the *most* likely identification.

Glucose = +	Sucrose = Neg	Lactose = +
Maltose = +	Fructose = Neg	

A. *Neisseria gonorrhoeae*
B. *Neisseria sicca*
C. *Neisseria flavescens*
D. *Neisseria lactamica*

Microbiology/GNC/3

45. Sputum from a patient with pneumonia produced many colonies of gram-negative diplococci on a chocolate plate that were also present in fewer numbers on MTM after 48 hours of incubation. Given the following results, what is the *most* likely identification?

Catalase = +	Oxidase = +
DNase = +	Tributyrin hydrolysis = +
Glucose = Neg	Sucrose = Neg
Lactose = Neg	Maltose = Neg
Fructose = Neg	

A. *Moraxella catarrhalis*
B. *Neisseria flavescens*
C. *Neisseria sicca*
D. *Neisseria elongata*

Microbiology/GNC/3

Answers to Questions 41–45

41. A Gram staining of urethral discharge (in men only) that shows typical gonococcal cells in polymorphonuclear leukocytes (PMNs) should be reported "presumptive *N. gonorrhoeae*, confirmation to follow." With female patients, the normal vaginal microbiota contains gram-negative cocci and diplococci resembling gonococci, and therefore, no presumptive identification should be reported for *N. gonorrhoeae* from the vaginal Gram-stained smear.

42. A *N. lactamica* utilizes lactose by producing the enzyme β-galactosidase. All other *Neisseria* spp. that grow on MTM media are lactose negative.

43. C CTA agar with 1% carbohydrate and phenol red pH indicator added is used for the identification of *Neisseria* species. CTA carbohydrates must be placed in an ambient air incubator because a high CO_2 concentration may reduce the pH, causing a false-positive (acid) result. The utilization of carbohydrates by some fastidious gonococcal strains may take up to 72 hours to produce a color change in the pH indicator; is rarely used because identifications are performed by rapid molecular diagnostic methods or rapid biochemical, immunologic, or enzymatic methods.

44. D *N. lactamica* is part of the normal vaginal and oral microbiota and is the only *Neisseria* species that grows on MTM medium that utilizes lactose. Other saprophytic *Neisseria* spp. may utilize lactose but do not grow on MTM media.

45. A *M. catarrhalis* is part of the normal upper respiratory microbiota but is implicated in lower respiratory infections, including pneumonia. It produces stunted growth on MTM and is DNase positive, characteristics that differentiate it from the other saprophytic *Neisseria* spp.

46. Showing resistance to which drug categorizes a strain of *S. aureus* as MRSA?
A. Cefoxitin
B. Colistin
C. SXT
D. Oxacillin
Microbiology/Antibiotic susceptibility/GPC/2

47. An oxacillin-disk screen test is used to detect *S. pneumoniae* resistance to penicillin. Using Mueller-Hinton agar with 5% sheep blood and a 1-µg oxacillin disk, what is the recommended inhibition zone size for penicillin susceptibility?
A. 5 mm or greater
B. 10 mm or greater
C. 15 mm or greater
D. 20 mm or greater
Microbiology/Antibiotic sensitivity/GPC/2

48. Which test is used for the determination of inducible clindamycin resistance in staphylococci and streptococci?
A. E-test
B. D-zone test
C. A-test
D. CAMP test
Microbiology/Antibiotic susceptibility/GPC/1

49. A wound specimen was obtained from an older patient with diabetes and identified as being positive for vancomycin-resistant *S. aureus* (VRSA). The method used to determine VRSA was the standard microdilution technique. To be considered VSRA positive, which MIC must have been reported?
A. MIC 16 µg/mL or greater
B. MIC of 8 to 16 µg/mL
C. MIC of 4 to 8 µg/mL
D. MIC 8 µg/mL or greater
Microbiology/Antibiotic sensitivity/GPC/2

50. "Scalded skin syndrome" was a suspected infection in a newborn. Gram-positive, catalase-positive white colonies that are β-hemolytic grew on blood agar. What is the *most* likely identification?
A. *Streptococcus pyogenes*
B. *Staphylococcus aureus*
C. *Enterococcus faecalis*
D. *Streptococcus agalactiae*
Microbiology/Biochemical/GPC/2

Answers to Questions 46–50

46. A Oxacillin is the drug used to screen staphylococci for resistance to antibiotics having the β-lactam ring. Included in this group are penicillin, cephalosporin, monobactam, and carbapenem. MRSA defines strains of staphylococci that are resistant to all these antibiotic groups. Cefoxitin is the recommended antibiotic for detecting MRSA.

47. D The standard Kirby-Bauer method used for disk diffusion susceptibility testing recommended by the Clinical and Laboratory Standards Institute (CLSI) is 20 mm. The test requires 20- to 24-hour incubation at 35°C in 5% to 7% CO_2. If the zone size is 19 mm, an MIC should be performed on isolates from CSF or blood.

48. B By using a 15-µg erythromycin disk adjacent to a 2-µg clindamycin disk in a disk diffusion procedure, a flattening of the clindamycin zone occurs in inducible clindamycin resistance, causing the zone to look like the letter "D." This is referred to as *being D-zone positive*. The CLSI recommends that inducible clindamycin-resistant strains be reported as resistant.

49. A *S. aureus* (VRSA) is determined if the MIC result is 16 µg/mL or greater. Strains showing high levels of resistance (MIC greater than 8 µg/mL) and intermediate resistance (MIC 4 to 8 µg/mL) are thought to have structural changes within the cell wall. Two new agents available to combat vancomycin-resistant strains are linezolid and daptomycin.

50. B Strains of *S. aureus* producing toxins A and B are the cause of "scalded skin syndrome," which refers to skin infections that can be manifested as small blisters or covering 90% or greater of the body surface in newborns. *S. aureus* on blood agar may appear as white to yellow pigmented colonies.

51. An emergency department physician ordered a culture and sensitivity test on a catheterized urine specimen obtained from a 24-year-old female patient. A colony count was performed, and the following results were obtained after 24 hours:

Blood agar plate = >100,000 col/mL of gram-positive cocci resembling staphylococci
MacConkey agar = No growth CNA plate = Inhibited growth
Hemolysis = Neg Catalase = +
Novobiocin = Resistant

This isolate is:
A. *Staphylococcus saprophyticus*
B. *Micrococcus luteus*
C. *Staphylococcus aureus*
D. *Streptococcus pyogenes*
Microbiology/GPC/3

52. An outbreak of *S. aureus* in the hospital nursery prompted the Infection Control Committee to proceed with an environmental screening procedure. From the list of media provided, which could be used for this purpose?
A. CNA agar
B. THIO broth
C. Mannitol salt agar
D. Phenylethyl alcohol (PEA) agar
Microbiology/Culture/GPC/1

53. When testing for coagulase properties, a staphylococci isolate from a 67-year-old patient with diabetes showed a positive tube test (free coagulase) result. The organism should be preliminarily identified as:
A. *Staphylococcus aureus*
B. *Staphylococcus haemolyticus*
C. *Staphylococcus saprophyticus*
D. *Micrococcus luteus*
Microbiology/Biochemical/GPC/2

54. An isolate recovered from a vaginal culture obtained from a 25-year-old female patient who is 8 months pregnant demonstrated gram-positive cocci, catalase negative, and β-hemolytic colonies on blood agar. Which traditional biochemical tests are needed for further identification?
A. Optochin, bile solubility, PYR
B. Bacitracin, CAMP, PYR
C. Methicillin, PYR, trehalose
D. Coagulase, glucose, PYR
Microbiology/GPC/3

55. Which organism is the *most* often recovered gram-positive coccus (catalase negative), displaying α-, β-, or γ-hemolysis on blood agar from a series of blood culture specimens obtained from patients with endocarditis?
A. *Streptococcus agalactiae*
B. *Clostridium perfringens*
C. *Enterococcus faecalis*
D. *Pediococcus* spp.
Microbiology/GPC/3

Answers to Questions 51–55

51. A CNA inhibits most strains of *S. saprophyticus*. Routine blood agar should be used when culturing catheterized urine samples from young female patients. Most *S. saprophyticus* isolates are obtained from female patients ages 20 to 30 years.

52. C The high concentration of NaCl (7.5%) in mannitol salt agar allows for the recovery of *S. aureus* from heavily contaminated specimens while inhibiting other organisms. Furthermore, *S. aureus* ferments mannitol, thus allowing for easy detection of yellow-haloed colonies of *S. aureus* on red mannitol salt agar.

53. A *S. aureus* is an opportunistic human pathogen. A wound or ulcer infected with *S. aureus* that is left untreated is especially detrimental to a patient with diabetes.

54. B Group B streptococci (*S. agalactiae*) are important pathogens and can cause serious neonatal infections. Females heavily colonized vaginally with *S. agalactiae* pose a threat to the newborn, especially within the first few days after delivery. The infection acquired by the infant is associated with pneumonia.

55. C *Enterococcus faecalis* is associated with bacterial endocarditis and is one of the commonly isolated species in this condition.

56. A presumptive diagnosis of gonorrhea can be made from an exudate from a 20-year-old emergency department patient if which of the following criteria are present?

A. Smear of urethral exudate from a male patient demonstrates gram-negative, intracellular diplococci; growth of oxidase-positive, gram-negative diplococci on selective agar (MTM)

B. Smear from vaginal sample demonstrates gram-negative diplococci; colonial growth on blood agar

C. Smear from rectum demonstrates gram-negative diplococci; no growth on chocolate agar

D. Growth of gram-negative cocci on MacConkey agar and blood agar

Microbiology/GNC/2

57. Which method is *most* useful to confirm that a culture isolate is group B *Streptococcus*?

A. Southern blotting

B. PCR

C. Direct hybridization

D. Probe capture assay

Microbiology/Molecular/GPC/1

58. What gene(s) must be amplified in PCR to differentiate methicillin-resistant *Staphylococcus aureus* from methicillin-resistant coagulase-negative *Staphylococcus*?

A. *mecA/orfX*

B. *pncA/katG*

C. *VanA*

D. *iles-2*

Microbiology/Molecular/GPC/2

59. A pregnant female arrives at the emergency department with contractions that indicate delivery of the fetus is imminent. The patient indicates she has not been completing proper prenatal care. What action should the primary provider take to ensure the fetus does not contract group B streptococci during delivery?

A. Collect a vaginal culture to determine necessary antibiotic treatment

B. Perform a NAAT to determine colonization and treatment

C. Perform both culture and NAAT to determine treatment

D. Deliver the fetus via cesarean section if prenatal care cannot be determined

Microbiology/GPC/3

Answers to Questions 56–59

56. A *N. gonorrhoeae* can be presumptively identified from a male patient from Gram staining and growth on selective agar. In female patients, the normal microbiota from a urethral swab may appear to be *N. gonorrhoeae* (gram-negative diplococci) but may be part of the normal microbiota, such as *Veillonella* spp. (anaerobic gram-negative cocci resembling *N. gonorrhoeae*).

57. C In direct hybridization, a specific labeled probe reacts directly with the sample. Because a colony or pure broth culture of a primary isolate represents the progeny of a single bacterium, there is no need to use Southern blotting. The quantity of DNA available for testing is sufficient that amplification methods, such as PCR or probe capture hybridization, are unnecessary.

58. A The *mecA* is one of the genes that codes for resistance to methicillin in *S. aureus* and coagulase-negative *Staphylococcus*. The other gene included in molecular assays to detect methicillin-resistant *S. aureus* is *mecC*. To differentiate *mecA*-positive *S. aureus* from coagulase-negative *Staphylococcus*, such as *Staphylococcus epidermidis*, which are often present together in clinical specimens, the *orfX* gene specific for *S. aureus* is also amplified by multiplex PCR.

59. D If there is no record of prenatal care and delivery of the fetus is imminent, the provider will likely recommend a cesarean section to avoid potential exposure of the fetus to group B streptococcus. Neither a culture nor NAAT should be used to effectively treat colonization immediately prior to delivery.

60. **A vancomycin-resistant gram-positive coccobacillus resembling the *S. viridans* group was isolated from the blood of a 42-year-old patient undergoing bone marrow transplantation. The PYR and leucine aminopeptidase (LAP) tests were negative. The following results were noted:**

Catalase = Neg	CAMP = Neg
Esculin hydrolysis = Neg	Gas from glucose = +
Hippurate hydrolysis = Neg	6.5% salt broth = Neg

What is the correct identification?
A. *Leuconostoc* spp.
B. *Enterococcus* spp.
C. *Staphylococcus* spp.
D. *Micrococcus* spp.
Microbiology/Bacterial/3

61. **A catalase-negative, gram-positive coccus resembling staphylococci (clusters on the Gram-stained smear) was recovered from three different blood culture specimens obtained from a 60-year-old patient diagnosed with endocarditis. The following test results were noted:**

PYR = Neg	LAP = Neg (V)
Esculin hydrolysis = Neg	6.5% Salt broth = Neg
Vancomycin = Sensitive	CAMP test = Neg

What is the correct identification?
A. *Leuconostoc* spp.
B. *Gemella* spp.
C. *Enterococcus* spp.
D. *Micrococcus* spp.
Microbiology/Bacterial/3

62. **Several clinical culture specimens obtained from an immunocompromised patient with prior antibiotic treatment grew aerobic gram-positive cocci. The organism was vancomycin resistant and catalase negative. Additional testing proved negative for enterococci. What other groups of organisms might be responsible?**
A. *Leuconostoc* spp. and *Pediococcus* spp.
B. *Streptococcus pyogenes* and *Streptococcus agalactiae*
C. *Micrococcus* spp. and *Gemella* spp.
D. *Clostridium* spp. and *Streptococcus gallolyticus*
Microbiology/GPC/3

63. **A catalase-positive, gram-positive coccus (clusters on the Gram-stained smear) grew pale yellow, creamy colonies on 5% sheep blood agar. The specimen was recovered from pustules on the face of a 5-year-old child with impetigo. The following test reactions indicate which organism?**

Glucose = + (fermentation)	Oxidase = Neg
PYR = Neg	Bacitracin = Sensitive
Lysostaphin = Sensitive	

A. *Micrococcus* spp.
B. *Streptococcus* spp.
C. *Enterococcus* spp.
D. *Staphylococcus* spp.
Microbiology/GPC/3

64. **A wound (skin lesion) specimen obtained from a newborn grew predominantly β-hemolytic colonies of gram-positive cocci on 5% sheep blood agar. The newborn infant was covered with small skin eruptions that gave the appearance of a "scalding of the skin." The gram-positive cocci proved to be catalase positive. Which tests should be performed *next* for appropriate identification?**
A. Optochin, bile solubility, PYR
B. Coagulase, glucose fermentation, DNase
C. Bacitracin, PYR, 6.5% salt broth
D. CAMP, bile esculin, 6.5% salt broth
Microbiology/GPC/3

Answers to Questions 60–64

60. A *Leuconostoc* spp. are vancomycin-resistant opportunistic pathogens, and infection with them occurs after invasive procedures. The organisms are often recovered from positive neonatal blood culture specimens following colonization during delivery.

61. B *Gemella* spp. are often recovered from patients with endocarditis and meningitis. In the Gram-stained smear, they resemble staphylococci morphologically but are catalase negative.

62. A *Leuconostoc* spp. and *Pediococcus* spp. are vancomycin-resistant, catalase-negative, gram-positive aerobic organisms recovered from immunosuppressed patients.

63. D *S. aureus* is a usual cause of skin infections and a common cause of cellulitis, impetigo, postsurgical wounds, and scalded skin syndrome in infants.

64. B *S. aureus* is the cause of "scalded skin" syndrome in newborn infants. The production of a potent exotoxin (exfoliatin) causes the epidermis to slough off, leaving the newborn's skin with a red, raw texture or a burned, scalded look.

65. **A 20-year-old patient presented to the emergency department complaining of abdominal pain, fever, and a burning sensation during urination. An above-normal WBC count, along with pus cells and bacteria in the urine specimen, prompted the physician to order a urine culture. The colony count reported for this patient revealed greater than 100,000 col/mL of a nonhemolytic, catalase-negative, gram-positive organism on 5% sheep blood agar. The following test results indicate which organism?**

PYR = +	Bile esculin = +
6.5% salt broth = + growth	
Bacitracin = Neg	Optochin = Neg

A. *Enterococcus faecalis*
B. *Streptococcus pyogenes*
C. *Streptococcus agalactiae*
D. *Streptococcus bovis*

Microbiology/GPC/3

66. **A sputum specimen from an 89-year-old patient with suspected bacterial pneumonia grew a predominance of gram-positive cocci displaying α-hemolysis on 5% sheep blood agar. The colonies appeared donut shaped, mucoid and catalase negative. The *most* appropriate tests for a final identification are:**

A. Coagulase, glucose fermentation, lysostaphin
B. Penicillin, bacitracin, CAMP
C. Optochin, bile solubility, PYR
D. Bile esculin, hippurate hydrolysis

Microbiology/GPC/3

Answers to Questions 65–66

65. **A** *E. faecalis* gives a positive reaction to the PYR test and is often implicated in UTIs. It is part of the normal flora of the female genitourinary tract and the human gastrointestinal tract. On 5% sheep blood agar, *E. faecalis* colonies may appear as nonhemolytic, α-hemolytic, or β-hemolytic colonies, depending on the strain.

66. **C** *S. pneumoniae* colonies appear as α-hemolytic donut-shaped colonies on 5% sheep blood agar. The mucoid colonies may appear "wet" or "watery" because of the capsule surrounding the organism. The Gram stain smear reveals lancet-shaped gram-positive cocci in pairs surrounded by a clear area (the capsule). To differentiate the viridans streptococci from *S. pneumoniae*, the most appropriate test is the optochin disk test. *S. pneumoniae* on blood agar are susceptible to optochin, but viridans streptococci are resistant.

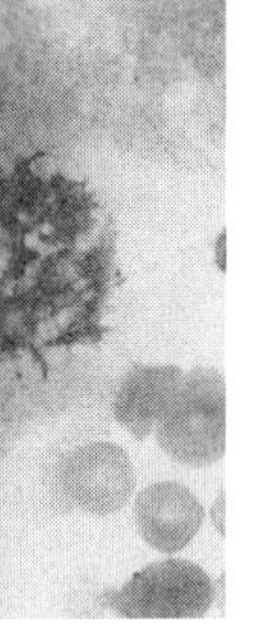

9.8

Aerobic Gram-Positive Rods, Spirochetes, Mycoplasmas, Ureaplasmas, and Chlamydia

1. **Large, gram-positive, spore-forming rods growing on blood agar as large, raised, β-hemolytic dry colonies are *most* likely:**
   A. *Pseudomonas* spp.
   B. *Bacillus* spp.
   C. *Corynebacterium* spp.
   D. *Listeria* spp.
   Microbiology/Phenotypic characteristics/GPR/2

2. ***Bacillus anthracis* and *Bacillus cereus* can *best* be differentiated by which traditional biochemical tests?**
   A. Motility and β-hemolysis on a blood agar plate
   B. Oxidase and β-hemolysis on a blood agar plate
   C. Lecithinase and glucose
   D. Lecithinase and catalase
   Microbiology/Biochemical/GPR/2

Answers to Questions 1–2

1. **B** The only spore former listed is the *Bacillus* spp., which grow as large, spreading colonies on blood agar plates. *Pseudomonas* spp. are gram-negative rods; *Corynebacterium* spp. appear as small, very dry colonies on BAP; *Listeria* spp. appear as very small β-hemolytic colonies on BAP, resembling *Streptococcus* spp.

2. **A** Both species of *Bacillus* are catalase and lecithinase positive and produce acid from glucose. *B. cereus* is β-hemolytic and motile, but *B. anthracis* is neither. See the following chart.

	β Hemolysis	Motility	Oxidase	Catalase	Lecithinase	Glucose
B. cereus	+	+	Neg	+	+	+
B. anthracis	Neg	Neg	Neg	+	+	+

3. Which is the specimen of choice for proof of food poisoning by *B. cereus*?
A. Sputum
B. Blood
C. Stool
D. Food
Microbiology/Specimen collection/GPR/2

4. A suspected *B. anthracis* culture obtained from a wound specimen produced colonies that had many outgrowths (Medusa-head appearance) but were not β-hemolytic on sheep blood agar. Which test should be performed next to rule out *B. anthracis*?
A. Penicillin (10-unit) susceptibility test
B. Lecithinase test
C. Glucose test
D. Motility test
Microbiology/Phenotypic characteristics/GPR/2

5. Which of the following rapid tests should be performed for initial differentiation of *L. monocytogenes* from group B streptococci?
A. Gram stain, motility at room temperature, catalase
B. Gram stain, CAMP test, H_2S/TSI
C. Oxidase, CAMP test, glucose
D. Oxidase, bacitracin
Microbiology/Biochemical/GPR/2

6. Culture of a wound specimen from a meat packer's finger produced short gram-positive, non–spore-forming bacilli on a blood agar plate showing no hemolysis. Given the following test results at 48 hours incubation, what is the *most* likely identification?

Catalase = Neg
H_2S/TSI = +
Motility (wet prep) = Neg Pos
Motility (gel media 22 °C) = + (bottle-brush growth in stab culture)

A. *Bacillus cereus*
B. *Listeria monocytogenes*
C. *Erysipelothrix rhusiopathiae*
D. *Bacillus subtilis*
Microbiology/GPR/3

7. Non–spore-forming, slender, gram-positive, rod-forming palisades and chains were recovered from a vaginal culture and grew well on 5% sheep blood agar as pinpoint, α-hemolytic colonies. The *most* likely identification is:
A. *Lactobacillus* spp.
B. *Bacillus* spp.
C. *Neisseria* spp.
D. *Streptococcus* spp.
Microbiology/Phenotypic characteristics/GPR/2

Answers to Questions 3–7

3. D The best specimen is the suspected food itself. Stool cultures are not useful because *B. cereus* is part of the normal fecal microbiota. The suspected food can be the source of food poisoning by *B. cereus* if 100,000 or greater organisms per gram of infected food are demonstrated.

4. D *B. anthracis* will appear as large gram-positive bacilli. Phenotypically the colonies on blood agar have a ground glass appearance, are nonpigmented and gamma hemolytic. *B. anthracis* does not grow on MacConkey or eosin methylene blue agar. If the organism meets all of the phenotypic characteristics noted, and is catalase positive and nonmotile, then *B. anthracis* cannot be ruled out and the isolate should be sent to a reference laboratory for further identification.

5. A *Streptococcus* spp. are catalase negative, and *L. monocytogenes* is catalase positive. *L. monocytogenes* appears on the Gram-stained smear as gram-positive short, thin, diphtheroidal shapes, whereas streptococci usually appear as short, gram-positive cocci in chains. The reactions shown in the following chart differentiate *L. monocytogenes* from the group B streptococci.

	Catalase	Motility	CAMP	H_2S	Bile Esculin
L. monocytogenes	+	+ (umbrella) Wet prep = tumbling	+	Neg	+
Group B streptococci	Neg	Neg	+	Neg	Neg

6. C *E. rhusiopathiae* is catalase negative, whereas the other three organisms are catalase positive. *E. rhusiopathiae* is seen primarily as a skin infection on the fingers of workers handling fish, meat, and poultry, as well as in farmers. Colonies growing on blood agar are small and transparent, may be either smooth or rough, and are often surrounded by a green tinge. *E. rhusiopathiae* is characterized by H_2S production in the butt of a TSI slant, which differentiates it from other catalase-negative, gram-positive rods. Motility observation notes a "bottle-brush" appearance in gel media at 22°C.

7. A *Lactobacillus* spp. produce both long, slender rods or short coccobacilli that form chains. *Lactobacillus* spp. are part of the normal vaginal microbiota (are not considered pathogens) and are sometimes confused with the streptococci. *Lactobacillus* spp. are absent or few when bacterial vaginosis is present with *G. vaginalis.*

8. A presumptive diagnosis of *Gardnerella vaginalis* can be made using which of the following findings?
A. Oxidase and catalase negative
B. Pleomorphic cocci heavily colonized on vaginal epithelium
C. Hippurate hydrolysis negative
D. α-Hemolytic on blood agar
Microbiology/Biochemical/GPR/2

9. A gram-positive branching filamentous organism recovered from a sputum specimen was found to be positive with a modified acid-fast stain method. What is the *most* likely presumptive identification?
A. *Bacillus* spp.
B. *Nocardia* spp.
C. *Corynebacterium* spp.
D. *Listeria* spp.
Microbiology/Phenotypic characteristics/GPR/2

10. Routine laboratory screening tests for *Treponema pallidum* (syphilis) involves:
A. Culturing
B. Serological analysis
C. Acid-fast staining
D. Gram staining
Microbiology/Spirochetes/1

11. Spirochetes detected in the hematology laboratory while scanning a blood film, even before the primary care provider suspects the infection, are:
A. *Borrelia* spp.
B. *Treponema* spp.
C. *Campylobacter* spp.
D. *Leptospira* spp.
Microbiology/Microscopy/Spirochetes/1

12. Which of the following organisms is the cause of Lyme disease?
A. *Treponema pallidum*
B. *Neisseria meningitidis*
C. *Babesia microti*
D. *Borrelia burgdorferi*
Microbiology/Spirochetes/1

13. The diagnostic method *most* used for the identification of Lyme disease is:
A. Serology
B. Culture
C. Gram staining
D. Acid-fast staining
Microbiology/Spirochetes/1

14. Primary atypical pneumonia is caused by:
A. *Streptococcus pneumoniae*
B. *Mycoplasma pneumoniae*
C. *Klebsiella pneumoniae*
D. *Mycobacterium tuberculosis*
Microbiology/Pathogenicity/Bacterial/1

Answers to Questions 8–14

8. A A Gram-stained smear from a vaginal secretion showing many squamous epithelial cells loaded with pleomorphic gram-variable (positive and negative) bacilli is considered presumptive for *G. vaginalis*. Such cells are called *clue cells*. Other important findings are:

β-Hemolysis on BAP Pos	Catalase = Neg
Oxidase = Neg	Hippurate hydrolysis Pos

9. B *Nocardia* spp. should be suspected if colonies that are partially acid-fast by the traditional method are positive with the modified acid-fast method using Kinyoun stain and 1% sulfuric acid as the decolorizing agent. The other organisms listed are negative or considered non-acid-fast. Depending on the secondary stain used in the procedure, non-acid-fast organisms will appear blue (methylene blue) or green (malachite green).

10. B Serological tests of the patient's serum for evidence of syphilis are routinely performed, but culturing is not because research animals must be used for inoculation of the suspected spirochete. *T. pallidum* stains poorly or not at all by either the Gram or acid-fast technique. Darkfield microscopy for direct visualization, phase contrast, or indirect immunofluorescence using fluorescein-conjugated antihuman globulin may be used for visualization of spirochetes but is no longer routinely performed in a clinical laboratory. Tests for specific antibodies to *T. pallidum* are available in a wide range of immunoassay formats, including chemiluminescence and point-of-care immunochromatography. Therefore, a reverse algorithm that screens with a specific test for treponemal antibody is often used.

11. A *Borrelia* spp. are often seen on Wright-stained smears of peripheral blood as helical bacteria with 3 to 10 loose coils. They are gram negative but stain well with Giemsa stain. *B. recurrentis* is the cause of relapsing fever, a louse-borne epidemic. The use of thick and thin smears is helpful in observing the organism.

12. D Lyme disease may result in acute arthritis and meningitis and is caused by *B. burgdorferi*. This spirochete is carried by the deer tick belonging to the *Ixodes* genus (*I. dammini* in the eastern and north-central United States and *I. pacificus* in the northwest United States).

13. A Although PCR has been used for the diagnosis of early and late-stage Lyme disease, serology continues to be the standard for the diagnosis. Serological analysis is available commercially in a variety of formats including IFA, EIA, CIA, immunoblots, and Western blots. Titers of IgM remain high throughout the infection.

14. B A common cause of respiratory tract illness, *M. pneumoniae* generally causes a self-limited infection (3–10 days) and usually does not require antibiotic therapy.

15. Which organism typically produces "fried egg" colonies on agar within 1 to 5 days of culture obtained from a genital specimen?
A. *Mycoplasma hominis*
B. *Borrelia burgdorferi*
C. *Leptospira interrogans*
D. *Treponema pallidum*
Microbiology/Phenotypic characteristics/Bacteria/1

16. A gram-positive (gram-variable), beaded organism with delicate branching was recovered from the sputum of a 20-year-old patient with leukemia. The specimen produced orange, glabrous, waxy colonies on Middlebrook agar that showed partial acid-fast staining with the modified Kinyoun stain. What is the *most* likely identification?
A. *Rhodococcus* spp.
B. *Actinomadura* spp.
C. *Streptomyces* spp.
D. *Nocardia* spp.
Microbiology/Bacteria/3

17. A direct smear from a nasopharyngeal swab stained with Loeffler methylene blue showed various letter shapes and deep blue, metachromatic granules. The *most* likely identification is:
A. *Corynebacterium* spp.
B. *Nocardia* spp.
C. *Listeria* spp.
D. *Gardnerella* spp.
Microbiology/Microscopy/Bacteria/2

18. Which is the test of choice for the confirmation of *Chlamydia trachomatis* infection in urine?
A. Enzyme immunoassay antigen testing
B. Nucleic amplifcation
C. Culture using McCoy and Hela cells
D. Microimmunofluorescence (MIF) test
Microbiology/Chlamydia/2

19. Identify the following bacterium–specimen pairing that is *mismatched* (specimen not appropriate for isolation):
A. *Chlamydia psittaci*–fecal swab
B. *Chlamydia trachomatis*–first voided urine
C. *Chlamydia trachomatis*–endocervical swab
D. *Chlamydia pneumoniae*–throat swab or sputum
Microbiology/Specimen collection/Chlamydia/1

20. Which of the following organisms are transmitted to animals and humans after a tick bite?
A. *Leptospira spp.*
B. *Chlamydia* and *Mycoplasma* spp.
C. *Neisseria sicca*
D. *Ehrlichia* and *Anaplasma* spp.
Microbiology/Pathogenicity/Bacteria/1

Answers to Questions 15–20

15. A Genital mycoplasmas (*M. hominis*) is grown on specific agars. *M. hominis* is grown on "M" agar containing arginine and phenol red. Colonies of mycoplasma are 50 to 300 μm in diameter and display a "fried egg" appearance with red holes.

16. D All of the listed organisms produce mycelium (aerial or substrate), causing them to appear branched with Gram staining, but only the *Nocardia* spp. are positive for modified acid-fast stain. *Nocardia* is an opportunistic pathogen.

17. A *Corynebacterium* spp. are part of the normal upper respiratory tract microbiota. Organisms display typical pleomorphic shapes often resembling letters, such as "Y" or "L," and metachromatic granules.

18. B EIA and MIF tests, which are performed on serum, detect antibodies to *C. trachomatis* but may also detect antibodies that cross-react with other organisms. Cell culture is time consuming and dependent on the quality of the specimen and is rarely performed. A variety of platforms are FDA approved for nucleic acid testing and are both sensitive and specific and may be performed on urine.

19. A *Chlamydia psittaci* is found naturally in psittacine birds and other avian species. Psittacosis, the human infection, is the result of contact with pet birds and imported nonquarantined birds or from occupational contact in poultry farming or processing. Inhalation of the organisms from aerosols, fecal material, or feather dust causes a respiratory infection, and the specimen of choice is a throat swab or sputum.

20. D *Ehrlichia* and *Anaplasma* spp. are intracellular bacteria and are the causative agents of human monocytotropic ehrlichiosis (HME) and human granulocytotropic anaplasmosis (HGA). The organisms infect humans, dogs, and cattle through the bite of an infected *Ixodes* tick (named the Lone-Star tick transmitting *Ehrlichia* spp.), which also transmits *Borrelia* spp., causing Lyme disease.

21. A patient presented to the primary care provider with a circular, "bull's eye" rash on the ankle. The patient indicated that they had identified a tick there while walking in the woods 2 weeks prior. Which specimen(s) should be obtained to establish a diagnosis of Lyme borreliosis?

A. Lymph node biopsy, skin scraping
B. Blood, CSF, skin biopsy
C. Hair, fingernails
D. Saliva, sputum

Microbiology/Specimen collection/Bacterial/2

22. Partially acid-fast, gram-positive, filamentous-branching bacteria that fragmented into rods and cocci were seen in a sputum sample from a patient with human immunodeficiency virus (HIV) infection. Which of the following is the *most* likely presumptive identification?

A. *Rhodococcus equi*
B. *Streptococcus* spp.
C. *Bacillus subtilis*
D. *Corynebacterium* spp. (diphtheroids)

Microbiology/Phenotypic characteristics/Bacterial/3

23. An asymptomatic 25-year-old female patient with persistent nongonococcal urethritis (NGU) and pelvic inflammatory disease (PID) was suspected of being infected with *Mycoplasma genitalium*. Which category of testing should *not* be utilized to establish a final identification?

A. NAAT
B. Real-time PCR
C. PCR
D. Culture

Microbiology/Mycoplasma/2

24. A 1-month-old infant underwent a spinal tap to rule out bacterial meningitis. The CSF was cloudy, and the smear showed many WBCs and short gram-positive rods. After 18 hours, many colonies appeared on blood agar that resembled *Streptococcus* spp. or *L. monocytogenes*. Which of the following preliminary biochemical tests differentiate *L. monocytogenes* from *Streptococcus* spp.?

A. Hanging-drop motility (25°C) and catalase
B. PYR and bacitracin
C. Oxidase and glucose
D. Coagulase and catalase

Microbiology/Biochemical/Bacterial/3

25. Laboratory diagnosis for a *Chlamydia trachomatis* infection is typically performed by this method.

A. Cytology
B. Culture
C. NAAT
D. Antigen detection

Microbiology/Chlamydia/2

Answers to Questions 21–25

21. B Whole blood in EDTA can be used to perform culture or nucleic amplification during the early stages of disseminated disease. Serum should be collected in the acute and convalescent phase for antibody testing. CSF may be useful if the patient is experiencing neurological symptoms. Tissue biopsy and synovial fluid are useful if the patient is experiencing arthritic symptoms and for monitoring treatment.

22. A *R. equi* are facultative intracellular organisms that are found within macrophages. They are found in soil and animal feces. *R. equi* is usually opportunistic and infects immunocompromised individuals as well as farm workers through inhalation of the organisms.

23. D Culture techniques are time consuming and difficult to use as a screening procedure. The fastidious *M. genitalium* are difficult to grow. Molecular NAAT testing using conventional PCR will take 2 to 3 days for results, whereas real-time PCR will yield results in 1 day. *M. genitalium* has been implicated in the sexual transmission of HIV.

24. A *L. monocytogenes* is catalase positive and displays a "tumbling" motility at room temperature. *Streptococcus* spp. are catalase negative and nonmotile.

25. C *C. trachomatis* can be detected using multiple different diagnostic methods including culture, cytology, direct antigen detection, serologic testing, and molecular amplification tests. The most common method utilized in the diagnostic laboratory is molecular direct detection or nucleic acid amplification.

26. A PCR analysis of a vaginal sample for *Chlamydia trachomatis* gives a negative result (optical density of biotinylated reaction product below the cutoff). The internal control result is also below the cutoff. Positive and negative controls produced acceptable results. What action should be taken?

A. The test should be reported as negative
B. The sample should be diluted and the test repeated
C. The result should not be reported, and the sample should be repeated
D. A preliminary result of negative should be reported but should be confirmed by further testing using a different method of analysis

Microbiology/Molecular/Chlamydia/3

27. A catalase-positive, gram-positive short rod was recovered from the blood of a prenatal patient. The organism appeared on 5% sheep blood as white colonies surrounded by a small zone of β-hemolysis. The following tests were performed, indicating the patient was infected with which organism?

Motility = + (tumbling on wet prep) room temperature
Motility = + (umbrella-shape on semisolid agar) room temperature
Glucose = + (fermentation)
Bile esculin = +
Voges-Proskauer = +

A. *Listeria monocytogenes*
B. *Streptococcus agalactiae*
C. *Streptococcus pyogenes*
D. *Lactobacillus* spp.

Microbiology/Bacterial/3

28. An emergency department physician suspected *C. diphtheriae* when examining the sore throat of an exchange student from South America. What is the appropriate medium for the culture of the nasopharyngeal swab obtained from the patient?

A. Chocolate agar
B. Thayer-Martin agar
C. Tinsdale medium
D. MacConkey agar

Microbiology/GPR/2

Answers to Questions 26–28

26. C The internal control in PCR is an oligonucleotide sequence that differs from that of the target but binds the same primers. Its product is detected using a different probe than is used for the target sequence. If the internal control is not amplified, this indicates an invalid test. Causes include the presence of a PCR inhibitor, denaturation of the polymerase, hybridization failure, or error in the detection system (e.g., improper pH preventing enzyme-conjugated streptavidin from acting on the substrate). The assay of this sample must be repeated, and a new sample may be required.

27. A *L. monocytogenes* colonies recovered from blood and CSF display a narrow zone of β-hemolysis on 5% sheep blood agar, which often mimics group B β-hemolytic streptococci. A catalase test and Gram staining will differentiate between the two organisms. *L. monocytogenes* are catalase positive, motile (tumbling motility at room temperature), and rod shaped instead of being coccus shaped.

28. C *C. diphtheriae*, unlike other *Corynebacterium* spp., are not part of the normal flora of the human nasopharynx. Exposure through direct contact (respiratory or cutaneous lesions) is the most likely mode of transmission. Underdeveloped countries are the prime areas where exposure to *C. diphtheriae* occurs. The diagnosis is made more rapidly when the examining provider alerts the laboratory that diphtheria is suspected so that Tinsdale agar or other media containing tellurite salts can be used for culture. *Corynebacterium* will grow on blood and chocolate agars, but Tinsdale agar is the preferred culture medium because the potassium tellurite in the agar causes *C. diphtheriae* to produce brown colonies surrounded by a brown halo. The halo effect is seen with *C. diphtheriae*, *C. ulcerans*, and *C. pseudotuberculosis*, but not with other *Corynebacterium* or with other pigmented colonies growing on Tinsdale agar, such as *Streptococcus* or *Staphylococcus* spp.

29. A 25-year-old pregnant patient complained of vaginal irritation. Cultures taken for sexually transmitted diseases (STDs) proved negative. The Gram-stained vaginal smear revealed many epithelial cells with gram-variable short rods (coccobacilli) covering the margins. What is the *most* likely cause of the vaginosis?

A. Group B streptococci
B. *Gardnerella vaginalis*
C. *Staphylococcus aureus*
D. *Staphylococcus saprophyticus*

Microbiology/Bacterial/3

30. A 50-year-old transplant recipient was experiencing neurological difficulties after a pulmonary infection. A spinal tap revealed a cloudy CSF with the Gram-stained smear revealing gram-positive long-beaded bacilli. An acid-fast smear showed filamentous partially AFB. What is the *most* likely identification of the organism?

A. *Nocardia asteroides*
B. *Mycobacterium avium*
C. *Mycobacterium bovis*
D. *Legionella* spp.

Microbiology/Bacterial/3

31. A 22-year-old pregnant individual (third trimester) presented to the emergency department complaining of diarrhea, fever, and other flu-like symptoms. Blood culture, along with a urine culture, were ordered. After 24 hours, the urine culture was negative, but the blood culture revealed a gram-positive, short rod that grew aerobically on blood agar. The colonies were small and smooth, resembling a *Streptococcus* spp. with a small narrow zone of β-hemolysis. The following test results indicate which organism?

Motility = + (wet mount = tumbling)	Catalase = +
Glucose = + (acid)	Esculin hydrolysis = +

A. *Listeria monocytogenes*
B. *Streptococcus pneumoniae*
C. *Streptococcus agalactiae*
D. *Corynebacterium* spp.

Microbiology/Bacterial/3

Answers to Questions 29–31

29. B *G. vaginalis* is part of the normal flora (anorectal) of adults and children. Clue cells (vaginal epithelial cells with gram-variable coccobacilli on the cell margins) are seen in vaginal washings and the organism grows slowly on chocolate agar, 5% sheep blood agar, and V factor agar.

30. A *N. asteroides* is a gram-positive, beaded, long bacillus and is partially acid-fast. It is an intracellular pathogen that grows in human cells. Immunocompromised patients are susceptible to infections, especially pulmonary infections, which then disseminate to other organs, often proving fatal.

31. A Early detection in the pregnant individual is very important when dealing with *L. monocytogenes*. If it is not detected and treated, infection of the fetus, resulting in stillbirth, abortion, or premature birth, may result. Detection can also be made postpartum by culturing the CSF, blood, amniotic fluid, and respiratory secretions of the neonate.

9.9

Anaerobic Bacteria

1. Obligate anaerobes, facultative anaerobes, and microaerophiles are terms referring to bacteria that require:

A. Increased nitrogen
B. Decreased CO_2
C. Increased O_2
D. Decreased O_2

Microbiology/Culture/Anaerobes/1

2. Which of the following *most* affects the oxidation–reduction potential (Eh, or redox potential) of media for anaerobic bacteria?

A. Oxygen
B. Nitrogen
C. pH
D. Glucose

Microbiology/Culture/Anaerobes/1

3. Which of the following is the medium of choice for the selective recovery of gram-negative anaerobes?

A. Kanamycin–vancomycin–anaerobe (KVA) agar
B. PEA agar
C. Cycloserine cefoxitin fructose agar (CCFA)
D. THIO broth

Microbiology/Culture/Anaerobes/2

4. Anaerobic bacteria are routinely isolated from all the following types of infections *except:*

A. Lung abscesses
B. Brain abscesses
C. Dental infections
D. Urinary tract infections

Microbiology/Specimen collection/Anaerobes/1

5. A gram-positive spore-forming bacillus growing on sheep blood agar anaerobically produces a double zone of β-hemolysis and is positive for lecithinase. What is the presumptive identification?

A. *Bacteroides ureolyticus*
B. *Bacteroides fragilis*
C. *Clostridium perfringens*
D. *Clostridioides difficile*

Microbiology/Biochemical/Anaerobic bacteria/2

Answers to Questions 1–5

1. D In general, anaerobic organisms lack superoxide dismutase (SOD) and catalase enzymes. The anaerobic bacteria are subdivided based on their O_2 requirement. Obligate anaerobes are killed by exposure to atmospheric O_2 for 10 minutes or longer. Facultative anaerobes grow under aerobic or anaerobic conditions. Microaerophilic organisms do not grow in an aerobic incubator on solid media and only minimally under anaerobic conditions. However, they will grow in minimal O_2 (5% O_2). SOD is produced by many anaerobes and catalyzes the conversion of superoxide radicals to less toxic H_2O_2 and molecular O_2.

2. C Eh is most affected by pH and is expressed at pH 7.0. In cultivating anaerobic bacteria, reducing agents, such as thioglycollate and L-cysteine, are added to anaerobic transport and culture media to maintain a low Eh. Certain anaerobes do not grow in the media above a specific critical Eh level.

3. A KVA allows growth of *Bacteroides* spp., *Prevotella* spp., and *Fusobacterium* spp. and inhibits most facultative anaerobic gram-negative rods and gram-positive bacteria (both aerobic and anaerobic). PEA inhibits facultative gram-negative bacteria but will support gram-positive aerobes and anaerobes and gram-negative obligate anaerobes. CCFA is selective for *C. difficile* from stool, whereas THIO broth supports gram-positive and gram-negative aerobes and anaerobes.

4. D The incidence of anaerobic bacteria recovered from the urine is approximately 1% of isolates. The other three types of infection are associated with a 60% to 93% incidence of anaerobic recovery. Urine is not cultured routinely under anaerobic conditions unless the specimen has been obtained surgically (e.g., suprapubic aspiration).

5. C *C. perfringens* produces a double zone of β-hemolysis on blood agar, which makes identification relatively easy. The inner zone of complete hemolysis is caused by a θ-toxin, and the outer zone of incomplete hemolysis is caused by an α-toxin (lecithinase activity). The *Bacteroides* spp. are gram-negative bacilli, and *C. difficile* is lecithinase negative and does not produce a double zone of β-hemolysis.

6. Egg yolk agar is used to detect which enzyme produced by several *Clostridium* species?
A. Lecithinase
B. β-Lactamase
C. Catalase
D. Oxidase
Microbiology/Biochemical/Anaerobes/1

7. Which of the following organisms will display lipase activity on egg yolk agar?
A. *Clostridium argentinense*
B. *Clostridium ramosum*
C. *Clostridioides difficile*
D. *Clostridium sporogenes*
Microbiology/Biochemical/Bacterial/2

8. Which spore type and location is found on *Clostridium tetani*?
A. Round, terminal spores
B. Round, subterminal spores
C. Ovoid, subterminal spores
D. Ovoid, terminal spores
Microbiology/Microscopy/Anaerobes/1

9. Gram-positive bacilli recovered from two blood cultures from a 60-year-old patient with diabetes demonstrated the following results:

Spores seen = Neg	Hemolysis = + (double zone)
Motility = Neg	Lecithinase = +

What is the *most* likely identification?
A. *Clostridium tetani*
B. *Clostridium perfringens*
C. *Clostridium novyi*
D. *Clostridium sporogenes*
Microbiology/Anaerobes/3

10. Which mode of transmission responsible for botulism in infants caused by *C. botulinum*?
A. Ingestion of spores in food or liquid
B. Ingestion of preformed toxin in food
C. Inhalation of toxin
D. Open wound contamination
Microbiology/Pathogenicity/Anaerobes/2

11. The classic form of foodborne botulism is characterized by the ingestion of:
A. Spores in food
B. Preformed toxin in food
C. Toxin H
D. Spores in the environment
Microbiology/Pathogenicity/Anaerobes/2

Answers to Questions 6–11

6. A Egg yolk agar (modified McClung or neomycin egg yolk agar) is used to determine the presence of lecithinase activity, which causes an insoluble, opaque, whitish precipitate within the agar. Lipase activity is indicated by an iridescent sheen or pearly layer on the surface of the agar.

7. D Lipase is produced by some *Clostridium* spp. and is seen as an iridescent pearly layer on the surface of the colonies that extend onto the surface of the egg yolk agar medium surrounding them. *C. sporogenes* can be associated with wound infections, enteritis, and bacteremia and is lipase positive. *C. perfringens*, the most frequently isolated *Clostridium* species, is negative for lipase production.

8. A Spore appearance and location, along with Gram stain morphology, aids in distinguishing the *Clostridium* spp. Round, terminal spores (drumstick spores) are demonstrated when *C. tetani* is grown in chopped meat with glucose broth.

9. B Spores are generally not demonstrated from clinical specimens containing *C. perfringens*, which is the only species producing a double zone of hemolysis. Nucleic acid amplification testing for *C. perfringens* identification is available.

10. A Infant botulism is the most frequent form occurring in the United States. Epidemiological studies have demonstrated that infant botulism results from the ingestion of spores via breastfeeding or exposure to honey. Preformed toxin has not been detected in food or liquids taken by the infants. *C. botulinum* multiplies in the gut of the infant and produces the neurotoxin *in situ.*

11. B Foodborne botulism in adults and children is caused by ingestion of the preformed toxin (botulinum toxins A, B, E, and F) in food. The neurotoxins of *C. botulinum* are protoplastic proteins made during the growing phase and released during lysis of the organisms.

12. Which test is performed to confirm an infection with *C. botulinum*?
A. Toxin detection
B. Spore-forming test
C. Lipase test
D. Gelatin hydrolysis test
Microbiology/Biochemical/Anaerobes/2

13. Which organism causes pseudomembranous colitis or antibiotic-associated colitis?
A. *Clostridium ramosum*
B. *Clostridioides difficile*
C. *Clostridium perfringens*
D. *Clostridium sporogenes*
Microbiology/Pathogenicity/Anaerobes/1

14. A reliable method for the identification of *C. tetani* is:
A. Gram stain of the wound site
B. Anaerobic culture of the wound site
C. MALDI-TOF MS
D. Clinical findings
Microbiology/Anaerobes/2

15. Obligate anaerobic gram-negative bacilli that do not form spores, grow well in 20% bile (*Bacteroides* bile esculin [BBE] agar), and are resistant to penicillin two-unit disks are most likely:
A. *Porphyromonas* spp.
B. *Bacteroides* spp.
C. *Fusobacterium* spp.
D. *Prevotella* spp.
Microbiology/Biochemical/Anaerobes/2

16. Which gram-negative bacilli produce brown to black pigment on KVA agar and brick red fluorescence when exposed to an ultraviolet (UV) light source?
A. *Porphyromonas* spp. and *Prevotella* spp.
B. *Fusobacterium* spp. and *Actinomyces* spp.
C. *Bacteroides* spp. and *Fusobacterium* spp.
D. All the organisms listed
Microbiology/Phenotypic characteristics/Anaerobes/2

17. The following characteristics of an obligate anaerobic gram-negative bacillus *best* describe which of the listed genera?

Gram staining = Long, slender rods with pointed ends
Colonial appearance = Dry bread crumbs or fried egg appearance
Penicillin two-unit disk test = Susceptible

A. *Bacteroides* spp.
B. *Fusobacterium* spp.
C. *Prevotella* spp.
D. *Porphyromonas* spp.
Microbiology/Phenotypic characteristics/Anaerobes/2

Answers to Questions 12–17

12. A There are more than 40 different botulinum neurotoxins that can be produced by *C. botulinum, C. butyricum, C. barattii,* and *C. argentinense.* Acceptable specimens include serum, feces, enema fluid, vomitus, tissue, exudates, gastric aspirates, or postmortem samples. All specimens should be kept at 4°C and sent to the Centers for Disease Control and Prevention (CDC) for culture and toxin assays.

13. B *C. difficile* is also implicated in health care–acquired diarrhea and colitis. Suspected infection requires the collection of freshly passed stool for culture, nucleic acid amplification, and toxin assays.

14. C The culture and Gram staining of the puncture wound site usually does not produce any evidence of *C. tetani.* Clinical findings associated with infection are characterized by spastic muscle contractions, lockjaw, and backward arching of the back caused by muscle contraction. *C. tetani* can be directly detected by NAATs. Matrix-assisted laser desorption/ionization time-of-flight mass spectrometry (MALDI-TOF MS) has been used to identify *Clostridium* species effectively.

15. B The *Bacteroides* group grows well in 20% bile (primary anaerobic plates include BBE agar or bile esculin plates) and is resistant to penicillin two-unit disks. Most *Prevotella* spp. are also resistant to penicillin two-unit disks, but most *Fusobacterium* spp. and *Porphyromonas* spp. are sensitive.

16. A Pigmenting *Porphyromonas* spp. and *Prevotella* spp. also show hemolysis on anaerobic blood agar and do not grow on BBE agar.

17. B *Fusobacterium* spp. are usually spindle-shaped, slim rods, whereas the other genera are small rods (variable length for *Bacteroides* spp. and tiny coccoid rods for *Prevotella* and *Porphyromonas* spp.). *Fusobacterium* spp. and *Porphyromonas* spp. are susceptible to penicillin two-unit disks, whereas most *Bacteroides* spp. and *Prevotella* spp. are resistant.

18. All the following genera are anaerobic cocci that stain gram positive *except:*
A. *Peptococcus* spp.
B. *Peptostreptococcus* spp.
C. *Streptococcus* spp.
D. *Veillonella* spp.
Microbiology/Microscopy/Anaerobes/1

19. The gram-positive non–spore-forming, anaerobic, short, pleomorphic rods *most* frequently recovered from blood cultures as a contaminant are:
A. *Cutibacterium acnes*
B. *Clostridium perfringens*
C. *Staphylococcus intermedius*
D. *Veillonella parvula*
Microbiology/Phenotypic characteristics/Anaerobes/2

20. Which *Clostridium* species is most often recovered from a wound infection with gas gangrene?
A. *Clostridium sporogenes*
B. *Clostridium sordellii*
C. *Clostridium novyi*
D. *Clostridium perfringens*
Microbiology/Pathogenicity/Anaerobes/1

21. Gram staining of a smear taken from the periodontal pockets of a 30-year-old patient with poor dental hygiene showed sulfur granules containing non–acid-fast, gram-positive rods (short diphtheroids and some unbranched filaments). Colonies on blood agar resembled "molar teeth." The *most* likely organism is:
A. *Actinomyces israelii*
B. *Cutibacterium acnes*
C. *Staphylococcus intermedius*
D. *Peptostreptococcus anaerobius*
Microbiology/Phenotypic characteristics/Anaerobes/3

22. Antimicrobial susceptibility testing of *Bacteroides* and *Clostridium* spp. is routinely performed by which of the following methods?
A. Broth microdilution
B. Agar dilution
C. E-test
D. Not routinely performed
Microbiology/Antimicrobial susceptibility/Anaerobes/2

Answers to Questions 18–22

18. D *Veillonella* spp. are gram-negative cocci. All four genera are part of the normal human microbiota and are the anaerobic cocci most frequently isolated from blood cultures, abscesses, wounds, and body fluids. The *Streptococcus* spp. are facultative anaerobes.

19. A *C. acnes* is a non–spore former and is described as a diphtheroid-shaped rod. It is part of the normal skin, nasopharynx, genitourinary tract, and gastrointestinal tract microbiota but is implicated as an occasional cause of endocarditis and is seen in the inflammatory process of acne. *C. acnes* is referred to as the "anaerobic diphtheroid."

20. D Wounds infected with clostridia are characterized by invasion and liquefactive necrosis of muscle tissue with gas formation. The most frequently isolated organism is *C. perfringens. C. ramosum* may also cause gas gangrene or necrotizing fasciitis. *C. perfringens* is also seen in food poisoning with the release of the toxin when large numbers of the organism are ingested.

21. A *A. israelii* is part of the normal microbiota of the mouth and tonsils but may cause upper or lower respiratory tract infections. The sulfur granules are granular microcolonies with a purulent exudate. Like *Nocardia, Actinomyces* produces unbranched mycelia and is sometimes (erroneously) considered a fungus. It has also been implicated in pelvic infection associated with intrauterine contraceptive devices (IUDs).

22. D Although all three methods of antimicrobial susceptibility testing may be used for anaerobic bacteria, the fastidious nature and labor insensitivity prevent the routine performance on clinical isolates. AST is recommended when therapy fails, or an organism persists at a site of infection. It may also be useful in very serious infections. The three methods listed use *Brucella* blood agar or broth, at 35°C to 37°C incubation (anaerobically), and take up to 48 hours for results.

23. An abdominal postoperative wound specimen grew catalase-positive, indole-negative, nonpigmented, nonfluorescent, gram-negative, pleomorphic bacilli (safety pin–shaped) on 20% bile agar media. The colonies also grew on KVA agar (resistant to kanamycin, vancomycin, and colistin). What is the *most* likely identification?

A. *Fusobacterium nucleatum*
B. *Bacteroides fragilis*
C. *Prevotella* spp.
D. *Porphyromonas* spp.

Microbiology/Anaerobes/3

24. Large gram-positive bacilli (boxcar-shaped) recovered from a blood culture specimen taken from a 70-year-old patient with diabetes demonstrated the following results:

Aerobic growth = Neg	Anaerobic growth = +
Spores = Neg	Motility = Neg
Lecithinase = +	Hemolysis = β (double zone)
GLC – gas liquid chromotography (volatile acids) = Acetic acid and butyric acid	

What is the *most* likely identification?

A. *Clostridium perfringens*
B. *Fusobacterium* spp.
C. *Bacteroides* spp.
D. *Clostridium sporogenes*

Microbiology/Anaerobes/3

25. Anaerobic gram-negative rods were recovered from the blood of a patient after gallbladder surgery. The bacteria grew well on agar containing 20% bile but were resistant to kanamycin and vancomycin. What is the *most* likely identification?

A. *Clostridium perfringens*
B. *Bacteroides fragilis* group
C. *Prevotella* spp.
D. *Porphyromonas* spp.

Microbiology/Anaerobes/3

26. When attempting to identify a suspected *Clostridium* spp. from a culture using MALDI-TOF MS, how should the sample be treated prior to testing?

A. Colony is spotted directly to the target
B. Following spotting, formic acid treatment is recommended
C. Tube extraction methods are required to properly identify the organism
D. MALDI-TOF MS cannot be used to identify anaerobic bacteria

Microbiology/Anaerobes/2

27. Anaerobic gram-positive, spore-forming bacilli were recovered from the feces of a chemotherapy patient with severe diarrhea. The patient had undergone antibiotic therapy 1 week earlier. The fecal culture produced growth only on the CCFA plate. No aerobic growth of normal flora was seen after 48 hours. The following results were noted:

Kanamycin = Sensitive	Vancomycin = Sensitive
Colistin = Resistant	Lecithinase = Neg
Lipase = Neg	Nitrate = Neg
Indole = Neg	Urease = Neg
Catalase = Neg	Spores = +
CCFA agar = Growth of yellow, "ground-glass" colonies that fluoresce chartreuse (yellow-green)	

What is the correct identification?

A. *Clostridium perfringens*
B. *Clostridium tetani*
C. *Clostridium sordellii*
D. *Clostridioides difficile*

Microbiology/Anaerobes/3

Answers to Questions 23–27

23. B *B. fragilis* infections usually occur below the diaphragm and are the most encountered anaerobic infections. The Gram-stained smear showing "safety pin" and pleomorphic bacilli is often seen as a preliminary clue in abdominal fluids.

24. A *C. perfringens* is an anaerobic gram-positive rod that is often isolated from the tissue of patients with gas gangrene (myonecrosis). Spore production is not usually seen with this organism, which may also stain gram negative.

25. B *B. fragilis* is the most frequently isolated gram-negative anaerobic bacillus. It is resistant to many antibiotics. A good screening agar is a 20% bile plate that does not support the growth of *Prevotella* spp. or *Porphyromonas* spp.

26. B MALDI-TOF MS is more reliable for the identification of *Clostridum* spp. in comparison to biochemical methods. Following spotting of the pure colony on the target plate, it is recommended that formic acid be utilized for optimal extraction prior to attempting to identify the organism.

27. D The overgrowth of *C. difficile* in the bowel is the cause of antimicrobial-associated colitis. Culturing for *C. difficile* is less specific for infection than toxin testing, but is the more sensitive method, along with NAAT, to detect possible disease related to *C. difficile*. A characteristic "horse stable" odor is noted on CCFA growing *C. difficile*.

28. Anaerobic gram-positive diphtheroids (non–spore formers) were cultured from two separate blood culture bottles (at 5 days) obtained from a 25-year-old patient admitted to the hospital with dehydration, diarrhea, and other flu-like symptoms. Four other blood culture bottles did not grow any organisms at 7 days and were discarded. The following results were obtained from the recovered anaerobe:

Indole = +	Nitrate = +	Catalase = +
Kanamycin = Sensitive	Vancomycin = Sensitive	
Colistin = Resistant	Major acid from PYG broth by GLC = Propionic acid	

What is the correct identification?

A. *Eggerthella lenta*
B. *Cutibacterium acnes*
C. *Actinomyces* spp.
D. *Peptostreptococcus* spp.

Microbiology/Anaerobes/3

29. Anaerobic gram-positive bacilli with subterminal spores were recovered from several blood cultures obtained from a patient diagnosed with a malignancy of the colon. The following results were recorded:

Indole = Neg	Urease = Neg	Lipase = Neg
Catalase = Neg	Lecithinase = Neg	Double-zone of β-hemolysis = Neg
Growth on blood agar = Swarming colonies		

What is the correct identification?

A. *Clostridium septicum*
B. *Clostridium perfringens*
C. *Clostridium sordellii*
D. *Cutibacterium acnes*

Microbiology/Anaerobes/3

30. Anaerobic gram-negative bacilli were recovered from fluid obtained from drainage of a postsurgical abdominal wound. The following test results were recorded:

Kanamycin = Resistant	Vancomycin = Resistant
Colistin = Resistant	
Growth on 20% bile plate = +	Pigment = Neg
Indole = V (Neg)	Nitrate = Neg
Urease = Neg	Lipase = Neg

What is the correct identification?

A. *Prevotella* spp.
B. *Bacteroides fragilis* group
C. *Porphyromonas* spp.
D. *Clostridium* spp.

Microbiology/Anaerobes/3

31. Anaerobic, nonpigmented, gram-negative rods were recovered from an anaerobic blood agar plate after 48 hours of incubation. The Gram-stained smear showed thin bacilli with pointed ends. The colonies on blood agar had the appearance of dry, irregular, white breadcrumb-like morphology with greening of the agar. The following reactions were noted:

Kanamycin = Sensitive	Vancomycin = Resistant
Colistin = Sensitive	Nitrate = Neg
Indole = +	Catalase = Neg
Lipase = Neg	Urease = Neg
Growth on 20% bile agar = Neg	

What is the correct identification?

A. *Fusobacterium nucleatum*
B. *Bacteroides fragilis*
C. *Clostridium perfringens*
D. *Peptostreptococcus* spp.

Microbiology/Anaerobes/3

Answers to Questions 28–31

28. B *C. acnes* is a diphtheroid (pleomorphic rod) that may appear to branch on the Gram-stained smear. It is one of the most common organisms isolated from blood cultures and is often a contaminant. Abundant propionic acid is produced by GLC.

29. A *C. septicum* is often recovered from patients with malignancies or other diseases of the colon, especially the cecum. The following chart defines the swarming *Clostridium* spp.

	Indole	Urease	Spores
C. septicum	Neg	Neg	Subterminal
C. tetani	–/+	Neg	Terminal
C. sordellii	+	+	Subterminal

30. B The *B. fragilis* group is a dominant part of the indigenous flora of the large bowel and is recovered most from postoperative abdominal fluids. The *B. fragilis* group is more resistant to antibiotics and is not pigmented. *Prevotella* and *Porphyromonas* spp. are pigmented.

31. A A slender gram-negative rod with pointed ends that does not grow on 20% bile agar rules out *B. fragilis* group and indicates *F. nucleatum*.

9.10
Mycobacteria

1. **The *best* specimen for recovery of the mycobacteria from a sputum sample is the:**
   A. First morning specimen
   B. 10-hour evening specimen
   C. 12-hour pooled specimen
   D. 24-hour pooled specimen

   Microbiology/Specimen collection/Mycobacteria/1

2. **What concentration of sodium hydroxide (NaOH) is used to prepare a working decontamination solution for the processing of not normally sterile specimens for mycobacteria?**
   A. 1% NaOH
   B. 4% NaOH
   C. 8% NaOH
   D. 12% NaOH

   Microbiology/Specimen processing/Mycobacteria/2

3. **Which is the *most* appropriate nonselective medium for recovery of mycobacteria from a heavily contaminated specimen?**
   A. Löwenstein-Jensen agar
   B. Middlebrook 7H10 agar
   C. Petragnani agar
   D. Middlebrook 7H11 agar

   Microbiology/Culture/Mycobacteria/2

4. **Mycobacteria stained by using the Ziehl-Neelsen or Kinyoun methods with methylene blue counterstain are seen microscopically as:**
   A. Bright red rods against a blue background
   B. Bright yellow rods against a yellow background
   C. Orange-red rods against a black background
   D. Bright blue rods against a pink background

   Microbiology/Microscopy/Mycobacteria/2

5. **Acid-fast staining of a smear prepared from digested sputum demonstrated slender, slightly curved, beaded, red rods. Growth on the Middlebrook 7H10 medium produced buff-colored microcolonies with a serpentine pattern after 14 days at 37°C. Niacin and nitrate reduction test results were positive. What is the *most* probable presumptive identification of the organism?**
   A. *Mycobacterium tuberculosis*
   B. *Mycobacterium ulcerans*
   C. *Mycobacterium kansasii*
   D. *Mycobacterium avium* complex

   Microbiology/Mycobacteria/3

Answers to Questions 1–5

1. A Contamination by fungi and other bacteria contributes to lower yields of mycobacteria in a 24-hour sample. The first morning specimen collected by expectoration or nebulization produces the highest concentration of mycobacteria in sputum.

2. B A strong decontamination solution (6% NaOH or greater) may kill or severely damage the mycobacteria. A 4% NaOH solution is mixed with an equal volume of *N*-acetyl-L-cysteine (NALC), a digestant or mucolytic agent, to yield a final working concentration of 2% NaOH. The exposure time of the specimen to the digestion/decontamination solution must be monitored because overtreatment may result in reduced viability and recovery of the organism in culture.

3. C All four media contain malachite green as an inhibitory agent of non-mycobacteria, but the Petragnani medium contains a higher concentration (0.052 g/dL) compared with the Löwenstein-Jensen (0.025 g/dL) or Middlebrook 7H10/7H11(0.0025 g/dL) medium. A combination of solid and a liquid media is recommended for optimal recovery.

4. A Carbolfuchsin (fuchsin with phenol) stains mycobacteria red and does not decolorize after the acid–alcohol is added. The background and any other bacterial elements will decolorize and are counterstained blue by the methylene blue. A fluorescent staining procedure may be used as an alternative to acid-fast staining.

5. A *M. tuberculosis* is positive for niacin accumulation, whereas the other three species are niacin negative. *M. ulcerans* is associated with skin infections (in the tropics), does not grow at 37°C (optimal temperature is 33°C), and is not recovered from sputum. A serpentine pattern of growth indicates production of cording factor, a virulence factor for *M. tuberculosis.*

6. Which organism, associated with tuberculosis in cattle, causes tuberculosis in humans, especially in regions where dairy farming is prevalent?
A. *Mycobacterium avium* complex
B. *Mycobacterium kansasii*
C. *Mycobacterium marinum*
D. *Mycobacterium bovis*
Microbiology/Pathogenicity/Mycobacteria/1

7. Which of the following organisms are used as controls for rapid growers and slow growers, respectively?
A. *Mycobacterium fortuitum* and *Mycobacterium tuberculosis*
B. *Mycobacterium avium* complex and *Mycobacterium tuberculosis*
C. *Mycobacterium chelonae* and *Mycobacterium fortuitum*
D. *Mycobacterium kansasii* and *Mycobacterium tuberculosis*
Microbiology/Culture/Mycobacteria/2

8. Which of the following *Mycobacterium* spp. produces pigmented colonies in the dark (is a scotochromogen)?
A. *M. szulgai*
B. *M. kansasii*
C. *M. tuberculosis*
D. *M. marinum*
Microbiology/Phenotypic characteristics/Mycobacteria/2

9. All the following mycobacteria are associated with skin infections *except:*
A. *M. marinum*
B. *M. haemophilum*
C. *M. ulcerans*
D. *M. kansasii*
Microbiology/Pathogenicity/Mycobacteria/1

10. All the following *Mycobacterium* spp. produce the enzyme required to convert niacin to niacin ribonucleotide *except:*
A. *M. kansasii*
B. *M. tuberculosis*
C. *M. avium* complex
D. *M. szulgai*
Microbiology/Biochemical/Mycobacteria/2

11. The catalase test for mycobacteria differs from that used for other types of bacteria by using:
A. 1% H_2O_2 and 10% Tween 80
B. 3% H_2O_2 and phosphate buffer, pH 6.8
C. 10% H_2O_2 and 0.85% saline
D. 30% H_2O_2 and 10% Tween 80
Microbiology/Biochemical/Mycobacteria/2

Answers to Questions 6–11

6. D *M. bovis* is also called the *bovine tubercle bacillus*. A nonvirulent strain, bacillus Calmette-Guérin (BCG), is used as a tuberculosis vaccine throughout the world. Infections with *M. bovis* resemble infections caused by *M. tuberculosis* and are seen in circumstances where there is close contact between humans and cattle.

7. A When utilizing traditional culture methods for the identification of *Mycobacterium* spp., growth rates of mycobacteria can be used along with biochemical tests as an aid to identification. *M. fortuitum* grows within 3 to 5 days at 37°C and is used as the control for rapid growers. *M. tuberculosis* grows in 12 to 25 days at 37°C and is a control organism for slow growers. In addition to *M. fortuitum*, *M. chelonei* is a rapid grower (3–5 days at 28°C–35°C). In addition to *M. tuberculosis*, *M. avium* and *M. kansasii* are slow growers (10–21 days at 37°C).

8. A *M. tuberculosis* does not produce pigmentation in the dark or after exposure to light (photochromogen). *M. szulgai*, *M. gordonae,* and *M. scrofulaceum* are potentially pathogenic scotochromogens. *M. kansasii* and *M. marinum* are potentially pathogenic photochromogen-producing organisms. The bacteria produce a yellow pigment following exposure to light and red β-carotene crystals after long incubation periods.

9. D *M. kansasii* is a photochromogen that causes chronic pulmonary disease (classic tuberculosis). The other three species cause cutaneous or subcutaneous disease.

10. B Niacin production is common to all mycobacteria. However, the niacin accumulates as a water-soluble metabolite in the culture medium when the organism cannot form niacin ribonucleotide. *M. tuberculosis*, *M. simiae*, and some strains of *M. marinum*, *M. chelonae*, and *M. bovis* lack the enzyme and therefore are called *niacin positive* because of the accumulation of niacin detected in the test medium.

11. D One milliliter of an equal mixture of 30% H_2O_2 (Superoxol) and Tween 80 (a strong detergent) is added to a 2-week-old subculture on the Löwenstein-Jensen medium and placed upright for 5 minutes. Catalase activity is determined semiquantitatively by measuring the height of the column of bubbles produced above the culture surface.

12. Growth inhibition by thiophene-2-carboxylic hydrazide (TCH) can be used to differentiate *M. tuberculosis* from which other *Mycobacterium* species?
A. *M. bovis*
B. *M. avium* complex
C. *M. kansasii*
D. *M. marinum*

Microbiology/Biochemical/Mycobacteria/2

13. Which of the following *Mycobacterium* spp. can be differentiated by the rapid hydrolysis of Tween 80?
A. *M. fortuitum*
B. *M. chelonae*
C. *M. kansasii*
D. *M. gordonae*

Microbiology/Biochemical/Mycobacteria/2

14. Mycobacteria isolated from the hot water system of a hospital grew at 42°C. Colonies on the Löwenstein-Jensen medium were not pigmented after exposure to light and were negative for niacin accumulation and nitrate reduction. The *most* likely identification is:
A. *M. xenopi*
B. *M. marinum*
C. *M. ulcerans*
D. *M. haemophilum*

Microbiology/Mycobacteria/3

15. A *Mycobacterium* species recovered from a patient with AIDS gave the following results:

Niacin = Neg	TCH = +
Tween 80 hydrolysis = Neg	Nitrate reduction = Neg
Heat-stable catalase (68°C) = ±	
Nonphotochromogen	

What is the *most* likely identification?
A. *M. gordonae*
B. *M. bovis*
C. *M. avium* complex
D. *M. kansasii*

Microbiology/Mycobacteria/3

16. The urease test can be used to differentiate *M. scrofulaceum* from which of the following mycobacteria?
A. *M. gordonae*
B. *M. kansasii*
C. *M. avium* complex
D. *M. bovis*

Microbiology/Biochemical/Mycobacteria/2

Answers to Questions 12–16

12. A *M. bovis* and *M. tuberculosis* are very similar biochemically, and some strains of *M. bovis* also accumulate niacin. The TCH inhibition test differentiates *M. tuberculosis* from *M. bovis*. However, some strains of *M. bovis* that are resistant to isoniazid may also be resistant to TCH. *M. tuberculosis* is not inhibited by TCH.

13. C The hydrolysis of Tween 80 is usually positive when testing the clinically insignificant mycobacteria. *M. fortuitum*, *M. chelonae*, and *M. gordonae* are saprophytic (and opportunistic) species, but *M. kansasii* is a pathogen. *M. kansasii* hydrolyses Tween 80 more rapidly than the other species (within 3–6 hours). A positive reaction is indicated by a change in the color of neutral red from yellow to pink.

14. A *M. xenopi* causes a pulmonary infection resembling *M. tuberculosis* and is frequently isolated from patients with an underlying disease, such as alcoholism, AIDS, diabetes, or malignancy. It is often recovered from hot water taps and contaminated water systems and is a possible source of nosocomial infection. The other three species cause skin infections and grow on artificial media at a much lower temperature than *M. xenopi* (below 32°C).

15. C With the exception of *M. tuberculosis*, *M. avium* complex is the *Mycobacterium* species most often isolated from patients with AIDS. It is biochemically inert, which is a distinguishing factor for identification.

16. A Both pathogenic and saprophytic mycobacteria may produce urease, and urease production can be used to differentiate several mycobacteria species. Biochemically, *M. scrofulaceum* is identical to *M. gordonae*, except for the urease reaction for which *M. scrofulaceum* is positive and *M. gordonae* is negative. Urease reactions for the other pathogenic mycobacteria are:

M. tuberculosis = +	*M. kansasii* = +	*M. bovis* = +
M. avium complex = Neg		

17. Culture of a skin (hand) wound from a manager of a tropical fish store grew on Löwenstein-Jensen agar slants at 30°C in 10 days but did not grow on the same medium at 37°C in 20 days. Given the following results, what is the *most* likely identification?

Photochromogen = +	Niacin = Neg	Urease = +
Heat-stable catalase (68°C) = Neg		
Nitrate reduction = Neg	Tween 80 hydrolysis = +	

A. *Mycobacterium marinum*
B. *Mycobacterium kansasii*
C. *Mycobacterium avium* complex
D. *Mycobacterium tuberculosis*

Microbiology/Mycobacteria/3

18. Which typically nonpathogenic *Mycobacterium* species is isolated most often from clinical specimens and is called the "tap water bacillus"?
A. *M. kansasii*
B. *M. avium* complex
C. *M. leprae*
D. *M. gordonae*

Microbiology/Mycobacteria/1

19. How long should *M. tuberculosis*–positive cultures be kept by the laboratory after identification and antibiotic susceptibility testing have been performed?
A. 1 to 2 months
B. 2 to 4 months
C. 5 to 6 months
D. 6 to 12 months

Microbiology/Antibiotic susceptibility/Mycobacteria/2

20. According to the reporting standards, one or more AFB per oil immersion field (1,000×) are reported as:
A. Numerous or 3+
B. Few or 2+
C. Rare or 1+
D. Indeterminate; a new specimen should be requested

Microbiology/Microscopy/Mycobacteria/1

21. Which of the following *Mycobacterium* spp. would *most* likely grow on a MacConkey agar plate?
A. *M. avium* complex
B. *M. smegmatis*
C. *M. haemophilum*
D. *M. tuberculosis* complex

Microbiology/Culture/Mycobacteria/2

Answers to Questions 17–21

17. A *M. marinum* is typically recovered from cutaneous wounds resulting from infection when the skin is traumatized and exposed to inadequately chlorinated fresh water or salt water, such as in swimming pools or fish aquariums. The other three species are slow growers at 37°C. *M. tuberculosis* and *M. avium* complex are nonphotochromogens. *M. avium* complex is urease negative, *M. tuberculosis* is positive for niacin and nitrate, and *M. kansasii* is positive for nitrate and catalase.

18. D *M. gordonae* is generally considered a nonpathogen, scotochromogen, and rapid grower (7 days at 37°C). The organism may be associated with pulmonary pneumonitis and other hypersensitivity lung disease in immunocompromised patients. The other three species are pathogenic mycobacteria.

19. D Standard therapy using isoniazid and rifampin for classic, uncomplicated pulmonary tuberculosis is 9 months. The patient may not respond to therapy, even when the organism is susceptible to the antibiotics *in vitro*; therefore, cultures must be kept for up to 1 year to facilitate testing of additional antibiotics should the infection become refractory to therapy.

20. C Acid-fast smears are standardized for reporting the number of AFB seen. The following criteria should be used to uniformly report results when evaluating an acid-fast smear at 1,000× total magnification:

1–9/100 fields	1+/rare
1–9/10 fields	2+/few
1–9/field	3+/moderate
>9/field	4+/many

21. D *Mycobacteria* spp. growing on MacConkey agar and other routine media are usually nonpathogens. *M avium* complex may grow on MacConkey agar and often cause infections in immunocompromised patients.

22. Rapid methods for identifying classic infection with *M. tuberculosis* include:
A. Nucleic acid amplification
B. Nucleic acid probes
C. Acid-fast and fluorochrome-stained smears
D. MALDI-TOF MS
Microbiology/Mycobacteria/2

23. Individuals showing a positive purified protein derivative (PPD) skin test for *M. tuberculosis* are usually:
A. Infective
B. Symptomatic of pulmonary disease
C. Latently infected
D. Falsely positive
Microbiology/Mycobacteria/2

24. Which of the following *Mycobacterium* species cannot be identified using traditional culture methods?
A. *M. leprae*
B. *M. bovis*
C. *M. canettii*
D. *M. avium*
Microbiology/Culture/Mycobacteria/1

25. Which *M. avium* complex organism is the *most* frequently isolated mycobacterium in disseminated disease from patients with AIDS?
A. *M. avium* subsp. *avium*
B. *M. intracellulare* subsp. *intracellulare*
C. *M. scrofulaceum*
D. *M. bovis*
Microbiology/Pathogenicity/Mycobacteria/2

26. Which two mycobacteria commonly isolated from subcutaneous skin have an optimal growth temperature of 30°C?
A. *M. haemophilum* and *M. ulcerans*
B. *M. kansasii* and *M. xenopi*
C. *M. gordonae* and *M. avium*
D. *M. simiae* and *M. avium*
Microbiology/Culture/Mycobacteria/2

27. Which mycobacterium may be associated with Crohn disease?
A. *M. marinum*
B. *M. avium* subsp. *paratuberculosis*
C. *M. fortuitum*
D. *M. gordonae*
Microbiology/Pathogenicity/Mycobacteria/1

Answers to Questions 22–27

22. A *M. tuberculosis* is a slow grower with a prolonged culture time of 12 to 25 days and requires 3 to 6 weeks for definitive identification and antibiotic susceptibility testing. DNA probes and NAATs are widely used for the rapid identification of *M. tuberculosis*. DNA probe testing requires cultivation of the organism prior to testing; however, amplification assays provide a more rapid identification directly from a patient's respiratory specimen. Mass spectrometry (MALDI-TOF) is used for early culture identification when there is moderate culture growth.

23. C A positive PPD test result indicates a person who is latently infected with *M. tuberculosis*. These individuals are generally asymptomatic and not infectious but have a 10% risk of developing tuberculosis during their lifetime.

24. A *M. leprae* cannot be cultured in vitro. Biopsies from nodules and plaques of skin that show numerous AFB are presumptively diagnosed as positive for *M. leprae*. Confirmatory identification is made by NAAT.

25. A *M. avium* subsp. *avium* has been identified to include three additional subspecies with identical complete 16s rRNA gene sequences. *M. avium* is often associated with pulmonary disease in adults and disseminated infection in HIV patients. *M. intracellulare* subsp. *intracellulare*, although also associated with pulmonary disease, is rarely associated with disseminated infection in HIV patients.

26. A *M. haemophilum*, *M. ulcerans*, and *M. marinum* grow optimally at 27°C to 30°C. *M. xenopi* grows optimally at 42°C to 45°C and is frequently isolated from hot water systems and storage tanks. All other mycobacteria are cultured at 35°C to 37°C.

27. B *M. avium* subsp. *paratuberculosis* is known to cause an ulcerative intestinal disease with chronic diarrhea in cattle known as *Johne disease*. Although *M. paratuberculosis* has been isolated from the intestines of humans with Crohn disease with significantly greater frequency than from control subjects, the organism has not yet been proved to cause ileitis in humans.

28. Which incubation temperature range is ideal for the recovery of *M. marinum*?

A. 24°C to 26°C
B. 30°C to 32°C
C. 42°C to 44°C
D. 44°C to 48°C

Microbiology/Culture/Mycobacterial/2

29. The traditional key biochemical tests used to identify *M. tuberculosis* include:

A. Niacin, nitrate reduction, growth on TCH (10 mg/mL)
B. Light and dark incubation, Tween 80 hydrolysis
C. Heat resistance, catalase (68°C)
D. Growth on MacConkey and blood agars

Microbiology/Biochemical/Mycobacterial/2

30. What report should be given for the results of the following AFB smear?

Number of AFB seen = 2 per 300 fields (1,000× magnification)

A. 1+
B. 2+
C. 3+
D. Indeterminate; repeat with new specimen

Microbiology/Microscopy/Mycobacterial/2

31. What vaccine against tuberculosis is available, and what is the source of the vaccine?

A. No vaccine is available
B. BCG—source *M. bovis*
C. MAC—source *M. avium* complex
D. INH—source CDC

Microbiology/Mycobacterial/1

32. Acid-fast–positive bacilli were recovered from the sputum of a 79-year-old patient who had been treated for pneumonia. Which of the following test reactions after 3 weeks of incubation on Löwenstein-Jensen agar are consistent with *M. tuberculosis*?

A. Niacin = + Nitrate reduction = + Photochromogenic = Neg
B. Niacin= Neg Optochin = + Catalase = +
C. PYR = + Urease = + Bacitracin = +
D. Ampicillin = Resistant Penicillin = Resistant

Microbiology/Mycobacterial/3

33. Which statement *best* describes real-time PCR testing for *Mycobacterium tuberculosis*?

A. The test is positive only in cases of smear-positive and culture-positive infections
B. The test has a sensitivity of greater than 99% on all specimen types when compared to culture
C. The test can detect 85% to 90% of smear-negative, culture-positive infections
D. The test sensitivity is near 100%, but specificity is approximately 80%

Microbiology/Molecular/Mycobacterial/2

Answers to Questions 28–33

28. B *M. marinum* is usually recovered from skin lesions that have been in contact with underchlorinated freshwater, saltwater, or tropical fish aquariums.

29. A *M. tuberculosis* tests positive in the niacin (nicotinic acid) accumulation test, which is performed after sufficient cultural growth is observed. Even though all other species produce niacin, *M. tuberculosis* produces the most, which is tested directly on the Löwenstein-Jensen slant, provided sufficient numbers of the typical buff-colored, slow-growing, rough colonies (serpentine) are observed.

30. D This smear cannot be reported as positive or negative because only two AFB were observed per 300 fields. The two AFB observed could be contaminants in the oil immersion or on the lens of the microscope from a previous positive AFB smear. A new specimen should be requested.

31. B Presently, BCG (an attenuated strain of *M. bovis*) has been used in many parts of the world to vaccinate susceptible individuals against tuberculosis.

32. A *M. tuberculosis* is niacin positive and nonphotochromogenic. This organism takes up to 3 weeks to grow on selective agar.

33. C PCR detection is dependent on having at least a minimal number of organisms present in the specimen, and sensitivity is 90% or less when the specimen is negative for AFB smear but positive for culture. Specificity of PCR is approximately 98%.

9.11
Mycology

1. For which clinical specimens is the KOH direct mount technique for examination of fungal elements used?
A. Skin
B. CSF
C. Blood
D. Bone marrow
Microbiology/Microscopy/Mycology/1

2. The India ink stain is used as a presumptive test for the presence of which organism?
A. *Aspergillus niger* in blood
B. *Cryptococcus neoformans* in CSF
C. *Histoplasma capsulatum* in CSF
D. *Candida albicans* in blood or body fluids
Microbiology/Microscopy/Mycology/2

3. Cutaneous disease involving skin, hair, and nails usually indicates an infection with a:
A. Dimorphic fungus
B. Dermatophyte
C. Mucorales
D. *Candida* species
Microbiology/Pathogenicity/Mycology/2

4. What is the first step to be performed in a traditional identification algorithm of an unknown yeast isolate?
A. Gram staining
B. India ink staining
C. Catalase test
D. Germ tube test
Microbiology/Microscopy/Mycology/2

5. An isolate produced a constriction that was interpreted as a positive germ tube, but *C. albicans* was ruled out when biochemical tests were performed. Which of the following fungi is the *most* likely identification?
A. *Candida tropicalis*
B. *Cryptococcus neoformans*
C. *Candida glabrata*
D. *Rhodotorula rubra*
Microbiology/Microscopy/Mycology/2

Answers to Questions 1–5

1. A A solution of 10% KOH is used for contaminated specimens, such as skin, nail scrapings, hair, and sputum, to clear away background debris that may resemble fungal elements.

2. B The India ink test is not diagnostic for cryptococcal meningitis caused by *C. neoformans* because positive staining results are demonstrated in less than 50% of confirmed cases. In other words, a negative test does not exclude cryptococcal meningitis. A positive India ink test shows yeast cells in CSF with a surrounding clear area (the capsule) because the capsule of *C. neoformans* is not penetrated by ink particles.

3. B Superficial dermatophytes rarely invade deeper tissues and are the cause of most cutaneous fungal infections. Fungal infections of the skin are most often caused by *Microsporum* spp., *Trichophyton* spp., and *Epidermophyton* spp., although *Candida* spp. are sometimes implicated as the cause of nail infections.

4. D When performing traditional, phenotypic identification of a yeast isolate, a microscopic examination that would include a germ tube test is performed. The true germ tube (filamentous extension from a yeast cell) is approximately one-half the width and three to four times the length of the cell with no true hyphae constriction at the point of origin. *C. albicans* complex (*C. albicans, C. dublinensis,* and *C. Africana)* produce germ tubes.

5. A *C. tropicalis* forms pseudohyphae that resemble true germ tubes by producing a constriction at the point of origin of the yeast cell. Germ tubes represent true hyphae without constriction, and therefore, the test should have been repeated along with carbohydrate tests using a traditional phenotypic identification algorithm before making a presumptive identification. The other three species of yeast listed do not form hyphae.

6. Cornmeal agar with Tween 80 is used to identify the following characteristics of an unknown yeast isolate *except*:
A. Hyphae (true and pseudo)
B. Blastoconidia and arthroconidia
C. Chlamydoconidia
D. Conidiophores
Microbiology/Phenotypic characteristics/Mycology/1

7. Blastoconidia are the beginning of which structures?
A. Arthroconidia
B. Germ tubes
C. Pseudohyphae
D. True hyphae
Microbiology/Phenotypic characteristics/Mycology/1

8. An isolate from CSF growing on cornmeal agar produces the following structures:

Blastoconidia = +	Pseudohyphae = Neg
Chlamydoconidia = Neg	Arthroconidia= Neg

Which phenotypic tests should be performed next?
A. Bird seed agar and urease
B. Germ tube and glucose
C. India ink and germ tube
D. Rapid nitrate and glucose
Microbiology/Biochemical/Mycology/2

9. Which of the following yeast enzymes is detected using bird seed (niger seed) agar?
A. Phenol oxidase
B. Catalase
C. Urease
D. Nitrate reductase
Microbiology/Biochemical/Mycology/2

10. Which of the following yeasts is characteristically positive for germ tube production?
A. *Candida tropicalis*
B. *Candida kefyr*
C. *Cryptococcus neoformans*
D. *Candida albicans*
Microbiology/Microscopy/Mycology/1

11. Arthroconidia production is used to differentiate which two yeast isolates?
A. *Candida albicans* and *Candida dubliniensis*
B. *Cutaneotrichosporon cutaneum* and *Cryptococcus neoformans*
C. *Candida albicans* and *Candida tropicalis*
D. *Saccharomyces cerevisiae* and *Candida glabrata*
Microbiology/Phenotypic characteristics/Mycology/2

12. Presumptive identification from primary culture media that includes the urease test, niger seed agar test, and the germ tube test can be used for the identification of:
A. *Rhodotorula rubra*
B. *Cryptococcus neoformans*
C. *Trichosporon cutaneum*
D. *Candida albicans*
Microbiology/Biochemical/Mycology/2

Answers to Questions 6–12

6. D Cornmeal agar with Tween 80 (polysorbate) reduces the surface tension and allows for enhanced formation of hyphae, blastospores, and chlamydoconidia. Conidiophores are structures identified on filamentous molds, not yeast isolates.

7. C Pseudohyphae are the result of a pinching-off process, blastoconidiation, with the growth of filaments with constrictions. Germ tubes are the beginning of true hyphae (no constrictions). Arthrospores are the result of a breaking-off process of true septate hyphae resulting in square conidia.

8. A A yeast that is isolated from CSF and is producing blastospores is most likely to be *C. neoformans*, which is positive for urease and produces brown colonies on bird seed agar.

9. A Most isolates of *C. neoformans* produce phenol oxidase when grown on *Guizotia abyssinica* medium (bird seed medium), producing brown to black pigmented colonies. *C. neoformans* is the only *Cryptococcus* species that oxidizes *o*-diphenol to melanin, which is responsible for the color.

10. D *C. albicans*, *C. africana,* and *C. dubliniensis* produce germ tubes within 1 to 3 hours of incubation at 37°C. *C. tropicalis* produces pseudohyphae after incubation for 3 hours, which may be mistaken for germ tubes. A careful evaluation of the tube origin for constriction is required to avoid a false-positive interpretation.

11. B *C. cutaneum* and *C. neoformans* are both urease positive, but organisms in the genera *Trichosporon* and *Cutaneotrichosporon* produce arthroconidia, and *C. neoformans* does not. In addition, arthroconidia are produced by *Geotrichum* spp.

12. B Germ tube–negative isolates producing dark brown to black colonies on niger seed agar and a positive urease test are presumptive of *C. neoformans*. A positive germ tube test result is a presumptive identification for *C. albicans* and *C. africana* as well as for *C. dubliniensis.*

13. Which of the following yeasts is positive for the production of blastoconidia and negative for pseudohyphae or arthroconidia on cornmeal Tween 80 agar?

A. *Candida* spp.
B. *Trichosporon* spp.
C. *Geotrichum* spp.
D. *Cryptococcus* spp.

Microbiology/Phenotypic characteristics/Mycology/2

14. Ascospores are formed by which yeast isolate?

A. *Saccharomyces cerevisiae*
B. *Candida albicans*
C. *Cryptococcus neoformans*
D. *Schizophyllum radiatum*

Microbiology/Phenotypic characteristics/Mycology/2

15. A germ tube–negative, pink yeast isolate was recovered from the respiratory secretions and urine of a patient with AIDS. Given the following results, what is the *most* likely identification?

CORNMEAL TWEEN 80 AGAR	
Blastoconidia = +	Pseudohyphae = Neg
Arthroconidia= Neg	Urease = +

A. *Candida albicans*
B. *Rhodotorula* spp.
C. *Cryptococcus* spp.
D. *Trichosporon* spp.

Microbiology/Mycology/3

16. Terminal chlamydoconidia production is demonstrated by which *Candida* species?

A. *Candida glabrata*
B. *Candida krusei*
C. *Candida albicans*
D. *Candida tropicalis*

Microbiology/Phenotypic characteristics/Mycology/1

17. Yeast recovered from the urine of a catheterized patient receiving chemotherapy for cancer demonstrated the following results:

CORNMEAL TWEEN 80 AGAR	
Germ tube = +	Blastoconidia = +
Pseudohyphae = +	Arthroconidia = Neg
Terminal chlamydoconidia = +	

What further phenotypic testing would be recommended for the identification of the isolate?

A. Carbohydrate assimilation and urease
B. Urease and niger seed
C. Nitrate reductase and carbohydrate fermentation
D. No further testing is needed for identification

Microbiology/Mycology/3

18. A blood agar plate inoculated with sputum from a patient with diabetes mellitus grew very few bacterial colonies and a predominance of yeast. Given the following results, what is the *most* likely identification of the yeast isolate?

CORNMEAL TWEEN 80 AGAR	
Germ tube = Neg	Pseudohyphae = +
Arthroconidia = Neg	Blastoconidia = + (arranged along pseudohyphae)
Chlamydoconidia = Neg	

A. *Candida tropicalis*
B. *Candida kefyr*
C. *Cutaneotrichosporon cutaneum*
D. *Geotrichum candidum*

Microbiology/Mycology/3

Answers to Questions 13–18

13. D *Cryptococcus* spp. do not form either pseudohyphae or arthroconidia. *Candida* spp. produce blastoconidia or pseudohyphae. *Trichosporon* and *Cutaneotrichosporon* spp. produce pseudohyphae, blastoconidia, and arthroconidia. Arthroconidia are generally not visible on young cultures.

14. A Sexual spore production is a characteristic of the *Ascomycotina*, which produce an ascus (saclike structure) after the union of two nuclei. The resulting spore is termed an *ascospore*. *S. cerevisiae* produces ascospores when grown on ascospore agar for 10 days at 25°C. *Schizophyllum radiatum* is a basidiomycete and produces basidiospores.

15. B *Rhodotorula* spp. produces pink- to coral-colored colonies on Sabouraud agar and cornmeal agar. It is usually considered a contaminant but is an opportunistic pathogen and must be identified when found in specimens from immunosuppressed patients.

16. C Cornmeal Tween 80 agar supports the growth of *C. albicans* and the formation of its distinctive thick-walled, usually single, terminal chlamydoconidia.

17. D This isolate is most likely *C. albicans*, which also produces some true hyphae along with pseudohyphae. A positive germ tube is a presumptive identification along with the production of blastoconidia, terminal chlamydoconidia, and pseudohyphae.

18. A *C. tropicalis* and *C. kefyr* differ in their arrangement of blastoconidia along the pseudohyphae. *C. kefyr* forms elongated blastoconidia arranged in parallel clusters that simulate logs in a stream. *Cutaneotrichosporon* spp. and *Geotrichum* spp. form arthroconidia.

19. Dimorphic molds are found in infected tissue in which form?
A. Mold phase
B. Yeast phase
C. Encapsulated
D. Latent

Microbiology/Phenotypic characteristics/Mycology/2

20. The mycelial form of which dimorphic mold produces thick-walled, rectangular, or barrel-shaped alternate arthroconidia?
A. *Coccidioides immitis/C. posadasii*
B. *Sporothrix schenckii*
C. *Histoplasma capsulatum*
D. *Blastomyces dermatitidis*

Microbiology/Phenotypic characteristics/Mycology/2

21. The yeast form of which dimorphic fungus appears as oval or elongated cigar shapes?
A. *Coccidioides immitis/C. posadasii*
B. *Sporothrix schenckii*
C. *Histoplasma capsulatum*
D. *Blastomyces dermatitidis*

Microbiology/Phenotypic characteristics/Mycology/2

22. The mycelial form and macroconidia of *H. capsulatum* seen on agar resembles:
A. *Sepedonium* spp.
B. *Penicillium* spp.
C. *Sporothrix* spp.
D. *Coccidioides* spp.

Microbiology/Phenotypic characteristics/Mycology/2

23. The yeast form of which dimorphic mold shows a large parent yeast cell surrounded by smaller budding yeast cells?
A. *Paracoccidioides brasiliensis*
B. *Sporothrix schenckii*
C. *Coccidioides immitis*
D. *Histoplasma capsulatum*

Microbiology/Phenotypic characteristics/Mycology/2

24. Which group of molds can be ruled out when septate hyphae are observed in a culture?
A. Dematiaceous molds
B. Mucorales
C. Dermatophytes
D. Dimorphic molds

Microbiology/Phenotypic characteristics/Mycology/1

25. Tinea versicolor is a skin infection caused by:
A. *Malassezia furfur*
B. *Trichophyton rubrum*
C. *Trichophyton schoenleinii*
D. *Microsporum gypseum*

Microbiology/Pathogenicity/Mycology/1

Answers to Questions 19–25

19. B Dimorphic molds are in the yeast form in infected tissues because they are thermodimorphic and convert to a yeast form at 37°C. Specimens are cultured and incubated at both room temperature and 35°C to 37°C. To prove that a mold growing at room temperature (or 30°C) is a dimorphic fungus, conversion to the yeast form is demonstrated via subculture and incubation at 37°C.

20. A The mold form of *C. immitis* shows barrel-shaped arthroconidia separated by empty cells (ghost or disjunctor cells) that cause an uneven staining effect when they are examined under a microscope. *S. schenckii*, *H. capsulatum*, and *B. dermatitidis* produce conidia that are round or oval in the mold phase.

21. B *S. schenckii* is usually acquired by humans through thorns or splinters because it is commonly found on living or dead vegetation. It is called "rose gardener's disease" because gardeners, florists, and farmers are most often infected. *S. schenckii* is often recovered from exudates of unopened subcutaneous nodules or open draining lesions.

22. A *Sepedonium* spp. are saprophytic molds that do not have a yeast phase and produce large spherical tuberculate macroconidia, similar to *H. capsulatum*, but do not produce microconidia. *Sepedonium* spp. also grow poorly or not at all at 37°C.

23. A *P. brasiliensis* yeast forms are sometimes seen as a "mariner's wheel" because multiple budding cells surround the periphery of the parent cell.

24. B Mucorales commonly recovered from clinical specimens are *Rhizopus* spp. and *Mucor* spp. Both display aseptate hyphae, whereas the other groups listed display septate hyphae. *Rhizopus* spp. may demonstrate rare septa.

25. A *M. furfur* has a worldwide distribution and causes a superficial, brownish, dry, scaly patch on the skin of light-skinned persons and lighter patches on persons with dark skin. The lesions typically occur on the smooth surfaces of the body including the trunk, shoulders, arms, and face.

26. Which of the following structures are invaded by the genus *Microsporum*?
A. Hair and skin
B. Nails and skin
C. Nails and hair
D. Hair, skin, and nails
Microbiology/Pathogenicity/Mycology/1

27. An organism cultured from the skin produces colonies displaying a cherry-red color on Sabouraud dextrose agar after 3 to 4 weeks and teardrop-shaped microconidia along the sides of the hyphae. The *most* likely identification is:
A. *Trichophyton rubrum*
B. *Trichophyton tonsurans*
C. *Trichophyton schoenleinii*
D. *Trichophyton violaceum*
Microbiology/Phenotypic characteristics/Mycology/2

28. Which *Microsporum* species causes an epidemic form of tinea capitis in children?
A. *Microsporum canis*
B. *Microsporum audouinii*
C. *Nannizzia gypsea* complex
D. *Paraphyton cookei* species complex
Microbiology/Pathogenicity/Mycology/2

29. Microscopic examination of a fungus cultured from a patient with athlete's foot showed large, smooth-walled, club-shaped macroconidia appearing singly or in clusters of two or three from the tips of short conidiophores. The colonies did not produce microconidia. What is the *most* likely identification?
A. *Trichophyton* spp.
B. *Alternaria* spp.
C. *Epidermophyton* spp.
D. *Microsporum* spp.
Microbiology/Pathogenicity/Mycology/2

30. Which *Trichophyton* species causes the favus type of tinea capitis?
A. *T. verrucosum*
B. *T. violaceum*
C. *T. tonsurans*
D. *T. schoenleinii*
Microbiology/Phenotypic characteristics/Mycology/2

Answers to Questions 26–30

26. A *Trichophyton* spp., *Microsporum* spp., and *Epidermophyton* spp. are the organisms causing human dermatomycoses or cutaneous infections. *Trichophyton* spp. infect hair and nails, as well as skin. Infections with members of the genus *Microsporum* are confined to the hair and skin, whereas infections caused by the genus *Epidermophyton* are seen only on skin and nails.

27. A *T. rubrum* can be differentiated from the other members of the genus by its distinctive cherry-red color. *Trichophyton mentagrophytes* may also produce a red pigment, but it is usually rose colored or orange, or deep red. *T. tonsurans* produces white-tan to yellow, suedelike colonies. *T. schoenleinii* produces white to cream-colored colonies, and *T. violaceum* produces port wine to deep violet colonies.

28. B *M. audouinii* and *M. canis* cause tinea capitis in children. *M. audouinii* causes a chronic infection transmitted directly via infected hairs on caps, hats, combs, upholstery, and hair clippers and is associated with widespread epidemics in children. *Nannizzia gypsea* species complex, formerly *Miacrosporum gypseum* species complex, is geophilic and only occasionally infects the scalp and the skin. *Paraphyton cookei* is also geophilic and rarely infects humans.

29. C *Epidermophyton* spp. do not produce microconidia; this differentiates them from *Trichophyton* spp. and *Microsporum* spp. *Alternaria* is not a dermatophyte. *Epidermophyton floccosum* is the most frequently isolated member of the genus and infects skin, but not hair.

30. D *T. schoenleinii* is identified microscopically by its characteristic antler-shaped hyphae and chlamydoconidia in the absence of conidia.

31. The hair penetration test is used to differentiate which two species of *Trichophyton* that produce red colonies on Sabouraud agar plates?

A. *Trichophyton mentagrophytes* and *Trichophyton rubrum*
B. *Trichophyton tonsurans* and *Trichophyton schoenleinii*
C. *Trichophyton tonsurans* and *Trichophyton violaceum*
D. *Trichophyton verrucosum* and *Trichophyton rubrum*

Microbiology/Phenotypic characteristics/Mycology/2

32. A mold that produces colonies with a dark brown, green-black, or black appearance of both the surface and reverse side is classified as a:

A. Dematiaceous mold
B. Dermatophyte
C. Hyaline mold
D. Dimorphic fungus

Microbiology/Phenotypic characteristics/Mycology/1

33. A rapidly growing hyaline mold began as a white colony but soon developed a "black pepper" effect on the agar surface. The older colony produced a black matte, making it resemble a dematiaceous mold. What is the *most* likely identification?

A. *Penicillium notatum*
B. *Aspergillus niger*
C. *Paecilomyces* spp.
D. *Scopulariopsis* spp.

Microbiology/Phenotypic characteristics/Mycology/2

34. Which dematiaceous mold forms flask-shaped phialides, each with a flask-shaped collarette?

A. *Phialophora* spp.
B. *Exophiala jeanselmei* species complex
C. *Exophilia dermatitidis* spp.
D. *Phialemonium* spp.

Microbiology/Phenotypic characteristics/Mycology/2

35. Which *Aspergillus* species, recovered from sputum or bronchial mucus, is most often associated with disseminated aspergillosis?

A. *A. niger*
B. *A. versicolor*
C. *A. fumigatus*
D. *A. ustus*

Microbiology/Pathogenicity/Mycology/1

36. A hyaline mold recovered from a patient with AIDS produced rose-colored colonies with lavender centers on Sabouraud dextrose agar. Microscopic examination showed multiseptate macroconidia appearing as sickles or canoes. What is the *most* likely identification?

A. *Fusarium* spp.
B. *Phialemonium* spp.
C. *Exophiala* spp.
D. *Phialophora* spp.

Microbiology/Mycology/3

Answers to Questions 31–36

31. A *T. mentagrophytes* may produce a deep red pigment seen through the reverse side of the agar plate that resembles the cherry-red pigment produced by *T. rubrum*. However, *T. mentagrophytes* can be differentiated by the ability to invade the hair shaft. *T. rubrum* grows on the surface of hair but does not penetrate the shaft.

32. A The dematiaceous molds are easily recognized and confirmed by observing dark yellow or brown septate hyphae upon microscopic examination.

33. B *A. niger* is the only species listed producing black conidia, which causes a "pepper" effect as the colony grows. The reverse side of the agar plate remains buff or cream colored, which differentiates it from the dematiaceous (dark) molds.

34. A All the genera listed produce phialides. *Exophilia* and *Phialemonium* spp. form phialides without a collarette, as opposed to the flask-shaped phialides of *Phialophora*, which contain clusters of conidia at the tips.

35. C *A. fumigatus* is most often associated with compost piles and is found in the soil of potted plants and is most often the common cause of invasive disseminated aspergillosis and frequently associated with sinusitis. *A. niger* is the cause of cavitary fungus ball lesions of the lungs and nasal passages and often associated with ear infections. *A. versicolor* is only occasionally involved in pulmonary infections. *A. ustus* is only occasionally involved in infections in various body sites.

36. A *Fusarium* spp. are usually a contaminant but are sometimes seen as a cause of mycotic eye, nail, or skin infection in debilitated patients. *Fusarium* is a hyaline (light) mold and grows on Sabouraud agar plates at 30°C within 4 days. The other three organisms are members of the Dematiaceae family (dark molds).

37. Material from a fungus-ball infection produced colonies with a green surface on Sabouraud agar in 5 days at 30°C. Microscopic examination showed club-shaped vesicles with sporulation from the top half of the vesicle. This hyaline mold is *most* probably which *Aspergillus* sp.?
A. *A. niger*
B. *A. fumigatus*
C. *A. flavus*
D. *A. terreus*
Microbiology/Mycology/3

38. A rapidly growing nonseptate mold produced colonies with a gray surface resembling cotton candy that covered the entire plate. Microscopic examination revealed sporangiophores arising between, not opposite, the rhizoids and producing pear-shaped sporangia. What is the *most* likely identification?
A. *Lichtheimia* spp.
B. *Penicillium* spp.
C. *Rhizopus* spp.
D. *Aspergillus* spp.
Microbiology/Mycology/3

39. An India ink test was performed on CSF from a patient with HIV infection. Many encapsulated yeast cells were seen in the centrifuged sample. Further testing revealed a positive urease test and growth of brown colonies on niger seed agar. The diagnosis of meningitis was caused by which yeast?
A. *Candida albicans*
B. *Cryptococcus neoformans* species complex
C. *Cryptococcus gattii* species complex
D. *Candida tropicalis*
Microbiology/Mycology/3

40. A bone marrow sample obtained from an immunocompromised patient revealed small intracellular cells using a Wright stain preparation. Growth on Sabouraud–dextrose agar plates of a mold phase at 25°C and a yeast phase at 37°C designates the organism as thermally dimorphic. The mold phase produced thick, spherical tuberculated macroconidia. What is the *most* likely identification?
A. *Histoplasma capsulatum*
B. *Sepedonium* spp.
C. *Sporothrix schenckii*
D. *Coccidioides immitis*
Microbiology/Mycology/3

Answers to Questions 37–40

37. B *A. fumigatus* is the most common cause of aspergillosis. It is characterized by sporulation from the upper half or two-thirds of the vesicle. Colonies of *A. niger* are white with black pepper growth and produce phialides over the entire vesicle, forming the classic "radiate" head. *A. flavus* colonies are yellow to yellow-green and produce phialides that cover the entire vesicle and point out in all directions. *A. terreus* produces brown colonies and phialides that cover the entire vesicle.

38. A *Lichtheimia* spp. are similar to *Rhizopus* spp. except for the location of rhizoids (rootlike hyphae). The rhizoids of *Rhizopus* spp. are located at the point where the stolons and sporangiophores meet, whereas those of *Lichtheimia* spp. arise at a point on the stolon between the rhizoids. *Penicillium* spp. and *Aspergillus* spp. do not form rhizoids.

39. B Immunocompromised patients are at risk for invasion of *C. neoformans*. The polysaccharide capsule of *C. neoformans* is not recognized by phagocytes, which cause patients with impaired cell-mediated immunity to become readily infected with *C. neoformans*. Infections in the lungs and brain are more commonly caused by *C. gattii* species complex in immunocompetent individuals.

40. A Thermally dimorphic *H. capsulatum* produce microconidia and hyphal fragments at 37°C (yeast phase), whereas at 25°C (mold phase), the organism displays large, thick-walled, round macroconidia with knobby or knoblike projections. The yeast form can survive within circulating monocytes or tissue macrophages that can be demonstrated with Giemsa or Wright stain.

41. A lung biopsy obtained from an immunocompromised patient showed many "cup-shaped" cysts (gray to black) in a foamy exudate (green background) using Gomori methenamine silver (GMS) stain. The organism cannot be cultured because it does not grow on routine culture media for molds. The patient was diagnosed with pneumonia resistant to antibiotic treatment. The *most* likely identification is:

A. *Pneumocystis jirovecii*
B. *Histoplasma capsulatum*
C. *Sporothrix schenckii*
D. *Scopulariopsis* spp.

Microbiology/Mycology/3

42. Upon direct examination of a sputum specimen, several spherules that contained endospores were noted. Growth on Sabouraud–dextrose agar showed aerial mycelial elements. The septate hyphae produced barrel-shaped arthroconidia. What is the *most* likely identification?

A. *Talaromyces marneffei*
B. *Scopulariopsis* spp.
C. *Cryptococcus neoformans*
D. *Coccidioides immitis*

Microbiology/Mycology/3

43. A bone marrow specimen was obtained from an immunocompromised patient who tested positive for HIV. The organism grew rapidly in 3 days, showing a mold form (at 25°C), displaying conidiophores with four to five terminal metulae with each having four to six phialides. The conidia at the end of the phialides were oval and in short chains. They appear fan- or broom-like under 10× and 40× magnification. At 37°C, the yeast form grew more slowly, showing conidia that formed hyphal elements breaking at the septa to produce oval arthroconidia. This thermal dimorphic mold is *most* likely:

A. *Paecilomyces* spp.
B. *Talaromyces marneffei*
C. *Rhizomucor* spp.
D. *Aspergillus fumigatus*

Microbiology/Mycology/3

44. What is the specimen of choice for the initial diagnosis of *Pneumocystis jirovecii* in an immunocompromised patient?

A. Induced sputum
B. Open-thorax lung biopsy
C. CSF
D. Urine

Microbiology/Specimen collection/Mycology/2

Answers to Questions 41–44

41. A *P. jirovecii* is classified as a fungus but formerly was classified as a parasite. It is best recovered by bronchoalveolar lavage or induced sputum in immunocompromised patients. Open lung biopsy sample was the specimen of choice before the AIDS epidemic. GMS stain is used to identify the organism, which stains the cyst form in lung tissue, but not the trophic form. By using hematoxylin and eosin (H&E) staining on a smear, an eosinophilic, foamy material can be detected that is formed from the successful replication of the organism in alveolar lining fluid.

42. D *C. immitis* endospores are often confused with yeast cells, but they do not bud. *C. immitis* is endemic in the southwestern United States.

43. B *Talaromyces marneffei* are seen as yeast at 35°C to 37°C on 5% sheep blood agar or in BHI broth. *T. marneffei* are recovered from the blood, skin, lymph nodes, bone marrow, and internal organs of immunocompromised patients.

44. A Open lung biopsy is *not* recommended for immunocompromised patients because of the increased risk of death, infection, and complications associated with this surgical procedure. Immunocompromised individuals with *P. jirovecii* pneumonia (PCP) can be diagnosed with chest radiography, special stains, and nucleic acid amplification methods from specimens obtained by bronchoalveolar lavage (BAL). Immunocompetent patients have a much lower yield or number of infectious organisms, and therefore, besides BAL, tracheal aspiration, endoscopic lung biopsy, cellular material from bronchial brushings, and open lung biopsy specimens are more often indicated.

45. A transplant patient is suspected of having invasive aspergillosis based on clinical and radiological findings. Which specimen is *best* for the initial identification of aspergillosis by soluble galactomannan antigen testing?
A. Blood culture
B. Lung biopsy
C. Serum or urine
D. Sputum
Microbiology/Specimen collection/Mycology/2

46. What is the *most* common cause of mucormycosis infection in humans?
A. *Penicillium* spp.
B. *Candida albicans*
C. *Scopulariopsis* spp.
D. *Rhizopus* spp.
Microbiology/Pathogenicity/Mycology/1

47. A thermally dimorphic fungus shows a filamentous mold form with tuberculate macroconidia at room temperature and a yeast form above 35°C. Which organism *best* fits this description?
A. *Histoplasma capsulatum*
B. *Paracoccidioides brasiliensis*
C. *Candida albicans*
D. *Coccidioides immitis*
Microbiology/Phenotypic characteristics/Mycology/2

48. After a vacation to the southwestern United States, a patient complained of flu-like symptoms with fever, chills, nonproductive cough, and chest pain. Microscopic examination of sputum revealed large, thick-walled spherules containing endospores. Upon culture, the mold phase showed septate hyphae and alternating barrel-shaped arthroconidia. Which organism is *most* likely the cause of this pneumonia?
A. *Coccidioides immitis*
B. *Histoplasma capsulatum*
C. *Paracoccidioides brasiliensis*
D. *Talaromyces marneffei*
Microbiology/Mycology/3

49. Skin scraping from a patient showed many yeast cells of oval and bottle-shapes with monopolar budding. The direct microscopic examination also showed hyphal elements with a "spaghetti and meatball" morphological appearance. The *most* likely organism is:
A. *Malassezia furfur*
B. *Candida glabrata*
C. *Candida albicans*
D. *Cryptococcus neoformans*
Microbiology/Mycology/2

Answers to Questions 45–49

45. C To determine an early diagnosis, soluble antigens (the galactomannan assay targets antigens of *Aspergillus* spp.) are detected by using methods such as ELISA, latex agglutination, and immunoblotting using serum or body fluids. Blood and sputum cultures are usually negative, and tissue biopsy is associated with a significantly higher risk of complications. NAATs, multiplex amplification, and reverse transcription PCR (RT-PCR) have been developed, which detect systemic aspergillosis in respiratory specimens. MALDI-TOF MS methodology has proved successful in old and young cultures, with 98.6% correct identification.

46. D Vascular invasion, followed by thrombosis, tissue infarction, and necrosis, are the most common clinical manifestations of cutaneous infections caused by *Rhizopus* spp. Infections occur mainly in patients who are already being treated for other conditions, including lymphoma, leukemia, neutropenia, renal failure, and diabetic ketoacidosis.

47. A The yeast phase of *H. capsulatum* develops as small oval budding cells seen in macrophages. The yeast phase of *P. brasiliensis* develops large cells that bud creating a structure resembling a mariner's wheel, and *C. immitis* produces very large spherules. At 25°C *P. brasiliensis* produces small single conidia, and *C. immitis* produces arthroconidia. *Candida* spp. are not dimorphic.

48. A *C. immitis* is a soil fungus and is endemic to the southwestern United States. Infection results from inhaling the arthroconidia, which form endospore-forming spherules, and leads to infection within 1 to 3 weeks. Immunocompetent individuals usually do not require treatment and are immune to reinfection. However, immunodeficient individuals may develop symptomatic pulmonary and multiorgan infections.

49. A *M. furfur*, the cause of tinea versicolor, is often diagnosed with a direct skin scraping specimen. The classic "spaghetti and meatball" formations of the yeast and hyphal cells are distinct.

50. Microscopically, *Scopulariopsis* spp. resemble *Penicillium* spp. Which of the following *best* differentiates the organisms?
A. Nonseptate hyphae and foot cells
B. Brush-like conidiophores and large echinulate conidia
C. No hyphae and no phialides
D. Growth at 45°C

Microbiology/Phenotypic characteristics/Mycology/2

51. A fast-growing (2–5 days) culture of fluffy white to blue-green colonies from a respiratory specimen obtained from an immunocompromised intensive care unit (ICU) patient showed septate hyphae with many conidiophores. The tips of the conidiophores expand into large dome-shaped vesicles with bottle-shaped phialides covering the upper half or two-thirds of its surface. Long chains of small conidia form a columnar mass on the surface. At the base of the conidiophore, a "foot cell" is seen attaching the conidiophore to the septate hyphae. The *most* likely organism is:
A. *Penicillium* spp.
B. *Scopulariopsis* spp.
C. *Aspergillus fumigatus*
D. *Paecilomyces* spp.

Microbiology/Mycology/3

52. A 2-month-old infant in good health was scheduled for a checkup at the pediatrician's office. After arriving for the appointment, the mother noted white patches on the baby's tongue and in his mouth. The baby constantly used a pacifier. What is the *most* likely organism causing the white patches?
A. *Cryptococcus neoformans*
B. *Candida albicans*
C. *Aspergillus fumigatus*
D. *Sporothrix schenkii*

Microbiology/Mycology/3

53. A 69-year-old patient who was a cigarette smoker visited the clinic complaining of a cough and congestion of the lungs. Routine cultures of early morning sputum for bacteria and AFB revealed no pathogens. A fungal culture grew the following on Sabouraud dextrose agar after 3 days:

Hyphae = Septate with dichotomous branching
Spores = Produced by conidial heads with numerous conidia
Colonies = Velvety or powdery, white at first, then turning dark greenish to gray (reverse = white to tan)
Vesicle = Holding phialides usually on upper two-thirds only

What is the most likely identification?
A. *Aspergillus niger*
B. *Absidia* spp.
C. *Mucor* spp.
D. *Aspergillus fumigatus*

Microbiology/Mycology/3

Answers to Questions 50–53

50. B Microscopically, *Scopulariopsis* spp. resemble *Penicillium* spp. except for the following: *Scopulariopsis* spp. produce annellophores with flask-shaped annelides bearing large lemon-shaped, rough-walled conidia in chains; *Penicillium* spp. display brush-like conidiophores producing metulae with flask-shaped phialides, resulting in chains of small, smooth-walled conidia.

51. C A "foot cell" is characteristic of *Aspergillus fumigatus*. The presence of a foot cell, which is a T- or L-shaped cell at the base of the conidiophore (it is not a separate cell), is characteristic and distinct for *A. fumigatus*, which is thermotolerant, growing at temperatures up to 45°C.

52. B *C. albicans* is the common cause of oral thrush involving the mucocutaneous membranes of the mouth. *C. albicans* is part of the normal flora of skin, mucous membranes, and the gastrointestinal tract.

53. D *A. fumigatus* is the cause of aspergillosis and involves the organism colonizing the mucus plugs in the lung. This is called *allergic aspergillosis* and is characterized by a high titer of IgE antibody to *Aspergillus*. Invasive aspergillosis seen in patients with neutropenia exhibits sinusitis and is disseminated throughout the body.

54. A young patient with a fungus of the feet visited the podiatrist seeking relief from the itching. A culture specimen was sent to the microbiology laboratory that grew after 8 days on Sabouraud dextrose agar. Colonies were powdery pink with concentric and radial folds, with the reverse side showing brownish tan to red. Other observations were as follows:

Hyphae = Septate   Urease = +
Macroconidia = Cigar shaped, thin walled with 1 to 6 cells
Microconidia = Round and clustered on branched conidiophores
Red pigment on cornmeal (1% dextrose) = Neg
In vitro hair perforation = +

The *most* likely identification is:
A. *Trichophyton mentagrophytes*
B. *Trichophyton rubrum*
C. *Candida albicans*
D. *Aspergillus niger*
Microbiology/Mycology/3

55. A 79-year-old nursing home patient was admitted to the hospital with a fever and central nervous system dysfunction. Routine blood work and blood cultures were ordered. After 48 hours, the blood culture showed budding yeasts. The following tests performed from Sabouraud dextrose agar (after 3 days of growth) showed:

Germ tube = Neg growth	Bird seed agar = Brown
Urease = +	Pseudohyphae = Neg
Blastospores =+	Chlamydoconidia (spores) = Neg

Arthrospores = Neg
Assimilation agar = + (dextrose, sucrose, maltose)

What is the *most* likely identification?
A. *Candida albicans*
B. *Cryptococcus laurentii*
C. *Cryptococcus neoformans*
D. *Candida tropicalis*
Microbiology/Mycology/3

56. Identification of yeasts and yeast like isolates using MALDI-TOF MS is highly dependent on what?
A. The skill of the technologist
B. The concentration of the formic acid and age of the culture
C. The extraction method
D. The age of the culture and the extraction method
Microbiology/Detection/Mycology/2

57. The T2Candida system utilizes what technology to detect organisms directly in blood samples?
A. Nucleic acid amplification
B. Mass spectroscopy and nucleic acid amplification
C. Magnetic resonance, nanotechnology, and nucleic acid amplification
D. Nanotechnology and next-generation sequencing
Microbiology/Mycology/2

Answers to Questions 54–57

54. A *T. mentagrophytes*, a common cause of athletes' foot, is sometimes confused with *T. rubrum*, the most common dermatophyte to infect humans. The differential tests are shown in the following chart.

	Urease	***In Vitro* Hair Perforation Test**	**Red Pigment on Cornmeal Agar**
T. mentagrophytes	+	+	Neg
T. rubrum	Neg or weak	Neg	+

55. C *C. neoformans* produces brown colonies on bird seed agar, is urease positive, and produces only blastospores. Immunosuppressed patients are susceptible to this organism.

56. D MALDI-TOF MS can identify most species of *Candida* and other yeasts including *Trichosporon* and related genera. Variation does occur based on the age of culture and the extraction method used.

57. C The T2Candida system (T2 Biosystems, Lexington, KY) utilizes magnetic resonance combined with nanotechnology and nucleic acid amplification to identify infectious agents. The system has a low limit of detection and can identify an organism typically within 5 hours.

58. A patient presented to the emergency department with a subcutaneous infiltrative lesion on their left arm. They had recently traveled to Latin America. A biopsy of the tissue stained with hematoxylin and eosin demonstrated yeastlike cells that were uniform in size with a thick outer membrane. The cells appeared to be chaining and connected with small tubules. What is the *most* likely etiologic agent of the infection?

A. *Lagenidium* spp.
B. *Paracoccidioides loboi*
C. *Paracoccidioides brasiliensis*
D. *Pneumocystis jirovecii*

Microbiology/Mycology/3

Answer to Question 58

58. B The organism is most likely *Paracoccidioides loboi* and is transmitted through contact with contaminated water. Morphologically, the organism resembles *Paracoccidioides brasiliensis*. The organism causes a rare granulomatous fungal infection that predominantly infects the skin and subcutaneous tissues where *P. brasiliensis* is more often associated with lung infections or infections of the face, nasal, and oral mucocutaneous borders.

9.12
Virology

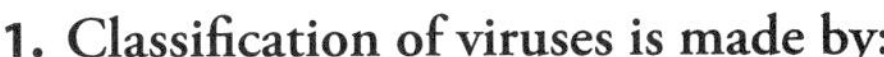

1. **Classification of viruses is made by:**
   A. Complement fixation serology
   B. Electron microscopy
   C. Nucleic acid composition
   D. Cellular inclusion bodies

   Microbiology/Taxonomy and classification/Viruses/1

2. **Which virus is a common etiological agent of viral respiratory diseases in infants and children?**
   A. Respiratory syncytial virus (RSV)
   B. Measles virus
   C. Coxsackie A virus
   D. Coxsackie B virus

   Microbiology/Disease/Viruses/1

3. **Which of the following viruses is implicated along with Epstein-Barr virus (EBV) as a cause of infectious mononucleosis?**
   A. Cytomegalovirus (CMV)
   B. Enterovirus
   C. SARS-CoV-2 (severe acute respiratory syndrome coronavirus 2)
   D. Hepatitis B virus

   Microbiology/Disease/Viruses/1

4. **Which of the following viruses are common causes of pneumonia in adults?**
   A. Influenza and adenovirus
   B. Hepatitis A and B viruses
   C. Enteroviruses (coxsackie virus B2[CVB2])
   D. Herpes simplex and CMV

   Microbiology/Disease/Viruses/1

5. **Which virus belonging to the Reoviridae group causes gastroenteritis in infants and young children but typically an asymptomatic infection in adults?**
   A. Enterovirus (coxsackie virus B [CVB])
   B. Rotavirus
   C. Respiratory syncytial virus
   D. Rhabdovirus

   Microbiology/Disease/Viruses/1

Answers to Questions 1–5

1. C Viruses are classified according to the type of nucleic acid that is either RNA or DNA and single- or double-stranded. Virus homology is linked by "type genomic sequences." Members of these classes are further divided into groups that cause human disease based on host range, mode of transmission, tissues invaded, diseases produced, and antigenic characteristics.

2. A These viruses are most often identified in young children. RSV is associated with croup, bronchitis, bronchiolitis, and interstitial pneumonia. Hospitalized children less than 1 year of age are the most susceptible.

3. A CMV infection in a previously healthy individual causes self-limiting mononucleosis syndrome. CMV is an opportunistic pathogen that may produce lifelong infections and causes a variety of diseases, including congenital and neonatal infection, hepatitis, pneumonia, and disseminated infection in immunocompromised patients.

4. A Influenza and adenoviruses cause respiratory infections, including the common cold, tracheobronchitis, and pneumonia. Adenoviruses also cause conjunctivitis, keratitis, cystitis, and gastroenteritis and are transmitted by aerosolized droplet, contaminated respiratory secretions, stool, or fomites.

5. B Rotaviruses have been implicated in both nosocomial infections and epidemic gastroenteritis. Children ages 6 to 24 months are most affected. Diarrhea begins after an incubation period of 3 days, lasts for 2 to 10 days, and is associated with vomiting and dehydration. In immunosuppressed children, rotavirus causes a chronic infection.

6. A very small, single-stranded DNA virus that causes a febrile illness with a rash and is called the *fifth childhood disease* or erythema infectiosum is:

A. Rotavirus
B. Adenovirus type 40
C. Coxsackie A virus
D. Parvovirus B19

Microbiology/Disease/Viruses/1

7. Hepatitis B virus can be transmitted by all the following *except*:

A. Acupuncture
B. Perinatally
C. Sexual contact
D. Ingestion of food and water

Microbiology/Transmission/Viruses/1

8. Which virus has been implicated in adult gastroenteritis resulting from ingestion of contaminated food and water?

A. Noroviruses (Norwalk-like viruses)
B. Rotavirus
C. Hepatitis C virus
D. Coronavirus

Microbiology/Transmission/Viruses/1

9. Which virus is associated with venereal and respiratory tract warts and produces lesions of skin and mucous membranes?

A. Polyomavirus
B. Poxvirus
C. Adenovirus
D. Papillomavirus

Microbiology/Disease/Viruses/1

10. Which technique is used for the confirmation of infection with HIV-1 and HIV-2?

A. Western blot (immunoblot) assay
B. ELISA
C. FDA-approved nucleic acid amplification testing (NAAT)
D. p24 antigen testing

Microbiology/Detection/Viruses/2

Answers to Questions 6–10

6. D Parvovirus causes a fever and characteristic "slapped cheek" rash in young children. Adults are usually immune, but immunocompromised individuals may exhibit arthritis or anemia (the virus infects immature RBCs in bone marrow).

7. D Although the most common mode of transmission of hepatitis B is via needle puncture, it may also be transmitted by other parenteral means, including through sexual transmission and contact with contaminated blood via broken skin or mucous membranes. HBV is not transmitted by casual contact such as coughing or sneezing, hugging, or physical touching, or by ingestion of food and water.

8. A Noroviruses are small RNA viruses that have been implicated in epidemics of community gastroenteritis as well as sporadic infections. Unlike rotaviruses, which cause gastroenteritis in infants and young children, noroviruses produce infections in all age groups. Norovirus is highly contagious and is often associated with outbreaks that occur in closed community settings as a result of ingestion of contaminated food or water or from fomites (inanimate surfaces).

9. D Human papillomaviruses (HPVs) cause genital warts, the most prevalent sexually transmitted viral disease in the United States. Several strains are associated with penile, cervical, and vaginal neoplasia. There are 14 high risk-HPV types that are detected by most clinically validated HPV assays, including the 12 types that are considered oncogenic.

10. C The Western blot assay is no longer used to confirm a positive serological test of antibodies to HIV. Western blot detects antibodies, but it may miss people in the window phase of infection, is not confirmatory for neonatal infections because of the presence of maternal antibodies, and has a long turnaround time resulting in loss of contact with the patient. For these reasons, the CDC recommends using a simultaneous test for antibodies to both HIV-1 and HIV-2 and p24 antigen to screen for infection by immunoassay. Positive specimens would be tested by separate immunoassays to identify whether the infection is HIV-1 or HIV-2. Samples that test negative in suspected cases should be tested by a nucleic acid amplification method, such as PCR for viral RNA for definite identification.

11. A 13-year-old patient was admitted to the hospital with a diagnosis of viral encephalitis. History revealed that the patient had been caring for wild raccoons from the nearby woods. What is the *best* method to determine whether the boy has contracted rabies?

A. Remove the brainstems from all the raccoons and examine for cytopathic effects
B. Request immunofluorescent test for antibody on the saliva from all the raccoons
C. Request immunofluorescent test for antigen in cutaneous nerve specimen obtained by nuchal biopsy
D. Isolate the virus from the saliva of both the animals and the patient

Microbiology/Viruses/3

12. A 65-year-old individual was admitted to the hospital with acute respiratory distress, fever, myalgia, and headache. Influenza A or B was suspected after ruling out bacterial pneumonia. Which of the following methods is commonly used to confirm influenza infection?

A. Cell culture
B. ELISA
C. Direct examination of nasal epithelium for virus using fluorescent antibody stain
D. MALDI-TOF MS

Microbiology/Detection/Viruses/1

13. The most rapid definitive diagnosis of a genital herpes simplex virus (HSV-2) infection in a 20-year-old patient is made by using which method?

A. Direct immunofluorescence test for viral antigen in vesicle fluid
B. Nucleic acid amplification
C. Detection of anti–herpes simplex in seminal fluid
D. Cell culture of vesicle fluid

Microbiology/Detection/Viruses/2

14. A 20-year-old college student complained of a sore throat and extreme fatigue. The primary care provider noted lymphadenopathy and ordered a rapid test for infectious mononucleosis antibodies, which was negative. Bacterial cultures were negative, as were serological tests for influenza A and B, HIV-1, CMV, hepatitis B, and anti-streptolysin O. What would be the next line of viral testing to establish a diagnosis?

A. Herpes simplex
B. Rubella
C. EBV
D. West Nile

Microbiology/Virology/3

Answers to Questions 11–14

11. C Using direct immunofluorescence microscopy (DIF), rabies antigen can be detected in the cutaneous nerves surrounding the hair follicles of the posterior region of the neck (nuchal biopsy). Antibodies to rabies can be detected in the serum and CSF of infected persons within 8 to 10 days of illness; however, infection usually occurs several months before the onset of symptoms. The saliva and the skin sample are both tested by real-time reverse transcription PCR (RT-PCR). The serum and CSF are analyzed using the rapid fluorescent focus inhibition test (RFFIT) and for rabies virus–specific IgG and IgM using rabies-infected cells and IFA tests.

12. C Direct fluorescent and enzyme immunoassays by using monoclonal antibodies to nucleoprotein antigens in infected nasal epithelium are used for rapid diagnosis of both influenza A and influenza B infections. Real-time PCR assays are also used for the detection of influenza in either a monoplex or multiplex format.

13. B PCR or other DNA amplification procedures provide improved sensitivity and the most rapid method for direct detection in most clinical laboratories. Immunostaining techniques require less expertise and are less expensive but also demonstrate decreased sensitivity.

14. C EBV serological testing for IgM-VCA (viral capsid antigen) during the illness may or may not be positive. Patients who present with an infectious mononucleosis–like syndrome should be tested for both EBV and CMV. Both viruses cause the same symptoms during the acute phase of the illness. Nucleic acid amplification methods are the most important and widely used technique for the detection of EBV in clinical specimens.

15. A 60-year-old gardener from New York State was hospitalized with flu-like symptoms and was eventually diagnosed with encephalitis. While working in his garden, the individual noticed several dead birds around the bird feeder. The region is known for heavy mosquito infestation. What is the *most* likely cause of the patient's illness?
A. West Nile virus
B. EBV
C. Parvovirus
D. Hantavirus
Microbiology/Virology/3

16. A 30-year-old patient, who was a contractor and building inspector in the southwestern United States, complained of difficulty breathing and was admitted to the hospital with severe respiratory disease. The primary care provider noted a high fever and cough. Two days earlier, the patient had inspected an old, abandoned warehouse that was infested by rodents. The patient was given IV antibiotics, but 2 days into therapy, the pneumonia worsened, leading to pulmonary edema. Which organism should be suspected of causing this illness?
A. Hantavirus
B. Rotavirus
C. West Nile virus
D. Norovirus
Microbiology/Virology/3

17. A 3-year-old child was admitted to the hospital following a 2-day visit with relatives over the Christmas holidays. Vomiting and diarrhea left the patient severely dehydrated. No other members of the family were affected. All bacterial cultures proved negative. A stool sample should be tested for which virus?
A. CMV
B. EBV
C. Hepatitis D
D. Rotavirus
Microbiology/Disease/Virology/3

18. A 6-month-old infant was hospitalized with a respiratory infection. The infant was diagnosed with apnea and bronchiolitis. Further testing revealed congenital heart disease. Bacterial cultures were negative for *S. pneumoniae* and *H. influenzae*. What is the likely etiology of the infection?
A. RSV
B. Rotavirus
C. Norovirus
D. HIV
Microbiology/Disease/Viruses/3

Answers to Questions 15–18

15. A West Nile virus causes neurological diseases with meningitis and encephalitis at the top of the list. The animal reservoirs are birds, with humans being accidental hosts. Transmission of West Nile virus is from mosquito to bird.

16. A Hantavirus is transmitted by a rodent host, the deer mouse; it was originally endemic in the southwest United States, but has been discovered throughout the country. The name of the hantavirus responsible for outbreaks in the southwest is the Sin Nombre virus. Inhalation of mice excrement is the most common mode of infection, and the lung is the site of initial infection, causing labored breathing or hantavirus pulmonary syndrome (HPS).

17. D Rotavirus is one of the most common causes of gastroenteritis in infants and young children (ages 6 months to 2 years). Vomiting and diarrhea are also common symptoms of norovirus infections, but the prevalence of rotavirus during the winter months and the absence of illness in other family members point to rotavirus being a more likely cause. Commercial availability of immunoassays for rotavirus makes its diagnosis easier to establish and rule out than infection with norovirus.

18. A RSV is spread by large particles, such as dust, and is one of the most common causes of hospitalization for respiratory illness in infants age less than 1 year. RSV causes bronchiolitis, pneumonia, and croup in infants and upper respiratory illness in children. It has also been found to cause nosocomial infection in long-term health-care facilities.

19. A hunter encountered a fox during a walk in the woods. The fox was staggering but appeared nonthreatening. The hunter tried to avoid contact but was attacked and bitten on the leg. The bite broke the skin but was not deep. Wildlife officials were unable to locate the fox for testing. What test or procedure is warranted to properly care for the hunter?

A. Spinal tap with CSF testing for rabies virus (within 2 months)
B. Administration of hyperimmune anti-rabies globulin and rabies vaccine
C. Biopsy of the wound site
D. Throat culture and blood culture (weekly)

Microbiology/Virology/3

20. A 40-year-old individual presented with a respiratory infection after returning home from a visit to China. Rapid onset of pneumonia in the lower respiratory tract prompted the provider to place the patient in isolation. The patient was diagnosed presumptively with SARS and placed on a respirator. What type of testing should be performed to identify the infectious agent?

A. RT-PCR
B. Latex agglutination test
C. Blood culture
D. Complement fixation

Microbiology/Virology/3

21. A 25-year-old pregnant female with genital lesions delivered a premature newborn with complications. The baby tested negative for bacterial infection (cultures of blood and urine). Antigen testing of the baby's urine proved negative for group B streptococci and *S. pneumoniae*. The mother tested negative for bacterial STDs and for group B streptococci. The baby was treated with acyclovir but failed to survive. What was the *most* likely cause of death?

A. CMV
B. HIV
C. RSV
D. HSV

Microbiology/Virology/3

22. A parent of two small children complained of a rash on the torso of their body. The children had been diagnosed with chickenpox and confined to their home. The parent experienced chickenpox as a child and felt the rash was not the same as the children's rash. What is the *most* likely cause of the parent's rash?

A. HSV-1
B. Varicella-zoster virus
C. HSV-2
D. EBV

Microbiology/Virology/3

23. The organs of a 65-year-old individual were donated soon after a fatal auto collision. Three recipients of the person's corneas and kidneys died within weeks after receiving them. Which of the following viruses *most* likely caused the death of the transplant recipients?

A. HIV
B. Rabies
C. Norovirus
D. Rotavirus

Microbiology/Virology/3

Answers to Questions 19–23

19. B Rabies virus can be detected by FA staining and PCR testing. The virus replicates at the site of the bite and penetrates the surrounding tissue, finding its way to the central nervous system. Because the source cannot be tested, the best immediate course of action is to initiate postexposure prophylaxis with antirabies globulin and to immunize the patient with the rabies vaccine.

20. A SARS virus was first identified in China in November 2002 when it caused a worldwide outbreak that was finally contained by July 2003. The virus belongs to the group of coronaviruses causing the common cold and is easily transmitted to health care workers who have close contact with infected individuals. This virus is the cause of a severe lower respiratory infection that can be fatal. Laboratory confirmation is performed by RT-PCR testing, which is available commercially.

21. D HSV-2 infections produce genital lesions. Infants born prematurely with disseminated infection of HSV-2 from HSV-positive mothers have a mortality rate of 50% to 60%. Testing of pregnant females for HSV and cesarean section delivery can prevent most neonatal HSV infections because the virus enters the fetus during the delivery process.

22. B Varicella-zoster virus is the cause of an infection with chickenpox. As an adult, the parent is experiencing shingles, a reactivation of the virus. The virus lies dormant in the sensory (dorsal root) ganglia of the spinal nerves, and its reactivation produces a nonweeping, blister-like rash on an inflamed skin base that follows the path of the underlying nerves.

23. B Transmission of rabies (rhabdovirus) occurs primarily from the bite of a rabid animal, but in 20% of human rabies cases, there is no known exposure to rabid animals. Donor tissues are not routinely tested for rabies.

24. While on a 7-day cruise to Vancouver and Alaska, several passengers reported to the ship's medical staff complaining of vomiting and diarrhea. Which is the *most* likely virus to have infected the passengers?
A. Rotavirus
B. Parainfluenza virus
C. RSV
D. Norovirus
Microbiology/Disease/Virology/2

25. A pregnant patient was seen by the obstetrician with signs of flu-like illness during the second trimester. NAAT was ordered for *Toxoplasma gondii*, rubella, CMV, and HSV-1 and -2. All test results were negative. However, after delivery, the newborn exhibited signs of an infection and failed to survive. Which virus in the mother demonstrates a high transplacental infection rate?
A. Hepatitis A
B. Hepatitis B
C. Hepatitis D
D. Hepatitis G
Microbiology/Virology/3

26. An immunocompromised patient was admitted to the hospital with a diagnosis of hemorrhagic cystitis. Which virus and specimen would be the *most* likely specimen and etiology for the disorder?
A. BK virus–urine
B. Human papillomavirus–skin
C. Hepatitis B virus–serum
D. EBV–serum
Microbiology/Disease/Virology/2

27. Which of the following genera and RNA viruses listed is the cause of viral hemorrhagic fever, displaying many branching "6" and circular forms while being viewed under the electron microscope?
A. Filovirus: Ebola virus
B. Flavivirus: West Nile virus
C. Picornavirus: poliovirus
D. Toga virus: western equine encephalitis virus
Microbiology/Disease/Virology/2

28. Which of the following RNA flaviviruses is responsible for Guillain-Barre syndrome and birth defects of the brain (microcephaly, absent forehead, and triangular face shape) or poor outcomes in pregnant individuals and was first recognized in 2015 in Brazil?
A. West Nile virus
B. Hepatitis C virus
C. Zika virus
D. Dengue fever virus
Microbiology/Disease/Virology/2

Answers to Questions 24–28

24. D Adult gastroenteritis caused by norovirus follows a 1- to 2-day incubation. Diagnosis is usually made based on clinical criteria and confirmed by EIA or RT-PCR.

25. B Tests for toxoplasmosis, German measles (rubella), CMV, and HSV comprise a panel of infectious agents known as the *TORCH panel*. The TORCH panel consists of serological tests for antibodies to these organisms and has largely been replaced by more sensitive NAAT when infection is suspected. The "O" in TORCH stands for "other," and other viruses that cause transplacental infection, such as HBV and HIV, are usually tested prenatally.

26. A BK virus, a polyomavirus, is transmitted by direct contact with infected respiratory secretions. It has tropism for the urinary system and often causes a latent, asymptomatic infection in the kidneys. However, in immunocompromised patients, the virus is often implicated in renal and bladder infections. Kidney failure caused by BK virus is a significant concern in bone marrow and renal transplant recipients.

27. A The Ebola RNA virus is endemic in the Democratic Republic of the Congo with a high human case fatality rate. The virus is transmitted from person to person or to caregivers through body fluids and respiratory droplets. Transmission of the virus to humans is from monkeys or other wild animals. It is speculated that bats harbor the virus as carriers or reservoirs. Although not utilized in the clinical laboratory for diagnosis, the virus can be visualized using electron microscopy.

28. C The Zika virus is transmitted by the bite of the *Aegypti* mosquito, and the virus disappears from blood after 2 weeks; however, the virus can linger in sperm for 2 months. Zika virus outbreaks were seen in Brazil and southern Mexico. According to the Pan-American Health Organization (PAHO), reports of local transmission of Zika virus occurred throughout Mexico, with a peak in number of infections occurring in October 2016. To curb the transmission of the virus, genetically modified mosquitoes were used; after mating, the offspring would die before reaching adulthood. Spraying with insecticides kills the adults and larvae, and this was one way used to control outbreaks that occurred in Miami in 2016.

29. Which of the following diseases, which are spread through direct contact and aerosols of the (RNA) coronavirus genera, caused a severe acute respiratory illness that led to a worldwide outbreak?
A. SARS
B. Encephalitis
C. Gastroenteritis
D. Liver necrosis
Microbiology/Disease/Virology/2

30. A pregnant patient presented with symptoms similar to hepatitis A but tested negative. She had traveled to India most recently. Which of the following is the cause of a hepatitis infection with a high mortality rate (10%–20%) in pregnant females and is transmitted via the fecal–oral route?
A. Hepatitis B
B. Hepatitis E
C. Hepatitis C
D. Hepatitis D
Microbiology/Virology/3

31. How can PCR be applied to the detection of HIV and other RNA viruses?
A. The virus must be inserted into human DNA by viral integrase prior to PCR
B. Substitute deoxyuridine triphosphate in place of deoxythymidine triphosphate in the master mix
C. Add a heat-stable reverse transcriptase enzyme to the master mix
D. Substitute ribonucleotide triphosphates for deoxyribonucleotide triphosphates in the master mix
Microbiology/Molecular/Virology/2

32. *In situ* hybridization (ISH) tests for human papillomavirus (HPV) using cervical smears differ from immunochemical staining of tissue in which regard?
A. ISH has lower analytical sensitivity
B. ISH has lower analytical specificity
C. ISH differentiates subtypes more easily
D. ISH differentiates cervical neoplasia from genital warts
Microbiology/Molecular/Virology/2

33. Which method is *most* sensitive for detection of viral meningitis?
A. Viral culture
B. CSF WBC count
C. Specific antibody testing of CSF for viral antigens
D. Real-time RT-PCR
Microbiology/Molecular/Virology/2

Answers to Questions 29–33

29. A There have been two well-documented outbreaks of SARS caused by coronaviruses. Both originated in China, one in 2002 and the second in 2019, COVID-19. SARS virus is detected with RT-PCR. Low levels of the virus early in the infection pose a problem in diagnosing SARS.

30. B Hepatitis E virus (HEV) is transmitted by the fecal–oral route and mimics hepatitis A, except that HEV has a high rate of fatality (10%–20%) among pregnant females. It is not endemic in the United States or in other developed areas of the world. Fulminant hepatitis, with a fatality rate of 30%, results if an infection occurs during the third trimester.

31. C Reverse transcriptase PCR (RT-PCR) is used to detect RNA viruses and to amplify RNA transcription products by converting the template to DNA. The master mix contains the same components needed for PCR with the addition of a heat-stable reverse transcriptase (enzyme that transcribes RNA to DNA, such as *rTth* DNA polymerase), manganese (a cofactor for this enzyme), and a primer to mRNA.

32. C ISH using probes that anneal with specific subtypes of HPV are able to distinguish the subtype of virus most commonly responsible for sexually transmitted warts and associated with neoplasia. Positive reactions can be detected with light microscopy by using probes conjugated to biotin. Sensitivity is approximately 88% and specificity 99% (higher than for histochemical immunoperoxidase staining). HPV is present in normal-appearing cells as well as in those demonstrating intraepithelial neoplastic lesions. However, individuals testing positive for HPV types associated with cervical cancer, such as type 16, are at higher risk for cervical neoplasia.

33. D Enterovirus is the most common cause of viral meningitis, accounting for greater than 85% of cases. Viral culture is positive in 50% to 70%, whereas the sensitivity of real-time PCR is above 95%. Enterovirus strains show significant homology at the 5′ end, making it possible to detect several different enterovirus serotypes using a single primer pair. The PCR reaction is not inhibited by antiviral therapy and can be done in hours versus days for viral culture. Multiplex PCR panels that include parechovirus and herpes simplex increase diagnostic sensitivity for meningitis. Expanded meningitis/encephalitis panels include additional viruses, *Cryptococcus*, and the most frequently implicated bacteria.

34. A dehydrated 25-year-old patient was admitted to the hospital with symptoms similar to chronic fatigue syndrome. Serological testing proved negative for recent streptococcal infection, EBV, and hepatitis. Which of the following viral serological tests should help with a possible diagnosis?
A. CMV
B. Echovirus
C. RSV
D. Measles virus

Microbiology/Virology/3

35. A nursing student working in the emergency department accidentally suffered a needlestick after removing an IV set from a suspected drug user. The *best* course of action, after reporting the incident to her supervisor, is to:
A. Test the student for HIV if flu-like symptoms develop in 2 to 4 weeks
B. Immediately test the patient and the student for HIV by using an EIA or ELISA test
C. Perform a Western blot assay on the student's serum
D. Draw blood from the student only and freeze it for further testing

Microbiology/Virology/3

36. A 30-year-old patient complained of vaginal irritation and symptoms (fever, dysuria, and inguinal lymphadenopathy) associated with STDs. Examination showed extensive lesions in the genital area. *Chlamydia* spp. testing, *N. gonorrhoeae*, and *Gardnerella vaginalis* cultures were negative. Rapid plasma reagin (RPR) testing was also negative. What is the next line of testing?
A. Darkfield examination
B. HSV testing
C. *Trichomonas* spp. testing
D. Group B streptococci testing

Microbiology/Virology/3

37. Prion disease or transmissible spongiform encephalopathies can be transmitted by:
A. Eating contaminated meat and respiratory droplets
B. Protein spontaneous mutations
C. Protein mutations, zoonotic or iatrogenic transmission
D. Zoonotic or human contact

Microbiology/Virology/2

Answers to Questions 34–37

34. A CMV infection in young adults causes a self-limiting mononucleosis syndrome. CMV infections are common and usually self-limiting, except in neonates and immunosuppressed patients, in whom they may cause a life-threatening situation.

35. B With the permission of the patient (state law may require the student to sign a consent form) and after counseling, the appropriate course of action is to test the patient for HIV by using a screening test (EIA or ELISA). The student should also be tested for baseline values. If the HIV test result is positive for the patient, the student is administered the appropriate antiviral drug(s) immediately or within 2 hours of the incident. Confirmatory testing should be performed after an initial positive HIV test result. The CDC algorithm recommends follow-up testing using NAAT to determine whether the virus is HIV1 or HIV2.

36. B Herpes genitalis is an infection caused by HSV-2. Symptomatic primary herpes by HSV-2 is responsible for about 85% of herpes infections. HSV-1 (causing the other 15%) does not involve recurring infections of herpes and causes fever blisters. HSV-2 causes 99% of recurrent genital herpes.

37. C Prion disease is caused by spontaneous mutations in the *PRNP* gene or by zoonotic or iatrogenic transmission.

9.13

Parasitology

1. **The *incorrect* match between organism and the appropriate procedure is:**
   A. *Onchocerca volvulus*—examination of skin snips
   B. *Cryptosporidium* spp.—modified acid-fast stain
   C. *Enterobius vermicularis*—routine ova and parasite examination
   D. *Schistosoma haematobium*—examination of urine sediment
   Microbiology/Specimen processing/Parasitology/2

2. **Charcot-Leyden crystals in a stool specimen may be associated with an immune response and are thought to be formed from the breakdown products of:**
   A. Neutrophils
   B. Eosinophils
   C. Monocytes
   D. Lymphocytes
   Microbiology/Microscopy/Parasitology/1

3. **Parasitic organisms that may be transmitted sexually *do not* include:**
   A. *Entamoeba gingivalis*
   B. *Dientamoeba fragilis*
   C. *Trichomonas vaginalis*
   D. *Dibothriocephalus latus*
   Microbiology/Transmission/Parasitology/1

4. **The *incorrect* match between the organism and one method of acquiring the infection is:**
   A. *Trypanosoma brucei rhodesiense*—bite of sand fleas
   B. *Giardia duodenalis*—ingestion of water contaminated with cysts
   C. Hookworm—skin penetration of larvae from soil
   D. *Toxoplasma gondii*—ingestion of infected raw or rare meats
   Microbiology/Transmission/Parasitology/1

5. **Upon examination of a stool specimen for *Cystoisospora belli*, one would expect to see:**
   A. Cysts containing sporozoites
   B. Precysts containing chromatoidal bars
   C. Oocysts that are modified acid-fast positive
   D. Sporozoites that are hematoxylin positive
   Microbiology/Morphology/Parasitology/1

6. **Which specimen is the *least* likely to provide recovery of *Trichomonas vaginalis*?**
   A. Urine
   B. Urethral discharge
   C. Vaginal discharge
   D. Feces
   Microbiology/Specimen collection/Parasitology/2

7. **Which of the following is the *best* technique to recover and identify *Dientamoeba fragilis* in stool?**
   A. Formalin concentrate
   B. Trichrome-stained smear
   C. Modified acid-fast–stained smear
   D. Giemsa stain
   Microbiology/Microscopy/Parasitology/2

Answers to Questions 1–7

1. C The appropriate procedure for the identification of *E. vermicularis* would involve the microscopic examination of a series of consecutive cellulose tape preps. Typical eggs and/or a rare adult pinworm could be identified under the microscope.

2. B When eosinophils disintegrate, the granules reform into Charcot-Leyden crystals.

3. D Of the organisms listed, *Dibothriocephalus latus* cannot be transmitted sexually; this infection is acquired from the ingestion of infected raw or poorly cooked freshwater fish.

4. A East and West African trypanosomiasis (*T. brucei rhodesiense* and *T. brucei gambiense*) are acquired when infective forms are introduced into the human body through the bite of the tse-tse fly, not sand fleas.

5. C *C. belli* oocysts in various stages of maturity would be seen in the concentrated stool sediment or possibly the direct, wet preparation; these oocysts would stain positive with modified acid-fast stains.

6. D *T. vaginalis* is site specific. The organisms are found in the urogenital tract; thus, the intestinal tract is not the normal site for these organisms.

7. B The best technique to recover and identify *D. fragilis* trophozoites and rare cysts would be the trichrome-stained smear.

8. One of the following protozoan organisms has been implicated in waterborne and foodborne outbreaks within the United States. The suspect organism is:
A. *Pentatrichomonas hominis*
B. *Dientamoeba fragilis*
C. *Giardia duodenalis*
D. *Balantioides coli*
Microbiology/Transmission/Parasitology/1

9. Gram staining of a sample from a gum lesion showed what appeared to be amoebae. A trichrome smear showed amoebae with a single nucleus and partially digested PMNs. The correct identification is:
A. *Trichomonas tenax*
B. *Entamoeba histolytica*
C. *Entamoeba gingivalis*
D. *Entamoeba polecki*
Microbiology/Microscopy/Parasitology/2

10. An *E. histolytica* (true pathogen) trophozoite has the following characteristics:
A. Compact karyosome in the nucleus, ingested RBCs, and clear pseudopodia
B. Ingested RBCs, clear pseudopodia, and uneven chromatin on the nuclear membrane
C. Ingested RBCs, clear pseudopodia, and large glycogen vacuoles in cytoplasm
D. Large, blotlike karyosome, ingested WBCs, and granular pseudopods
Microbiology/Microscopy/Parasitology/2

11. A 12-year-old is brought to the emergency department with meningitis and a history of swimming in a warm-water spring. Motile amoebae that measure 10 μm are seen in CSF and are *most* likely:
A. *Iodamoeba bütschlii* trophozoites
B. *Endolimax nana* trophozoites
C. *Dientamoeba fragilis* trophozoites
D. *Naegleria fowleri* trophozoites
Microbiology/Transmission/Parasitology/2

12. Characteristics of the rhabditiform (noninfective) larvae of *Strongyloides stercoralis* include a:
A. Short buccal capsule and large genital primordium
B. Long buccal capsule and pointed tail
C. Short buccal capsule and small genital primordium
D. Small genital primordium and notch in tail
Microbiology/Microscopy/Parasitology/1

13. Visceral larva migrans is associated with which of the following organisms and diagnostic method?
A. *Toxocara*—tissue biopsy
B. *Onchocerca*—skin snips
C. *Dracunculus*—skin biopsy
D. *Angiostrongylus*—CSF examination
Microbiology/Disease/Parasitology/1

14. The following organisms are linked with specific, relevant information. The *incorrect* combination is:
A. *Strongyloides stercoralis*—internal autoinfection
B. *Echinococcus granulosus*—hydatid examination
C. *Toxoplasma gondii*—serology
D. *Balantioides coli*—common in the United States
Microbiology/Epidemiology/Parasitology/1

Answers to Questions 8–14

8. C *G. duodenalis* has been implicated in both waterborne and foodborne outbreaks from the ingestion of infective cysts within contaminated water and food.

9. C *E. gingivalis* is known to be an inhabitant of the mouth and is characterized by morphology that resembles *E. histolytica*. However, *E. gingivalis* tends to ingest WBCs, and fragments may be present inside vacuoles of the protozoan.

10. A The trophozoite of *E. histolytica* has evenly arranged chromatin on the nuclear membrane; a central, compact karyosome in the nucleus; and clear pseudopodia; and may have ingested RBCs in the cytoplasm.

11. D *N. fowleri* are free-living soil and water amoebae that cause primary amebic meningoencephalitis (PAM). The number of cases reported is few; however, the infection is very acute and almost always fatal.

12. A The rhabditiform larvae of *S. stercoralis* are characterized by the short buccal capsule (mouth) and large genital primordium, whereas hookworm larvae have a long buccal capsule and very small genital primordium.

13. A *Toxocara* spp. are the cause of visceral larva migrans, which occurs when humans accidentally ingest the infective eggs of the dog or cat ascarid. The larvae migrate through the deep tissues, including the eye. The test of choice is a skin biopsy and the identification of migrating larvae. Although serology has been used, antibody titers vary and may be cross-reactive with other helminth infections.

14. D *B. coli* is a ciliate that can cause watery diarrhea in humans; however, it is not commonly found within the United States. It is the largest of the intestinal protozoa and can be found in proficiency testing specimens. Therefore, although it is not common, laboratories must still be able to identify these organisms.

15. Examination of 24-hour unpreserved urine specimen is sometimes helpful in the recovery of:
A. *Trichomonas vaginalis* trophozoites
B. *Schistosoma haematobium* eggs
C. *Enterobius vermicularis* eggs
D. *Strongyloides stercoralis* larvae
Microbiology/Specimen collection/Parasitology/1

16. The examination of sputum may be necessary to identify an infection with:
A. *Paragonimus westermani*
B. *Trichinella spiralis*
C. *Wuchereria bancrofti*
D. *Fasciola hepatica*
Microbiology/Specimen collection/Parasitology/1

17. Two helminth eggs that may resemble one another are:
A. *Dibothriocephalus latus* and *Paragonimus westermani*
B. *Clonorchis sinensis* and *Fasciolopsis buski*
C. *Taenia saginata* and *Hymenolepis nana*
D. *Ascaris lumbricoides* and *Trichostrongylus*
Microbiology/Microscopy/Parasitology/2

18. Eating poorly cooked infected pork can lead to an infection with:
A. *Taenia solium* and *Trichinella spiralis*
B. *Taenia saginata* and *Hymenolepis nana*
C. *Trichuris trichiura* and *Hymenolepis diminuta*
D. *Dibothriocephalus latus* and *Ascaris lumbricoides*
Microbiology/Transmission/Parasitology/1

19. An operculated cestode egg that can be recovered from human feces is:
A. *Clonorchis sinensis*
B. *Dibothriocephalus latus*
C. *Paragonimus westermani*
D. *Dipylidium caninum*
Microbiology/Microscopy/Parasitology/1

20. The adult tapeworm of *Echinococcus granulosus* is found in the intestine of:
A. Dogs
B. Sheep
C. Humans
D. Cattle
Microbiology/Epidemiology/Parasitology/1

21. In infections with *Taenia solium*, humans can serve as the:
A. Definitive host
B. Intermediate host
C. Either the definitive or the intermediate host
D. None of the above
Microbiology/Life cycle/Parasitology/2

22. Humans acquire infections with *Dibothriocephalus latus* adult worms by:
A. Ingestion of freshwater crabs
B. Skin penetration of cercariae
C. Ingestion of water chestnuts
D. Ingestion of raw freshwater fish
Microbiology/Transmission/Parasitology/1

Answers to Questions 15–22

15. B *S. haematobium* blood flukes reside in the veins over the bladder. When the eggs are passed from the body, they are often found in urine.

16. A *P. westermani* adult worms are found in the lung, and eggs may be coughed up in the sputum. Consequently, both sputum and stool (if the sputum containing the eggs is swallowed) are the recommended specimens for examination for the eggs.

17. A Both *D. latus* and *P. westermani* eggs are operculated and approximately the same size. The morphology is similar, although *D. latus* has a knob at the abopercular end and *P. westermani* has a thickened abopercular end and shoulders into which the operculum fits.

18. A Both *T. solium* (pork tapeworm) and *T. spiralis* can be acquired from the ingestion of raw or poorly cooked infected pork.

19. B *D. latus* is the only operculated cestode egg that is found in humans; the infection is acquired from the ingestion of infected raw or poorly cooked freshwater fish.

20. A Although hydatid cysts are found in sheep or in humans (accidental intermediate host), the adult tapeworms of *E. granulosus* are found in the intestine of the dog.

21. C If humans ingest *T. solium* cysticerci in uncooked or rare pork, the adult tapeworm will mature within the intestine (human will serve as definitive host); if eggs from the adult tapeworm are ingested, then the cysticerci will develop in human tissues (accidental intermediate host), causing cysticercosis.

22. D The ingestion of raw freshwater fish containing the encysted larvae of *D. latus* will result in the development of an adult tapeworm within the human intestine.

23. Humans can serve as both the intermediate and definitive host in infections caused by:
A. *Enterobius vermicularis*
B. *Hymenolepis nana*
C. *Schistosoma japonicum*
D. *Ascaris lumbricoides*
Microbiology/Life cycle/Parasitology/1

24. *Babesia* is an organism that is implicated in disease from both splenectomized and nonsplenectomized patients. Morphologically, the parasites resemble:
A. *Plasmodium falciparum* rings
B. *Leishmania donovani* amastigotes
C. *Trypanosoma cruzi* trypomastigotes
D. Microsporidian spores
Microbiology/Microscopy/Parasitology/2

25. Organisms that under normal conditions *cannot* be transmitted in the laboratory are:
A. *Cryptosporidium*—cryptosporidiosis
B. *Taenia solium*—cysticercosis
C. *Ascaris lumbricoides*—ascariasis
D. *Enterobius vermicularis*—pinworm infections
Microbiology/Transmission/Parasitology/2

26. *Toxoplasma gondii* is characterized by:
A. Possible congenital infection and ingestion of oocysts
B. Cosmopolitan distribution and possible difficulties with interpretation of serological results
C. Paroxyms and reinfection
D. Both A and B
Microbiology/Disease/Parasitology/2

27. Oocysts of *Cryptosporidium* spp. can be detected in stool specimens by using:
A. Modified acid-fast stain
B. Gram stain
C. Methenamine silver stain
D. Trichrome stain
Microbiology/Microscopy//Parasitology/1

28. Which microfilariae are usually *not found* circulating in peripheral blood?
A. *Brugia malayi*
B. *Wuchereria bancrofti*
C. *Onchocerca volvulus*
D. *Loa loa*
Microbiology/Life cycle/Parasitology/1

Answers to Questions 23–28

23. B In infections with *H. nana*, humans serve as both intermediate and definitive hosts. When ingested, the oncosphere penetrates the intestinal mucosa, develops into the mature cysticercoid (human is intermediate host), and returns to the gut, where the adult tapeworm matures (human is definitive host). Thus, the life cycle can go from egg to adult tapeworm within the human host.

24. A *Babesia* is an intracellular parasite that closely resembles the ring forms (early trophozoites) of *P. falciparum*. Often in babesiosis, there are more rings per cell and the ring form is the only stage seen.

25. C *A. lumbricoides* eggs require a period of development in the soil before they are infective for humans. The other organisms listed can be transmitted within the laboratory or in the hospital setting.

26. D Infection with *T. gondii* is acquired through the ingestion of infected rare or raw meats, infective oocysts from cat feces, or as a congenital transmission. The organism has a cosmopolitan distribution and although serological testing is generally the test of choice, the results may be very difficult to interpret in certain situations (e.g., congenital infection and immunocompromised patients).

27. A Oocysts of *Cryptosporidium* spp. can be identified using microscopic examination of fecal smears stained with modified acid-fast stains. They appear as purple-red-pink round objects, measuring approximately 4 to 6 µm. Often, the four sporozoites and residual body can be seen within the oocyst wall.

28. C *O. volvulus* microfilariae are normally found in the fluid right under the outer layer of skin. Therefore, the skin snip is the proper specimen to examine.

29. Massive hemolysis, blackwater fever, and central nervous system involvement are *most* common with:
A. *Plasmodium vivax*
B. *Plasmodium falciparum*
C. *Plasmodium ovale*
D. *Plasmodium malariae*
Microbiology/Disease/Parasitology/2

30. Organisms that should be considered in a nursery school outbreak of diarrhea include:
A. *Endolimax nana*, *Giardia duodenalis*, and *Entamoeba coli*
B. *Giardia duodenalis*, *Dientamoeba fragilis*, and *Cryptosporidium parvum*
C. *Cryptosporidium* spp., *Trichomonas vaginalis*, and *Entamoeba coli*
D. *Trichomonas hominis*, *Dientamoeba fragilis*, and *Endolimax nana*
Microbiology/Transmission/Parasitology/2

31. The *incorrect* match between disease and symptoms is:
A. Paragonimiasis—hemoptysis
B. Cryptosporidiosis—watery diarrhea
C. Toxoplasmosis in compromised host—central nervous system symptoms
D. Enterobiasis—dysentery
Microbiology/Disease/Parasitology/2

32. The formalin-ether (ethyl acetate) concentration procedure for feces is used to demonstrate:
A. Motility of helminth larvae
B. Protozoan cysts and helminth eggs
C. Formation of amoebic pseudopods
D. Trophozoites
Microbiology/Specimen processing/Parasitology/2

33. Cysts of *Iodamoeba bütschlii* typically have:
A. Chromatoidal bars with rounded ends
B. A heavily vacuolated cytoplasm
C. A large glycogen vacuole
D. Many ingested bacteria and yeast cells
Microbiology/Microscopy/Parasitology/1

34. Organisms that should be considered in a waterborne outbreak of diarrhea include:
A. *Giardia lamblia* (*G. intestinalis*, *G. duodenalis*) and *Cryptosporidium* spp.
B. *Endolimax nana* and *Entamoeba histolytica*
C. *Blastocystis* spp. and *Trichomonas vaginalis*
D. *Toxoplasma gondii* and *Schistosoma mansoni*
Microbiology/Transmission/Parasitology/2

Answers to Questions 29–34

29. B The pathogenic sequelae of malarial infections with *P. falciparum* are the most severe of the four species listed. They can include massive hemolysis, blackwater fever, and multiple organ involvement, including the central nervous system (cerebral malaria).

30. B *G. duodenalis*, *D. fragilis*, and *Cryptosporidium* have been implicated in nursery school outbreaks. Among the many protozoa and coccidia found in the human, these three organisms have become the most likely parasites in this type of setting.

31. D Infections with *E. vermicularis* (the pinworm) may cause anal itching, sleeplessness, and possibly some vaginal irritation or discharge; however, dysentery (bloody diarrhea) has not been associated with this infection.

32. B The ova and parasite examination includes three components: the direct wet film (demonstrates protozoan trophozoite motility), the formalin-ethyl acetate concentration (demonstrates protozoan cysts, coccidian oocysts, and helminth eggs), and the trichrome or iron hematoxylin–stained smear (confirms protozoan cysts and trophozoites).

33. C The cyst of *I. bütschlii* is characterized by a large glycogen vacuole that is seen on the wet smear (stains brown with iodine) and on the permanent stained smear (vacuole will appear clear). Occasionally the vacuole will be so large that the organism will collapse on itself.

34. A Both *G. duodenalis* and *Cryptosporidium* have been implicated in waterborne outbreaks of diarrheal disease. These infections would result from the ingestion of *Giardia* cysts and/or *Cryptosporidium* oocysts.

35. Fecal immunoassays can be used to diagnose infections with:
A. *Endolimax nana* and *Blastocystis* spp.
B. *Giardia duodenalis* and *Cryptosporidium* spp.
C. *Ascaris lumbricoides* and *Trichuris trichiura*
D. *Strongyloides stercoralis* and *Trichomonas vaginalis*
Microbiology/Detection/Parasitology/2

36. The most common infections with microsporidia often originate in:
A. The lung
B. The nervous system
C. The gastrointestinal tract
D. Mucocutaneous lesions
Microbiology/Life cycle/Parasitology/2

37. Eye infections with *Acanthamoeba* spp. have most commonly been traced to:
A. Use of soft contact lenses
B. Use of hard contact lenses
C. Use of contaminated lens care solutions
D. Failure to remove lenses while swimming
Microbiology/Transmission/Parasitology/2

38. The microsporidia are organisms (now classified with the fungi) that have been implicated in human disease primarily in:
A. Immunocompromised patients
B. Pediatric patients under age 5 years
C. Adult patients with congenital immunodeficiencies
D. Patients who have been traveling in the tropics
Microbiology/Epidemiology/Parasitology/2

39. When staining *Cystoisospora belli* oocysts with modified acid-fast stains, the important difference between these methods and the reagents used for AFB is:
A. The staining time is much longer with regular AFB acid-fast stains
B. The decolorizer is much weaker than acid alcohol used for AFB decolorizing
C. A counterstain must be used for the modified methods
D. The stain is more concentrated when staining for AFB
Microbiology/Microscopy/Parasitology/2

40. The *incorrect* match between symptoms and disease is:
A. Dysentery and amebiasis
B. Malabsorption syndrome and giardiasis
C. Cardiac involvement and chronic Chagas disease
D. Myalgias and trichuriasis
Microbiology/Disease/Parasitology/2

41. The *incorrect* match between organism and characteristic is:
A. *Chilomastix mesnili* and Shepherd's crook and lemon shape
B. *Plasmodium malariae* and "band trophozoite"
C. *Hymenolepis nana* and striated shell
D. *Wuchereria bancrofti* and sheathed microfilariae
Microbiology/Microscopy/Parasitology/2

Answers to Questions 35–41

35. B Fecal immunoassays have become more commonly used for the diagnosis of infections with *Giardia* and *Cryptosporidium*. These tests are available in EIA, FA, or rapid cartridge formats.

36. C With the possible exception of direct inoculation infection in the eye, the microsporidia are thought to initially infect the gastrointestinal (GI) tract through ingestion of the infective spores; infections in other body sites are thought to disseminate from the GI tract.

37. C The majority of eye infections with *Acanthamoeba* spp. have resulted from the use of contaminated eye care solutions, primarily the use of homemade saline. It is recommended that all solutions be discarded at the expiration date. Continued use may increase the risk of environmental contamination.

38. A Although the microsporidia have been known as pathogens in many groups of animals, their involvement in humans has primarily been in immunocompromised patients, especially those with AIDS. Microsporidia can be found in different tissues, and currently, there are several genera implicated in human disease.

39. B The decolorizer in modified acid-fast stains (Kinyoun cold method, modified hot method) is usually 1% to 3% sulfuric acid rather than the much stronger acid alcohol used in the routine AFB stains.

40. D *T. trichiura* (whipworm) may cause diarrhea and occasionally dysentery in very heavy infections; however, the worms are confined to the intestine, and myalgias are not seen in this helminth infection.

41. C *H. nana* has a thin eggshell containing a six-hooked embryo (oncosphere) and polar filaments that lie between the eggshell and the embryo. The striated eggshell is generally associated with the eggs of *Taenia* spp.

42. The *incorrect* match between method and objective is:

A. Direct wet examination and detection of organism motility
B. Knott concentration and the recovery of operculated helminth eggs
C. Baermann concentration and the recovery of *Strongyloides*
D. Permanent stained fecal smear and confirmation of protozoa

Microbiology/Detection/Parasitology/2

43. The *incorrect* match between organism and characteristic or diagnostic method is:

A. *Dientamoeba fragilis* and tetrad karyosome in the nucleus
B. *Toxoplasma gondii* and diagnostic serology
C. *Echinococcus granulosus* and daughter cysts
D. *Schistosoma mansoni* and egg with terminal spine

Microbiology/Parasitology/2

44. There are few procedures considered *STAT* in parasitology *except*:

A. Ova and parasite examination for giardiasis
B. Baermann concentration for strongyloidiasis
C. Blood films for malaria
D. Culture of amebic keratitis

Microbiology/Detection/Parasitology/2

45. An immunosuppressed patient has several episodes of pneumonia, intestinal pain, sepsis with gram-negative rods, and a history of military service in Southeast Asia 20 years earlier. The *most* likely etiological agent of the infection is:

A. *Trypanosoma cruzi*
B. *Strongyloides stercoralis*
C. *Naegleria fowleri*
D. *Paragonimus westermani*

Microbiology/Parasitology/3

46. In a pediatric patient, the recommended clinical specimens for recovery of *Enterobius vermicularis* is:

A. Stool specimens
B. Sigmoidoscopy scrapings
C. Duodenal aspirates
D. Series of cellophane tape preparations

Microbiology/Specimen collection/Parasitology/1

47. Protozoan cysts were seen in a concentration sediment and tentatively identified as *Entamoeba coli*. However, the organisms were barely visible on the permanent stained smear because:

A. The organisms were not present in the concentration sediment
B. There were too few cysts to allow identification on the stained smear
C. *Entamoeba coli* cysts were present but poorly fixed due to the thick cyst wall
D. The concentrate and permanent stained smear were not from the same patient

Microbiology/Parasitology/3

Answers to Questions 42–47

42. B The Knott concentration is designed to allow the recovery of microfilariae from a blood specimen. Dilute formalin (2%) is used; blood is introduced into the formalin, the RBCs lyse, and the sediment can be examined as a wet preparation or permanent stained smear (Giemsa or hematoxylin-based stain) for the presence of microfilariae.

43. D The egg of *S. mansoni* is characterized by a large lateral spine; *S. haematobium* has the characteristic terminal spine.

44. C The request for blood films for malaria should always be considered a *STAT* request. In cases of *P. falciparum* malaria, any delay in diagnosing the infection could be fatal for the patient.

45. B A latent infection with *S. stercoralis* acquired years before may cause severe symptoms in the immunosuppressed patient ("autoinfective" capability of life cycle and migratory route through the body leading to the hyperinfection syndrome and disseminated disease).

46. D The collection of a series of consecutive Scotch/cellophane tape preparations is recommended for the diagnosis of infection with the pinworm *E. vermicularis*.

47. C As *E. coli* cysts mature, the cyst wall becomes more impenetrable to fixatives. Consequently, the cysts may be visible in the concentrated sediment but appear very distorted or pale on the permanent stained smear.

48. When humans have hydatid disease, the causative agent and host classification are:
A. *Echinococcus granulosus*—accidental intermediate host
B. *Echinococcus granulosus*—definitive host
C. *Taenia solium*—accidental intermediate host
D. *Taenia solium*—definitive host
Microbiology/Life cycle/Parasitology/2

49. A 45-year-old hunter developed fever, myalgia, and periorbital edema. The patient has a history of bear meat consumption. The *most* likely causative agent is:
A. *Toxoplasma gondii*
B. *Taenia solium*
C. *Hymenolepis nana*
D. *Trichinella spiralis*
Microbiology/Parasitology/3

50. In this condition resulting from the accidental ingestion of eggs, the human becomes the intermediate host, rather than the definitive host. The correct answer is:
A. Trichinosis
B. Cysticercosis
C. Ascariasis
D. Strongyloidiasis
Microbiology/Disease/Parasitology/2

51. An immunosuppressed transplant recipient developed increasing diarrhea. What is the *most* likely disease state and laboratory procedure to confirm the patient's condition?
A. Trichinosis and trichrome staining
B. Microsporidiosis and modified trichrome staining
C. Toxoplasmosis and Gram staining
D. Paragonimiasis and wet preparation
Microbiology/Parasitology/3

52. After returning from a 2-year stay in India, a patient has eosinophilia, an enlarged left spermatic cord, and bilateral inguinal lymphadenopathy. What specimen would be required for the identification of the potential etiological agent associated with the patient's condition?
A. Thin blood films and *Leishmania*
B. Urine and concentration for *Trichomonas vaginalis*
C. Thin blood films and *Babesia*
D. Thick blood films and microfilariae
Microbiology/Parasitology/3

53. Patients with severe diarrhea should use "enteric precautions" to prevent health care–associated infections with:
A. *Giardia duodenalis*
B. *Ascaris lumbricoides*
C. *Cryptosporidium* spp.
D. *Cystoisospora belli*
Microbiology/Transmission/Parasitology/2

54. A 60-year-old Brazilian patient with cardiac irregularities and congestive heart failure suddenly dies. Examination of the myocardium revealed numerous amastigotes, an indication that the cause of death was *most* likely:
A. Leishmaniasis with *Leishmania donovani*
B. Leishmaniasis with *Leishmania braziliense*
C. Trypanosomiasis with *Trypanosoma gambiense*
D. Trypanosomiasis with *Trypanosoma cruzi*
Microbiology/Parasitology/3

Answers to Questions 48–54

48. A The cause of hydatid disease is *E. granulosus*, and the human is classified as the accidental intermediate host. Infection occurs when humans accidentally ingest the eggs of *E. granulosus* and the hydatid cysts develop in the liver, lung, and other organs of the human instead of sheep (normal cycle).

49. D Bear meat is another excellent source of *T. spiralis*. In this case, the patient had evidently consumed poorly cooked infected bear meat, thus ingesting the encysted larvae of *T. spiralis*.

50. B The accidental ingestion of *T. solium* eggs can result in the disease called *cysticercosis*. The cysticerci will develop in several different tissues, including the brain, and humans are accidental intermediate hosts.

51. B The fact that the patient has received a transplant, is immunosuppressed, and has increasing diarrhea suggests infection with microsporidia; the most appropriate method would be the modified trichrome stain.

52. D The preparation and examination of thick blood films for the recovery and identification of microfilariae should be performed. The symptoms suggest early filariasis.

53. C *Cryptosporidium* oocysts (unlike those of *C. belli*) are immediately infective when passed in stool, and nosocomial infections have been well documented with this coccidian.

54. D *T. cruzi*, the cause of Chagas disease, exists in two forms within humans, the trypomastigote in the blood and the amastigote in the striated muscle (usually cardiac muscle and intestinal tract muscle).

55. When analysis of blood smears for malaria is requested, what patient information should be obtained?
A. Diet, age, gender
B. Age, antimalarial medication, gender
C. Travel history, antimalarial medication, date of return to United States
D. Fever patterns, travel history, diet
Microbiology/Parasitology/3

56. In an outbreak of diarrheal disease traced to a municipal water supply, the *most* likely causative agent is:
A. *Cryptosporidium* spp.
B. *Cystoisospora belli*
C. *Entamoeba histolytica*
D. *Dientamoeba fragilis*
Microbiology/Transmission/Parasitology/2

57. Within the United States, sporadic mini-outbreaks of diarrheal disease have been associated with the ingestion of contaminated imported strawberries, raspberries, fresh basil, mesclun (baby lettuce leaves), and snow peas. The *most* likely causative agent is:
A. *Dientamoeba fragilis*
B. *Cyclospora cayetanensis*
C. *Schistosoma mansoni*
D. *Cystoisospora belli*
Microbiology/Transmission/Parasitology/2

58. Which of the following statements is true regarding onchocerciasis?
A. The adult worm is present in blood
B. The microfilariae are in the blood during the late evening hours
C. The diagnostic test of choice is the skin snip
D. The parasite resides in the deep lymphatics
Microbiology/Life cycle/Parasitology/2

59. The *most* prevalent helminth to infect humans is:
A. *Enterobius vermicularis*, the pinworm
B. *Ascaris lumbricoides,* the large intestinal roundworm
C. *Taenia saginata,* the beef tapeworm
D. *Schistosoma mansoni,* one of the blood flukes
Microbiology/Disease/Parasitology/1

60. A helminth egg is described as having terminal polar plugs. The *most* likely helminth is:
A. Hookworm
B. *Trichuris trichiura*
C. *Fasciola hepatica*
D. *Diphyllobothrium latum*
Microbiology/Microscopy/Parasitology/1

61. Ingestion of which of the following eggs will result in infection?
A. *Strongyloides stercoralis*
B. *Schistosoma japonicum*
C. *Toxocara canis*
D. *Clonorchis sinensis*
Microbiology/Transmission/Parasitology/2

Answers to Questions 55–61

55. C Travel history (areas of drug resistance), the date of return to the United States (primary versus relapse case), and history of antimalarial medication and illness (severe illness, few organisms on smear) are very important questions to ask. Without this information, a malaria diagnosis can be missed or delayed with severe patient consequences.

56. A *Cryptosporidium* can be transmitted through contaminated municipal water sources. Such outbreaks are well documented.

57. B The coccidian *C. cayetanensis* has been linked to mini-outbreaks of diarrhea. Epidemiological evidence strongly implicates various berries, basil, mesclun, and snow peas as likely causes. These outbreaks are very sporadic and tend to occur primarily from imported foods.

58. C The adult *O. volvulus* reside in subcutaneous nodules, and the microfilariae are found in the fluids right under the outer layers of skin. The appropriate diagnostic test is the microscopic examination of skin snips for the presence of microfilariae.

59. A The pinworm, *E. vermicularis*, is the most common parasitic infection throughout the world, and the eggs are infective within just a few hours.

60. B The eggs of *T. trichiura* (the whipworm) have been described as barrel shaped, with a thick shell and two polar plugs, one at each end of the egg.

61. C The eggs of *T. canis* are infectious for humans and cause visceral and ocular larva migrans. These ascarid eggs of the dog can infect humans; the eggs hatch and the larvae wander through the deep tissues, occasionally the eye. In this case, the human becomes the accidental intermediate host.

62. *Plasmodium vivax* and *Plasmodium ovale* are similar because they:
A. Exhibit Schüffner dots and have a true relapse in the life cycle
B. Have no malarial pigment and multiple rings
C. Commonly have appliqué forms in the RBCs
D. Have true stippling, do not have a relapse stage, and infect old RBCs
Microbiology/Parasitology/2

63. The term *autoinfection* can be associated with the following parasites:
A. *Cryptosporidium* spp. and *Giardia duodenalis*
B. *Cystoisospora belli* and *Strongyloides stercoralis*
C. *Cryptosporidium* spp. and *Strongyloides stercoralis*
D. *Giardia duodenalis* and *Cystoisospora belli*
Microbiology/Life cycle/Parasitology/2

64. Microsporidia have been identified as causing severe diarrhea, disseminated disease in other body sites, and ocular infections. Routes of infection have been identified as:
A. Ingestion
B. Inhalation
C. Direct contamination from the environment
D. Ingestion, inhalation, and direct contamination from the environment
Microbiology/Disease/Parasitology/2

65. An immunocompromised patient continues to have diarrhea after repeated ova and parasite (O&P) examinations (sedimentation concentration, trichrome permanent stained smear) were reported as negative; organisms that might be responsible for the diarrhea include:
A. *Cryptosporidium* spp., *Giardia duodenalis*, and *Cystoisospora belli*
B. *Giardia duodenalis*, microsporidia, and *Endolimax nana*
C. *Taenia solium* and *Endolimax nana*
D. *Cryptosporidium* spp. and microsporidia
Microbiology/Parasitology/3

66. Identification of microsporidia is evident by visualizing:
A. The oocyst wall
B. Sporozoites within the oocyst
C. Evidence of the polar tubule
D. Organisms stained with modified acid-fast stains
Microbiology/Microscopy/Parasitology/1

67. Early ring forms of the fifth human malaria parasite, *Plasmodium knowlesi*, resemble those of:
A. *Plasmodium vivax*
B. *Plasmodium ovale*
C. *Plasmodium malariae*
D. *Plasmodium falciparum*
Microbiology/Microscopy/Parasitology/2

68. Parasite stages that are immediately infective for humans on passage from the gastrointestinal tract include:
A. *Schistosoma* spp. eggs
B. *Toxoplasma gondii* bradyzoites
C. *Ascaris lumbricoides* eggs
D. *Cryptosporidium* spp. oocysts
Microbiology/Transmission/Parasitology/2

69. Trophozoites and schizonts of *Plasmodium knowlesi* resemble those of:
A. *Plasmodium vivax*
B. *Plasmodium ovale*
C. *Plasmodium malariae*
D. *Plasmodium falciparum*
Microbiology/Microscopy/Parasitology/2

Answers to Questions 62–69

62. A Both *P. vivax* and *P. ovale* infect young RBCs, have true stippling (Schüffner dots), contain malarial pigment, and have a true relapse stage in the life cycle.

63. C Both *Cryptosporidium* and *Strongyloides* have the capability for internal autoinfection in their life cycles. This means that the cycle and infection can continue even after the patient has left the endemic area.

64. D Infectious routes for microsporidial infections have been confirmed as ingestion and inhalation of the spores; direct transfer of infectious spores from environmental surfaces to the eyes has also been reported.

65. D Routine O&P examinations usually do not detect *Cryptosporidium* oocysts and microsporidial spores; special stains are required. Modified acid-fast stains for *Cryptosporidium* and modified trichrome stains for the microsporidia are recommended.

66. C Evidence of the cross/diagonal line polar tubules provides confirmation for microsporidial spores in the clinical specimen. Not all spores will contain visible polar tubules; the stain of choice is the modified trichrome stain (Ryan/blue or Weber/green).

67. D Early ring forms of the fifth human malaria, *P. knowlesi*, resemble ring forms of *P. falciparum*. However, in the early ring form stage, all human malaria species tend to look very similar.

68. D On passage in stool from the gastrointestinal tract, the oocysts of *Cryptosporidium* are immediately infective. The oocysts of other coccidia must undergo further development before they are infective.

69. C Developing trophozoites and schizonts of *P. knowlesi* tend to closely resemble those of *P. malariae* (band forms, "daisy head").

70. Autofluorescence requires no stain and can be used for the presumptive identification of:
A. *Entamoeba histolytica* cysts
B. *Toxoplasma gondii* tachyzoites
C. *Dientamoeba fragilis* trophozoites
D. *Cyclospora cayetanensis* oocysts
Microbiology/Detection/Parasitology/2

71. Key characteristics of infection with *Plasmodium knowlesi* include:
A. Rapid erythrocyte cycle (24 hours), will infect all ages of RBCs, and can cause serious disease
B. Erythrocytic cycle limited to young RBCs and causes a relatively benign disease
C. The possibility of a true relapse from the liver, infection in older RBCs, and causes serious disease
D. Extended life cycle (72 hours) will infect all ages of RBCs, and disease is similar to that caused by *Plasmodium ovale*
Microbiology/Life cycle/Parasitology/3

72. Microsporidial infections can be confirmed by using:
A. Light microscopy and modified trichrome staining
B. Phase contrast microscopy and routine trichrome staining
C. Electron microscopy and modified acid-fast staining
D. Fluorescence microscopy and hematoxylin staining
Microbiology/Detection/Parasitology/2

73. Although the pathogenicity of *Blastocystis* spp. remains controversial, newer information suggests that:
A. Most organisms are misdiagnosed as artifacts
B. Approximately 10 of 18 subtypes/strains are identified in humans, some of which are pathogenic, and some are nonpathogenic
C. The immune status of the host is solely responsible for symptomatic infections
D. The number of organisms present determines pathogenicity
Microbiology/Parasitology/3

74. Potential problems using EDTA anticoagulant and holding the blood too long prior to preparation of thick and thin blood films include all the following *except*:
A. Changes in parasite morphology, loss of organisms within several hours, and poor staining
B. Loss of Schüffner dots, and parasites beginning the vector cycle within the tube of blood
C. Poor adherence of the blood to the glass side
D. Improved staining and identification
Microbiology/Microscopy/Parasitology/3

75. Key characteristics of the thick film include:
A. The ability to visualize the parasite within the RBCs
B. The ability to identify the parasites to the species level
C. The examination of less blood than the thin blood film
D. The necessity to lake the RBCs during or prior to staining
Microbiology/Microscopy/Parasitology/2

Answers to Questions 70–75

70. D Autofluorescence can be used in preliminary testing for the presence of *C. cayetanensis* oocysts (8–10 μm). If positive, then the specimen can be stained using modified acid-fast stains for confirmation.

71. A Characteristics of *P. knowlesi* include a rapid erythrocytic cycle of 24 hours, possible infection of all ages of RBCs (as with *P. falciparum*), and the potential for serious disease similar to *P. falciparum*.

72. A The use of a modified trichrome stain (Ryan/blue, Weber/green; both with a very high dye content) and light microscopy (oil immersion using the 100× objective) can be used to confirm a microsporidial infection.

73. B Although the pathogenicity of *Blastocystis* spp. continues to be debated (some patients are symptomatic, and some are asymptomatic), it is known that the organisms we see microscopically comprise a number of subtypes/strains/subspecies. Approximately half these subtypes are pathogenic for humans, and half are nonpathogenic; however, morphologically they all look the same. Correct reporting of this infection should be *Blastocystis* spp.; numbers should also be reported (rare, few, moderate, many, packed).

74. D All the changes mentioned in A through C are seen in a tube of EDTA blood that has been held too long prior to blood film preparation. Many morphological changes of parasites, as well as lost organisms, occur under these conditions. These blood specimens should always be handled *STAT* (ordering, collection, processing, examination, and reporting).

75. D With thick blood films, the RBCs must be ruptured (laked) either prior to or during staining. Without rupturing the RBCs, the stained smears would be too thick or too dark to be able to visualize any morphology. In contrast, the thin blood film is fixed prior to/during staining to preserve the RBC morphology; the parasite morphology within the infected RBC can be reviewed for possible diagnosis to the species level. The thin film has a much smaller amount of blood than the thick blood film.

76. A patient is being seen in the emergency department for a low-grade fever, headache, and general malaise after returning from a photographic safari in Africa. The provider has requested blood analysis for malaria; the laboratory would like to have patient information regarding:

A. Specific travel history and body temperature every 4 hours
B. Liver function tests and prophylactic medication history
C. Transfusion history and body temperature every 4 hours
D. Prophylactic medication history and specific travel history

Microbiology/Parasitology/3

77. Examination of a modified acid-fast–stained fecal smear reveals round structures measuring approximately 8 to 10 μm, some of which are stained and some of which are not. They do not appear to show any internal morphology. The patient is symptomatic with diarrhea, and the cause may be:

A. *Blastocystis* spp.
B. Polymorphonuclear leukocytes
C. *Cyclospora cayetanensis*
D. Large yeast cells

Microbiology/Parasitology/3

78. A patient has been diagnosed as having amebiasis but continues to be asymptomatic. The provider has asked for an explanation and recommendations regarding follow-up. Suggestions should include:

A. Consideration of *Entamoeba histolytica* versus *Entamoeba dispar*
B. A request for an additional three stools for culture
C. Initiating therapy, regardless of the patient's asymptomatic status
D. Performance of barium x-ray studies

Microbiology/Parasitology/3

Answers to Questions 76–78

76. D If the patient has malaria and has been taking prophylaxis (often sporadically), the number of parasites on the blood smear will be reduced and examination of routine thick and thin blood films should be more exhaustive. Furthermore, specific geographic travel history may help to determine whether chloroquine-resistant *P. falciparum* may be a factor. Also, if the patient is immunologically naïve (no prior exposure to malaria), these patients usually come into an emergency department with a very low parasitemia and no periodicity; thus, malaria may not even be suspected.

77. C One of the coccidian parasites, *C. cayetanensis*, has been implicated in cases of human diarrhea. The recommended stains are modified acid-fast stains, and the organisms are quite variable in their staining characteristics. The color can range from clear (resembling wrinkled cellophane) to red-purple. The oocysts are immature when passed (no internal morphology) and they measure about 8 to 10 μm.

78. A It is now well established that *E. histolytica* is being used to designate the true pathogenic species, whereas *E. dispar* is typically considered a nonpathogenic species. Unless trophozoites containing ingested RBCs (*E. histolytica*) are seen, the two organisms cannot be differentiated based on morphology. Because this patient is asymptomatic, the organisms seen in the fecal smears are probably *E. dispar* (nonpathogen); the laboratory report should have said *"Entamoeba histolytica/ Entamoeba dispar,"*—unable to differentiate based on morphology unless trophozoites are seen to contain ingested RBCs (*E. histolytica*—true pathogen). Immunoassays and real-time PCR can differentiate the true pathogen, *E. histolytica*, from nonpathogenic species of *Entamoeba* and are more sensitive and specific than microscopic examination alone.

79. Although a patient is strongly suspected of having giardiasis and is still symptomatic, three routine stool examinations (O&P examination) have been performed correctly and reported as negative. Biopsy confirmed the patient had giardiasis. Reasons for these findings may include:

A. The patient was coinfected with several bacterial species
B. *G. duodenalis* tends to adhere to the mucosal surface and more than three stool examinations may be required to confirm a suspected infection
C. The organisms present did not stain with trichrome stain, and therefore the morphology is very atypical
D. Special diagnostic procedures, such as the Knott concentration and nutrient-free agar cultures, should have been used

Microbiology/Parasitology/3

80. A transplant recipient is currently receiving steroids. The patient is now complaining of abdominal pain and has symptoms of pneumonia and positive blood cultures with gram-negative rods. The individual has been living in the United States for 20 years but grew up in Central America. The *most* likely parasite causing these symptoms is:

A. *Trypanosoma brucei rhodesiense*
B. *Giardia duodenalis*
C. *Strongyloides stercoralis*
D. *Schistosoma japonicum*

Microbiology/Parasitology/3

Answers to Questions 79–80

79. B It is well known that *G. duodenalis* trophozoites adhere to the intestinal mucosal surface by means of the sucking disk. Although a patient may have giardiasis and be symptomatic, confirmation of the infection from stool examinations may require more than the routine three stools or may require the examination of duodenal contents. These organisms are shed very sporadically.

80. C Although an infection with *S. stercoralis* may have been acquired in Central America many years before, the patient may have remained asymptomatic while the infection was maintained at a low level in the body via the autoinfective life cycle. As the patient became more immunosuppressed (steroids), the life cycle began to reactivate with penetration of the larvae through the intestinal wall (abdominal pain) and larval migration through the lungs (pneumonia). The patient may have presented with evidence of sepsis (often with gram-negative bacteria carried with the larvae as they penetrate the intestinal wall). In patients who become immunosuppressed, the life cycle of *Strongyloides* may be reactivated, and this results in serious illness (e.g., hyperinfection syndrome, disseminated disease); this can occur many years after the initial infection and after the patient has left the endemic area.

BIBLIOGRAPHY

1. Bennett JE, Dolan R, Blaser MJ. *Mandell, Douglas, and Bennett's Principles and Practices of Infectious Diseases*. 9th ed. Elsevier; 2020.
2. Carroll KC, Pfaller MA, Karlowsky J, et al, eds. *Manual of Clinical Microbiology*. 13th ed. ASM Press; 2023.
3. Christie R, Atkins NE, Munch-Petersen E. A note on a lytic phenomenon shown by group B streptococci. *Aust J Exp Biol Med Sci*. 1944;22:197–200.
4. Leber AL, Burnham CD, eds. *Clinical Microbiology Procedures Handbook*. 5th ed. ASM Press; 2023.
5. Tille PM. *Bailey and Scott's Diagnostic Microbiology*. 16th ed. Elsevier; 2026.
6. Westbalde LF, Burd EM, Lockhart SR, Procop GW. *Larone's Medically Important Fungi: A Guide to Identification*. 7th ed. ASM Press; 2023.

CHAPTER 10

Immunohematology

10.1 *Genetics of Blood Groups*

10.2 *Immunology of Blood Groups*

10.3 *ABO Blood Group System*

10.4 *Rh Blood Group System*

10.5 *Testing for Antibodies*

10.6 *Compatibility Testing*

10.7 *Transfusion Reactions*

10.8 *Components*

10.9 *Donors*

10.10 *Hemolytic Disease of the Fetus and Newborn*

10.11 *Serological Testing of Blood Products*

10.12 *Transfusion Practice*

10.1

Genetics of Blood Groups

1. What type of serological testing does the blood bank technologist routinely perform when determining the ABO blood group of a patient?
A. Genotyping
B. Phenotyping
C. Both genotyping and phenotyping
D. Polymerase chain reaction
Immunohematology/Genetics/1

2. If anti-K reacts 3+ with a donor cell with a genotype KK and 2+ with a Kk cell, the antibody is demonstrating:
A. Dosage
B. Linkage disequilibrium
C. Homozygosity
D. Heterozygosity
Immunohematology/Genetics/3

3. Patient A expresses the blood group antigens Fy(a+b+). Patient B shows expressions of Fy(a−b−). What factor(s) may account for the absence of the Fy antigens in Patient B?
A. Gender
B. Race
C. Gender and race
D. Medication
Immunohematology/Genetics/2

4. Which of the following statements is true?
A. An individual with the *BO* genotype is homozygous for B antigen
B. An individual with the *BB* genotype is homozygous for B antigen
C. An individual with the *OO* genotype is heterozygous for O antigen
D. An individual with the *AB* phenotype is homozygous for A and B antigens
Immunohematology/Genetics/1

5. Which genotype is heterozygous for C?
A. *DCe/dce*
B. *DCE/DCE*
C. *Dce/dce*
D. *DCE/dCe*
Immunohematology/Genetics/2

6. Which genotype(s) will give rise to the Bombay phenotype?
A. *HH* only
B. *HH* and *Hh*
C. *Hh* and *hh*
D. *hh* only
Immunohematology/Genetics/1

Answers to Questions 1–6

1. B Phenotyping, or the physical expression of a genotype, is routinely performed in the blood bank. An individual, for example, may have the *AO* genotype but phenotypes as group A.

2. A Dosage is defined as an antibody reacting stronger with homozygous cells (e.g., KK) than with heterozygous cells (e.g., Kk). In addition to Kell, dosage effect is seen commonly with antigens of the Kidd, Duffy, and MNS and the antigens of the Rh system.

3. B The frequency of Duffy antigens Fy^a and Fy^b varies with race. The Fy(a−b−) phenotype occurs in almost 70% of African Americans and is rare in other populations.

4. B An individual having the *BB* genotype has inherited the *B* gene from both parents and, therefore, is homozygous for B antigen.

5. A The genotype *DCe/dce* contains one *C* and one *c* gene and is heterozygous for C and c antigens.

6. D The Bombay phenotype will be expressed only when no H substance is present. The O_h type is expressed by the genotype *hh*. Bombay phenotypes produce naturally occurring anti-H, and their serum agglutinates type A, B, AB, and O blood groups.

7. Which of the following correctly identifies the antigens found on a red blood cell (RBC) in an individual who has the *H, Le,* and *Se* genes?
A. *H, Le^a*
B. *H, Le^b*
C. *Le^a* only
D. *Le^b* only
Immunohematology/Genetics/2

8. Which of the following describes the expression of *most* blood group antigens?
A. Dominant
B. Recessive
C. Co-dominant
D. Co-recessive
Immunohematology/Genetics/1

9. What blood type is *not* possible for an offspring of an *AO* and *BO* mating?
A. *AB*
B. *A or B*
C. *O*
D. All are possible
Immunohematology/Genetics/2

10. The alleged father of a child in a disputed case of paternity is blood group O. The mother is group O, and the child is group B. What type of exclusion is this?
A. Direct/primary/first order
B. Probability
C. Random
D. Indirect/secondary/second order
Immunohematology/Genetics/2

11. If the frequency of gene *Y* is 0.4 and the frequency of gene *Z* is 0.5, one would expect that they should occur together 0.2 (20%) of the time. The genes are identified in close proximity 32% of the time. This is an example of:
A. Crossing over
B. Linkage disequilibrium
C. Polymorphism
D. Chimerism
Immunohematology/Genetics/2

12. In the Hardy-Weinberg formula, p^2 represents:
A. The heterozygous population of one allele
B. The homozygous population of one allele
C. The recessive allele
D. The dominant allele
Immunohematology/Genetics/1

13. Which of the following blood group systems is associated with the Fy(a−b−) phenotype, which provides resistance to malaria?
A. Kell
B. Duffy
C. MNS
D. Kidd
Immunohematology/Genetics/1

Answers to Questions 7–13

7. B H antigen is present due to the *H* gene. The *Le* gene encodes the Lewis antigens, *Le^a* and *Le^b*. The expression of these antigens depends on the interaction with the *Se* gene, which allows the expression of Lewis b antigen (Le^b). Because both the *Le* gene and the *Se* gene are present, the Le^b antigen is expressed on the RBCs.

8. C The inheritance of most blood group genes is co-dominant, meaning that no gene or allele is dominant over another. For example, a person who is group AB expresses both the A and B antigen on their RBCs.

9. D A mating between *AO* and *BO* persons can result in an offspring with blood type A, B, AB, or O.

10. D An indirect/secondary/second order, exclusion occurs when a genetic marker is absent in the child but should have been transmitted by the alleged father. In this case, the child should lack the B antigen and be type O.

11. B Linkage disequilibrium is a phenomenon in which alleles situated in close proximity on a chromosome associate with one another more than would be expected from individual allelic frequencies.

12. B In the Hardy-Weinberg formula ($p^2 + 2pq + q^2$), p^2 and q^2 represent homozygous expressions, and 2pq represents heterozygous expression. This formula is used in population genetics to determine the frequency of different alleles.

13. B *Plasmodium vivax* uses the Duffy antigens as a receptor to invade RBCs. Individuals with the Fy(a−b−) phenotype lack these antigens on their RBCs, preventing the parasite from gaining entry and providing resistance to malaria.

10.2

Immunology of Blood Groups

1. **Individuals with the following blood group have both anti-A and anti-B antibodies naturally in the serum:**
   A. Group A
   B. Group B
   C. Group O
   D. Group AB
   Immunohematology/Immunology/1

2. **Why do immunoglobulin M (IgM) antibodies, such as those formed against ABO antigens, directly cause visible agglutination of RBCs?**
   A. IgM antibodies are larger molecules and can bind more antigen
   B. IgM antibodies tend to clump together more readily to bind more antigen
   C. IgM antibodies are found in greater concentrations than IgG antibodies
   D. IgM antibodies are not limited by subclass specificity
   Immunohematology/Immunology/1

3. **Which of the following enhancement mediums decreases the zeta potential, allowing antibody and antigen to come closer together?**
   A. Low ionic strength solution (LISS)
   B. Polyethylene glycol
   C. Polybrene
   D. Dithiothreitol-papain (ZZAP)
   Immunohematology/Immunology/1

4. **Which immunoglobulin class is *most* effective in causing agglutination of non-ABO antigens?**
   A. IgA
   B. IgE
   C. IgG
   D. IgM
   Immunohematology/Immunology/1

5. **Which antibodies to a component of complement are contained in the rabbit polyspecific anti-human globulin (AHG) reagent for detection of *in vivo* sensitization?**
   A. Anti-IgG and anti-C3a
   B. Anti-IgG and anti-C3d
   C. Anti-IgM and anti-C3a
   D. Anti-IgM and anti-C3d
   Immunohematology/Immunology/2

Answers to Questions 1–5

1. C Individuals with group O blood lacks both A and B antigens on their RBCs. Their serum contains both anti-A and anti-B antibodies naturally and is unique to type O blood.

2. A An IgM molecule has the potential to bind up to 10 antigens compared with a molecule of IgG, which can bind only two.

3. A LISS contains a reduced concentration of NaCl (0.2%) and results in a reduction in charged ions within the ionic cloud, decreasing the zeta potential and facilitating antigen–antibody interaction.

4. C IgG is highly effective in causing agglutination of non-ABO antigens due to its strong antigen-antibody binding capabilities and ability to cross the placenta.

5. B In the direct antiglobulin test (DAT), rabbit polyspecific antisera contains both an anti-human IgG component and an antibody against the C3d component of complement.

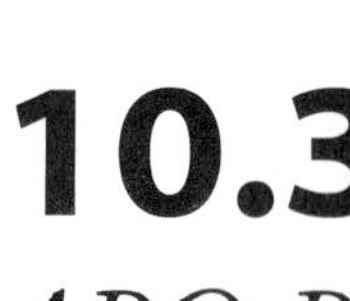

10.3
ABO Blood Group System

1. Which of the following distinguishes the A_1 blood group from the A_2 blood group?
A. A_2 antigen will not react with anti-A, A_1 will react strongly (4+)
B. An A_2 person may form anti-A_1; an A_1 person will not form anti-A_1
C. An A_1 person may form anti-A_2, an A_2 person will not form anti-A_1
D. A_2 antigen will not react with anti-A from a nonimmunized donor; A_1 will react with any anti-A
Immunohematology/ABO/2

2. A patient's serum is incompatible with O cells. The patient's RBCs give a negative reaction to anti-H lectin. What is the *most* likely cause of these results?
A. The patient may be a subgroup of A
B. The patient may have an immunodeficiency
C. The patient may be a Bombay phenotype individual
D. The patient may have developed alloantibodies
Immunohematology/ABO/3

3. What antibodies are formed by a Bombay phenotype individual?
A. Anti-A and anti-B
B. Anti-H
C. Anti-A, B
D. Anti-A, B, and H
Immunohematology/ABO/1

4. Acquired B antigens have been identified in:
A. Bombay phenotype individuals
B. Group O individuals
C. Persons of all blood groups
D. Group A individuals
Immunohematology/ABO/1

5. Blood is crossmatched on an A-positive person with a negative antibody screen. The patient received a transfusion of A-positive RBCs 3 years ago. The donors chosen for crossmatching were A-positive. Crossmatching was performed on the automated analyzer and yielded 3+ ABO incompatibility. How can these results be explained?
A. The patient has an antibody to a low-frequency antigen
B. The patient has an antibody to a high-frequency antigen
C. The patient is an A_2 subgroup with anti-A_1
D. The patient is an A_1 subgroup with anti-A_2
Immunohematology/ABO/3

Answers to Questions 1–5

1. B The group A_1 comprises both A_1 and A antigens. Anti-A will react with both A_1- and A_2-positive RBCs. A person who is group A_2 may form anti-A_1, but an A_1 person will not form anti-A_1 (which would cause autoagglutination).

2. C Bombay phenotype is the only ABO phenotype incompatible with O cells. The RBCs of a Bombay phenotype individual show a negative reaction to anti-H because the cells contain no H substance.

3. D A Bombay phenotype individual does not express A, B, or H antigens; therefore, anti-A, -B, and -H are formed. Because a Bombay phenotype individual has three antibodies, the only compatible blood must be from another Bombay phenotype donor.

4. D The acquired B phenomenon is only seen in group A individuals.

5. C The patient is likely an A_2 subgroup with anti-A_1, which is causing reactivity in the crossmatching. A negative antibody screen rules out the possibility of an antibody to a high-frequency antigen, and two donor units' incompatibility rules out an antibody to a low-frequency antigen.

6. A patient's RBCs forward type as group O, the reverse type agglutinates B cells (4+) only. The *next* step in processing the sample would be:

A. Extend reverse typing for 15 minutes
B. Perform an antibody screen, including room-temperature incubation
C. Incubate washed RBCs with anti-A_1 and anti-A, B for 30 minutes at room temperature
D. Test patient's RBCs with *Dolichos biflorus*

Immunohematology/ABO/3

7. Which typing results are *most* likely to occur when a patient has an acquired B antigen?

A. Anti-A 4+, anti-B 3+, A_1 cells neg, B cells neg
B. Anti-A 3+, anti-B neg, A_1 cells neg, B cells neg
C. Anti-A 4+, anti-B 1+, A_1 cells neg, B cells 4+
D. Anti-A 4+, anti-B 4+, A_1 cells 2+, B cells neg

Immunohematology/ABO/2

8. Which blood group has the *least* amount of H antigen?

A. A_1B
B. A_2
C. B
D. A_1

Immunohematology/ABO/1

9. What type of RBCs can be transfused to an A_2 patient with anti-A_1?

A. A_1 only
B. A_2 or O
C. B
D. A_2B

Immunohematology/ABO/3

10. What procedure should be performed if all forward and reverse ABO results as well as the autocontrol are positive?

A. Wash the cells with warm saline, and autoadsorb the serum at 4°C
B. Retype the sample using a different lot of reagents
C. Use polyclonal typing reagents
D. Report the sample as group AB

Immunohematology/ABO/3

11. What follow-up or procedure should be performed if all forward and reverse ABO reactions are negative?

A. Perform additional testing, such as typing with anti-A_1 lectin and anti-A, B
B. Incubate at 22°C or 4°C to enhance weak expression
C. Repeat the test with new reagents
D. Run an antibody identification panel

Immunohematology/ABO/3

12. *N*-acetyl-D-galactosamine is the immunodominant carbohydrate that reacts with:

A. *Arachis hypogaea*
B. *Salvia sclarea*
C. *Dolichos biflorus*
D. *Ulex europaeus*

Immunohematology/ABO/2

Answers to Questions 6–12

6. C The strong 4+ reaction in reverse grouping suggests the discrepancy is in forward grouping. Incubating washed RBCs at room temperature with anti-A and anti-A,B will enhance reactions.

7. C In forward typing, a 1+ reaction with anti-B is suspicious because of the weak reaction and the normal reverse grouping that appears to be group A. This may be indicative of an acquired antigen. In the case of an acquired B antigen, the reverse grouping is the same for a group A individual.

8. A The A_1B blood group has the least amount of H antigen. This occurs because both A and B epitopes are present on RBCs, compromising the availability of H epitopes. Type O has the most H antigen present.

9. B The patient is an A_2 with anti-A_1 can be transfused with A_2 or O cells. A_2 RBCs lack A_1 antigens and thus will not react with anti-A_1 antibodies. O RBCs lack both A and B antigens and will not react with either anti-A or anti-B antibodies, including anti-A_1.

10. A These results point to a cold autoantibody. Washing the cells with warm saline may elute the autoantibody, allowing a valid forward type to be performed. The serum should be adsorbed using washed cells until the autocontrol is negative. Then, the adsorbed serum should be used for reverse typing.

11. B All negative reactions may be caused by weakened antigens or antibodies. Room temperature or lower incubation temperature may enhance expression of weakened antigens or antibodies.

12. C The immunodominant sugar *N*-acetyl-galactosamine confers A antigen specificity when present at the terminus of the type 2 precursor chain on the RBC membrane. Therefore, its presence would cause RBCs to react with anti-A_1 lectin, *Dolichos biflorus*.

13. A stem cell transplant recipient was retyped when the patient was transferred from another hospital. What is the *most* likely cause of the following results?

Patient cells:	Anti-A, neg	Anti-B, 4+
Patient serum:	A_1 cells, neg	B cells, neg

A. Viral infection
B. Alloantibodies
C. Immunodeficiency
D. Autoimmune hemolytic anemia

Immunohematology/ABO/3

14. What reaction would be the same for an A_1 and an A_2 individual?

A. Positive reaction with anti-A_1 lectin
B. Positive reaction with A_1 cells
C. Equal reaction with anti-H
D. Positive reaction with anti-A, B

Immunohematology/ABO/2

15. A pregnant patient at 28 weeks' gestation yields the following results:

Patient cells:	Anti-A, 3+	Anti-B, 4+	
Patient serum:	A_1 cells, neg	B cells, 1+	O cells, 1+

Which of the following could be causing the ABO discrepancy?

A. Hypogammaglobulinemia
B. Cold reacting alloantibody
C. Acquired B
D. Weak subgroup

Immunohematology/ABO/3

16. Which condition would *most* likely be responsible for the following typing results?

Patient cells:	Anti-A, neg	Anti-B, neg
Patient serum:	A_1 cells, neg	B cells, 4+

A. Immunodeficiency
B. Masking of antigens by the presence of massive amounts of antibody
C. Weak or excessive antigen(s)
D. Impossible to determine

Immunohematology/ABO/3

17. Which of the following results is *most* likely discrepant?

Anti-A, neg	Anti-B, 4+
A_1 cells, neg	B cells, neg

A. Negative B cells
B. Positive reaction with anti-B
C. Negative A_1 cells
D. No problem with this typing

Immunohematology/ABO/3

Answers to Questions 13–17

13. C The transplant recipient is probably taking immunosuppressive medication to increase graft survival. This can contribute to the loss of normal blood group antibodies as well as other types of antibodies.

14. D Anti-A,B should react positively with group A or B and any subgroup of A or B (with exception of A_m). An A_1 (not A_2) would react with anti-A_1 lectin; only an A_2 individual with anti-A_1 would give a positive reaction with A_1 cells; an A_2 would react more strongly with anti-H than A_1.

15. B The patient most likely has an AB blood type who has formed a cold-reacting alloantibody reacting with B cells and O cells. An identification panel should be performed. An acquired B patient or someone with hypogammaglobulinemia should not make antibody that would agglutinate O cells.

16. C Excessive A substance, as may be found in some types of tumors, may be neutralizing anti-A. Weak A subgroups may fail to react with anti-A and require additional testing techniques (e.g., room-temperature incubation) before their expression is apparent.

17. C The reverse typing should agree with the forward typing in this result. The 4+ reaction with anti-B indicates group B. A positive reaction is expected with A_1 cells in the reverse group.

18. A 61-year-old patient who is B positive with a history of multiple myeloma underwent stem cell transplantation 3 years ago. The donor was O positive. The patient is admitted to a community hospital for fatigue and nausea. Typing results reveal the following:

Anti-A = 0
Anti-B = 0
Anti-A, B = 0
Anti-D = 4+
A_1 cells = 4+
B cells = 0

How would you report this type?

A. O positive
B. B positive
C. A positive
D. Undetermined

Immunohematology/ABO/3

Answer to Question 18

18. D In a transplantation scenario, there are no methods to employ to solve the discrepancy. The medical laboratory scientist must rely on the patient history of donor type and recipient type and the present serological picture. Giving a B-positive recipient an O-positive transplant constitutes a minor ABO mismatch. The forward type resembles the donor. The reverse type still resembles the recipient. The ABO type reported does not fit a pattern, resulting in an undetermined type.

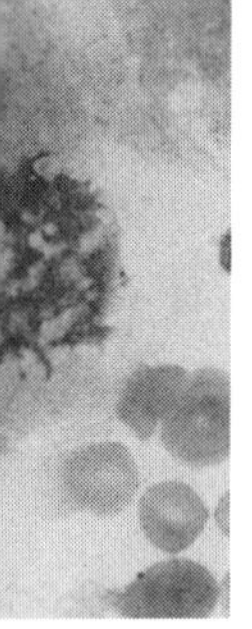

10.4
Rh Blood Group System

1. A complete Rh typing for antigens D, C, c, E, and e revealed negative results for D, C, and E. How is the individual designated?

A. Rh positive
B. Rh negative
C. Positive for c and e
D. Impossible to determine

Immunohematology/Rh/1

2. How is an individual with genotype *Dce/dce* classified?

A. Rh positive
B. Rh negative
C. Rh_{null}
D. Total Rh

Immunohematology/Rh/2

3. If a patient has a positive DAT, should a weak D test be performed on the cells?

A. No, the cells are already coated with antibody
B. No, the cells are Rh_{null}
C. Yes, the immunoglobulin will not interfere with the test
D. Yes, Rh reagents are enhanced in protein media

Immunohematology/Rh/3

4. Which donor unit is selected for a recipient with anti-c?

A. $r'r$
B. *ROR1*
C. $R2r'$
D. $r'r^y$

Immunohematology/Rh/3

5. Which genotype usually shows the strongest reaction with anti-D?

A. *DCE/DCE*
B. *Dce/dCe*
C. *dce/dCe*
D. *dCE/Dce*

Immunohematology/Rh/1

Answers to Questions 1–5

1. **B** Rh positive refers to the presence of D antigen; Rh negative refers to the absence of D antigen. These designations are for D antigen only and do not involve other Rh antigens.

2. **A** This individual has D antigen and is classified as Rh positive. Any genotype containing D antigen will be considered Rh positive.

3. **A** If a person has a positive DAT, the RBCs are coated with immunoglobulin. If a test for weak D were performed, the test would yield positive results independent of the presence or absence of D antigen on the RBCs.

4. **D** The designation r' is *dCe* and r^y is *dCE*, neither of which contains c antigen. The other three Rh types contain c antigen and could not be used in transfusion for a person with anti-c.

5. **A** *DCE/DCE* is homozygous for the D antigen. Both alleles carry the D antigen, resulting in a high density of D antigen sites on the RBCs to produce the strongest reaction.

6. Why is testing for Rh antigens and antibodies different from ABO testing?

A. ABO reactions are primarily caused by IgM antibodies and usually occur at room temperature; Rh antibodies are IgG, and agglutination usually requires a 37°C incubation and enhancement media

B. ABO antigens are attached to receptors on the outside of the RBC and do not require any special enhancement for testing; Rh antigens are loosely attached to the RBC membrane and require enhancement for detection

C. Both ABO and Rh antigens and antibodies have similar structures, but Rh antibodies are configured so that special techniques are needed to facilitate binding to Rh antigens

D. There is no difference between ABO and Rh testing; both may be conducted at room temperature with no special enhancement needed for reaction

Immunohematology/Rh/1

7. Testing reveals a weak D that reacts 1+ after indirect antiglobulin testing (IAT). How is this result classified?

A. Rh-positive

B. Rh-negative, Du-positive

C. Rh-negative

D. Rh-positive, Du-positive

Immunohematology/Rh/2

8. Which of the following Rh genotypes is possible for a patient who develops an anti-C antibody?

A. *R1r*

B. *R1R1*

C. *r′r*

D. *rr*

Immunohematology/Rh/2

9. A patient developed a combination of Rh antibodies: anti-C, anti-E, and anti-D. Can compatible blood be identified for this patient?

A. It is almost impossible to find blood lacking C, E, and D antigens

B. *rr* blood could be used without causing a problem

C. *R0R0* may be used because it lacks all three antigens

D. Although rare, $r^{y}r$ blood may be obtained from close relatives of the patient

Immunohematology/Rh/1

10. A patient tests positive for weak D but also appears to have anti-D in his serum. Assuming there are no testing errors, what may be the problem?

A. Mix up of the samples or testing error

B. Most weak D individuals make anti-D

C. The problem could be caused by a disease state

D. A D mosaic may make antibodies to the missing antigen parts

Immunohematology/Rh/2

11. Which offspring is *not* possible for a mother who is *R1R2* and a father who is *R1r*?

A. *DcE/DcE*

B. *Dce/DCe*

C. *DcE/DCe*

D. *Dce/dce*

Immunohematology/Rh/2

Answers to Questions 6–11

6. A Detection of ABO and Rh antigens and antibodies requires different reaction conditions. ABO antibodies are naturally occurring IgM molecules and react best at room temperature. Rh antibodies are generally IgG molecules that result from an immune response to transfusion or pregnancy. Detection may require 37°C incubation and/or enhancement techniques.

7. A Blood tested for weak D that shows 1+ reaction after IAT is classified as Rh positive. The weak D designation is not noted in the reporting of the result.

8. D Only *rr* (*dce/dce*) does not contain C antigen. A person will form alloantibodies only to the antigens the individual lacks.

9. B The genotype *rr* (*dce/dce*) lacks D, C, and E antigens and would be suitable for an individual who has developed antibodies to all three antigens. This is the most common Rh-negative genotype and is found in nearly 14% of blood donors who are Caucasian.

10. D The D antigen comprises different parts designated as a mosaic. If an individual lacks parts of the antigen, they may make antibodies to the missing parts if exposed to the whole D antigen.

11. A *DcE/DcE* (*R2R2*) is not possible because *R2* can be inherited only from the mother and is not present in the father.

12. Which of the following Rh antigens is the *most* immunogenic?
A. D
B. C
C. c
D. E
Immunohematology/Rh/1

13. What antibodies could an *R1R1* make if exposed to *R2R2* blood?
A. Anti-e and anti-C
B. Anti-E and anti-c
C. Anti-E and anti-C
D. Anti-e and anti-c
Immunohematology/Rh/2

14. What does the genotype —/— represent in the Rh system?
A. Rh negative
B. D mosaic
C. Rh_{null}
D. Bombay
Immunohematology/Rh/2

15. What techniques are necessary for weak D testing?
A. Saline + 22°C incubation
B. Albumin or LISS + 37°C incubation
C. Saline + 37°C incubation
D. 37°C incubation + IAT
Immunohematology/Rh/2

16. Which Rh antigen is considered the *most* clinically significant after the D antigen?
A. C
B. E
C. c
D. e
Immunohematology/Rh/1

17. According to the Wiener nomenclature and/or genetic theory of Rh inheritance:
A. There are three closely linked loci, each with a primary set of allelic genes
B. The alleles are named *R1, R2, R0, r, r′, r″*, R^z, and r^y
C. There are multiple alleles at a single complex locus that determine each Rh antigen
D. The antigens are named D, C, E, c, and e
Immunohematology/Rh/2

18. The Wiener nomenclature for the E antigen is:
A. hr′
B. hr"
C. rh″
D. Rh_0
Immunohematology/Rh/1

Answers to Questions 12–18

12. A The D antigen is the most immunogenic Rh antigen. It is a major antigen in the Rh blood group system and is highly effective at eliciting an immune response.

13. B The *R1R1* (*DCe/DCe*) individual does not have the E or c antigen and could make anti-E and anti-c antibodies when exposed to *R2R2* cells (*DcE/DcE*).

14. C An individual who is Rh_{null} shows no Rh antigens on their RBCs. The Rh_{null} phenotype can result from either genetic suppression of the *Rh* genes or inheritance of amorphic genes at the Rh locus.

15. D Weak D testing requires both 37°C incubation and the IAT procedure. Anti-D is an IgG antibody, and attachment of the D antigen is optimized at warmer temperatures. AHG in the IAT phase facilitates lattice formation by binding to the antigen–antibody complexes.

16. C The Rh antigen c is considered the most clinically significant after the D antigen because of its potential to cause hemolytic transfusion reactions and hemolytic disease of the fetus and newborn (HDFN) as well as its relatively high frequency in the population.

17. C Wiener proposed a single-locus theory for Rh, with multiple alleles determining surface molecules that embody numerous antigens.

18. C The Wiener designation for the E antigen is rh″. The Wiener designation hr′ denotes c, hr″ denotes e, and Rh_0 is D.

19. A provider orders 2 units of leukocyte-reduced RBCs. The patient is a 55-year-old adult with anemia. The blood type is AB negative, and the antibody screen is negative. There is only 1 unit of AB negative in inventory. What is the *next* blood type that should be administered to the patient?

A. AB positive
B. A negative
C. B negative
D. O negative

Immunohematology/Rh/3

20. Arrange the following Rh antigens in order of immunogenicity, from most to least immunogenic:

A. D, E, c, C, e
B. D, c, E, C, e
C. D, C, E, c, e
D. D, c, C, E, e

Immunohematology/Rh/2

Answers to Questions 19–20

19. B Although giving Rh-positive RBCs to an Rh-negative patient would not harm the patient in this case, giving A negative would be the first choice. The patient should not be exposed to the D antigen, if possible, and the residual anti-B in a unit of A-negative packed cells is less immunogenic than giving B or O RBCs.

20. B D, c, E, C, e reflects the descending order of immunogenicity among the Rh antigens. Understanding the immunogenicity of these antigens is crucial for ensuring safe blood transfusions and managing Rh incompatibility.

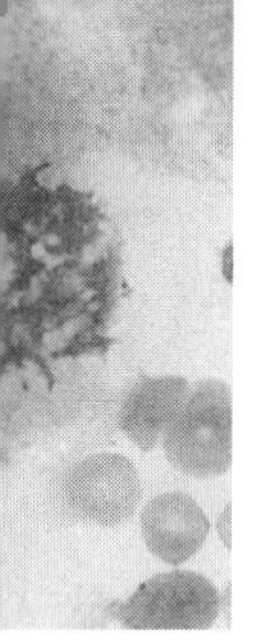

10.5
Testing for Antibodies

1. **A patient has the Lewis phenotype Le(a−b−). An antibody panel reveals the presence of anti-Le^a. Another patient with the phenotype Le(a−b+) has a positive antibody screen; however, a panel reveals no conclusive antibody. Should anti-Le^a be considered a possibility for the patient with the Le(a−b+) phenotype?**
   A. Anti-Le^a should be considered as a possible antibody
   B. Anti-Le^a may be a possible antibody, but further studies are needed
   C. Anti-Le^a is not a likely antibody because even Le^b individuals secrete some Le^a
   D. Anti-Le^a may be found in saliva but not detectable in serum

   Immunohematology/Antibodies/2

2. **A medical laboratory scientist is having difficulty resolving an antibody mixture. One of the antibodies is anti-Le^a. This antibody is not clinically significant in this situation, but it needs to be removed to reveal the possible presence of an underlying antibody of clinical significance. What step(s) should be performed *next*?**
   A. Perform an enzyme panel
   B. Neutralize the serum with saliva
   C. Neutralize the serum with hydatid cyst fluid
   D. Use dithiothreitol (DTT) to treat the panel cells

   Immunohematology/Antibodies/3

3. **What type of blood should be transfused to an individual who has anti-Le^b that reacts 1+ at the IAT phase?**
   A. Blood that is negative for Le^b antigen
   B. Blood that is negative for both Le^a and Le^b antigens
   C. Blood that is positive for Le^b antigen
   D. Lewis antibodies are not clinically significant, so any type of blood may be given

   Immunohematology/Antibodies/3

4. **Which of the following statements is true concerning the MNS blood group?**
   A. Antigens are destroyed using bleach-treated cells
   B. Dosage effect may be seen for both M and N antigens
   C. Both M and N antigens are impossible to detect because of cross-interference
   D. MN is a rare phenotype seldom found in routine antigen typing

   Immunohematology/Antibodies/2

Answers to Questions 1–4

1. **C** Anti-Le^a is produced primarily by persons with the Le(a−b−) phenotype because Le(a−b+) persons still have some Le^a antigen present in saliva. Although Le^a is not present on their RBCs, Le(a−b+) persons do not form anti-Le^a.
2. **B** Saliva from an individual with the *Le* gene contains the Le^a antigen. This combines with anti-Le^a, neutralizing the antibody.
3. **A** Lewis antibodies are generally not considered clinically significant unless they react at 37°C or at the IAT phase. The antibody must be honored in this scenario due to its reactivity at the IAT phase of testing.
4. **B** *Dosage effect* is the term used to describe the phenomenon of an antibody that reacts more strongly with homozygous cells than with heterozygous cells. Dosage effect is a characteristic of the *MNS blood group* because the M and N antigens are both present on the same cell.

5. Anti-M is sometimes found with reactivity detected at the immediate spin (IS) phase that persists in strength to the IAT phase. What is the concern in this instance with a strong anti-M?

A. Anti-M may not allow detection of a clinically significant antibody
B. Compatible blood may not be identified for the patient with a strongly reacting anti-M
C. Anti-M cannot be removed from serum
D. Anti-M may react with the patient's own cells, causing a positive autocontrol

Immunohematology/Antibodies/2

6. A patient is suspected of having paroxysmal cold hemoglobinuria (PCH). Which pattern of reactivity is characteristic of the Donath-Landsteiner antibody?

A. The antibody attaches to RBCs at 4°C and causes hemolysis at 37°C
B. The antibody attaches to RBCs at 37°C and causes agglutination at the IAT phase
C. The antibody attaches to RBCs at 22°C and causes hemolysis at 37°C
D. The antibody attaches to RBCs and causes agglutination at the IAT phase

Immunohematology/Antibodies/2

7. How can interfering anti-P_1 antibody be removed from a mixture of antibodies?

A. Neutralization with saliva
B. Agglutination with human milk
C. Combination with urine
D. Neutralization with hydatid cyst fluid

Immunohematology/Antibodies/1

8. Which antibody is frequently identified in patients with warm autoimmune hemolytic anemia (WAIHA)?

A. Anti-Jk^a
B. Anti-e
C. Anti-K
D. Anti-Fy^b

Immunohematology/Antibodies/2

9. A patient's antibody shows strong reactions in all test phases. All screen and panel cells are positive. Serum is then tested with a cord blood cell, and the reaction is negative. What antibody is suspected?

A. Anti-I
B. Anti-i
C. Anti-H
D. Anti-p

Immunohematology/Antibodies/2

10. Which group of antibodies is commonly identified as a cold agglutinin?

A. Anti-K, anti-k, anti-Js^b
B. Anti-D, anti-e, anti-C
C. Anti-M, anti-N
D. Anti-Fy^a, anti-Fy^b

Immunohematology/Antibodies/1

11. Which of the following antibodies characteristically demonstrates a refractile mixed-field appearance?

A. Anti-K
B. Anti-Di^a
C. Anti-Sd^a
D. Anti-s

Immunohematology/Antibodies/1

Answers to Questions 5–11

5. A Although anti-M may not be clinically significant, a strongly reacting anti-M that persists through to the IAT phase may interfere with detection of a clinically significant antibody that reacts only at IAT.

6. A The Donath-Landsteiner antibody has anti-P specificity with biphasic activity. The antibody attaches to RBCs at 4°C and then causes the RBCs to hemolyze when warmed to 37°C.

7. D Hydatid cyst fluid contains P_1 substance, which can neutralize anti-P_1 antibody.

8. B Anti-e is frequently implicated in cases of WAIHA. The corresponding antigen is characterized as high frequency in the Rh system and can mask the presence of other alloantibodies.

9. A Adult cells contain mostly I antigen, and anti-I would react with all adult cells included on the screen or panel cells. Cord blood cells, however, contain mostly i antigen and would test negative with anti-I.

10. C Antibodies to the M and N antigens are IgM antibodies, which are commonly cold agglutinins.

11. C Anti-Sd^a are known for their unique agglutination pattern. They cause a mixed-field appearance with small, refractile agglutinates. This is a distinctive feature that can help in their identification during antibody screening and identification tests.

12. What does the 3+3 rule ascertain?
A. An antibody is ruled in
B. An antibody is ruled out
C. 95% confidence that the correct antibody has been identified
D. 95% confidence that the correct antibody has not been identified

Immunohematology/Antibodies/1

13. The k (Cellano) antigen is a high-frequency antigen and is found on most RBCs. How often would one expect to find the corresponding antibody?
A. Often, because it is a high-frequency antibody
B. Rarely, because most individuals have the antigen and would not develop an antibody
C. Depends on the population, because certain racial and ethnic groups show a higher frequency of anti-k
D. Impossible to determine without consulting regional blood group antigen charts

Immunohematology/Antibodies/1

14. Which procedure would help to distinguish between anti-e and anti-Fy^a in an antibody mixture?
A. Lowering the pH of test serum
B. Running an enzyme panel
C. Using a thiol reagent
D. Running a LISS panel

Immunohematology/Antibodies/1

15. Which characteristics are true of all three of the following antibodies: anti-Fy^a, anti-Jk^a, and anti-K?
A. Detected at the IAT phase; may cause hemolytic disease of the fetus and newborn (HDFN) and hemolytic transfusion reactions
B. Not detected with enzyme-treated cells
C. Requires the IAT technique for detection; usually not associated with HDFN
D. Enhanced reactivity with enzyme-treated cells; may cause severe hemolytic transfusion reactions

Immunohematology/Antibodies/2

16. A patient is admitted to the hospital. Medical records indicate that the patient has a history of anti-Jk^a. A type and screen were performed. The blood type is O positive, and the antibody screen is negative. What should be the *next* step in the process?
A. Crossmatch using units negative for Jk^a antigen
B. Crossmatch random units, since the antibody is not demonstrating
C. Request a new sample
D. Repeat the screen with enzyme-treated screening cells

Immunohematology/Antibodies/3

17. A medical laboratory scientist performs an antibody screen and finds 1+ and weak positive reactions for several of the panel cells. The reactions do not fit a pattern. Several selected panels and a patient phenotype do not reveal any additional information. Serum is diluted and retested, but the same reactions persist. What type of antibody may be causing these results?
A. Biphasic antibody
B. Antibody to a low-frequency antigen
C. High titer low avidity (HTLA)
D. Anti-human leukocyte antigen (anti-HLA)

Immunohematology/Antibodies/3

Answers to Questions 12–17

12. C The 3+3 rule ascertains correct identification of antibody at a confidence level of 95%. For this level to be met, reagent RBCs are found containing target antigen to suspected antibody that react in test phase; likewise, reagent RBCs devoid of antigen will not react in test phase.

13. B k antigen is identified with a frequency of 99.8%; therefore, k-negative individuals are rare. Because of this, the occurrence of anti-k is also rare.

14. B Enzyme-treated cells will not react with Duffy antibodies. Rh antibodies react more strongly with enzyme-treated RBCs. An enzyme panel, therefore, would enhance reactivity of anti-e and destroy reactivity to anti-Fy^a.

15. A Anti-Fy^a, anti-Jk^a, and anti-K are usually detected at IAT and all may cause HDFN and transfusion reactions that may be hemolytic. Reactivity with anti-Fy^a is lost with enzyme-treated RBCs, but reactivity with anti-Jk^a is enhanced with enzyme-treated cells. Reactivity with anti-K is unaffected by enzyme-treated cells.

16. A The Kidd antibodies are notorious for disappearing from serum, yielding a negative result for the antibody screen. If a patient has a history of a Kidd antibody, blood must be crossmatched using antigen-negative units. If the patient is transfused with the corresponding antigen, an anamnestic response may occur with a subsequent hemolytic transfusion reaction.

17. C HTLA antibodies may persist in reaction strength, even when diluted. These antibodies are directed against high-frequency antigens (e.g., Ch^a). They are not clinically significant but, when present, are responsible for a high incidence of incompatible crossmatches.

18. An antibody is detected in a pregnant person and is suspected of being the cause of fetal distress. The antibody reacts at the IAT phase but does not react with DTT-treated cells. This antibody causes *in vitro* hemolysis. What is the *most* likely antibody specificity?

A. Anti-Le^a
B. Anti-Lu^a
C. Anti-Lu^b
D. Anti-Xg^a

Immunohematology/Antibodies/3

19. What sample is *best* for detecting complement-dependent antibodies?

A. Plasma stored at 4°C for no longer than 24 hours
B. Serum stored at 4°C for no longer than 48 hours
C. Either serum or plasma stored at 20°C to 24°C no longer than 6 hours
D. Serum heated at 56°C for 30 minutes

Immunohematology/Antibodies/2

20. Which antibody would *not* be detected by group O screening cells?

A. Anti-N
B. Anti-A_1
C. Anti-Di^a
D. Anti-k

Immunohematology/Antibodies/1

21. Refer to Panel 1. Which antibody is *most* likely implicated?

A. Anti-Fy^b
B. Anti-Jk^b
C. Anti-e
D. Anti-c and anti-K

Immunohematology/Antibodies/2

Answers to Questions 18–21

18. C Of the antibodies listed, only Lu^b is detected in the IAT phase, causes *in vitro* hemolysis, may cause HDFN, and does not react with DTT-treated cells.

19. B Serum stored at 4°C for no longer than 48 hours preserves complement activity. Plasma is inappropriate because most anticoagulants chelate calcium needed for activation of complement. Heating the serum to 56°C destroys complement.

20. B ABO antibodies are not detected by group O screening cells because O cells contain no A or B antigens.

21. B The pattern clearly fits that of anti-Jk^b, an antibody that usually reacts best at IAT. The weaker reactions are caused by the dosage effect found on cells that are heterozygous for the Jk^b antigen.

Panel 1

Cell	D	C	E	c	e	K	k	Kp^a	Kp^b	Js^a	Js^b	Fy^a	Fy^b	Jk^a	Jk^b	Xg^a	Le^a	Le^b	S	s	M	N	P_1	Lu^a	Lu^b	37°	IAT
1	+	+	O	O	+	O	+	O	+	O	+	O	+	O	+	+	+	O	O	+	O	+	O	O	+	O	2+
2	+	+	O	O	+	+	+	O	+	O	+	+	+	+	+	+	O	+	+	+	O	+	+	O	+	O	1+
3	+	O	+	+	O	O	+	O	+	O	+	+	O	+	+	O	O	+	+	+	+	+	+	O	+	O	1+
4	O	+	O	+	+	O	+	O	+	O	+	+	+	+	+	+	O	+	O	+	+	+	O	O	+	O	±
5	O	O	+	+	+	+	+	O	+	O	+	+	+	+	O	O	O	+	O	+	+	+	+	O	+	O	O
6	O	O	O	O	+	O	+	O	+	O	+	+	+	+	+	+	+	O	+	+	+	O	+	O	+	O	±
7	O	O	O	+	+	+	+	O	+	O	+	O	O	+	O	+	O	+	+	O	+	O	+	O	+	O	O
8	O	O	O	+	+	O	+	O	+	O	+	O	+	O	+	+	O	O	+	+	+	O	+	O	+	O	2+
9	+	+	O	O	+	O	+	O	+	O	+	+	+	+	+	+	+	O	O	+	+	+	+	O	+	O	1+
10	+	O	O	+	+	O	+	O	+	O	+	O	O	+	+	+	O	O	O	O	+	O	+	O	+	O	1+

22. Refer to Panel 2. Which antibody specificity is *most* likely present?
A. Anti-S and anti-E
B. Anti-E and anti-K
C. Anti-Le^a and anti-Fy^b
D. Anti-C and anti-K
Immunohematology/Antibodies/3

23. On Panel 2, which *best* describes the pattern for the K antigen on cell lines 2, 5, and 7?
A. High frequency
B. Low frequency
C. Homozygous
D. Heterozygous
Immunohematology/Antibodies/2

24. On Panel 2, which cells are homozygous for C?
A. 1, 2, 3
B. 1, 2, 9
C. 3, 4, 7
D. 7, 8, 10
Immunohematology/Antibodies/2

25. A 77-year-old patient is admitted to a community hospital after a cardiac arrest. History includes an abdominal aortic aneurysm 2 years ago for which they received 6 units of packed RBCs. Their blood type is A positive, and the antibody screen is positive at the AHG phase in screening cells II and III. A panel is performed by using LISS. In Panel 3, which antibodies are likely implicated?
A. C and K
B. Jk^a and c
C. E and c
D. Fy^a and M
Immunohematology/Antibodies/3

Answers to Questions 22–25

22. D The pattern fits anti-C at 37°C, which becomes stronger at the IAT phase. The additional antibody is anti-K, which appears only at the IAT phase.

23. B The reactivity pattern observed on the panel for cell lines 2, 5, and 7 suggests that the antibody to the K antigen could not be ruled out. The presence of the K antigen and k antigen indicates that the RBCs are heterozygous for the K antigen.

24. B On panel cells 1, 2, and 9, C antigen is present, and c antigen is absent, rendering the cells homozygous for C.

25. C The antibodies evident in Panel 3 are E and c. Every positive reaction at 37°C and IAT phases are positive for either the E antigen and/or for cells homozygous for c antigen.

Panel 2

Cell	D	C	E	c	e	K	k	Kp^a	Kp^b	Js^a	Js^b	Fy^a	Fy^b	Jk^a	Jk^b	Xg^a	Le^a	Le^b	S	s	M	N	P_1	Lu^a	Lu^b	37°	IAT
1	+	+	O	O	+	O	+	O	+	O	+	O	+	O	+	+	+	O	O	+	O	+	O	O	+	1+	2+
2	+	+	O	O	+	+	+	O	+	O	+	+	+	+	+	+	O	+	+	+	O	+	+	O	+	1+	2+
3	+	O	+	+	O	O	+	O	+	O	+	+	O	+	+	O	O	+	+	+	+	+	+	O	+	O	O
4	O	+	O	+	+	O	+	O	+	O	+	+	+	+	+	+	O	+	O	+	+	+	O	O	+	±	+
5	O	O	+	+	+	+	+	O	+	O	+	+	+	+	O	O	O	+	O	+	+	+	+	O	+	O	2+
6	O	O	O	O	+	O	+	O	+	O	+	+	+	+	+	+	+	O	+	+	+	O	+	O	+	O	O
7	O	O	O	+	+	+	+	O	+	O	+	O	O	+	O	+	O	+	+	O	+	O	+	O	+	O	2+
8	O	O	O	+	+	O	+	O	+	O	+	O	+	O	+	+	O	O	+	+	+	O	+	O	+	O	O
9	+	+	O	O	+	O	+	O	+	O	+	+	+	+	+	+	+	O	O	+	+	+	+	O	+	1+	1+
10	+	O	O	+	+	O	+	O	+	O	+	O	O	+	+	+	O	O	O	O	+	O	+	O	+	O	O

26. Refer to Panel 3. What observation is apparent with one of the antibodies present on Panel 3?
A. One antibody is only reacting with heterozygous cells
B. Both antibodies are only reacting with homozygous cells
C. One antibody is only reacting with homozygous cells
D. Both antibodies are exhibiting dosage
Immunohematology/Antibodies/3

27. What corrective action should be taken when rouleaux causes positive test results?
A. Perform a saline replacement technique
B. Perform an autoabsorption
C. Run a panel
D. Perform an elution
Immunohematology/Antibodies/3

28. All the following are reasons for performing an adsorption *except*:
A. Separation of mixtures of antibodies
B. Removal of interfering substances
C. Confirmation of weak antigens on RBCs
D. Identification of antibodies causing a positive DAT
Immunohematology/Antibodies/2

29. A patient's serum contains a mixture of antibodies. One of the antibodies is identified as anti-D. Anti-Jk^a or anti-Fy^a and possibly another antibody is present. What technique(s) may be helpful to identify the additional antibody(s)?
A. Enzyme panel; select cell panel
B. Thiol reagents
C. Lowering the pH and increasing the incubation time
D. Using albumin as an enhancement medium in combination with selective adsorption
Immunohematology/Antibodies/3

Answers to Questions 26–29

26. C Anti-c is only reacting with homozygous cells.

27. A Rouleaux may be dispersed or lessened by using the saline replacement technique. This involves recentrifuging the tube, then withdrawing serum and replacing it with equal amount of saline. The tube is respun and examined for hemolysis.

28. D Antibodies causing a positive DAT would be coating RBCs and would require elution, not adsorption, to identify the antibodies.

29. A An enzyme panel would help to distinguish between anti-Jk^a (reaction enhanced) and anti-Fy^a (destroyed). Anti-D, however, would also be enhanced and may mask reactions that may distinguish another antibody. A select panel of cells negative for D may help to reveal an additional antibody or antibodies.

Panel 3

Cell	D	C	E	c	e	K	k	Kp^a	Kp^b	Js^a	Js^b	Fy^a	Fy^b	Jk^a	Jk^b	Xg^a	Le^a	Le^b	S	s	M	N	P_1	Lu^b	37°	IAT
1	0	+	0	+	+	0	+	0	+	0	+	+	+	+	0	+	0	+	+	+	+	+	0	+	0	0
2	+	0	0	+	+	+	+	0	+	0	+	0	+	0	+	+	+	0	0	+	0	0	0	+	+	+
3	+	+	+	0	0	0	+	0	+	0	+	0	0	+	+	0	0	+	+	+	+	+	0	+	+	+
4	+	+	0	0	+	+	+	0	+	0	+	+	+	+	+	+	+	+	0	0	+	+	+	+	0	0
5	+	+	0	+	+	0	+	0	+	0	+	0	+	0	+	0	0	+	+	+	+	+	+	+	0	0
6	0	+	+	+	+	0	+	0	+	0	+	+	0	0	+	+	+	+	+	+	+	+	0	+	+	+
7	0	+	0	0	+	+	+	0	+	0	+	+	+	+	+	+	+	0	0	+	0	+	+	+	0	0
8	0	+	+	0	+	0	+	0	+	0	+	0	+	0	+	+	+	+	+	+	+	+	+	+	+	+
9	0	0	0	+	+	0	+	0	+	0	+	+	+	+	+	+	+	0	0	+	+	+	+	+	+	+
10	+	+	0	+	+	+	+	0	+	0	+	+	+	0	+	+	0	+	+	+	+	+	+	+	0	0

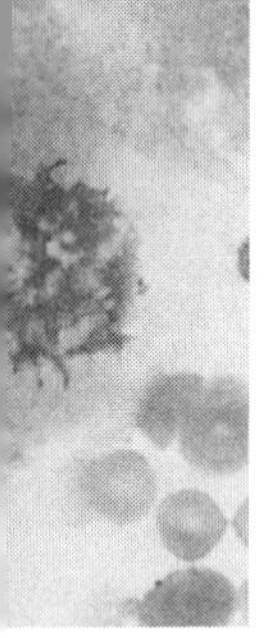

10.6

Compatibility Testing

1. An emergency trauma patient requires transfusion. Six units of blood are ordered *STAT.* There is no time to draw a patient sample. O-negative blood is issued. When will compatibility testing be performed?

A. Compatibility testing must be performed before blood is issued
B. Compatibility testing will be performed when a patient sample is available
C. Compatibility testing may be performed immediately by using donor serum
D. Compatibility testing is not necessary when blood is issued in emergency situations

Immunohematology/Compatibility/3

2. How would autoantibodies affect pretransfusion testing?

A. No effect
B. Only the antibody screen will be affected
C. ABO, Rh, antibody screen, and crossmatching may show abnormal results
D. Results would depend on the specificity of autoantibody

Immunohematology/Compatibility/3

3. An antibody screen is reactive at the IAT phase of testing with all three-cells of a three-cell screen, and the autocontrol is negative. What is a possible explanation for these results?

A. A cold alloantibody
B. High-frequency alloantibody or a mixture of alloantibodies
C. A warm autoantibody
D. A cold and warm alloantibody

Immunohematology/Compatibility/3

4. What does a routine crossmatch consist of?

A. Recipient plasma and recipient RBCs
B. Recipient plasma and donor RBCs
C. Recipient RBCs and donor plasma
D. Donor plasma and donor RBCs

Immunohematology/Compatibility/1

5. Can routine crossmatching be performed on the 14th day of the month for a same-day transfusion using a patient sample drawn on the 12th day of the month?

A. Yes, a new sample would not be needed
B. Yes, but only if the previous sample has no alloantibodies
C. No, a new sample is needed because the 2-day limit has expired
D. No, a new sample is needed for each individual compatibility testing

Immunohematology/Compatibility/2

Answers to Questions 1–5

1. B When a patient sample is available, it will be cross-matched with donor cells. Patient serum might contain antibodies against antigens on donor cells that may destroy donor cells. If an incompatibility is discovered, the problem will be reported immediately to the patient's physician.

2. C Autoantibodies may cause positive reactions with screening cells, panel cells, donor cells, and patient cells at all levels of pretransfusion testing.

3. B High-frequency alloantibodies or a mixture of alloantibodies may cause all three screening cells to be positive. A negative autocontrol would rule out autoantibodies.

4. B A routine crossmatch consists of donor RBCs and recipient serum or plasma to ensure compatibility prior to transfusion.

5. A Routine compatibility testing may be performed on a patient sample that has been collected within 3 days of the scheduled transfusion.

6. A type and screen is performed on a 32-year-old patient and is typed as AB negative. There are no AB-negative units in the blood bank. What is the *next* step?

A. Order AB-negative units from a blood supplier
B. Check inventory of A-, B-, and O-negative units
C. Ask the patient to make a preoperative autologous donation
D. Nothing—the blood will probably not be used

Immunohematology/Compatibility/2

7. What ABO type(s) is(are) considered the universal donor?

A. A negative, B negative, AB negative, O negative
B. O negative
C. AB negative
D. AB negative, A negative, B negative

Immunohematology/Compatibility/1

8. What type(s) of RBC(s) is (are) acceptable to transfuse to an O-negative patient?

A. A negative, B negative, AB negative, or O negative
B. O negative
C. AB negative
D. AB negative, A negative, B negative

Immunohematology/Compatibility/1

9. A medical laboratory scientist removed 4 units of blood from the blood bank refrigerator and placed them on the counter. A clerk was waiting to take the units for transfusion. As the clerk checked the paperwork, the clerk noticed that one of the units was leaking onto the counter. What should the clerk do?

A. Issue the unit if the RBCs appear normal
B. Reseal the unit
C. Discard the unit
D. Call the medical director and ask for an opinion

Immunohematology/Compatibility/3

10. Which of the following is the primary purpose of the immediate spin (IS) phase of crossmatching?

A. Detecting ABO incompatibilities
B. Identifying unexpected antibodies
C. Measuring hemoglobin levels
D. Checking for hemolysis

Immunohematology/Compatibility/1

11. Which of the following is *not* a requirement for electronic crossmatching?

A. The computer system contains logic to prevent assignment and release of ABO-incompatible blood
B. There are concordant results of at least two determinations of the recipient's ABO type on record, one of which is from the current sample
C. Critical elements of the system have been validated on site
D. There are concordant results of at least one determination of the recipient's ABO type on file

Immunohematology/Compatibility/1

12. A patient showed positive results with screening cells and 4 donor units at the IAT phase. The patient's sample autocontrol was negative. What is the *most* likely antibody?

A. Anti-H
B. Anti-S
C. Anti-Kp^a
D. Anti-k

Immunohematology/Compatibility/3

Answers to Questions 6–12

6. B An individual with an AB blood type is the universal recipient and may receive any blood type. In this scenario, because only a type and screen were ordered and blood may not be used, the inventory should be checked for A-, B-, and O-negative units.

7. B An O-negative individual has no A, B, or D antigens and may donate RBCs to any other ABO type.

8. B An O-negative individual may receive only O-negative RBCs.

9. C Leaking may indicate a broken seal or a puncture, which indicates possible contamination of the unit, even if the RBCs appear normal. The unit should be discarded.

10. A The IS phase is designed to quickly identify any agglutination that would indicate an ABO mismatch between the donor and recipient. Identifying unexpected antibodies is typically done in the IAT phase, which follows the immediate spin phase.

11. D ABO determinations must be concordant on at least two occasions, including the current sample.

12. D Anti-k (Cellano) is a high-frequency alloantibody that would react with screening cells and most donor units. The negative autocontrol rules out autoantibodies. Anti-H and anti-S are cold antibodies, and anti-Kp^a is a low-frequency alloantibody.

13. Screening cells and major crossmatch are positive on IS only, and the autocontrol is negative. Identify the problem.
A. Cold alloantibody
B. Cold autoantibody
C. Abnormal protein
D. Antibody mixture

Immunohematology/Compatibility/3

14. What is the primary reason for performing the autocontrol during an antibody screen and identification?
A. Check for ABO incompatibility
B. Identify the recipient's blood type
C. Detect autoantibodies in the recipient's serum
D. Measure hemoglobin level

Immunohematology/Compatibility/1

15. An incompatible donor unit is found to have a positive result on DAT. What should the laboratory do with the donor unit?
A. Discard the unit
B. Antigen type the unit for high-frequency antigens
C. Wash the donor cells and use the washed cells for testing
D. Perform a panel on the incompatible unit

Immunohematology/Compatibility/3

16. Screening cells, major crossmatch, and patient autocontrol are positive in all phases. Identify the problem.
A. Specific cold alloantibody
B. Specific cold autoantibody
C. Abnormal protein or nonspecific autoantibody
D. Cold and warm alloantibody mixture

Immunohematology/Compatibility/3

17. A panel study has revealed the presence of patient alloantibody(ies). What is the *next* step to confirm?
A. Perform a DAT on patient cells and donor units
B. Antigen type patient cells
C. Adsorb any antibodies from patient serum
D. Obtain a different enhancement medium for testing

Immunohematology/Compatibility/3

18. What is the likely result if a recipient has an anti-K antibody, and the donor RBCs are K-positive?
A. Positive ABO compatibility
B. Positive Rh compatibility
C. Positive major crossmatch
D. Negative antibody screen

Immunohematology/Compatibility/2

19. Given a situation where screening cells, major crossmatch, autocontrol, and DAT (anti-IgG) are all positive, what procedure should be performed *next*?
A. Adsorption using rabbit stroma
B. Antigen typing of patient cells
C. Elution followed by a cell panel on the eluate
D. Selected cell panel

Immunohematology/Compatibility/3

20. A major crossmatch and screening cells are 2+ at the IS phase, 1+ at 37°C, and negative at the IAT phase. Identify the *most* likely concern.
A. Combination of antibodies
B. Cold alloantibody
C. Rouleaux
D. Test error

Immunohematology/Compatibility/3

Answers to Questions 13–20

13. A A cold alloantibody would show a reaction with screening cells and donor units only at the IS phase. The negative autocontrol rules out autoantibodies and abnormal protein.

14. C The primary reason is to help differentiate between these possibilities by confirming or ruling out the presence of autoantibodies in the recipient's serum.

15. A The incompatible unit may have RBCs coated with antibody and/or complement. If RBCs are sensitized, then some problem exists with the donor. Discard the unit.

16. C An abnormal protein or nonspecific autoantibody would cause the antibody screen, crossmatch, and patient autocontrol to be positive. Alloantibodies would not cause a positive patient autocontrol.

17. B The next step after identifying patient alloantibody(ies) in a panel study is to antigen type the patient's cells. This step helps to confirm the specific antigens present are absent on the patient's RBCs and guides the selection of compatible donor blood that will not react with the alloantibodies.

18. C If a recipient has anti-K antibodies and the donor RBCs are K positive, the likely result is a positive major crossmatch, indicating incompatibility.

19. C A positive DAT using anti-IgG indicates that antibodies are coating the patient's cells. An eluate would be helpful to remove the antibody, followed by a cell panel to identify it.

20. B The reaction pattern fits that of a cold antibody reacting at the IS phase and of sufficient titer to persist at 37°C incubation. The reactions disappear in the IAT phase.

21. How long must a recipient sample be kept in the blood bank after compatibility testing?
A. 3 days
B. 5 days
C. 7 days
D. 10 days
Immunohematology/Compatibility/1

22. What is the crossmatching protocol for platelets and/or plasma?
A. Perform a reverse grouping on donor plasma
B. No testing is required
C. Perform a reverse grouping on recipient plasma
D. Full crossmatch through IAT phase
Immunohematology/Compatibility/2

23. What are the compatibility requirements for an autologous unit?
A. ABO and Rh typing
B. Type and screen
C. Major crossmatch
D. All the responses are correct
Immunohematology/Compatibility/1

24. A patient is typed as AB positive. Two units of blood have been ordered by the provider. The present inventory includes no AB units, 10 A-positive units, 1 A-negative unit, 5 B-positive units, and 20 O-positive units. Which units should be selected first for the major crossmatch?
A. A-positive units
B. O-positive units
C. B-positive units
D. Call another blood supplier for type-specific blood
Immunohematology/Compatibility/2

25. Which of the following comprises an abbreviated crossmatch?
A. ABO, Rh, and antibody screen
B. ABO, Rh, antibody screen, IS crossmatch
C. Type and screen
D. ABO, Rh, IS crossmatch
Immunohematology/Compatibility/2

26. When should IS crossmatching be performed?
A. When a patient is being massively transfused
B. When there is no history of antibodies, and the current antibody screen is negative
C. When blood is being emergency released
D. When a patient has not been transfused in the past 3 months
Immunohematology/Compatibility/1

Answers to Questions 21–26

21. C According to the American Association of Blood Banks (AABB) standards, the recipient sample must be kept for 7 days after compatibility testing. This duration ensures that the sample is available for any necessary follow-up testing during the immediate post-transfusion period.

22. B For transfusion of platelets and plasma, there is no required protocol for routine crossmatching. ABO/Rh compatibility is preferred.

23. A The only requirement for transfusing an autologous unit is a confirmation check of the ABO and Rh types.

24. A The type chosen should be A-positive RBC units. Although all choices would be compatible, the first choice should be A-positive because this unit will contain residual plasma anti-B. Anti-B is less immunogenic than anti-A, which would be present, albeit in small amounts, in B-positive and O-positive units.

25. B The abbreviated crossmatch usually consists of a type and screen and an IS crossmatch.

26. B IS crossmatching may be performed when the patient has no history of antibodies, and the current antibody screen is negative.

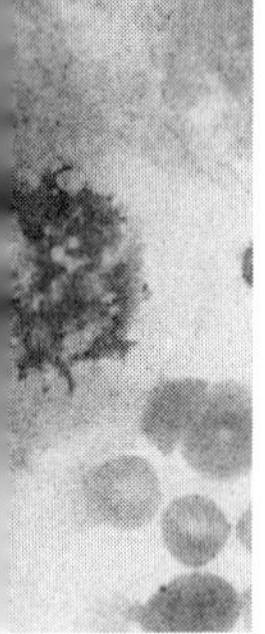

10.7
Transfusion Reactions

1. A patient had a transfusion reaction to packed RBCs. The medical laboratory scientist began the laboratory investigation of the transfusion reaction by assembling pre- and post-transfusion specimens and related documentation. What is the *next* step?
A. Perform a DAT on the post-transfusion sample
B. Check for clerical error(s)
C. Repeat ABO and Rh typing of patient and donor units
D. Perform an antibody screen on the post-transfusion sample
Immunohematology/Transfusion reactions/2

2. What is the pathophysiological cause that is associated with anaphylactic and anaphylactoid reactions?
A. Antibody in patient's serum is detected 3 to 7 days after transfusion and is attached to donor RBCs
B. Donor plasma has reagins (IgE or IgA) that combine with allergens in patient's plasma
C. Patient develops IgE antibodies via sensitization as a result of transfusion or pregnancy
D. Patient develops IgA antibodies via sensitization as a result of transfusion or pregnancy
Immunohematology/Transfusion reactions/2

3. A patient has a hemolytic reaction to a blood transfusion from 8 days ago. What is the *most* likely cause?
A. Immediate, nonimmunologic, probably because of volume overload
B. Delayed immunologic, probably because of an antibody such as anti-Jk^a
C. Delayed nonimmunologic, probably because of iron overload
D. Immediate, immunologic, probably because of clerical error, ABO incompatibility
Immunohematology/Transfusion reactions/2

4. What may be identified in the serum of a patient who is exhibiting signs of transfusion-related acute lung injury (TRALI)?
A. RBC alloantibody
B. IgA antibody
C. Anti-HLA antibody
D. Allergen
Immunohematology/Transfusion reactions/2

5. Which type of transfusion reaction occurs in about 1% of all transfusions, results in a temperature rise of greater than 1°C above 37°C associated with blood components, and is not related to the patient's medical condition?
A. Immediate hemolytic
B. Delayed hemolytic
C. Febrile nonhemolytic transfusion reaction (FNHTR)
D. TRALI
Immunohematology/Transfusion reactions/2

Answers to Questions 1–5

1. B Over 90% of transfusion reactions are caused by some type of clerical error. The most time-saving approach would be to check all paperwork before performing any laboratory testing.

2. D Anaphylactic or anaphylactoid reactions are the most severe form of allergic transfusion reaction and are associated with the formation of anti-IgA. These patients must be transfused with washed cellular products where the plasma has been removed.

3. B A transfusion reaction that occurs several days after a transfusion of blood products is probably a delayed immunologic reaction because of an antibody formed against donor antigens. This is a classic example of a reaction caused by an antibody, such as anti-Jk^a.

4. C TRALI is associated with antibodies to HLA or neutrophil antigens, which react with the patient's granulocytes and cause acute respiratory insufficiency.

5. C FNHTR is defined as a rise in temperature of greater than 1°C above 37°C, associated with transfusion and unexplained by other causes. The patient has formed antibodies to HLA, which reacted with donor cells and resulted in the release of pyrogens.

6. What is the consequence of group A blood administered to a group O patient?
A. Nonimmune transfusion reaction
B. Immediate hemolytic transfusion reaction
C. Delayed hemolytic transfusion reaction
D. FNHTR

Immunohematology/Transfusion reactions/2

7. Patient X received 2 units of group A-positive RBCs 2 days ago. Today, the patient developed a fever and appeared jaundiced. The patient's blood type is A positive. A transfusion reaction workup is ordered. No clerical errors were detected. A post-transfusion specimen was collected and a DAT performed. The DAT result is positive with monospecific anti-IgG. The plasma is also hemolyzed. An antibody screen and panel reveals the presence of anti-Jk^b in the post-transfusion specimen. The antibody screen on the pretransfusion specimen was negative. Which of the following explains the positive DAT?
A. The donor cells had a positive DAT
B. The donor cells were polyagglutinable
C. The donor cells were likely positive for the Jk^b antigen
D. The recipient cells were likely positive for the Jk^b antigen

Immunohematology/Transfusion reactions/3

8. Which transfusion reaction is *most* often associated with the rapid infusion of large volumes of blood products?
A. Transfusion-associated circulatory overload (TACO)
B. TRALI
C. Delayed hemolytic transfusion reaction (DHTR)
D. FNHTR

Immunohematology/Transfusion reactions/2

9. A 68-year-old patient diagnosed with neutropenia and inflammation of the left hand was typed as A positive and received 1 packed RBC unit. The antibody screen was negative, and the crossmatch was compatible. During the transfusion, the patient's pulse was 94 bpm, and blood pressure (BP) rose from 114/59 mm Hg to 132/64 mm Hg. Temperature rose from 37.1°C before transfusion to 37.8°C 60 minutes after beginning the transfusion and then to 38.3°C upon completion. A post-transfusion specimen yielded plasma that was not hemolyzed or icteric. The specimen also was DAT negative. Post-transfusion urinalysis showed 1+ blood and protein with 10 RBCs/high-power field (hpf) microscopically. The clerical check result was acceptable. What type of reaction *most* likely occurred?
A. Allergic
B. Circulatory overload
C. Febrile nonhemolytic
D. Delayed hemolytic

Immunohematology/Transfusion reactions/3

Answers to Questions 6–9

6. B Group A blood administered to a group O patient would cause an immediate hemolytic transfusion reaction because a group O patient has anti-A and anti-B antibodies and would destroy the A cells due to ABO incompatibility.

7. C This is an example of an anamnestic reaction, in which the patient was most likely exposed to the Jk^b antigen at some point in their life, and the antibody titer was below datable limits during the pretransfusion antibody screen and crossmatch. Upon reexposure to the antigen, the antibody titer rose to detectable levels. This resulted in positive DAT and post-transfusion antibody screen results.

8. A TACO occurs when a large volume of blood products is infused rapidly, leading to fluid overload. This can cause symptoms such as dyspnea (shortness of breath), hypertension, pulmonary edema, and heart failure. TACO is more common in patients with preexisting cardiac or renal conditions and in the elderly patient.

9. C The temperature rose from 37.1°C to 38.3°C. The DAT result was negative, and although blood was identified in the urinalysis, microscopic RBCs were also noted. Because intact RBCs are not caused by a transfusion reaction, the cause of hematuria was not likely transfusion related. A febrile nonhemolytic reaction is highly consistent with both symptoms and post-transfusion test results.

10. A 92-year-old patient diagnosed with anemia and episodes of frequent falling was typed as B negative and transfused with 1 unit of packed B negative RBCs. The patient had not been recently transfused, and the antibody screen was negative. During the transfusion, the patient's temperature rose from 36.2°C to 36.4°C, pulse from 96 to 124 bpm, respirations from 18 to 20, and BP from 127/81 mm Hg to 174/83 mm Hg. The patient was transfused with 205 mL before a reaction was called by the transfusionist. The post-transfusion specimen DAT result was negative, and the clerical check result was acceptable. Urinalysis showed 1+ blood with 5 RBCs microscopically. Other symptoms included tachycardia and flushing. What reaction had *most* likely taken place?

A. Febrile nonhemolytic
B. Acute hemolytic
C. Anaphylactic
D. Volume overload

Immunohematology/Transfusion reactions/3

11. A 76-year-old patient diagnosed with urosepsis was transfused with 2 units of AB positive packed RBCs. The patient's blood type is AB positive and had a negative result on antibody screen. Upon receiving the second unit, the patient became hypoxic with tachypnea. The clerical check result was acceptable, and the DAT was negative. The patient received 269 mL from the second unit before a reaction was called. Their temperature fell from 38°C to 36.4°C, pulse increased from 72 to 90 bpm, and respirations rose from 35 to 41. The BP was 110/70 mm Hg. The patient died approximately 12 hours following the reaction. What type of reaction was *most* likely present?

A. Febrile
B. Symptoms not related to transfusion
C. Allergic
D. TRALI

Immunohematology/Transfusion reactions/3

12. A 52-year-old patient received 2 units of packed RBCs as an outpatient in the IV therapy unit. The patient experienced head trauma 20 years ago and was quadriplegic. They had recurrent pneumonia and hematuria upon removal of a Foley catheter. The patient's blood type is A positive, with previously identified anti-Fy^a. There was an ABO discrepancy, in that reverse typing with reagent A_1 cells was positive. The medical laboratory scientist attributed this reaction to Fy^a antigen present on the reagent A_1 cells. The patient also had a cold autoantibody. Two units of A-positive packed cells were crossmatched that were Fy^a negative and were compatible. One unit was transfused at 11:30 a.m. without incident. The second unit was transfused at 2:16 p.m. and stopped at 3:55 p.m. because of reddish brown–tinged urine noted in the patient's collection bag. A post-transfusion specimen yielded a positive DAT and plasma that was grossly hemolyzed. A prewarm crossmatch was incompatible in both the pre- and post-transfusion specimens. Anti-E and anti-c were present in the post-transfusion specimen. What reaction was *most* likely present?

A. Acute hemolytic
B. Febrile
C. Allergic
D. TRALI

Immunohematology/Transfusion reactions/3

Answers to Questions 10–12

10. D The tachycardia, increased pulse, and volume transfused before a reaction was called are consistent with volume overload. The temperature change did not meet criteria for a febrile reaction, and evidence for a hemolytic reaction is lacking.

11. B This case emphasizes the statistic that not all causes of death are related to transfusion. The temperature dropped, ruling out a febrile reaction; there was no evidence of pulmonary edema or hypotension seen with TRALI (and plasma products are more associated with TRALI compared with RBCs); and there was no sign of hives or itching, which are often associated with an allergic reaction.

12. A This case represents an acute hemolytic reaction in which the patient had previous sensitization to E and c antigens. Given the history of anti-Fy^a, an assumption was made that anti-Fy^a was the cause of the positive reverse type with A_1 cells, even though this antibody does not react at the IS phase. This brings to light the importance of running a panel whenever the patient has a positive antibody screen, regardless of previous results. Hemoglobinuria, a positive DAT, and the hemolyzed post-transfusion specimen all are consistent with an acute hemolytic reaction.

13. An 82-year-old patient was admitted for renal failure. The patient's blood type is B positive, and the antibody screen is negative. Two units of RBCs were ordered. The first unit was transfused at 1:00 p.m. without incident. The second was started at 4:15 p.m. and stopped at 5:12 p.m. after the nurse observed that the patient had expired. Vital signs were taken at 4:30 p.m. with no abnormalities. A transfusion reaction was called, and the blood unit, tubing, and documentation were sent to the blood bank. There were no clinical manifestations noted in the documentation, and no post-transfusion specimen was sent to the blood bank. What type of reaction *most* likely occurred?

A. Unable to determine
B. Acute hemolytic reaction
C. Anaphylactic reaction
D. Volume overload

Immunohematology/Transfusion reactions/3

Answer to Question 13

13. A This example represents a situation in which the pathologist was not provided with all information needed to interpret the reaction. There was no information on patient symptoms, the patient had received another unit of RBCs hours previously with no problems, and a postreaction specimen was not collected. Therefore, any serological abnormalities could not be identified. The Food and Drug Administration (FDA) recommends collecting a postmortem specimen if a reaction is called so that the investigation of transfusion reaction can be completed.

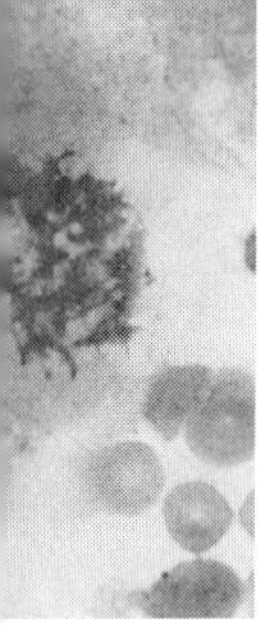

10.8
Components

1. **A patient with cancer was admitted to the hospital with acute abdominal pain and a hemoglobin level of 6 g/dL. Small bowel resection was indicated, but the attending provider wanted to raise the patient's hemoglobin level to 12 g/dL before surgery. How many units of RBCs would *most* likely be required to accomplish this?**
   - **A.** 2
   - **B.** 3
   - **C.** 6
   - **D.** 8

   Immunohematology/Components/2

2. **Which of the following is *not* a viable method for removing leukocytes from RBCs to achieve $<5 \times 10^6$?**
   - **A.** Pre-storage filtration
   - **B.** Bedside filtration
   - **C.** Post-storage filtration
   - **D.** Buffy coat removal

   Immunohematology/Components/1

3. **Four units of packed RBCs were brought to the nurses' station at 10:20 a.m. Two units were transfused immediately, and 1 unit was transfused at 10:40 a.m. The remaining unit was returned to the blood bank at 11:00 a.m. The units were not refrigerated after leaving the blood bank. What problem(s) is (are) present in this situation?**
   - **A.** The only problem is with the returned unit; the 30-minute limit has expired, and the unit cannot be used
   - **B.** The unit should not have been transfused at 10:40 a.m. because the time limit had expired; this unit and the remaining unit should have been returned to the blood bank
   - **C.** The returned unit may be held for this patient for 48 hours but cannot be used for another patient
   - **D.** No problems; all actions were performed within the allowable time limits

   Immunohematology/Components/3

4. **A unit of whole blood is collected at 10:00 a.m. and stored at 20°C to 24°C. How many hours is the unit viable to process platelet concentrate?**
   - **A.** 4 hours
   - **B.** 6 hours
   - **C.** 8 hours
   - **D.** 24 hours

   Immunohematology/Components/1

Answers to Questions 1–4

1. C One unit of RBCs will raise the hemoglobin level by approximately 1.0 to 1.5 g/dL, and the hematocrit by 3% to 4%. Results vary, depending on the age of the blood and the patient's blood volume and hydration status. Six units will raise the hemoglobin level to at least 12 g/dL.

2. D Removal of the buffy coat, which contains both platelets and white blood cells (WBCs), is not an approved method for leukocyte reduction of RBCs. The other methods can be employed to achieve a leukocyte reduction of less than 5×10^6.

3. A There is a 30-minute time limit for a unit of RBCs that is not kept under proper storage conditions (1°C–6°C).

4. C Platelet preparation from whole blood must be performed within 8 hours of collection.

5. Which of the following is acceptable according to the AABB standards?

A. Rejuvenated RBCs may be made within 3 days of the outdate and transfused or frozen within 24 hours of rejuvenation
B. Frozen RBCs must be prepared within 30 minutes of collection and may be used within 10 years
C. Irradiated RBCs must be treated within 8 hours of collection and transfused within 6 hours
D. Leukocyte-reduced RBCs must be prepared within 6 hours of collection and transfused within 6 hours of preparation

Immunohematology/Components/2

6. Which of the following is true regarding apheresis platelets?

A. The minimum platelet count must be 3.0×10^{11}, pH must be 6.0 or greater
B. The minimum platelet count must be 3.0×10^{10}, pH must be 6.2 or less
C. The minimum platelet count must be 3.0×10^{11}, pH must be 6.2 or greater
D. The minimum platelet count must be 5.5×10^{10}, pH must be 6.0 or less

Immunohematology/Components/1

7. What is the component of choice for a patient with chronic granulomatous disease (CGD)?

A. Fresh frozen plasma (FFP)
B. Granulocyte concentrates
C. Cryoprecipitate
D. Packed RBCs

Immunohematology/Components/3

8. Which blood component is frequently used to treat patients with a deficiency in clotting factors?

A. RBCs
B. FFP
C. Platelets
D. Cryoprecipitate

Immunohematology/Components/1

9. What is the primary purpose of transfusing washed RBCs?

A. Removing clotting factors
B. Reducing the risk of allergic reactions in sensitive patients
C. Increasing oxygen transport capacity
D. Enhancing blood volume

Immunohematology/Components/1

Answers to Questions 5–9

5. A Rejuvenated RBCs may be prepared within 3 days of the outdate of the unit and washed and transfused or frozen within 24 hours. A unit of RBCs may be frozen within 6 days of collection. An RBC unit can be irradiated any time prior to the expiration date; once irradiated, the unit must be transfused within 28 days of irradiation or the original outdate, whichever comes first. Leukocyte-reduced RBCs should be prepared within 6 hours of collection, but must be given within 24 hours, if prepared using an open system. Leukocyte-reduced RBCs prepared using a closed system may be kept until the original date of expiration.

6. C Single-donor platelets prepared by apheresis must contain a minimum of 3.0×10^{11} platelets, and pH must be 6.2 or higher throughout the shelf life of the product.

7. B Patients with CGD cannot fight bacterial infections because of dysfunctional phagocytic enzymes; granulocyte concentrates are the product of choice for these patients.

8. B FFP is a frequently used blood component to treat patients with deficiencies in clotting factors because it contains all the necessary clotting factors needed for proper blood coagulation. It is especially useful in conditions in which multiple clotting factors are deficient or dysfunctional.

9. B The primary purpose of transfusing washed RBCs is to reduce the risk of allergic reactions in patients who are sensitive to plasma proteins. The washing process removes the plasma proteins and other immunogenic substances that can trigger allergic reactions, making the transfusion safer for these individuals.

10. What process can be utilized to reduce the possibility of a transfusion reaction if administering RBCs to a patient with cold agglutinin disease?
  A. Irradiate to prevent graft-versus-host-disease (GVHD)
  B. Wash with 0.9% saline
  C. Warm to 37°C with a blood warmer
  D. Transport so that temperature is maintained at 20°C to 24°C

Immunohematology/Components/2

11. A unit of packed RBCs is split using the open system. One of the half units is used. What happens with the second half of the unit?
  A. Must be issued within 24 hours
  B. Must be issued within 48 hours
  C. Must be irradiated
  D. Must retain the original expiration date

Immunohematology/Components/2

12. A noticeable clot is found in an RBC unit. What is the correct required follow-up or action?
  A. Issue the unit; the blood will be filtered
  B. Issue the unit; note the presence of a clot on the release form
  C. Filter the unit in the blood bank before issue
  D. Do not issue the unit

Immunohematology/Components/2

13. Cryoprecipitate may be used to treat all the following *except*:
  A. von Willebrand disease
  B. Hypofibrinogenemia
  C. Idiopathic thrombocytopenic purpura (ITP)
  D. Factor XIII deficiency

Immunohematology/Components/3

14. What is the primary reason for performing irradiation on blood components?
  A. To increase the concentration of hemoglobin
  B. To prevent transfusion-associated graft-versus-host disease (TA-GVHD)
  C. To reduce the risk of allergic reactions
  D. To enhance clotting factor activity

Immunohematology/Components/2

15. What component(s) is (are) indicated for patients who have anti-IgA antibodies?
  A. FFP
  B. Packed RBCs
  C. Washed or deglycerolized RBCs
  D. Granulocytes

Immunohematology/Components/1

16. What is the expiration date for pooled cryoprecipitate (pooled before freezing)?
  A. 12 months from latest date of collection of products included in the pool
  B. 12 months from the earliest date of collection of products in pool
  C. 4 hours
  D. 6 hours

Immunohematology/Components/1

17. All the following are true regarding washed RBCs *except*:
  A. RBCs are washed with 1 to 2 L of normal saline
  B. Volume is 180 mL
  C. Shelf life is extended
  D. Leukocytes are removed

Immunohematology/Components/1

Answers to Questions 10–17

10. C A patient having cold agglutinins might have a reaction to a cold blood product. The product should be warmed to 37°C before transfusion.

11. A The other half unit must be issued within 24 hours, if an open system is used to split the unit.

12. D A unit having a noticeable clot should not be issued for transfusion to a patient. The clot may be an indication of contamination or bacterial growth.

13. C Cryoprecipitate may be used to treat von Willebrand disease, hypofibrinogenemia, and factor XIII deficiency, but is not indicated in ITP. IV immunoglobulin (IVIG) is the product of choice for ITP.

14. B The primary reason for performing irradiation on blood components is to prevent TA-GVHD by inactivating any residual lymphocytes in the blood products. This process helps ensure the safety of transfusions, particularly in immunocompromised patients or those at high risk for TA-GVHD.

15. C Patients with anti-IgA antibodies should not receive components containing plasma. Washed or deglycerolized RBCs can be issued.

16. B Expiration of pooled cryoprecipitate must consider that there may be units that make up the pool with differing collection dates where 12 months from the earliest date is used to determine the expiration date.

17. C Washed RBCs render the system "open" and shorten the expiration time to 24 hours.

18. What is the special condition for the storage of platelets?
A. Storage temperature 1°C to 4°C
B. No other components may be stored with platelets
C. Platelets must be stored upright in separate containers
D. Platelets require constant agitation at 20°C to 24°C

Immunohematology/Components/1

19. Transfusion of an irradiated product is indicated in all the following conditions *except*:
A. Exchange transfusion
B. Bone marrow transplantation
C. Severe combined immunodeficiency syndrome (SCIDS)
D. Warm autoimmune hemolytic anemia

Immunohematology/Components/2

20. What percentage of RBCs must be retained in leukocyte-reduced RBCs?
A. 75%
B. 80%
C. 85%
D. 100%

Immunohematology/Components/1

21. Which patient population is *most* likely to benefit from granulocyte concentrate transfusions?
A. Patients with sickle cell anemia
B. Patients with aplastic anemia and severe neutropenia
C. Patients undergoing hemodialysis
D. Patients with thrombocytopenia

Immunohematology/Components/2

22. What course of action should be taken if a medical laboratory scientist inadvertently irradiates a unit of RBCs twice?
A. Issue the unit
B. Discard the unit
C. Change the expiration date; then issue the unit
D. Note on the irradiation sticker that the unit was irradiated twice, and then issue the unit

Immunohematology/Components/2

23. What components(s) may be shipped together with FFP?
A. Frozen RBCs and cryoprecipitate
B. Platelets
C. Packed RBCs and granulocytes
D. Double RBC units

Immunohematology/Components/1

24. A blood supplier ships 3 units of pooled cryoprecipitate. Each pool consists of 5 units of cryoprecipitate. If 1 unit is thawed at 5:00 p.m., how many hours until it must be transfused?
A. 4 hours
B. 8 hours
C. 24 hours
D. 48 hours

Immunohematology/Components/1

25. How does irradiation prevent TA-GVHD?
A. Gamma rays and x-rays destroy the lymphocytes' ability to divide
B. X-rays cause lysis of lymphocytes
C. Gamma rays enhance lymphocyte reactivity
D. Ultraviolet radiation induces apoptosis of lymphocytes

Immunohematology/Components/1

Answers to Questions 18–25

18. D Platelets require constant agitation and are stored at temperatures between 20°C and 24°C. Cold-stored platelets (single donor [apheresis] platelets stored at 1°C to 6°C for up to 3 days) may be used for actively bleeding patients but are not approved for treating thrombocytopenia.

19. D WAIHA alone would not require irradiation unless the patient had an underlying immunosuppressive disorder.

20. C An RBC unit that has been leukocyte reduced must retain 85% of original RBCs.

21. B Patients with aplastic anemia and severe neutropenia are the most likely to benefit from granulocyte concentrate transfusions because their condition results in a significant reduction in neutrophils, making them highly susceptible to infections. Granulocyte transfusions provide the necessary immune cells to help combat these infections, especially when antibiotics alone are insufficient.

22. B If a medical laboratory scientist mistakenly irradiates a unit of RBCs more than once, the unit must be discarded because of subsequent potassium accumulation. This does not apply to platelets.

23. A FFP requires dry ice for shipment. Frozen RBCs and cryoprecipitate also require dry ice.

24. A A thawed unit of pooled cryoprecipitate must be dispensed within 4 hours unless a sterile connecting device was used, which would potentially extend expiration to 6 hours.

25. A Irradiation with gamma rays or x-rays will prohibit a lymphocyte's ability to divide, preventing TA-GVHD.

26. Which component has the longest expiration date when stored and shipped properly?
A. Cryoprecipitate
B. FFP
C. Frozen RBCs
D. Platelet concentrates

Immunohematology/Components/1

27. All the following are advantages of using single-donor platelets as opposed to random donor platelets *except*:
A. Less preparation time
B. Less antigen exposure for patients
C. May be HLA matched
D. No pooling is required

Immunohematology/Components/1

28. Which blood component is *most* appropriate for a patient with hemophilia B?
A. FFP
B. Cryoprecipitate
C. Factor IX concentrate
D. Platelets

Immunohematology/Components/2

29. What is the number of WBCs permitted in a unit of leukocyte-reduced RBCs?
A. Less than 5×10^{10}
B. Less than 5×10^{6}
C. Less than 8.3×10^{5}
D. Less than 8.3×10^{6}

Immunohematology/Components/1

30. A patient with cancer recently developed a severe infection. The patient's hemoglobin level is 8 g/dL resulting from chemotherapy with a drug known to cause bone marrow depression and immunodeficiency. Which blood products are indicated for this patient?
A. Liquid plasma and cryoprecipitate
B. Crossmatched platelets and washed RBCs
C. Factor IX concentrates and FFP
D. Irradiated RBCs, platelets, and granulocytes

Immunohematology/Components/3

Answers to Questions 26–30

26. C Frozen RBCs may be kept for up to 10 years or longer if the transfusion service or blood center has a policy for extension beyond 10 years. FFP and cryoprecipitate stored at −18°C or lower expire in 1 year. If FFP is kept at −65°C or lower, the expiration time is 7 years. Platelet concentrates expire from 24 hours to 5 days, depending on the collection system used.

27. A Single-donor platelets require more preparation time compared with random-donor platelets because they are prepared by apheresis, which may require 1 to 3 hours, depending on the instrumentation used. Pooling random donor platelets in equivalent amounts may require only a few minutes.

28. C The most appropriate blood component for a patient with hemophilia B is factor IX concentrate. This targeted therapy efficiently replaces the missing factor IX, allowing for effective management of bleeding episodes and prevention of complications associated with the disorder.

29. B RBCs that have been leukocyte reduced must have fewer than 5×10^{6} WBCs per unit.

30. D The patient is immunocompromised because of the medication; therefore, irradiated RBCs are indicated for the anemia. Platelets may be needed to control bleeding, and granulocytes may be indicated for short-term control of severe infection.

10.9 Donors

1. **Which of the following individuals is acceptable as a blood donor?**
   A. A 29-year-old male who received the hepatitis B vaccine last week
   B. A 21-year-old female who had her nose pierced last week
   C. A 30-year-old male who lived in Zambia for 3 years and returned last month
   D. A 54-year-old male who tested positive for hepatitis C last year but has no active symptoms of disease
   Immunohematology/Donors/2

2. **A 53-year-old individual donates blood at their place of employment. They weigh 150 lb and have a hemoglobin level of 13 g/dL. They are currently on warfarin and vitamin B_{12}. Is this individual an acceptable donor?**
   A. Yes
   B. No, they are on warfarin
   C. Yes, for RBCs only
   D. No, their hemoglobin is too low
   Immunohematology/Donors/2

3. **Which immunization has the longest deferral period?**
   A. Hepatitis B immune globulin (HBIG)
   B. Rubella vaccine
   C. Influenza vaccine
   D. Yellow fever vaccine
   Immunohematology/Donors/1

4. **The following whole blood donors regularly give blood. Which donor may donate on September 10?**
   A. A 40-year-old female who last donated packed RBCs on July 23
   B. A 28-year-old male who had plateletpheresis on August 24
   C. A 52-year-old male who made an autologous donation on September 9
   D. A 23-year-old female who donated whole blood on August 14
   Immunohematology/Donors/2

5. **Which of the following must be met for eligibility of a platelet pheresis donor?**
   A. Platelet count of 150×10^9/L in a donor who is a frequent platelet donor
   B. Plasma loss of 1,500 mL from plasmapheresis 1 week ago
   C. Plateletpheresis performed 24 hours ago
   D. Aspirin ingested that morning
   Immunohematology/Donors/1

Answers to Questions 1–5

1. **A** If the donor is symptom free, there is no deferral period for the hepatitis B vaccine. Persons who have had body piercing are given up to a 3-month deferral. Persons who lived in an area endemic for malaria or who received antimalarial drugs are deferred for 3 years. A positive test for the hepatitis C virus (HCV) is cause for indefinite deferral.

2. **C** The age and hemoglobin meet donor criteria. However, because they are currently on warfarin, only RBCs can be prepared from the donation.

3. **A** Deferral for HBIG injection is 12 months. Deferral for rubella vaccine is 4 weeks. The deferral period for influenza and yellow fever vaccines is 2 weeks.

4. **B** A plateletpheresis donor must wait at least 48 hours between donations. The waiting period following an autologous donation is at least 3 days. An 8-week interval must pass between all other types of donations.

5. **A** To be eligible for plateletpheresis, the platelet count should be greater than 150×10^9/L for a frequent platelet donor. Plasma loss exceeding 1,000 mL would be cause for rejection. A donor may donate 24 times a year, but not as frequent as after 24 hours. A donor cannot ingest aspirin within 36 hours of platelet donation.

6. Which of the following donors could be accepted for whole blood donation?
A. A construction worker who was incarcerated for IV opiate abuse
B. A triathlete with a pulse of 45 bpm
C. A male who is currently taking finasteride (Propecia)
D. A female in the 14th week of pregnancy
Immunohematology/Donors/2

7. Which physical examination result is cause for rejecting a whole blood donor?
A. Weight of 105 lb
B. Pulse of 75 bpm
C. Temperature of 37.4°C (99.3°F)
D. Diastolic blood pressure of 110 mm Hg
Immunohematology/Donors/1

8. Which situation is *not* a cause for indefinite deferral of a donor?
A. Male donor whose father has been diagnosed with Creutzfeldt-Jakob disease (CJD)
B. Donation of a unit of blood that transmitted hepatitis B virus (HBV) to a recipient
C. Donor tested reactive for HBV by nucleic acid testing (NAT)
D. Accidental needlestick 1 year ago; negative for infectious disease
Immunohematology/Donors/1

9. A whole blood donor currently on clopidogrel (Plavix) is precluded from donating which product?
A. Platelets
B. RBCs
C. FFP
D. Cryoprecipitate
Immunohematology/Donors/1

10. How much anticoagulant would have to be removed from the collection bag given a donor who weighs 90 lb?
A. 12 mL
B. 15 mL
C. 20 mL
D. 23 mL
Immunohematology/Donors/2

11. An 30 year old individual begins to breathe rapidly while donating blood. Choose the correct course of action.
A. Continue the donation; rapid breathing is not a reason to discontinue a donation
B. Withdraw the needle, raise their feet, and administer ammonia
C. Discontinue the donation, and provide a paper bag for the donor to breathe slowly into
D. Tell the individual to sit upright, and apply a cold compress to their forehead
Immunohematology/Donors/3

Answers to Questions 6–11

6. B Athletes may have a pulse below 50 and may still be acceptable as blood donors. IV drug use is cause for permanent deferral. Individuals taking Propecia are deferred from donating blood for 1 month after their last dose. After giving birth, mothers must wait a minimum of 6 weeks before they can donate blood.

7. D Diastolic pressure must not be higher than 100 mm Hg. Donors weighing less than 110 lb may donate up to 12% of their blood volume (volume = weight in kg/50 × 450 mL). Oral temperature must not be greater than 37.4°C (99.5°F). Blood pressure limits for donation are 180 mm Hg for systolic and 100 mm Hg for diastolic pressure.

8. D An accidental needlestick would not be a cause for indefinite deferral of a donor. The deferral period is 1 year.

9. A Clopidogrel (Plavix) renders platelets nonfunctional, and therefore, potential donors on this medication cannot donate platelets.

10. A To determine the amount of anticoagulant to remove when the donor is less than 110 lb, divide weight by 110 lb, and multiply by 450 mL; divide that number by 100, and multiply by 14 (this gives the anticoagulant volume needed); then subtract this from 63 mL, which is the standard volume of anticoagulant in a 450 mL bag. The result is the amount of anticoagulant to remove, which is 12 mL for this donor.

11. C This donor is hyperventilating; therefore, the donation should be discontinued. A paper bag should be provided to the donor to breathe into to increase the carbon dioxide in the donor's air.

12. A donor bag is half filled during donation when the blood flow stops. Select the correct course of action.
- **A.** Closely observe the bag for at least 3 minutes; if blood flow does not resume, withdraw the needle
- **B.** Remove the needle immediately, and discontinue the donation
- **C.** Check and reposition the needle, if necessary; if blood flow does not resume, withdraw the needle
- **D.** Withdraw the needle, and perform a second venipuncture in the other arm

Immunohematology/Donors/3

13. Who is the *best* candidate for an autologous donation?
- **A.** A 45-year-old who is having elective surgery in 2 weeks; they have alloanti-k
- **B.** A 23-year-old patient with leukemia and a hemoglobin level of 10 g/dL
- **C.** A 12-year-old who has hemophilia
- **D.** A 53-year-old who has septicemia

Immunohematology/Donors/2

14. Can an autologous donor donate blood on Monday if they are having surgery on Friday?
- **A.** Yes, they can donate up to 72 hours before surgery
- **B.** No, they cannot donate within 7 days of surgery
- **C.** Yes, they can donate, but only half a unit
- **D.** No, they cannot donate within 5 days of surgery

Immunohematology/Donors/2

15. Which of the following is an acceptable time in which a unit of whole blood is collected?
- **A.** 33 minutes
- **B.** 25 minutes
- **C.** 20 minutes
- **D.** 13 minutes

Immunohematology/Donors/1

16. Which of the following is true regarding acute normovolemic hemodilution?
- **A.** One or more units of blood are withdrawn from the patient and replaced with FFP
- **B.** Units removed may be stored in the operating room at room temperature for 8 hours
- **C.** Units removed may be stored in the operating room at room temperature for 24 hours
- **D.** Unused units can be added to the general donor blood inventory

Immunohematology/Donors/2

17. All the following apply to a double RBC unit apheresis collection *except*:
- **A.** The hematocrit must be at least 38%
- **B.** The weight for a female is at least 150 lb
- **C.** The height for a male is at least 5 ft 1 in
- **D.** The deferral period following collection is 16 weeks

Immunohematology/Donors/1

Answers to Questions 12–17

12. C If blood flow has stopped, check the needle first. If blood flow does not resume after repositioning, then withdraw the needle and discontinue the donation. Do not perform a second venipuncture on the donor.

13. A The 45-year-old adult with alloanti-k is the best candidate for predeposit autologous donation because compatible blood will be hard to find if the patient needs blood after surgery. The other candidates may not be good choices for donation because the process may prove harmful to them.

14. A An autologous donor can donate up to 72 hours before expected surgery.

15. D A unit of whole blood should be collected within 15 minutes.

16. B In acute normovolemic hemodilution, one or more units of blood are removed from the donor and replaced with crystalloid or colloid. Blood may be stored at room temperature for up to 8 hours or at 1°C to 6°C for up to 24 hours. Bleeding during surgery results in less RBC loss after hemodilution, and the autologous RBCs are infused after bleeding stops. Such units are for autologous transfusion only.

17. A The minimum hematocrit for a double RBC donation is 40%.

18. An autologous unit of whole blood was collected from a 33-year-old patient in preparation for a knee replacement procedure in 3 weeks. The whole blood unit was labeled with hyphenated last name, first name, and last four digits of the Social Security number for identification. The laboratory computer system, however, only had part of the hyphenated last name and first name, medical record number, and Social Security number. What action should be taken with this blood product?

A. Discard the unit
B. Make the unit available for transfusion
C. Confirm the name with the donor, have admissions make the correction in the computer system, and then make the unit available for transfusion
D. Ensure that Social Security numbers match, confirm the name with the donor, and have admissions make the correction in the computer system with the medical director's approval, and then make the unit available for transfusion

Immunohematology/Donors/3

19. What is the youngest age a person is permitted to provide an allogeneic whole blood donation?

A. 14 years
B. 15 years
C. 16 years
D. 17 years

Immunohematology/Donors/1

20. Which of the following donors is acceptable for whole blood donation?

A. A 15-year-old individual with parental consent
B. An individual who has had a tattoo within the past 3 months
C. An individual who weighs 45 kg (99 lb)
D. A healthy 18-year-old individual who meets all other eligibility criteria

Immunohematology/Donors/1

Answers to Questions 18–20

18. D This is a common scenario with individuals who have recently married and have not changed their license or other form of identification given to the collection facility. Checking that other demographic information matches is sufficient, if approved by the medical director, because an autologous unit is very difficult to replace in time for surgery.

19. C In most states, the youngest age a person can donate is 16 years with parental permission.

20. D A healthy 18-year-old individual who meets all other eligibility criteria is acceptable for whole blood donation. The minimum age for whole blood donation is typically 16 years old, with parental consent if required by state law. Individuals who have had a tattoo within the past 3 months are usually deferred from donating blood due to the risk of infection. The minimum weight requirement for whole blood donation is generally 50 kg (110 lb) to ensure the donor's safety.

10.10

Hemolytic Disease of the Fetus and Newborn

1. All the following are reasons for a positive DAT on cord blood cells of a newborn *except*:
A. High concentrations of Wharton jelly on cord blood cells
B. Immune anti-A from an O mother on the cells of an A baby
C. Immune anti-D from an Rh-negative mother on the cells of an Rh-positive baby
D. Immune anti-K from a K-negative mother on the cells of a K-negative baby
Immunohematology/HDFN/2

2. A fetal screen yielded negative results on a mother who is O negative and infant who is O positive. What course of action should be taken?
A. Perform a Kleihauer-Betke test
B. Issue one full dose of Rh immunoglobulin (RhIg)
C. Perform a DAT on the infant
D. Perform an antibody screen on the mother
Immunohematology/HDFN/3

3. What should be performed when a person who is 24 weeks pregnant has a positive antibody screen?
A. Perform an antibody identification panel and titer, if necessary
B. No need to do anything until 30 weeks' gestation
C. Administer RhIg
D. Adsorb the antibody onto antigen-positive cells
Immunohematology/HDFN/2

4. All the following are interventions for fetal distress caused by maternal antibodies attacking fetal cells *except*:
A. Intrauterine transfusion
B. Plasmapheresis on the mother
C. Transfusion of antigen-positive cells to the mother
D. Middle cerebral artery peak systolic velocity (MCA-PSV)
Immunohematology/HDFN/2

5. Cord blood cells are washed six times with saline, and the DAT result and negative control are still positive. What should be completed *next*?
A. Obtain a heel stick sample
B. Record the DAT result as positive
C. Obtain another cord blood sample
D. Perform elution on the cord blood cells
Immunohematology/HDFN/3

6. What is the process or follow-up required if HDFN is caused by maternal anti-K?
A. Give Kell immune globulin
B. Monitor the mother's antibody level
C. Prevent formation of K-positive cells in the fetus
D. Not a problem; anti-K is not known to cause HDFN
Immunohematology/HDFN/2

Answers to Questions 1–6

1. D Immune anti-K from the mother would not coat the baby's RBCs if they did not contain the K antigen; therefore, the DAT result would be negative.

2. B If the fetal screen has a negative result, indicating the fetal maternal blood is negligible in a possible RhIg candidate, standard practice is to issue one dose of RhIg.

3. A The identification of the antibody is very important at this stage of pregnancy. If the antibody is determined to be clinically significant, then a titer may determine the strength of the antibody and the need for clinical intervention.

4. C Transfusion of antigen-positive cells to the mother who already has an antibody might cause a transfusion reaction and/or evoke an even stronger antibody response, possibly causing more harm to the fetus.

5. A If the cord blood cells contain excessive Wharton jelly, then further washing or obtaining another cord blood sample will not solve the problem. A heel stick sample will not contain Wharton jelly and should give a valid DAT result.

6. B Anti-D is the only antibody for which prevention of HDFN is possible. If a pregnant individual develops anti-K, the patient will be monitored to determine if the antibody level and signs of fetal distress necessitate clinical intervention.

7. Should an O-negative pregnant patient receive RhIg if a positive DAT on an Rh-negative newborn is caused by immune anti-A?

A. No, the mother is not a candidate for RhIg because of the positive DAT result
B. Yes, if the baby's type is Rh negative
C. No, administering RhIg would not be necessary
D. No, the baby's problem is unrelated to Rh blood group antibodies

Immunohematology/HDFN/3

8. Should an A-negative patient who has a miscarriage in the second trimester receive RhIg?

A. Yes, but only if they do not have evidence of active anti-D
B. No, the type of baby is unknown
C. Yes, but only a minidose regardless of trimester
D. No, RhIg is given to patients at full-term pregnancies only

Immunohematology/HDFN/3

9. The automated blood bank analyzer reports a type of O negative on a patient who is 6 weeks pregnant with vaginal bleeding. The patient tells the emergency department they are O positive and presents a blood donor card. The medical laboratory scientist performs a test for weak D and observes a 1+ reaction in the AHG phase. The Kleihauer-Betke test result is negative. Is this patient a candidate for RhIg?

A. Molecular testing is indicated to ascertain the type of weak D
B. Yes, she is Rh positive
C. No, there is no evidence of a fetal bleed
D. Yes, based on the automated typing results

Immunohematology/HDFN/3

10. Which of the following patients would be a candidate for RhIg?

A. B-positive patient; B-negative baby; first pregnancy; no anti-D in patient
B. O-negative patient; A-positive baby; second pregnancy; no anti-D in patient
C. A-negative patient; O-negative baby; fourth pregnancy; anti-D in patient
D. AB-negative patient; B-positive baby; second pregnancy; anti-D in patient

Immunohematology/HDFN/2

11. The Kleihauer-Betke acid elution test identifies 40 fetal cells in 2,000 maternal RBCs. How many full doses of RhIg are indicated?

A. 1
B. 2
C. 3
D. 4

Immunohematology/HDFN/2

12. Kernicterus is caused by the effects of:

A. Anemia
B. Unconjugated bilirubin
C. Antibody specificity
D. Antibody titer

Immunohematology/HDFN/1

Answers to Questions 7–12

7. C The positive DAT is due to immune anti-A, which is related to ABO incompatibility, not Rh incompatibility. Therefore, administering RhIg would not be necessary or effective in this situation.

8. A When the fetus is Rh positive or the Rh status of the fetus is unknown, termination of a pregnancy from any cause presents a situation in which an Rh-negative patient should receive RhIg. A minidose is used if the pregnancy is terminated in the first trimester.

9. A The negative Kleihauer-Betke test result confirms that the positive reaction of the patient's RBCs with anti-D at the IAT phase is not the result of fetal bleeding. The patient is weak D positive and, therefore, requires molecular testing to discern whether they are a candidate for RhIg. Weak D types 1, 2, 3, and 4 do not make anti-D and do not require RhIg prophylaxis.

10. B An O-negative patient who gives birth to an A-positive baby and has no anti-D formed from a previous pregnancy would be a candidate for RhIg. A patient who already has active anti-D or a patient who gives birth to an Rh-negative baby is not a candidate for RhIg.

11. D To calculate the number of vials of RhIg to infuse, divide 40 by 2,000, and multiply by 5,000. This gives the estimated total blood volume of the mother in milliliters. Divide this number by 30 to obtain the number of doses. When the number to the right of the decimal point is less than 5, round down, and add one dose of RhIg. Conversely, when the number to the right of the decimal point is 5 or greater, round up, and add one dose of RhIg. In this example, the number of doses is 3.3. Rounding down and adding one vial gives an answer of four vials.

12. B Kernicterus occurs because of high levels of unconjugated bilirubin. High levels of this pigment cross into the central nervous system, causing brain damage to the infant.

13. Anti-E is detected in the serum of a patient in the first trimester of pregnancy. The first titer for anti-E is 32. Two weeks later, the antibody titer is 64 and then 128 after another 2 weeks. Clinically, there are beginning signs of fetal distress. What are the next steps?
A. Induce labor for early delivery
B. Perform plasmapheresis to remove anti-E from the patient
C. Administer RhIg to the patient
D. Perform an intrauterine transfusion using E-negative cells

Immunohematology/HDFN/3

14. What testing is performed for exchange transfusion when the patient's serum contains an alloantibody?
A. Crossmatching and antibody screen
B. ABO, Rh, antibody screen, and crossmatching
C. ABO, Rh, antibody screen
D. ABO and Rh only

Immunohematology/HDFN/1

15. Which blood type is the best to be transfused to an AB-positive infant who has HDFN caused by anti-D?
A. AB negative, CMV (cytomegalovirus) negative, hemoglobin S (Hgb S) negative
B. AB positive, CMV negative; irradiated or O positive, CMV negative
C. AB negative only
D. O negative, CMV positive, Hgb S negative

Immunohematology/HDFN/2

16. All the following are routinely performed on a cord blood sample *except*:
A. Forward ABO typing
B. Antibody screen
C. Rh typing
D. DAT

Immunohematology/HDFN/1

17. Why do Rh-negative patients with a record of a previous pregnancy tend to have a positive antibody screen compared with Rh-positive patients of childbearing age, without a history of pregnancy?
A. They have formed active anti-D
B. They have received RhIg
C. They have formed anti-K
D. They have a higher rate of transfusion

Immunohematology/HDFN/2

Answers to Questions 13–17

13. B Plasmapheresis removes excess anti-E from the patient and provides a temporary solution to the problem until the fetus is mature enough to be delivered. The procedure may need to be performed several times, depending on how quickly and how high the levels of anti-E rise. Administration of RhIg would not contribute to solving this problem caused by anti-E. Intrauterine transfusion would not be performed before week 20 and would be considered only if there is evidence of severe hemolytic disease.

14. B ABO (forward) and Rh are required. An antibody screen using either the neonatal serum or patient serum is required. Crossmatching is necessary as long as patient antibody persists in the infant's blood.

15. A The best blood type is AB negative OR O negative, CMV negative, Hgb S negative. This choice ensures compatibility with the baby's blood type, avoids further hemolysis due to anti-D antibodies, and reduces the risk of CMV infection and sickle cell complications.

16. B An antibody screen is not performed routinely on a cord blood sample because a baby does not make antibodies until about 6 months of age.

17. B The most common reason an Rh-negative patient has a positive antibody screen is because of previously receiving RhIg or passive anti-D.

18. An O-negative patient gave birth to a B-positive infant. The patient had no history of antibodies or transfusion. This was the individual's first pregnancy. The newborn was mildly jaundiced, and the DAT result was weakly positive with polyspecific antisera. What could have caused the positive DAT result?

A. Anti-D from the mother coating the infant RBCs
B. An alloantibody, such as anti-K, coating the infant RBCs
C. Maternal anti-B coating the infant RBCs
D. Maternal anti-A, B coating the infant RBCs

Immunohematology/HDFN/3

19. What is the mechanism of action of RhIg?

A. It binds to Rh-positive RBCs and marks them for destruction by the mother's immune system
B. It increases the production of anti-D antibodies in the mother
C. It neutralizes circulating anti-D antibodies in the mother's blood
D. It provides passive immunity to Rh-positive blood cells in the fetus

Immunohematology/HDFN/2

Answers to Questions 18–19

18. D Anti-A,B is a naturally occurring ABO IgG antibody and can cross the placenta and attach to infant cells. It is known as a single entity as opposed to separate antibodies. Anti-D would not be the cause because this is the first pregnancy. Anti-K is not the cause because there is no history of alloantibodies or past transfusions.

19. A RhIg contains anti-D antibodies that specifically target and bind the RhD antigen on the surface of Rh-positive RBCs and marks them for destruction. By clearing the Rh-positive RBCs from the mother's circulation (usually via the spleen), RhIg prevents the mother's immune system from recognizing and becoming sensitized to the RhD antigen. This prevents the production of maternal anti-D antibodies that could attack Rh-positive RBCs in future pregnancies.

10.11
Serological Testing of Blood Products

1. What protocol is followed when screening whole blood donors for HIV-1 and HIV-2 RNA?
- A. Whole blood donations are not screened for HIV-1 or HIV-2 RNA
- B. Pools of 20 are tested; if the pool is reactive, all blood is discarded
- C. Pools of up to 16 donors are tested; if pool is reactive, individual samples are screened
- D. All donors are screened individually; if samples are reactive, blood is discarded

Immunohematology/Serology/3

2. NAT is performed to detect which viruses?
- A. HIV-1/2 and human T-cell lymphotropic virus (HTLV-1)
- B. HTLV-1/2
- C. HIV-1/2, HCV, HBV, Zika, and West Nile virus (WNV)
- D. HIV-1/2, HBV, and WNV

Immunohematology/Serology/1

3. An individual comes in to donate a unit of whole blood at the collection center of the community blood supplier. The enzyme immunoassay (EIA) screen for anti-HIV-1/2 is nonreactive; however, the NAT HIV is reactive. After 8 weeks the same individual is tested again and identified as NAT nonreactive and EIA anti-HIV-1/2 nonreactive:
- A. This renders the individual eligible for donation
- B. Donation is deferred for 6 months
- C. Status is dependent on further confirmatory testing
- D. Donation is deferred for 12 months

Immunohematology/Serology/3

4. What marker is the first to appear in HBV infection?
- A. Hepatitis B core antibody (anti-HBc) IgM
- B. Hepatitis B surface antigen (HBsAg)
- C. Hepatitis B surface antibody (anti-HBs)
- D. Anti-HBc IgG

Immunohematology/Serology/1

5. What marker indicates immunity to hepatitis B infection?
- A. Anti-HBc IgM
- B. HBsAg
- C. Anti-HBs
- D. Anti-HBc IgG

Immunohematology/Serology/1

6. A patient with multiple myeloma is placed on daratumumab (Darzalex). What tests are affected by this medication, and what are typical recommendations for transfusion?
- A. Antibody screen/least incompatible RBCs
- B. ABO/washed RBCs
- C. Rh/leukocyte-poor RBCs
- D. All the above

Immunohematology/Serology/3

Answers to Questions 1–6

1. C Pools of up to 16 donors are tested by nucleic acid amplification technology. If the pool is reactive, samples from each individual donor are tested.

2. C According to the AABB standards, NAT testing is required for viruses HIV-1/2, HCV, HBV, Zika, and WNV. NAT also detects the presence of *Babesia microti* DNA, which helps prevent the transmission of babesiosis through blood transfusions.

3. A According to the FDA guidelines, donors who retest as NAT HIV nonreactive and negative for anti-HIV-1/2 are eligible to donate in the reentry program.

4. B The first viral marker of hepatitis B to appear in the serum once exposed is the HBsAg, which appears in as few as 5 days (5–28 days) after exposure.

5. C Anti-HBs is indicative of immunity or vaccination to hepatitis B. Anti-HBc IgM occurs in the early stage of infection; anti-HBc IgG follows and may persist for years following infection. HBsAg is a marker of HBV infection, not immunity.

6. A Daratumumab (Darzalex) is a monoclonal antibody directed against CD38, which shows enhanced expression on multiple myeloma tumor cells. Because CD38 is also expressed on RBCs, all screening cells will be positive. The serological workup appears as a warm autoantibody that cannot be resolved with adsorptions and often necessitates the transfusion of least incompatible RBCs.

7. A unit tests positive for syphilis with the rapid plasma reagin (RPR) test. The *Treponema pallidum* particle agglutination (TP-PA) test on the same unit is negative. What is the disposition of the unit?

A. The unit may be used to prepare components
B. The donor must be contacted and questioned further; if the RPR test result is most likely a false positive, then the unit may be used
C. The unit must be discarded
D. Cellular components may be prepared but must be irradiated before issue

Immunohematology/Serology/2

8. An individual donated a unit of whole blood in May. RBCs made from whole blood were transfused to a recipient at a community hospital in June, with no apparent complications. The blood supplier notified the medical director of the hospital that the donor had reported engaging in high-risk behavior in April, although viral tests remain negative, and the donor is healthy. What course of action should be taken?

A. No action should be taken
B. The recipient's physician should be notified
C. The recipient's physician and the recipient should be notified
D. The recipient should be notified

Immunohematology/Serology/3

9. All the following tests are required on donor blood *except*:

A. HBsAg
B. Anti-CMV
C. HIV-1/2
D. Anti-HTLV 1/2

Immunohematology/Serology/1

10. Which of the following is NOT a marker for HIV infection that is typically screened for in blood donations?

A. HIV p24 antigen
B. HIV-1/2 antibody
C. HIV-1/2 RNA
D. HIV-2 DNA

Immunohematology/Serology/2

Answers to Questions 7–10

7. A This is a case of a false-positive screening test result (RPR). The confirmatory test for treponemal antibodies was negative. The donor unit is acceptable and may be used to prepare blood components.

8. B The recipient's physician should be notified by the medical director to ensure that the recipient receives proper medical follow-up, counselling, and any necessary testing to monitor for infection.

9. B Testing of donor blood for antibodies to CMV is not required. However, testing may be performed on units intended for transfusion to low-birth-weight infants born to seronegative mothers or units used for intrauterine transfusion; units intended for immunocompromised patients who are seronegative; prospective transplant recipients who are seronegative; or transplant recipients who have received a seronegative organ. Leukocyte-reduced RBCs carry a reduced risk of transmitting CMV and are recommended for such patients when CMV testing has not been performed on donor units. The prevalence of anti-CMV in the population ranges from 40% to 90%.

10. D HIV-2 DNA is not a marker that is screened for in blood donations. Instead, screening focuses on HIV p24 antigen, HIV-1/2 antibodies, and HIV-1/2 RNA to ensure comprehensive detection of HIV infections and maintain the safety of the blood supply.

10.12

Transfusion Practice

1. Is there a discrepancy between the following blood type and secretor study results?

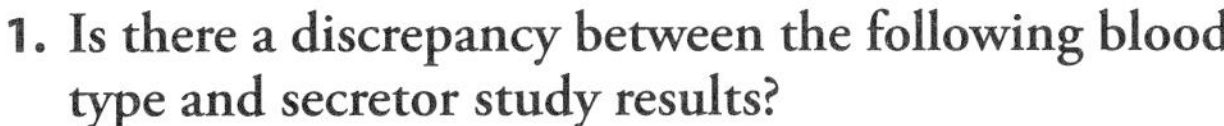

Blood typing results:	Anti-A	Anti-B	A_1 Cells	B Cells
	4+	0	0	4+
Secretor results:	Anti-A + saliva + A_1 cells = 0			
	Anti-B + saliva + B cells = 4+			
	Anti-H + saliva + O cells = 0			

A. No problem, the sample is from a group A secretor
B. Blood types as A and saliva types as B
C. Blood types as A, but the secretor study is inconclusive
D. No problem, the sample is from a group A nonsecretor

Immunohematology/Transfusion practice/3

2. What is the most likely cause of the following test result? (Assume the patient has not been transfused recently.)

Anti-A	Anti-B	A_1 cells	B cells
Mixed field	0	1+	4+

A. Nothing, typing is normal
B. Presence of cold agglutinins
C. Subgroup of B
D. Subgroup of A

Immunohematology/Transfusion practice/3

3. The following results were obtained on a 41-year-old patient:

Anti-A	Anti-B	A_1 cells	B cells	O cells
4+	0	3+	4+	3+

Because of the discrepant reverse grouping, a panel was performed on patient serum revealing the presence of anti-M. How can the reverse grouping be resolved?

A. Repeat the reverse grouping with a 10-minute incubation at room temperature
B. Repeat the reverse grouping using A_1 cells that are negative for M antigen
C. Repeat the reverse grouping using A_1 cells that are positive for M antigen
D. No further work is necessary

Immunohematology/Transfusion practice/3

Answers to Questions 1–3

1. A The blood typing result demonstrates A antigen on the RBCs and anti-B in serum. The secretor result reveals A antigen in the saliva. An antigen neutralized anti-A, preventing agglutination when A_1 cells were added. Each blood type (except a Bombay phenotype) contains some H antigen; therefore, H antigen in saliva would be bound by anti-H reagent. No agglutination would occur when O cells are added.

2. D Mixed-field agglutination in the anti-A test and weak agglutination with A_1 cells suggest the presence of an A subgroup. Subgroups of A, such as A_3, can show mixed-field reactions with anti-A and weak reactions with A_1 cells. The strong agglutination with B cells (4+) further supports that the patient is not group B.

3. B The scenario showed an antibody in the patient serum directed toward M antigen, and the M antigen happened to be on the A_1 cells in reverse grouping. To solve this problem, find A_1 cells negative for M antigen or enzyme treat the A_1 cells to resolve the ABO discrepancy.

4. A 59-year-old individual presented at the emergency department complaining of dizziness and fatigue. History included no transfusions and a positive rheumatoid factor 1 year ago. The complete blood count (CBC) confirmed anemia. A sample was sent to the blood bank for typing and crossmatching. Upon receipt of the sample in the blood bank, the medical laboratory scientist noticed the ethylenediaminetetraacetic acid (EDTA) sample appeared very viscous. Fearing that the sample would clog the automated instrument, testing was performed by using the tube method. The initial results revealed the following:

Anti-A	Anti-B	Anti-D	Rh Control	A_1 cells	B cells
0	0	4+	2+	4+	4+

The patient's RBCs were washed eight times with saline, and testing was repeated, giving the following results:

Anti-A	Anti-B	Anti-D	Rh Control	A_1 cells	B cells
0	0	4+	0	4+	4+

The antibody screen was negative at the IS, 37°C, and AHG phases; the check cells were positive. Crossmatch testing using two O-positive donor units revealed 1+ at IS, and negative results at the 37°C and AHG phases. The check cells were positive. In light of the crossmatching results, what is the next course of action?

A. Use other donor cells for crossmatching
B. Perform a saline replacement for crossmatching
C. Run the crossmatching test using the Gel system
D. Result the crossmatch as incompatible

Immunohematology/Transfusion practice/3

5. The following results were obtained on a 51-year-old patient with hepatitis C:

Anti-A	Anti-B	Anti-D	A_1 cells	B cells
4+	4+	3+	0	0

What should be performed next?

A. Retype the patient's sample to confirm group AB positive
B. Repeat the Rh typing
C. Run a saline control in forward grouping
D. Report the patient as group AB, Rh positive

Immunohematology/Transfusion practice/2

6. Rh phenotyping shows the following results:

Anti-D	Anti-C	Anti-E	Anti-c	Anti-e
4+	2+	0	0	0

What is the most likely Rh genotype?

A. *R1r"*
B. *R0r*
C. *R1R1*
D. *R1r*

Immunohematology/Transfusion practice/3

7. An obstetric patient, 34 weeks pregnant, shows a positive antibody screen at the IAT phase of testing in screening cells I and II; screening cell III was negative. The patient is group B, Rh negative. This is a first pregnancy, and the patient has no prior history of transfusion. What is the most likely explanation for the positive antibody screen?

A. Patient has developed an antibody to fetal RBCs
B. Recheck for technical error
C. The patient received an antenatal dose of RhIg
D. Impossible to determine without further testing

Immunohematology/Transfusion practice/3

8. An anti-M reacts strongly through all phases of testing. Which of the following techniques would *not* contribute to removing this reactivity so that more clinically significant antibodies may be revealed?

A. Acidifying the serum
B. Prewarmed technique
C. Adsorption with homozygous cells
D. Testing with enzyme-treated RBCs

Immunohematology/Transfusion practice/3

Answers to Questions 4–8

4. B The history of the patient correlates with abnormal plasma proteins causing a positive result with the Rh control. Perform a saline replacement technique to rectify the incompatible crossmatches at IS.

5. C Given the patient hepatitis C status, the most appropriate action would be to run a saline control in the forward grouping to rule out any nonspecific agglutination that might interfere with the results. This helps ensure the accuracy of the ABO and Rh typing before finalizing the report. If the saline control is negative and confirms the initial results, the patient can then be reported as group AB, Rh positive.

6. C The most likely genotype is *R1R1*. The possibilities are *DCe/DCe* or *DCe/dCe*, which translates to the more common *R1R1* or the less common *R1r'*.

7. C Because the patient has never been transfused or pregnant previously, they probably have not formed any atypical antibodies. Because the patient is Rh negative, they would have received a dose of RhIg at 28 weeks (antenatal dose) if the prenatal antibody screen had been negative. Although technical error cannot be ruled out, it is far less likely than RhIg administration to be the cause.

8. A Lowering the pH will actually enhance reactivity of anti-M. Prewarming (anti-M is a cold-reacting antibody), cold adsorption with homozygous M cells, and testing the serum with enzyme-treated RBCs (destroys M antigens) are all techniques to remove reactivity of anti-M.

9. The reactivity of an unknown antibody could be anti-Jk[a], but the antibody identification panel does not fit this pattern conclusively. Which of the following would *not* be effective in determining if the specificity is anti-Jk[a]?

A. Testing with enzyme-treated cells
B. Select panel of homozygous cells
C. Testing with 2-aminoethylisothiouronium bromide (AET)–treated cells
D. Increased incubation time

Immunohematology/Transfusion practice/3

10. A cold-reacting antibody is found in the serum of a recently transfused patient and is suspected to be anti-I. The antibody identification panel shows reactions with all cells at room temperature, including the autocontrol. The reaction strength varies from 2+ to 4+. What procedure would help to distinguish this antibody from other cold-reacting antibodies?

A. Autoadsorption technique
B. Neutralization using saliva
C. Autocontrol using ZZAP reagent-treated cells
D. Reaction with cord blood cells

Immunohematology/Transfusion practice/3

11. An antibody identification panel reveals the presence of anti-Le[b] and a possible second specificity. Saliva from which person would best neutralize the Le[b] antibody?

	Genes			
	Person	**Lewis**	**ABO**	**Secretor**
A.	Person A	Le	H	sese
B.	Person B	Le	Hh	Se
C.	Person C	Le	H	Se
D.	Person D	lele	Hh	sese

Immunohematology/Transfusion practice/3

12. A 29-year-old pregnant patient with a history of multiple blood transfusions presents for routine prenatal care. The initial Rh typing results are as follows:

IS	37°C	AHG	Rh Control
0	0	1+	0

Given the clinical history and these results, what is the most appropriate next step to confirm the Rh status and manage the pregnancy?

A. Report as Rh-negative and administer RhIg
B. Perform an antibody screen to detect alloantibodies
C. Use molecular genotyping to determine the RhD variant
D. Repeat the Rh typing using different monoclonal anti-D reagents

Immunohematology/Transfusion practice/3

Answers to Questions 9–12

9. C AET treatment does not affect Kidd antigens and would not be effective in determining if the specificity is anti-Jk[a]. The other methods (enzyme treatment, homozygous cells, and increased incubation time) can be useful in identifying anti-Jk[a] antibodies.

10. D Cord blood cells (newborn RBCs) lack the I antigen but express the i antigen. Testing the patient's serum with cord blood cells can help distinguish anti-I from other cold antibodies because anti-I will not react with cord blood cells, while other cold antibodies may still react.

11. C Lewis antibodies are usually not clinically significant but may interfere with testing for clinically significant antibodies. Lewis antibodies are most easily removed by neutralizing them with soluble Lewis substance. Lewis antigens are secreted into saliva and plasma and are adsorbed onto RBCs. Le[b] substance is made by adding an L-fucose to both the terminal and next to last sugar residue on the type 1 precursor chain. This requires the *Le*, *H*, and *Se* genes. Because some samples of anti-Le[b] react only with group O or A_2 RBCs, neutralization is best achieved if the saliva comes from a person who is group O.

12. C Given the initial Rh typing results and the patient's clinical history, the most appropriate next step is to use molecular genotyping to determine her RhD variant. This approach provides a definitive answer and helps in managing her pregnancy, particularly regarding RhIg administration.

13. The pregnant person's type is O negative. A cord blood workup was ordered for the infant, and the results are as follows:

Anti-A	Anti-B	Anti-A, B	Anti-D	DAT (poly)
4+	0	4+	0	2+

The test for weak D on the baby was positive at the AHG phase. Is the pregnant mother an RhIg candidate?

A. No, the infant is Rh positive
B. Yes, the mother is Rh negative, and the infant's Rh type cannot be determined
C. No, the infant is Rh negative
D. No, the pregnant mother is Rh negative, and the infant is Rh negative

Immunohematology/Transfusion practice/3

14. RBCs from a recently transfused patient were positive on DAT when tested with anti-IgG. Screen cells and a panel performed on the patient's serum showed very weak reactions with inconclusive results. What procedure could help to identify the antibody?

A. Elution followed by a panel on the eluate
B. Adsorption followed by a panel on the adsorbed serum
C. Enzyme panel
D. Antigen typing the patient's RBCs

Immunohematology/Transfusion practice/3

15. A patient types as O positive. All three screening cells and RBCs from two O-positive donor units show agglutination after incubation at 37°C and increase reactivity at the IAT phase of testing. What action should be taken next?

A. Perform an autocontrol and DAT on the patient
B. Perform an enzyme panel
C. Perform an elution
D. Choose another 2 units and repeat crossmatching

Immunohematology/Transfusion practice/3

16. Four units of blood are ordered for a patient. Blood bank records are checked and indicate that 5 years ago this patient had an anti-Jk^b. What is the next course of action?

A. Antigen type units for the Jk^b antigen, and only crossmatch units positive for Jk^b
B. Antigen type units for the Jk^b antigen, and only crossmatch units negative for Jk^b
C. Randomly pull 4 units of blood that are ABO compatible, and perform crossmatching
D. Perform IS crossmatching on 4 Jk^b-negative units

Immunohematology/Transfusion practice/3

17. A 56-year-old patient diagnosed with colon cancer demonstrates a positive antibody screen in all three screen cells at the AHG phase. The panel study shows 10 cells as positive as well as the autocontrol at the AHG phase. The reactions varied from 1+ to 3+. This patient had a history of receiving 2 units of blood approximately 1 month ago. What steps should be taken next?

A. Perform a DAT on patient cells
B. Perform an autoadsorption
C. Perform an alloadsorption
D. Issue O-negative cells

Immunohematology/Transfusion practice/3

Answers to Questions 13–17

13. B The infant forward types as an A, and the mother is O negative. It is possible that anti-A,B from the mother is attaching to the infant's RBCs, causing a positive DAT result. In the presence of a positive DAT, a weak test for D is not valid. Therefore, the infant's Rh type is unknown, and the motherwould be a candidate for RhIg.

14. A If the RBCs show a positive DAT result, then IgG antibody has coated incompatible, antigen-positive RBCs. If screening cells and panel cells show missing or weak reactions, most of the antibody is on the RBCs and would need to be eluted before it can be detected. An elution procedure followed by a panel performed on the eluate would help to identify the antibody.

15. A All screening cells and all units are positive at both 37°C and the IAT phase. This indicates the possibility of a high-frequency alloantibody or a warm autoantibody. An autocontrol would help make this distinction. A positive autocontrol indicates an autoantibody is present; a negative autocontrol and positive screen cells indicate an alloantibody. A DAT would be performed to determine whether an antibody has coated the patient's RBCs and is directed against screening cells and donor cells.

16. B A patient with a history of a significant antibody, such as anti-Jk^b, must receive blood that has been completely crossmatched and is negative for the corresponding antigen; otherwise, an anamnestic reaction may occur with subsequent lysis of donor cells.

17. C In this situation, an allogeneic adsorption must be performed to adsorb out the autoantibody and leave potential alloantibodies in the patient's serum that will need to be identified before transfusion of blood to the patient. An autoadsorption cannot be performed because any alloantibodies would be absorbed by circulating donor cells present from the previous month.

18. A 33-year-old obstetrics patient has blood drawn for a type and screen at 36 weeks' gestation. The following results were noted on the automated blood bank analyzer:

Anti-A	Anti-B	Anti-A,B	Anti-D	A_1 cells	B cells
3+	0	4+	4+	2+	4+
SC I	SC II	SC III	A_1 lectin		
0	0	0	3+		

The reference laboratory identified anti-P_1 in the patient's plasma by using enzyme techniques. How could the ABO discrepancy be solved?

A. Wash the patient's RBCs, and repeat the forward grouping
B. Test the patient's plasma against A_2 cells
C. Warm the patient's plasma at 37°C for 10 minutes, and repeat the reverse grouping
D. Treat the A_1 cells with DTT, and repeat the reverse grouping

Immunohematology/Transfusion practice/3

19. An O-negative patient with no record of any previous pregnancies gives birth to their first child, a B-positive newborn. The newborn's DAT is weakly positive, and the saline control is negative. The antibody screen is also negative. The infant appears healthy but after 2 days mild jaundice develops, which is treated with phototherapy. After 4 days in the hospital, the infant goes home, without complications. What is the *most* likely explanation for the weakly positive DAT result?

A. Technical error
B. A low-titer anti-D
C. Immune anti-B from the mother
D. A maternal antibody against a low-incidence antigen

Immunohematology/Transfusion practice/2

Answers to Questions 18–19

18. C Anti-P_1 is a cold-reacting antibody. Warming the plasma at 37°C will dissipate the antibody, preventing its reactivity with P_1 antigen on the A_1 cells.

19. C In this case, the pregnant person's anti-A,B is probably coating the infant's B cells, causing a positive DAT and jaundice. Anti-A,B from an O person is a single entity that cannot be separated. It is IgG and can cross the placenta. This antibody may attach to A, B, or AB RBCs.

BIBLIOGRAPHY

1. American Association of Blood Banks. *Standards for Blood Banks and Transfusion Services*. 34th ed. AABB; 2024.
2. Cohn CS, Delaney M, Johnson ST, Katz LM, eds. *Technical Manual*. 20th ed. AABB. 2020.
3. Cohn CS, Delaney M, Johnson ST, Katz LM, Schwartz J, eds. *Technical Manual*. 21st ed. AABB; 2023.
4. Harmening D. *Modern Blood Banking and Transfusion Practices*. 7th ed. F.A. Davis; 2019.
5. Murphy MF, Roberts DJ, Yazer MH, Dunbar NM, eds. *Practical Transfusion Medicine*. 6th ed. Wiley-Blackwell; 2022.
6. Reid ME, Lomas-Francis C, Olsson ML. *The Blood Group Antigen Facts Book*. 3rd ed. Elsevier; 2012.
7. Requirements for blood and blood components intended for transfusion or for further manufacturing use. 66 *Fed Regist*. 31,176. (June 11, 2001). https://www.ecfr.gov/current/title-21/chapter-I/subchapter-F/part-630

CHAPTER 11

Photomicrographs and Color Plate Examination

Refer to the photomicrographs and color plates that follow p. 482.

1. **Plate 1 is a photomicrograph of an antinuclear antibody test using human fibroblasts, fluorescein isothiocyanate (FITC)–conjugated antihuman serum, and transmitted fluorescence microscopy. Which pattern of immunofluorescence is demonstrated in this 400× field?**
   A. Homogeneous
   B. Peripheral
   C. Nucleolar
   D. Speckled

   Immunology/Immunologic techniques/2

2. **Plate 2 shows the electrophoresis of serum proteins on a high-resolution agarose gel at pH 8.6. Sample 1 (in lane 1) is a normal serum control. Which sample can be presumptively classified as a monoclonal gammopathy?**
   A. Sample 2
   B. Sample 4
   C. Sample 6
   D. Sample 8

   Chemistry/Protein electrophoresis/3

Answers to Questions 1–2

1. A Using FITC-conjugated antihuman serum, diffuse apple-green fluorescence seen over the entire nucleus characterizes the homogeneous pattern. At a significant titer, this pattern occurs in a variety of systemic autoimmune diseases, including systemic lupus erythematosus, rheumatoid arthritis (RA), systemic sclerosis, and Sjögren syndrome. The antibodies are directed against nucleoprotein; although they are mainly nonpathological, they are useful markers for active disease.

2. C A monoclonal gammopathy causes a band showing restricted electrophoretic mobility usually located in the γ- or the β-region. The band represents the accumulation of identical immunoglobulin (Ig) molecules or fragments secreted by a single malignant or benign clone of plasma cells.

3. Plate 3 shows a densitometric scan of a control serum for protein electrophoresis. The percentages of each fraction are shown below the scan. Given these results, what is the *most* appropriate initial corrective action?

A. Repeat the electrophoresis run using fresh control serum
B. Report the results, provided that the previous control run was acceptable
C. Move the fourth fraction mark to the right and redraw the scan
D. Calculate the concentration of each fraction in grams per deciliter

Chemistry/Protein electrophoresis/3

4. Plate 4 shows the electrophoresis of serum proteins on a high-resolution agarose gel at pH 8.6. Which band represents the β-lipoprotein?

A. A
B. B
C. C
D. D

Chemistry/Protein electrophoresis/2

5. Plate 5 is a densitometric scan of a serum protein electrophoresis sample. The relative and absolute concentrations of each fraction and reference limits are shown below the scan. What is the correct classification of this densitometric pattern?

A. Polyclonal gammopathy associated with chronic inflammation
B. Nephrotic syndrome
C. Acute inflammation
D. Hepatic cirrhosis

Chemistry/Protein electrophoresis/3

6. Plate 6 shows an agarose gel on which immunofixation electrophoresis (IFE) was performed at pH 8.6. The gel contains the same serum sample as number 6 shown in Plate 2. What is the heavy and light chain type of the monoclonal protein present in this sample?

A. Immunoglobulin A κ
B. Immunoglobulin G κ
C. Immunoglobulin G λ
D. Immunoglobulin M λ

Immunology/Immunologic techniques/3

7. Plate 7 shows the electrophoresis of hemoglobin (Hgb) samples performed on agarose gel, pH 8.8. The control sample is located in lanes 2 and 10 and contains Hgb A, S, and C. Which sample(s) is/are from neonates?

A. Samples 1 and 5
B. Sample 3
C. Sample 7
D. Samples 8 and 9

Hematology/Laboratory evaluation of anemia/3

Answers to Questions 3–7

3. C In this scan, the valley between the α_2-subfractions was selected incorrectly as the boundary between the α_2- and β-fractions. This fraction marker should be placed at the next valley to the right and the scan redrawn to determine the area under the α_2- and β-fractions correctly.

4. C Using high current, β-lipoprotein can be separated from transferrin and complement (C3). β-Lipoprotein migrates anodal to the transferrin band (labeled D) and appears as a thin wavy band. C3 migrates cathodal to the transferrin band. The band labeled A is α-antitrypsin and the band labeled B contains α_2-macroglobulin and haptoglobin.

5. C This pattern is characterized by significant relative increases in the α_1- and α_2-fractions and a decrease in serum albumin concentration. This pattern is most often caused by increased production of acute phase reactants, such as α_1-antitrypsin and haptoglobin, associated with acute inflammation.

6. B This IFE gel shows an insoluble immunoprecipitate restricted to a single band in lanes 2 (labeled IgG) and 5 (labeled κ). The proteins in lane 2 reacted with anti-γ (anti-IgG), and the proteins in lane 5 reacted with anti-κ. Lane 5 also contains a faint restricted band anodal to the IgG band. This band is not present in lane 2 and represents free κ–light chains.

7. A Neonates and infants up to age 6 months have Hgb F levels between 8% and 40%. The Hgb F level falls to below 2% in children age greater than 2 years. Hgb F is more acidic than Hgb S and less acidic than Hgb A. Therefore, at an alkaline pH, Hgb F has a greater net negative charge compared with Hgb S, but a lesser net negative charge compared with Hgb A, and migrates between Hgb A and Hgb S.

COLOR PLATE SECTION

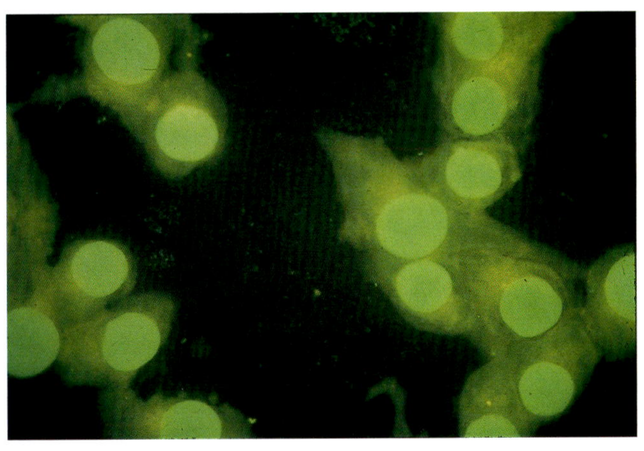

Plate 1

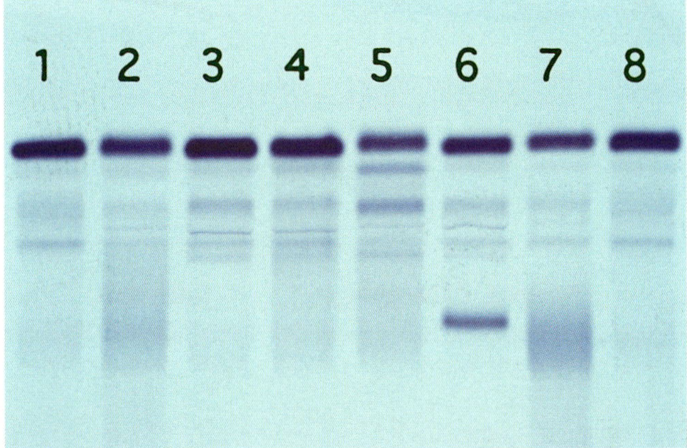

Plate 2

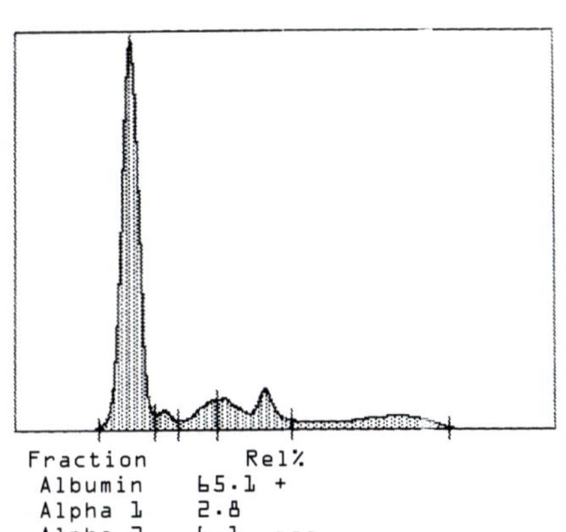

Fraction	Rel%	
Albumin	65.1	+
Alpha 1	2.8	
Alpha 2	6.1	---
Beta	13.5	
Gamma	12.4	

A/G: 1.87
Comments:

Reference Ranges:

Fraction	Rel%	G/dL
Albumin	51.7 – 62.5	3.10 – 5.00
Alpha 1	1.7 – 5.0	0.10 – 0.40
Alpha 2	10.0 – 12.5	0.60 – 1.00
Beta	10.0 – 16.3	0.60 – 1.30
Gamma	11.7 – 18.8	0.70 – 1.50

Plate 3

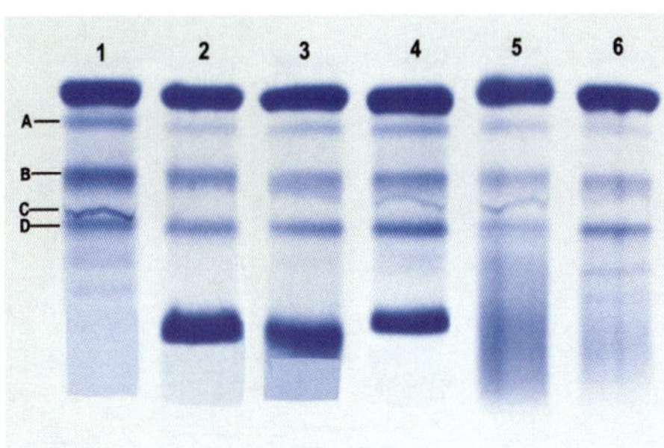

Plate 4

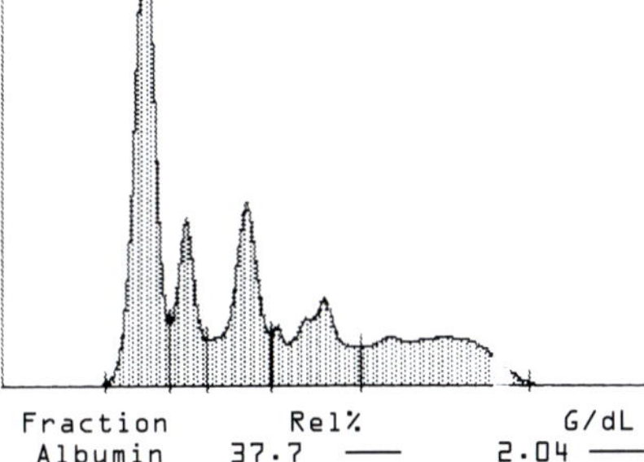

Fraction	Rel%		G/dL	
Albumin	37.7	——	2.04	——
Alpha 1	11.5	+++	0.62	+++
Alpha 2	17.5	+++	0.95	
Beta	14.8		0.80	
Gamma	18.5		1.00	

Total G/dL 5.40 A/G: 0.1
Comments:

Reference Ranges:

Fraction	Rel%	G/dL
Albumin	51.7 – 62.5	3.10 – 5.00
Alpha 1	1.7 – 5.0	0.10 – 0.40
Alpha 2	10.0 – 12.5	0.60 – 1.00
Beta	10.0 – 16.3	0.60 – 1.30
Gamma	11.7 – 18.8	0.70 – 1.50

Plate 5

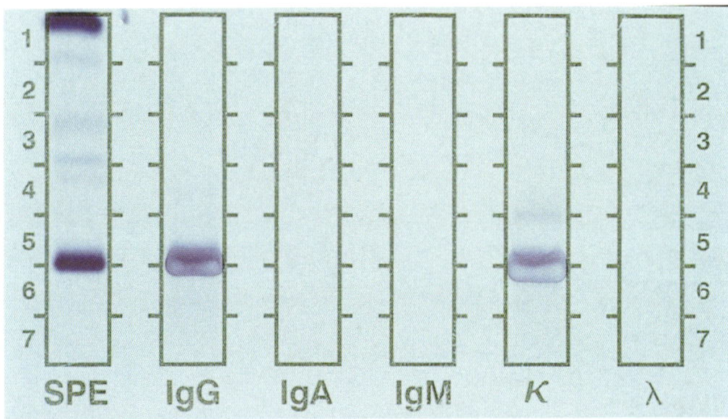

Plate 6

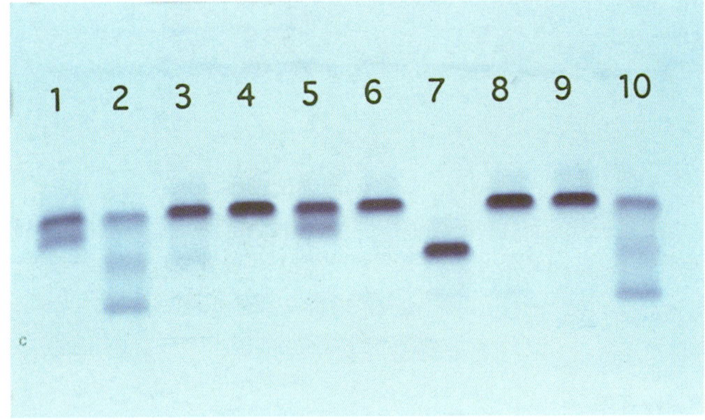

Plate 7

COLOR PLATE SECTION

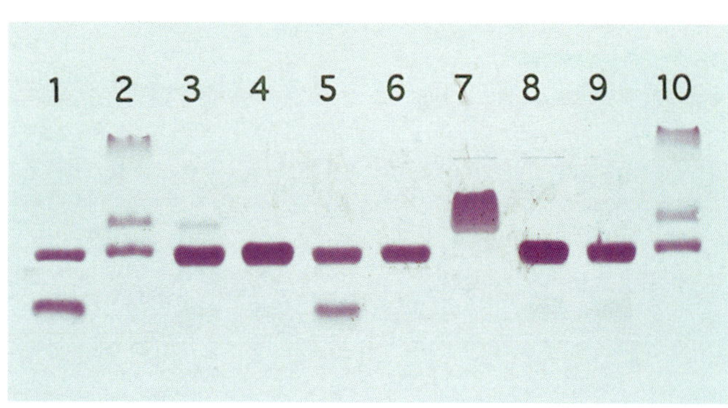

Plate 8

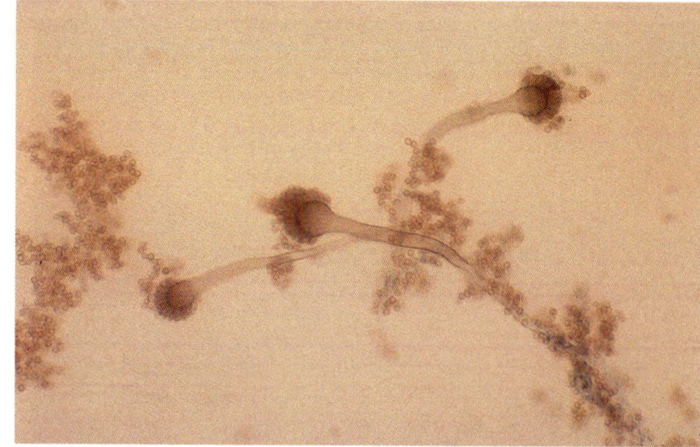

Plate 9

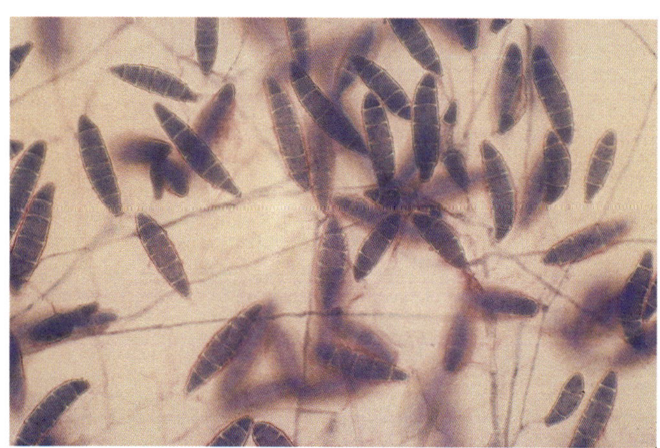

Plate 10

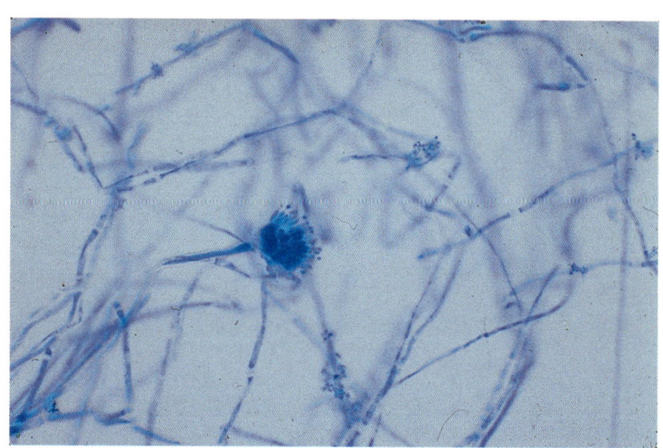

Plate 11

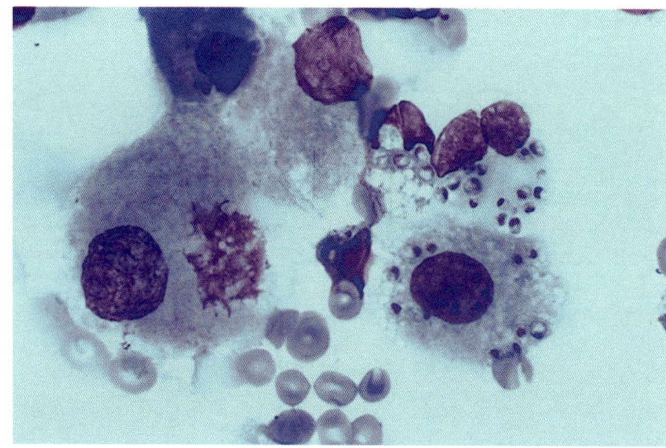

Plate 12

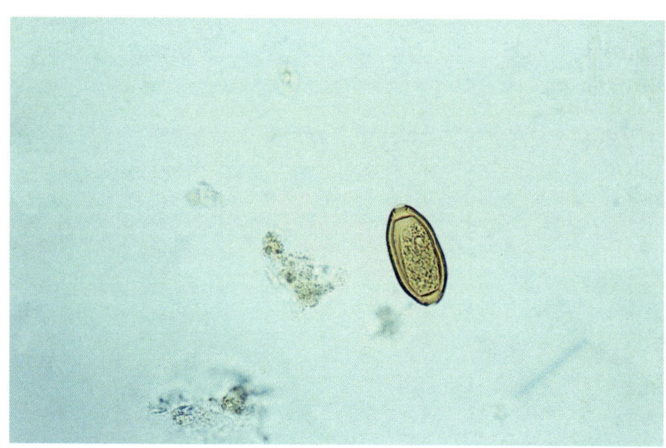

Plate 13

COLOR PLATE SECTION

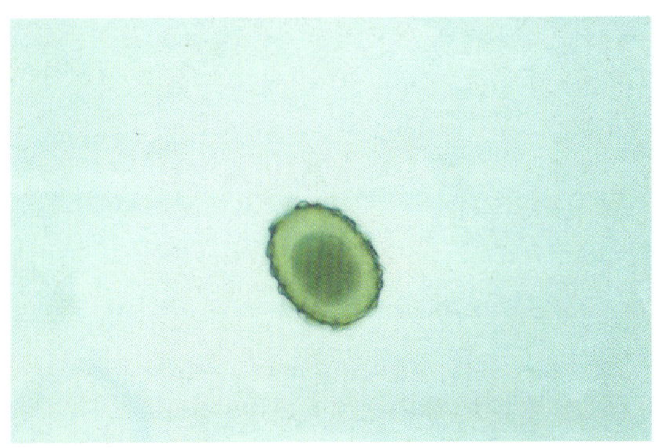

Plate 14

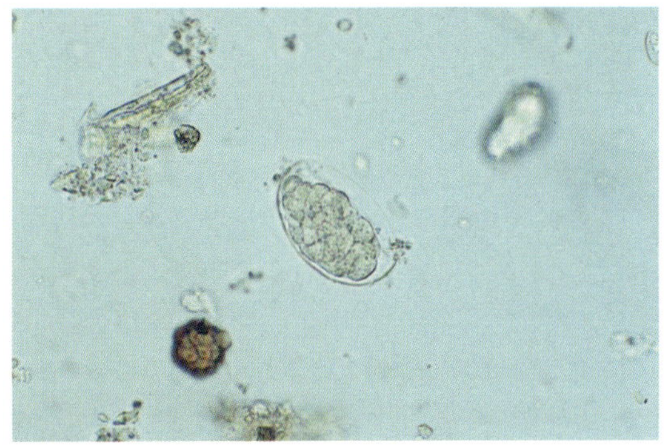

Plate 15

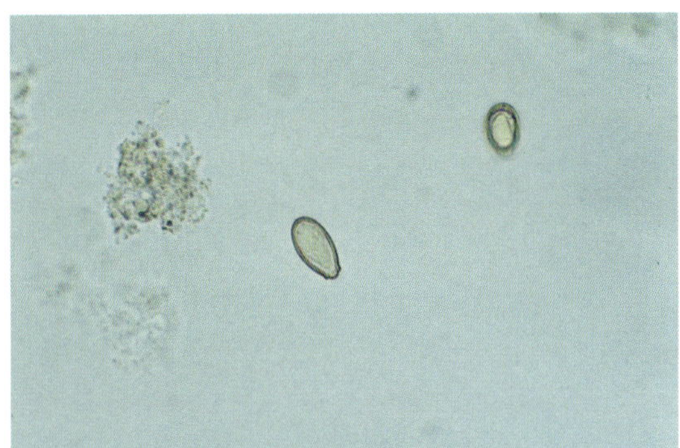

Plate 16

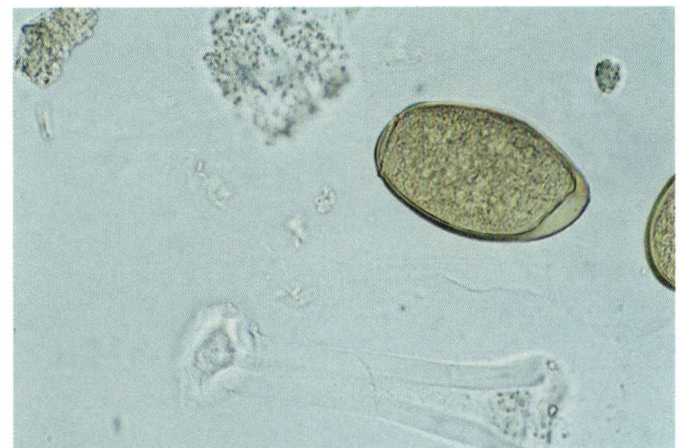

Plate 17

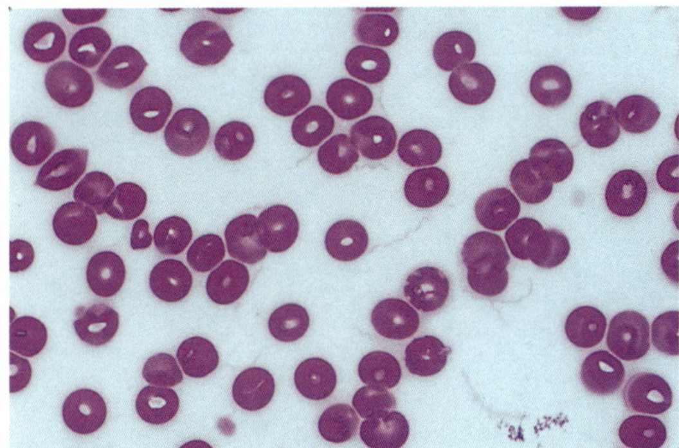

Plate 18

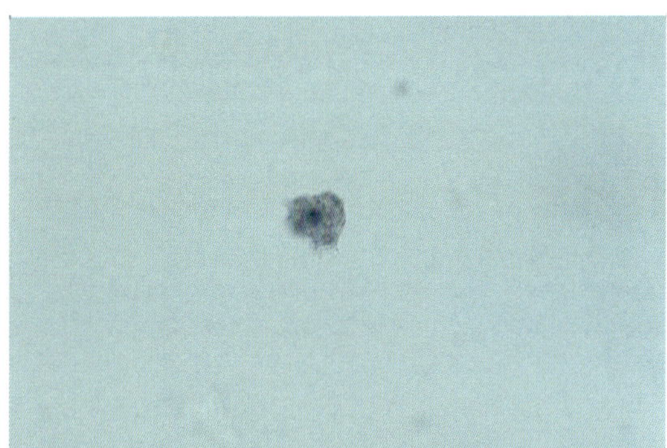

Plate 19

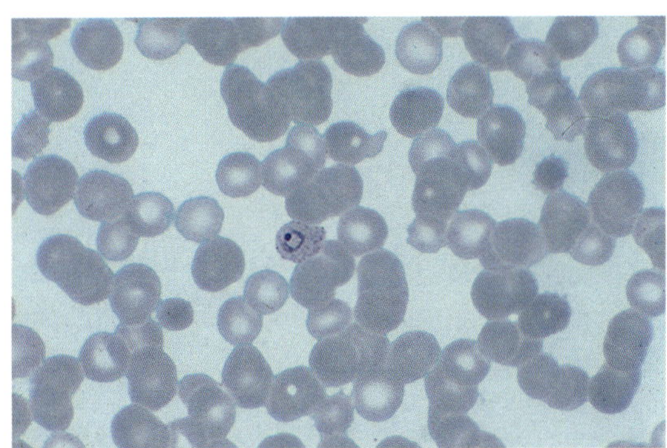

Plate 20

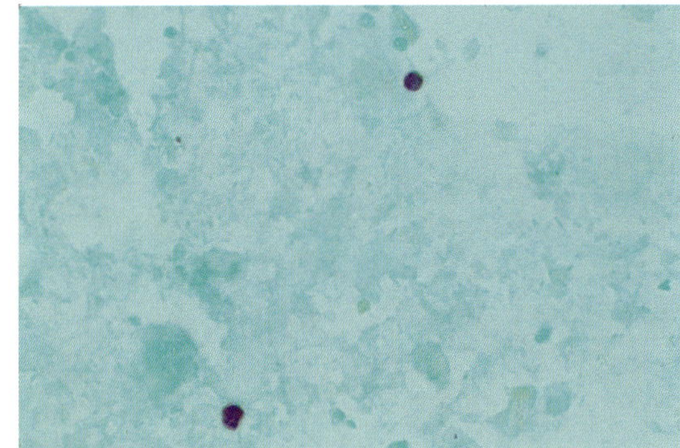

Plate 21

COLOR PLATE SECTION

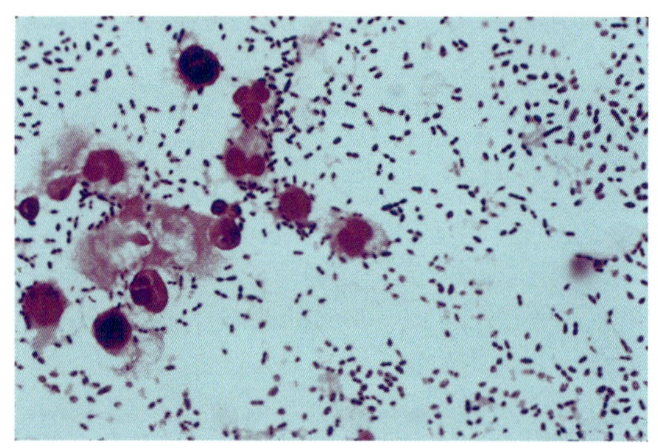

Plate 22

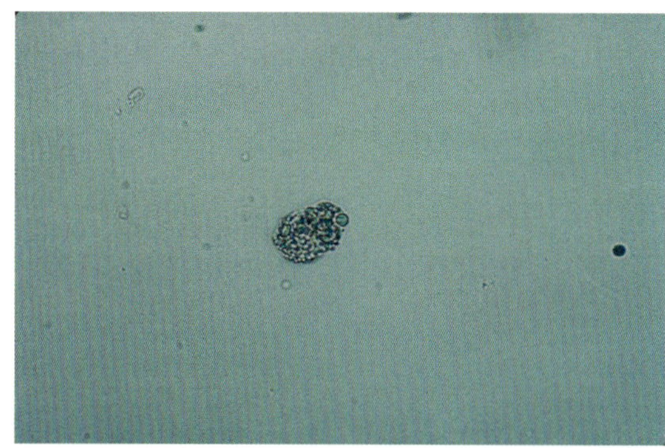

Plate 23

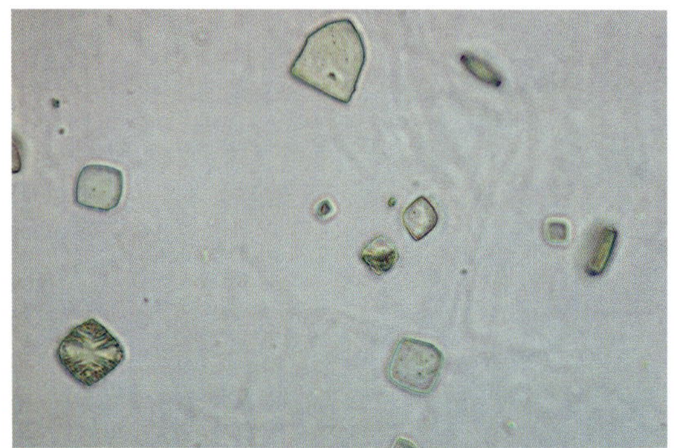

Plate 24

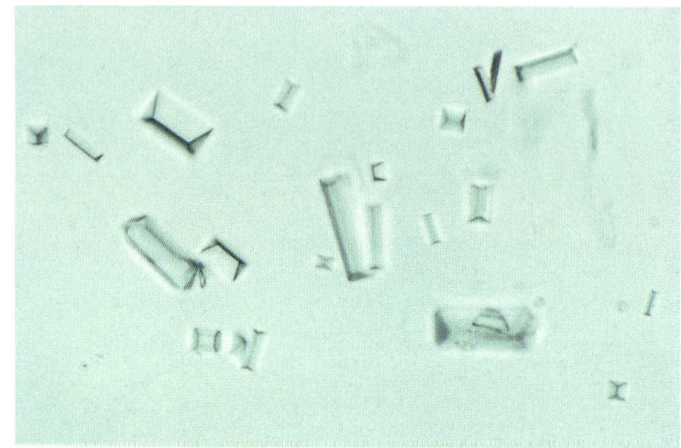

Plate 25

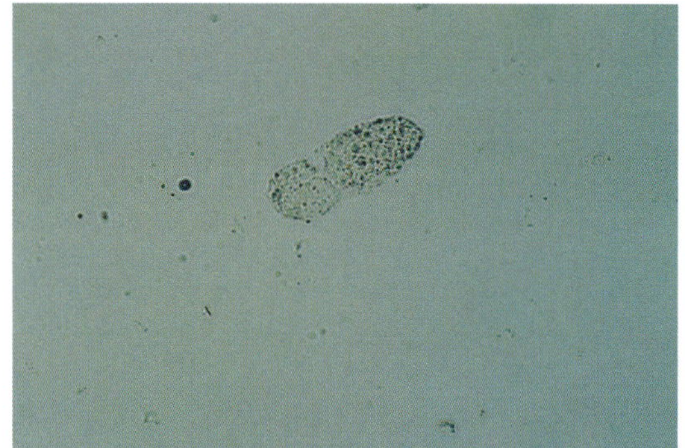

Plate 26

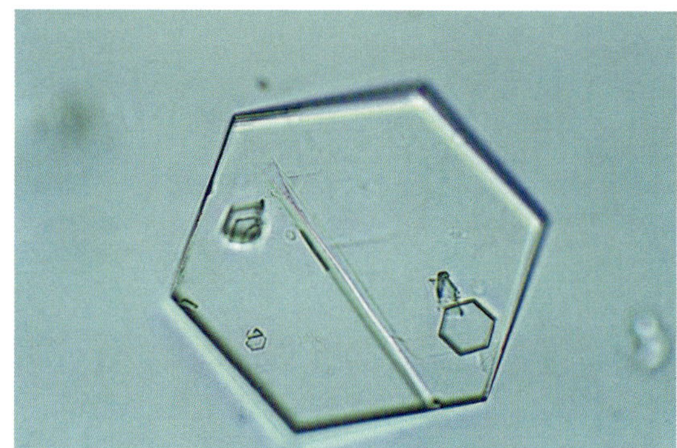

Plate 27

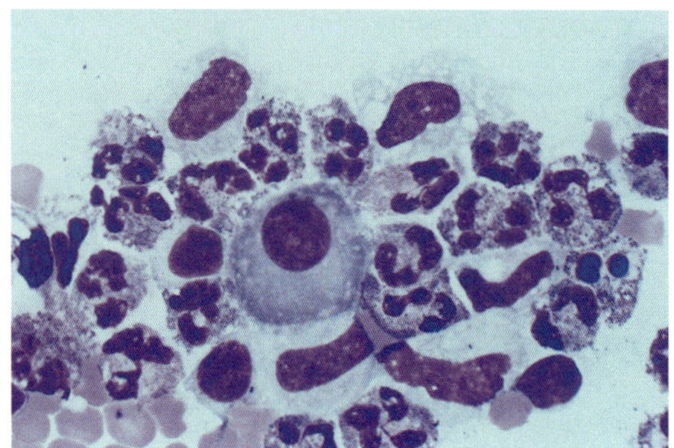

Plate 28

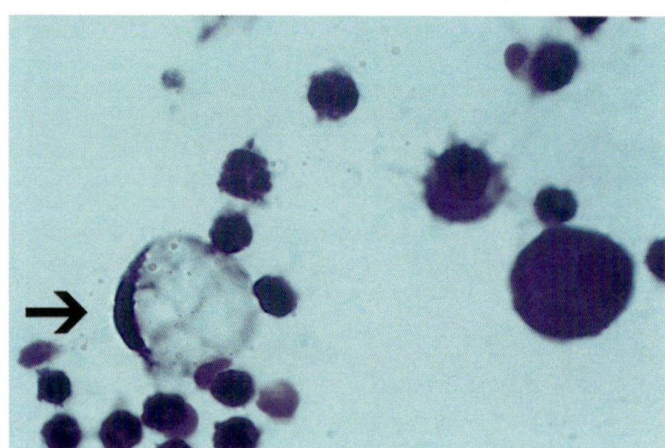

Plate 29

COLOR PLATE SECTION

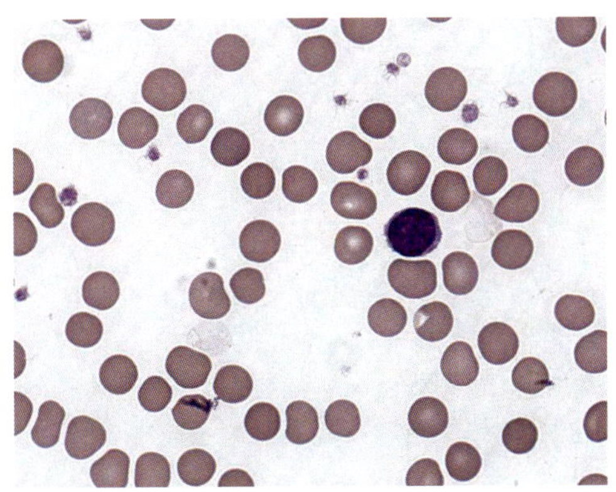

Plate 30

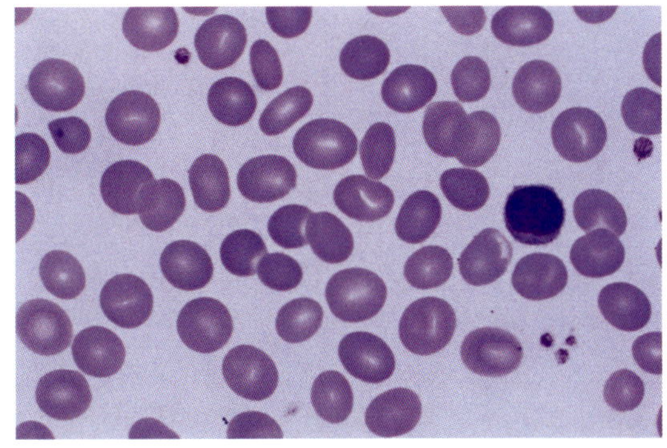

Plate 31

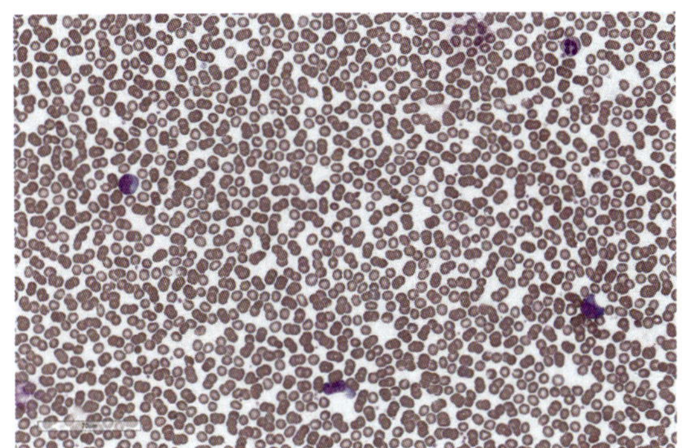

Plate 32

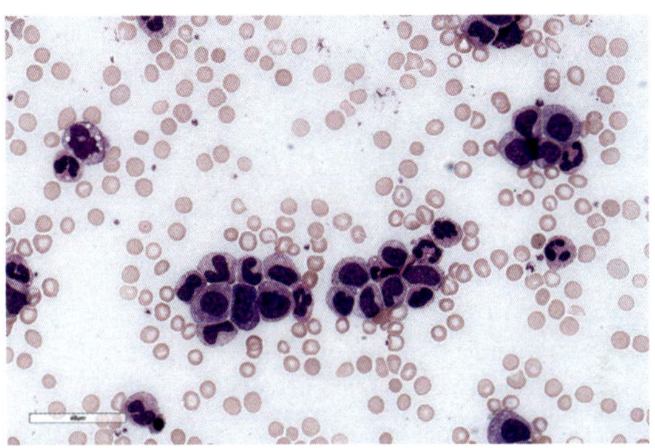

Plate 33

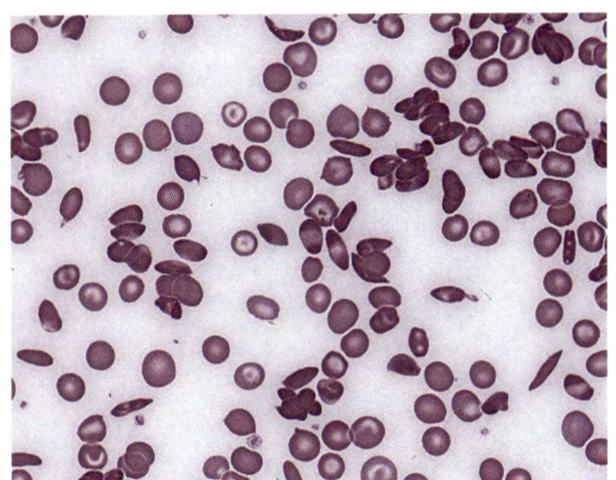

Plate 34

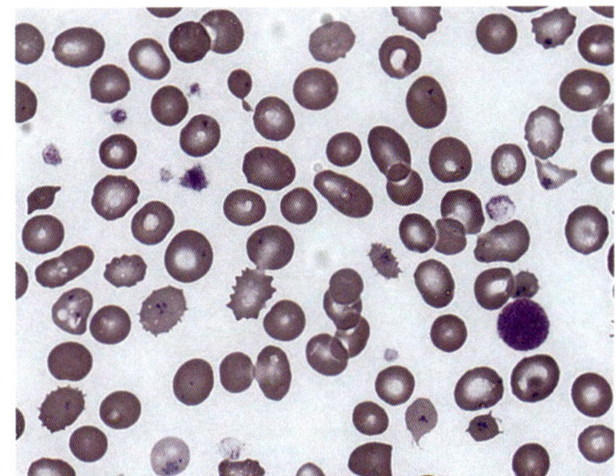

Plate 35

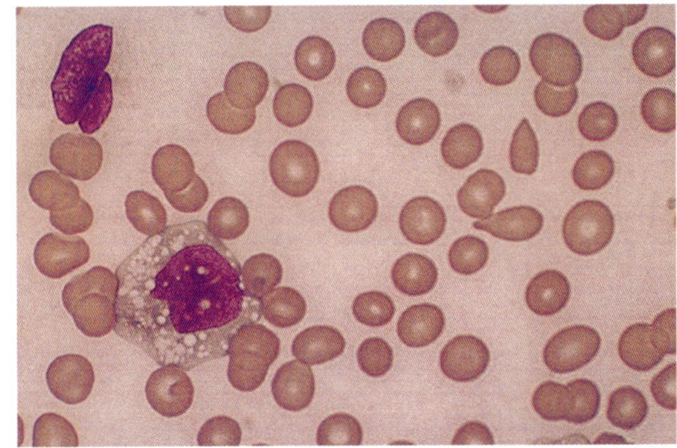

Plate 36

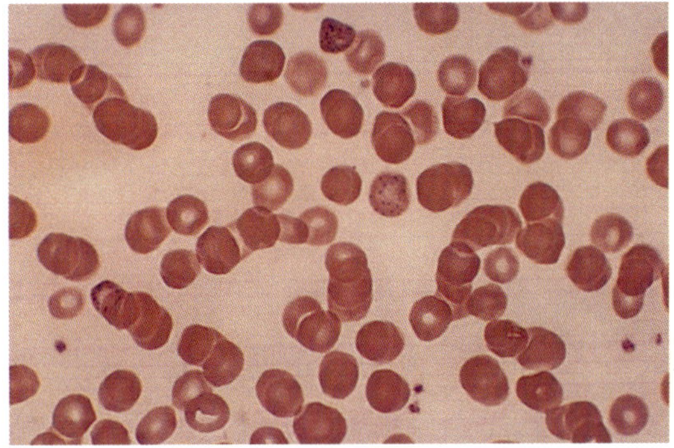

Plate 37

COLOR PLATE SECTION

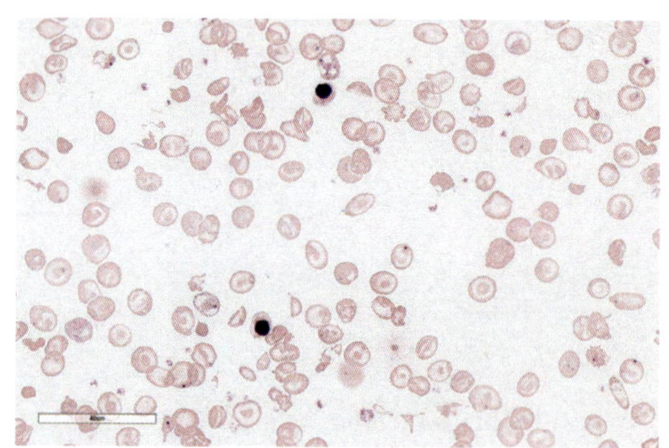

Plate 38

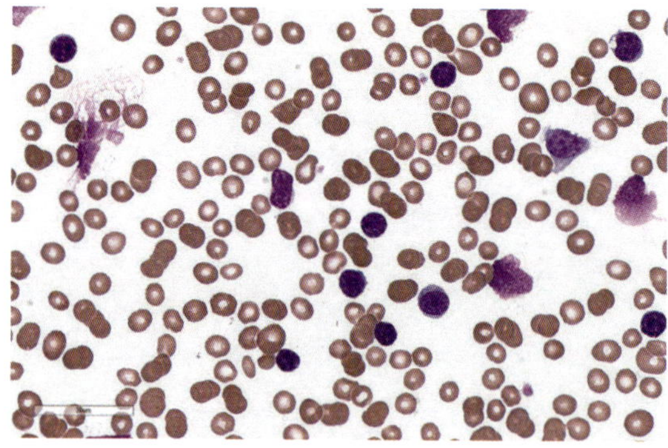

Plate 39

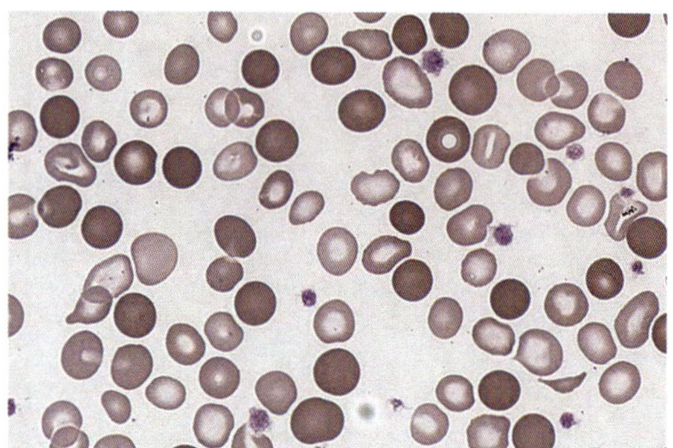

Plate 40

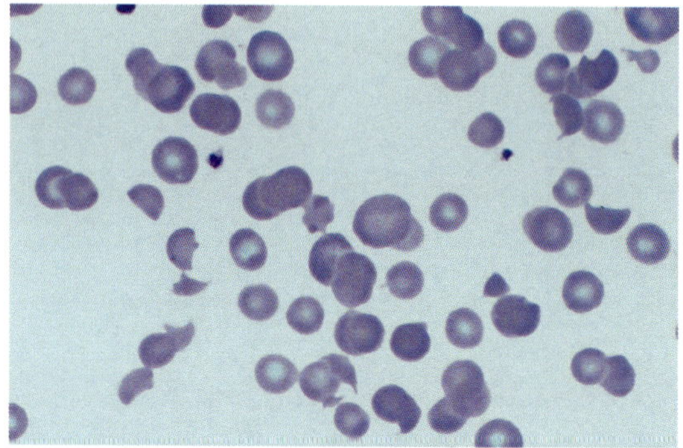

Plate 41

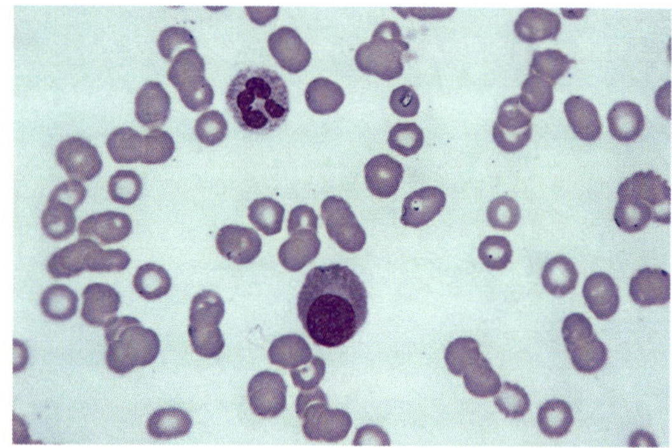

Plate 42

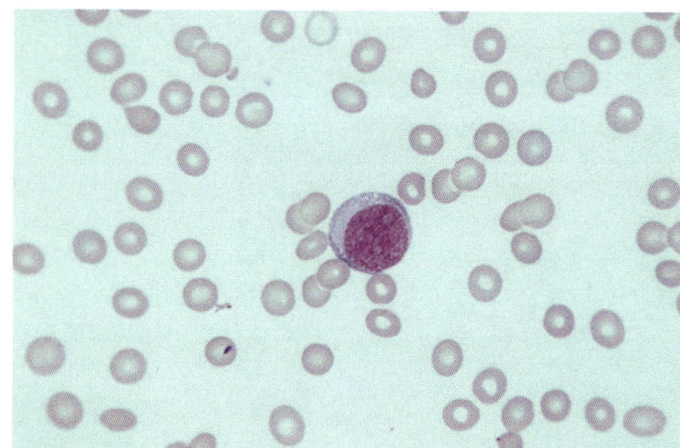

Plate 43

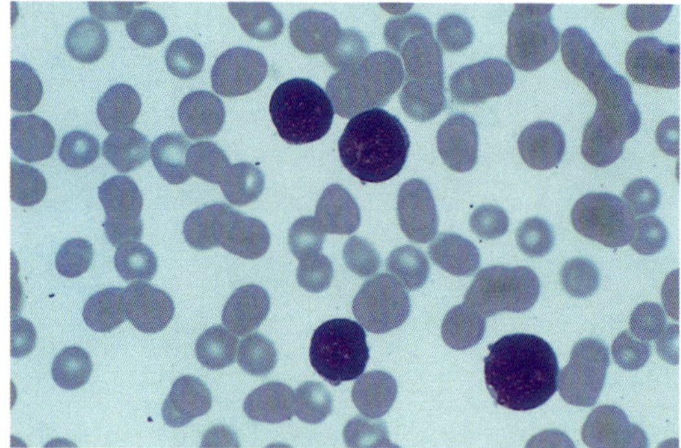

Plate 44

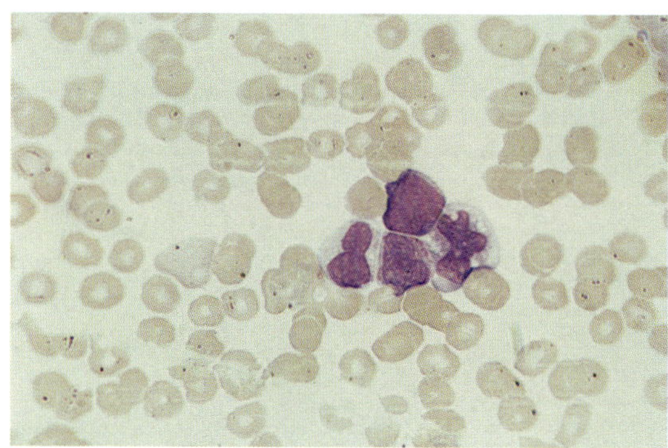

Plate 45

COLOR PLATE SECTION

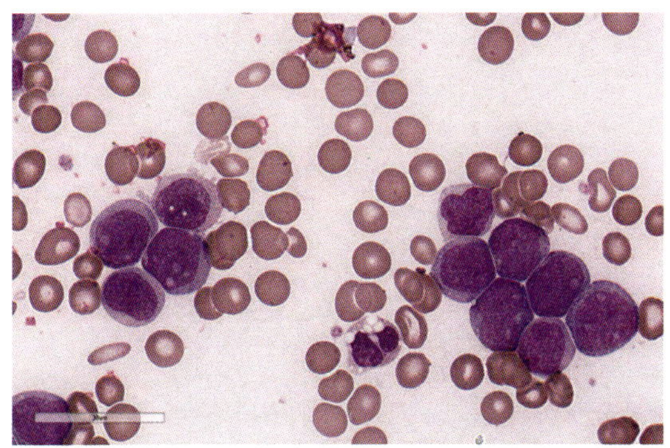

Plate 46

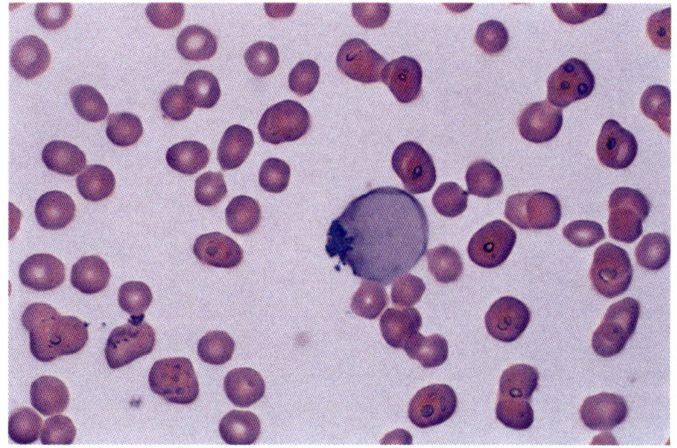

Plate 47A

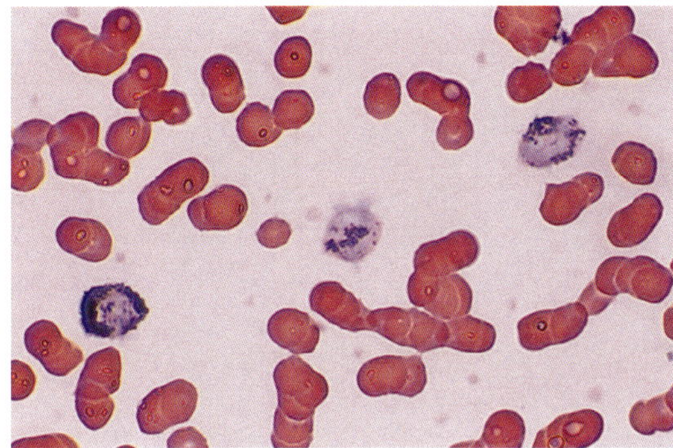

Plate 47B

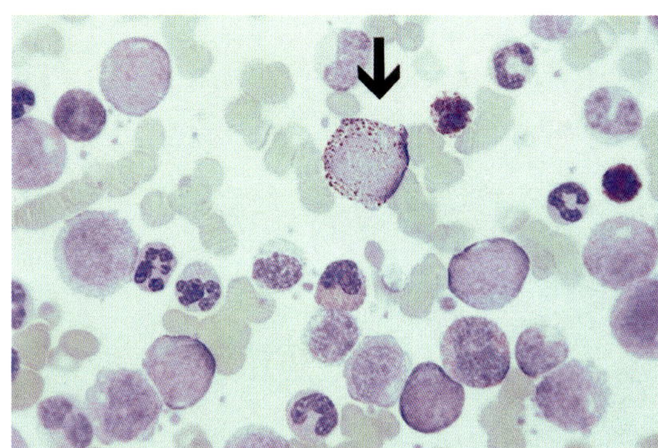

Plate 48

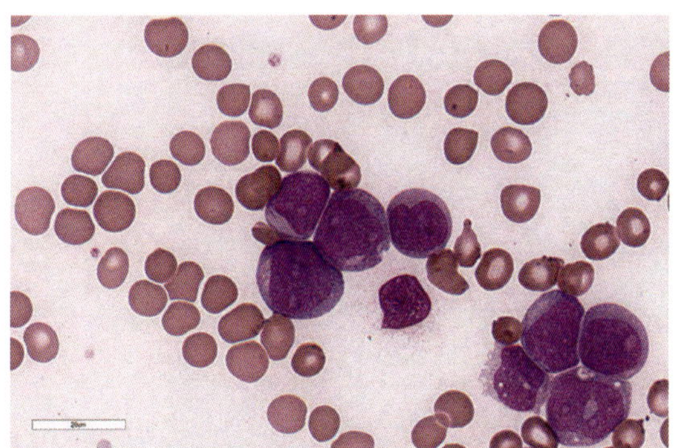

Plate 49

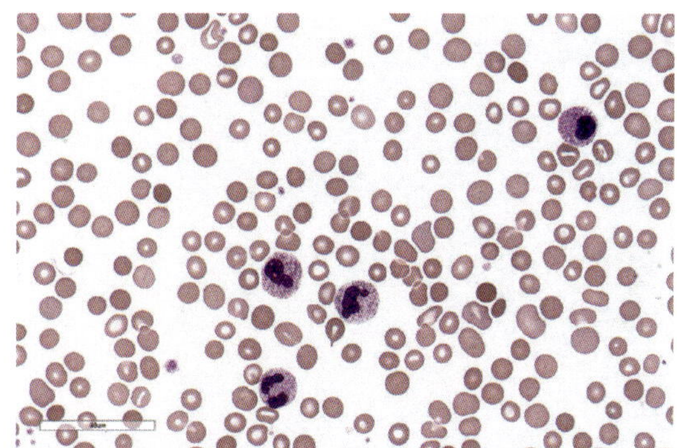

Plate 50

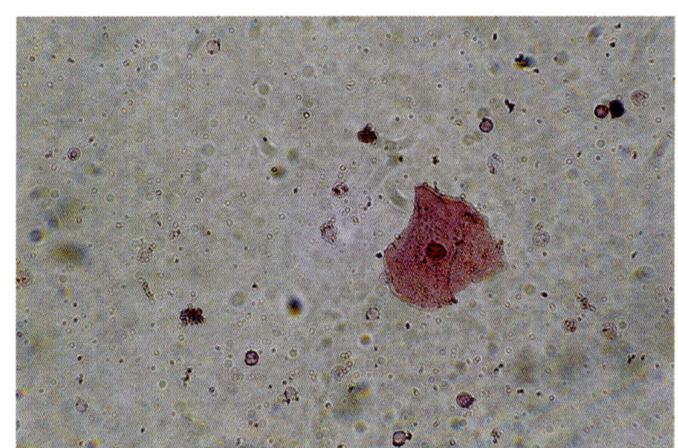

Plate 51

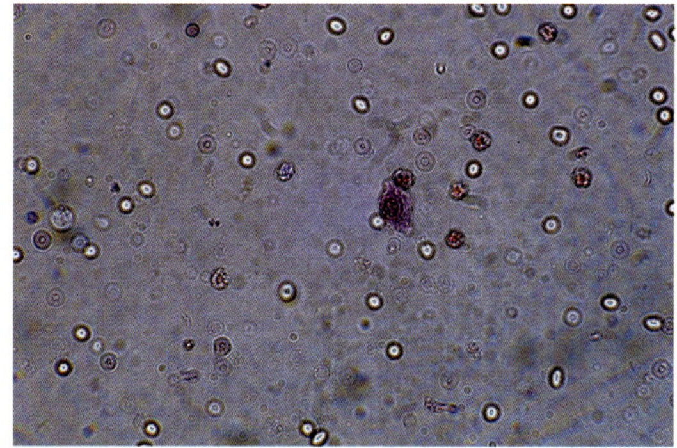

Plate 52

COLOR PLATE SECTION

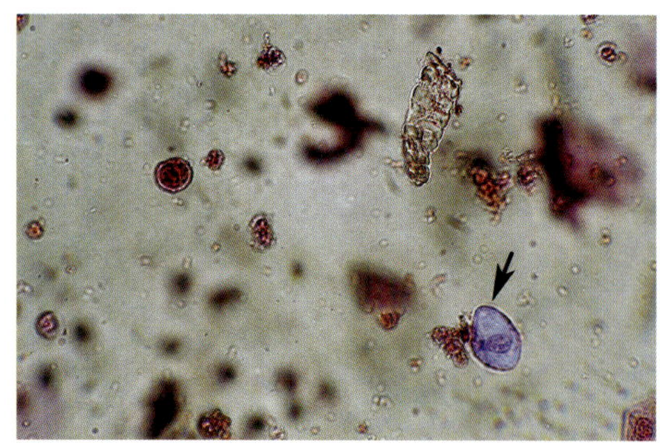

Plate 53

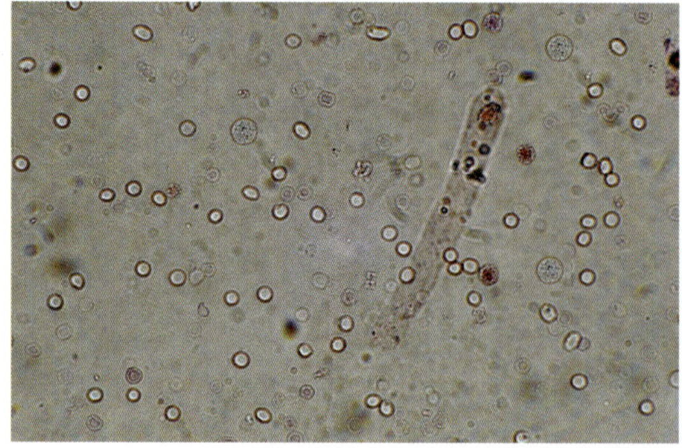

Plate 54

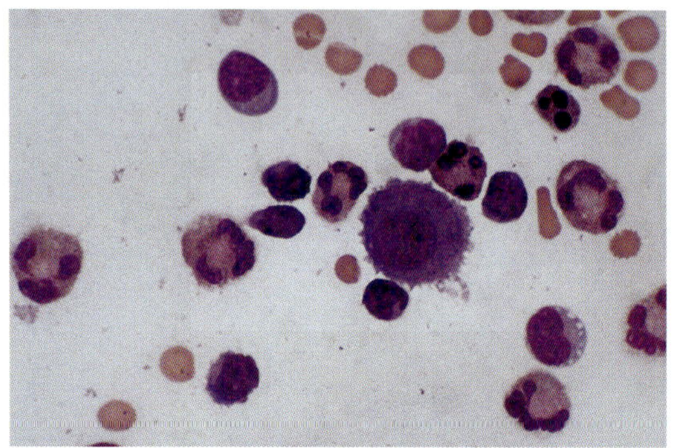

Plate 55

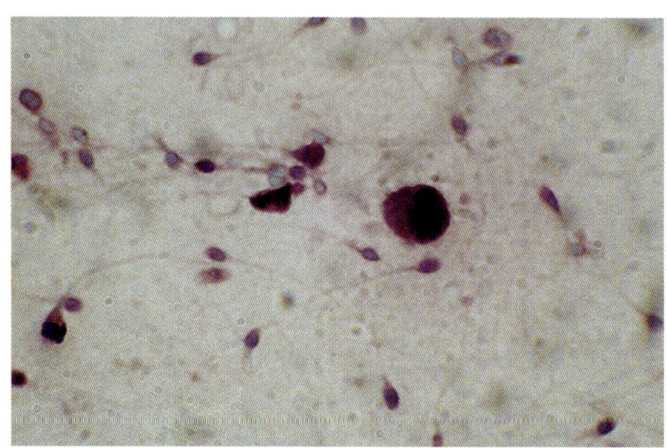

Plate 56

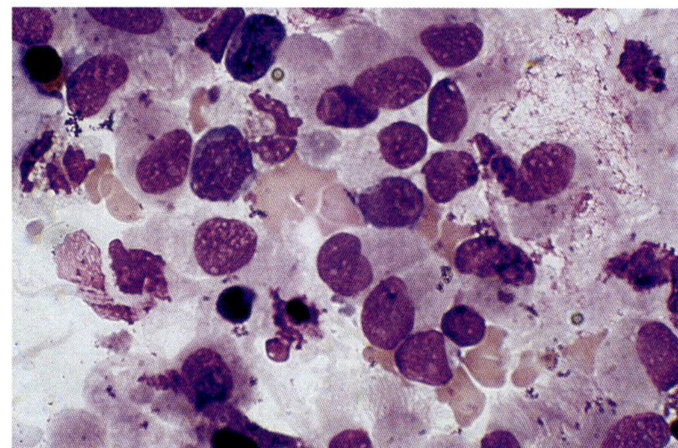

Plate 57

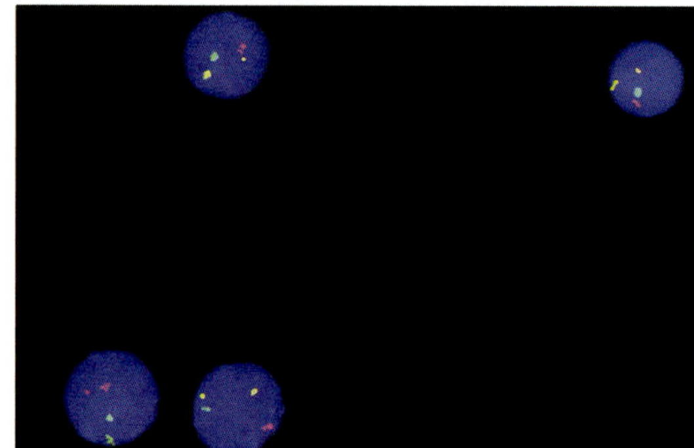

Plate 58

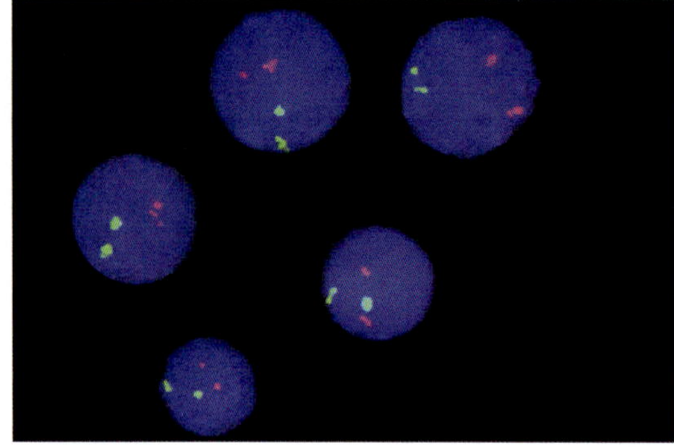

Plate 59

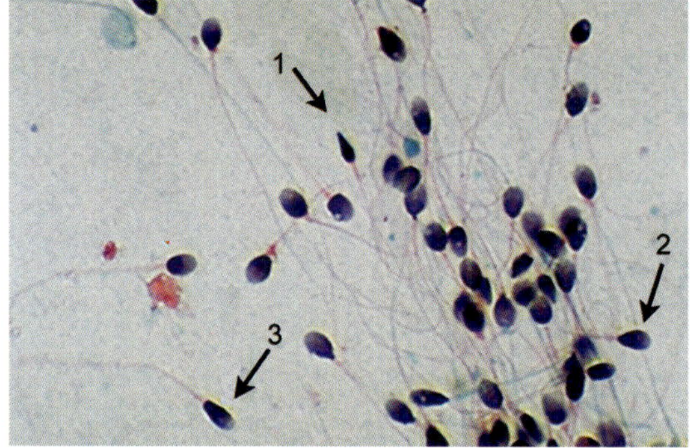

Plate 60

8. Plate 8 shows the electrophoresis of Hgb samples on acid agar gel, pH 6.0. Control hemolysate samples are in lanes 2 and 10 with A, S, C controls present. What is the patient's hemoglobin phenotype of sample 7?
A. SS
B. AS
C. SC
D. S-β-thalassemia

Hematology/Laboratory evaluation of anemia/3

9. Plate 9 is a photomicrograph of a fungal slide culture stained with lactophenol cotton blue, 400×. Which of the following fungi is present?
A. *Nannizzia gypsea*
B. *Microsporum canis*
C. *Aspergillus niger*
D. *Aspergillus fumigatus*

Microbiology/Mycology/2

10. Plate 10 is a photomicrograph of a fungal slide culture stained with lactophenol cotton blue, 400×. Which of the following fungi is present?
A. *Nannizzia gypsea*
B. *Microsporum canis*
C. *Trichophyton schoenleinii*
D. *Epidermophyton floccosum*

Microbiology/Mycology/2

11. Plate 11 is a photomicrograph of a fungal slide culture stained with lactophenol cotton blue, 400×. The morphology is *most* consistent with which fungus?
A. *Aspergillus* spp.
B. *Penicillium* spp.
C. *Scedosporium*
D. *Fusarium*

Microbiology/Mycology/2

12. Plate 12 is a bronchoalveolar lavage (BAL) sample concentrated by cytocentrifugation and stained with Wright stain, 1,000×. The sample was obtained from a patient with AIDS who resides in the midwestern United States. Which infectious agent is present?
A. *Pneumocystis jirovecii*
B. *Mycobacterium avium intracellulare*
C. *Histoplasma capsulatum*
D. *Cryptococcus neoformans*

Microbiology/Mycology/2

Answers to Questions 8–12

8. A Electrophoresis at an acidic pH (pH 6.0–6.4), as seen in plate 8, is considered confirmatory for a hemoglobin phenotype. The acidic pH allows for better separation of hemoglobin molecules that migrate to the same point in an alkaline pH (8.4–9.2). Sample 7 on plate 8 demonstrates one major band in the Hgb S position. Because Hgb A is not present, there is no normal β-gene, and the patient can be classified as a homozygote. On alkaline gels, Hgb S, D, and G migrate to the same point on the gel, but in acidic gel, Hgb S is alone and lines up with the control samples in lanes 2 and 10.

9. D *A. fumigatus* produces hyaline, septate hyphae, and dome-shaped vesicles, the upper one-half to two-thirds of which are covered with a row of phialides producing long chains of conidia. *A. niger* produces spherical vesicles that are completely covered with phialides. The phialides produce jet-black conidia that obscure the vesicle surface, forming a radiated head.

10. A *Nannizzia gypsea* (previously *Microsporum gypseum*) is now included in the *Nannizzia* species complex. It includes five species that are difficult to differentiate phenotypically. *N. gypsea* produces enormous numbers of symmetrical, rough macroconidia. These have thin walls with not more than six compartments and have rounded ends. The rounded ends differentiate this group from *M. canis*, which produces spindle-shaped macroconidia with usually more than six compartments and pointed ends.

11. A *Aspergillus* spp. has septate, branching hyphae and an unbranched conidiophore that arises from a specialized foot cell (not visible in this image). The conidiophore is present in the center and is enlarged and is covered with flask-shaped phialides. This species has a double row of phialides, which is considered biserate. The phialides produce chains of round conidia.

12. C This plate shows abundant *H. capsulatum* (yeast phase) within the cytoplasm of both the macrophage and histiocyte. Small oval yeast cells, 2 to 5 μm in diameter, are seen. All of the organisms listed may cause pulmonary pneumonia in patients with immunodeficiency.

13. Plate 13 is a fecal specimen seen under 400× using brightfield microscopy. The plate shows the ovum of which parasite?
A. *Necator americanus*
B. *Trichuris trichiura*
C. *Ascaris lumbricoides*
D. *Enterobius vermicularis*
Microbiology/Parasitology/2

14. Plate 14 is a fecal specimen unstained seen under 400× using brightfield microscopy. The plate shows the ovum of which parasite?
A. *Necator americanus*
B. *Trichuris trichiura*
C. *Ascaris lumbricoides*
D. *Enterobius vermicularis*
Microbiology/Parasitology/2

15. Plate 15 is an iodine-stained fecal specimen seen under 400× using brightfield microscopy. The plate shows the ovum of which parasite?
A. Pinworm
B. Threadworm
C. Hookworm
D. Whipworm
Microbiology/Parasitology/2

16. Plate 16 is an unstained fecal specimen seen under 400× using brightfield microscopy. The plate shows the ovum of which parasite?
A. *Clonorchis sinensis*
B. *Fasciola hepatica*
C. *Paragonimus westermani*
D. *Fasciolopsis buski*
Microbiology/Parasitology/2

17. Plate 17 is an unstained fecal specimen seen under 400× using brightfield microscopy. The plate shows the ovum of which parasite?
A. *Fasciola hepatica*
B. *Paragonimus westermani*
C. *Metagonimus yokogawai*
D. *Opisthorchis viverrini*
Microbiology/Parasitology/2

18. Plate 18 is a peripheral blood film stained with Giemsa stain, 1,000×. What condition is suspected from this field?
A. Macrocytic anemia
B. Agranulocytosis
C. Relapsing fever
D. Lead poisoning
Microbiology/Microscopy/2

Answers to Questions 13–18

13. B The ova of *T. trichiura* are brown and shaped like a football, with mucous plugs at both ends. Ova have a thick wall and measure about 50 μm long by 20 μm wide.

14. C *Ascaris* ova are large and oval, usually measuring 50 to 75 μm long by 35 to 50 μm wide. They are often bile stained and may have a thick shell with a coarse covering (corticated). This egg demonstrates a contracted embryo, leaving space between the shell and the embryo at the opposing poles. This indicates that the egg is fertilized.

15. C Hookworm ova are approximately 60 to 75 μm in length and 35 to 40 μm in width. They have a thin outer shell, usually containing an unembryonated or partly embryonated egg within. The ova of *Necator* and *Ancylostoma* cannot be differentiated from one another.

16. A *C. sinensis* produces small, bile-stained ova approximately 25 to 35 μm in length and 10 to 20 μm in width. Ova have a collar (shoulder) on both sides of the operculum and a knob at the end opposite the operculum.

17. B *P. westermani* produces large, operculated ova measuring approximately 80 to 100 μm in length and 50 to 70 μm in width. They are yellow-brown and nonembryonated. *Metagonimus* and *Opisthorchis* ova are small ova resembling *Clonorchis. Fasciola* produces ova that are also yellow-brown, operculated, and unembryonated. The ova are larger than *Paragonimus* and lack the small shoulders adjacent to the operculum of *Paragonimus* ova.

18. C This field shows long helical bacteria between RBCs of normal size and color. These spirochetes are sometimes seen in the blood of patients suffering from the febrile septic phase of infection with *Borrelia* or *Leptospira* spp. The former are more commonly encountered in differential examinations, especially in patients infected with *Borrelia recurrentis* and other species that cause relapsing fever.

19. Plate 19 shows an organism isolated from an eye wash from a patient who had a corneal infection and had been wearing contact lenses for the past 2 years. What is the name of the causative agent?

A. *Naegleria* spp.
B. *Acanthamoeba* spp.
C. *Entamoeba histolytica*
D. *Trichomonas vaginalis*

Microbiology/Parasitology/2

20. Plate 20 is a Wright-stained peripheral blood film, 1,000×. Which malarial stage is present in the red blood cell (RBC) in the center of the plate?

A. Ring trophozoite of *Plasmodium vivax*
B. Mature trophozoite of *Plasmodium malariae*
C. Macrogametocyte stage of *Plasmodium falciparum*
D. Mature gametocyte stage of *Plasmodium ovale*

Microbiology/Parasitology/3

21. Plate 21 is a modified acid-fast stain with malachite green counterstain of a stool specimen, 1,000×. The oocysts seen in this field are approximately 5 µm in diameter. Which organism is present?

A. *Cystoisospora belli*
B. *Cryptosporidium parvum*
C. *Cyclospora* spp.
D. *Sarcocystis* spp.

Microbiology/Parasitology/2

22. Plate 22 is a Gram-stained CSF sample concentrated by centrifugation, 1,000×. Although organisms cannot be identified solely using a Gram stain, which organism is likely present based on the microscopic morphology present?

A. *Neisseria meningitidis*
B. *Staphylococcus aureus*
C. *Streptococcus pneumoniae*
D. *Listeria monocytogenes*

Microbiology/Microscopy/2

23. Plate 23 is a urinary sediment sample viewed under 400× magnification by using a brightfield microscope. What is the object located in the center of the field?

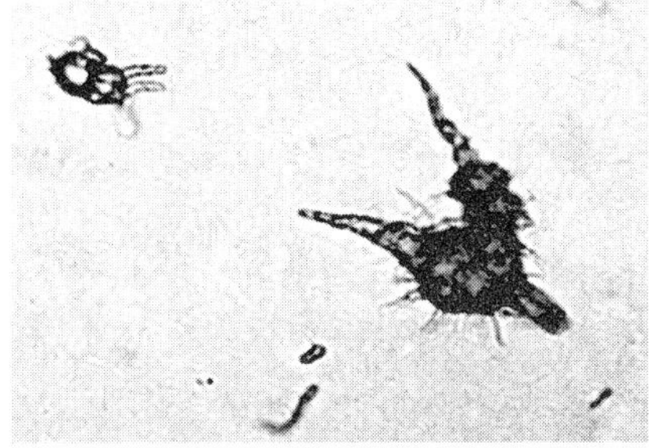

A. *Schistosoma haematobium* ovum
B. Ammonium biurate crystal
C. Glitter cell
D. Fecal contaminant

Urinalysis/Routine/2

Answers to Questions 19–23

19. B This is a large trophozoite with spiculated cytoplasm characteristic of *Acanthamoeba*. Eye infections caused by this organism have been documented in contact lens wearers who do not disinfect lenses properly. *Acanthamoeba* spp. are large trophozoites measuring 25 to 50 µm. They may also cause primary amoebic meningoencephalitis, although they are isolated less often than *Naegleria* in the cerebrospinal fluid (CSF) of patients with this disease.

20. A The infected RBC demonstrates enlarged ameba-like cytoplasm and Schüffner dots, which are characteristic of *P. vivax* and *P. ovale*. The parasite is at the ring-form trophozoite stage.

21. B All the organisms listed are coccidian parasites that cause diarrhea, especially in patients with immunodeficiency (e.g., those with AIDS). *Cryptosporidium* produces the smallest oocysts (half the size of *Cyclospora*, which is the next smallest) and is visible in stools with use of either acid-fast or immunofluorescent staining techniques. The oocysts are round, about 5 µm in diameter, and stain deep pink.

22. C This field shows abundant gram-positive diplococci with the lancet shape that is characteristic of *S. pneumoniae*.

23. B Ammonium biurate crystals are very rare in fresh urine; however, they are often present in urine that has been stored for a long period of time. When encountered, the integrity of the specimen should be questioned.

24. Plate 24 is a urinary sediment (pH 6.0) viewed under 400× magnification by using a brightfield microscope. Which crystals are seen?
A. Uric acid
B. Calcium oxalate
C. Triple phosphate
D. Hippuric acid
Urinalysis/Routine/2

25. Plate 25 is a urinary sediment (pH 7.5) viewed under 400× magnification by using a brightfield microscope. Which crystals are seen?
A. Uric acid
B. Calcium oxalate
C. Triple phosphate
D. Hippuric acid
Urinalysis/Routine/2

26. Plate 26 is a urinary sediment viewed under 400× magnification by using a brightfield microscope. Which type of cast is present?
A. Hyaline cast
B. Broad cast
C. Waxy cast
D. Coarse granular cast
Urinalysis/Routine/2

27. Plate 27 shows a urinary sediment (pH 6.0) viewed under 400× magnification by using brightfield microscopy. This colorless crystal is presumptively identified as:
A. Calcium phosphate
B. Acetaminophen
C. Cystine
D. Hippuric acid
Urinalysis/Routine/2

28. Plate 28 is a Wright-stained cytocentrifuge preparation of pleural fluid, 1,000×. What is the correct classification of the largest mononuclear cell located in the center of the plate?
A. Histiocyte
B. Macrophage
C. Lymphoblast
D. Mesothelial cell
Body fluids/Pleural fluid/2

29. Plate 29 is a Wright-stained smear of pleural fluid prepared by cytocentrifugation. The largest cell in this field (see arrow) is identified as a:
A. Signet ring macrophage
B. Reactive mesothelial cell
C. Foam cell
D. Metastatic cell from the breast
Body fluids/Pleural fluid/2

Answers to Questions 24–29

24. A Uric acid crystals are yellow to reddish brown and occur in acidic or neutral urine. Common forms include whetstones and rhombic plates (as seen here), as well as thin needles and rosettes. Calcium oxalate crystals are usually colorless octahedrons. Triple phosphate crystals are long, colorless, six-sided prisms, and hippuric acid crystals are colorless, long, flat, hexagonal plates.

25. C Triple phosphate crystals occur in alkaline or neutral urine. They are long, colorless hexagonal prisms that often resemble a "coffin lid." They may also occur in a feathery form that resembles a fern leaf. Triple phosphate crystals may form calculi in the renal pelvis appearing on an x-ray as an outline of the calyces and referred to as "staghorn" calculi.

26. D Coarse granular casts often form from degeneration of cellular casts. The finding of more than a rare granular cast is significant and helps identify the kidney as the source of urinary protein and cells. Coarse and fine granular casts usually have the same significance as cellular casts and point to glomerular damage.

27. C Cystine crystals form in acidic urine and appear as colorless, uniform, hexagonal plates in urinary sediment. Calcium phosphate crystals form in neutral to alkaline urine and appear as thin amorphous crystals resembling a sheet of ice or as flat needles that form a rosette. Acetaminophen crystals are cylinder shaped, with round edges. Hippuric acid crystals form long six-sided prisms in acidic urine. Cystine crystals must be differentiated from uric acid on the basis of solubility, polarized microscopy, or biochemical testing. Cystine crystals are less anisotropic than uric acid. Cystine crystals are soluble in dilute hydrochloric acid (HCl), but are insoluble in uric acid. Cystine causes a positive cyanide–nitroprusside test, and uric acid does not.

28. D Mesothelial cells are specialized epithelial cells that line the serous membranes, and they may be seen in small numbers in normal pleural, pericardial, and ascites fluids. They are often seen in increased numbers when there is an inflammatory injury involving the serous membranes. They are large mononuclear or binucleate cells with an open chromatin pattern and abundant agranular cytoplasm. Mesothelial cells may transform into phagocytic cells and undergo morphological changes that cause them to resemble malignant cells.

29. A Macrophages are frequently seen in serous fluids. They are present in increased numbers in exudative conditions. "Signet ring" forms result from compression of the nucleus against the cell wall, usually caused by large vacuoles that form after phagocytosis of erythrocytes or fat.

30. Plate 30 is from a Wright-stained peripheral blood film, 1,000×. Which of the following *best* describes the cells in this plate?

A. No aberrant morphology present
B. Macrocytic RBCs
C. Hypersegmented neutrophil present
D. Reduced platelets

Hematology/Normocytic normochromic anemia/2

31. Plate 31 is a Wright-stained peripheral blood film, 1,000×. What is the *most* appropriate classification of the RBC morphology seen in this field?

A. Microcytic, hypochromic
B. Microcytic, normochromic
C. Normocytic, normochromic
D. Macrocytic, normochromic

Hematology/Macrocytic normochromic anemia/3

32. Plate 32 is a Wright-stained peripheral blood film, 1,000×. What is the *most* appropriate classification of the white blood cells (WBCs) present in this field?

A. Reactive (atypical) lymphocytes
B. Large lymphoblasts exhibiting L2 morphology
C. The M4 subtype of acute granulocytic leukemia
D. Monocytes

Hematology/Qualitative and quantitative NM leukocyte disorders/3

33. Plate 33 is from a Wright-stained peripheral blood film, 400×. Which of the following tests may be performed to enable an accurate diagnosis?

A. Fluorescence *in situ* hybridization (FISH) or polymerase chain reaction (PCR) for *BCR/ABL*
B. Myeloid marker study by flow cytometry
C. Myeloperoxidase stain
D. Periodic acid–Schiff (PAS) stain

Hematology/Myeloproliferative disorders/3

Answers to Questions 30–33

30. A The central pallor of the erythrocytes are less than one-third of the diameter of the RBC, which equates to normochromic. There isn't a common lymphocyte for comparison to determine whether the RBC size is normocytic, but it can be inferred based on the normochromic color. Neutrophil in the field appears adequate in size, granularity, and lobularity. Platelets appear adequate in size and in distribution. If this is a representative image, an average of 10 to 30 platelets would provide an adequate platelet estimate.

31. D Many of the RBCs in this field are larger than the nucleus of the small lymphocyte, indicating that they are macrocytic. Several of the RBCs are elliptical and are classified as ovalocytes. The central pallor occupies less than one-third the diameter of the erythrocytes in the field, indicating they are normochromic. Macrocytic anemia (anemia with an increased mean cell volume [MCV]) is commonly seen in patients with chronic liver disease, vitamin B_{12} or folate deficiency, hypothyroidism, and alcoholism.

32. A These cells are atypical or reactive lymphocytes that are typically found in viral infections, such as infectious mononucleosis. In these conditions, the WBC count is increased (usually 15–25 × 10^3/μL), and lymphocytes account for the majority of the WBCs. When comparing common lymphocytes to reactive lymphocytes, the reactive lymphocytes are larger than normal due to increased cytoplasmic volume. The cytoplasm may have a rim of basophilia where it touches other cells (RBCs). The cytoplasm appears smooth in texture but may contain vacuoles or azurophilic granules. These are different from the granules found in monocytes, which contribute to the rough texture of the cytoplasm. The nucleus of the reactive lymphocytes has an open chromatin pattern due to the increased surface area and cellular volume.

33. A This plate shows a regenerative left shift, which is defined as an elevated WBC count (usually above 50,000/μL) with an increase in granulocytic precursors. There is also an accompanying thrombocytosis. Although not seen in the color plate, basophilia can also be present. Confirmation of these findings would involve a leukocyte alkaline phosphatase (LAP) score to differentiate between the true malignancy in chronic myelogenous leukemia (CML) and a leukemoid response to infection, inflammation, tissue damage, or malignancy. If the LAP score suggests CML, a FISH analysis testing for the Philadelphia chromosome would confirm the CML diagnosis. Ninety-five percent of patients with CML display the Philadelphia (Ph^1) chromosome in their granulocytes.

34. Plate 34 is from a Wright-stained peripheral blood film, 400×. The cells seen are diagnostic of which condition?

A. Intravascular hemolytic anemia
B. Sickle cell disease
C. Myelofibrosis
D. Erythroleukemia

Hematology/Normocytic normochromic anemia/3

35. Plate 35 is from a Wright-stained peripheral blood film, 1,000×. Which description of the RBC morphology and platelets is correct?

A. Microcytic, hypochromic with marked poikilocytosis and increased platelets
B. Macrocytic, hypochromic with marked anisocytosis and normal platelets
C. Normocytic, normochromic with mild poikilocytosis and increased platelets
D. Microcytic, hypochromic, with mild anisocytosis and normal platelets

Hematology/Laboratory evaluation of anemia/2

36. Plate 36 is a Wright-stained peripheral blood film, 1,000×. The RBCs in this plate are characteristic of:

A. Hemolytic anemia
B. Extramedullary hematopoiesis
C. Hemoglobin C discasc
D. Sideroblastic anemia

Hematology/Myeloproliferative disorders/2

37. Plate 37 is a Wright-stained peripheral blood film, 1,000×. The inclusions seen in this plate are associated with:

A. Lead poisoning
B. Aplastic anemia
C. Iron-deficiency anemia
D. Intravascular hemolysis

Hematology/Normocytic normochromic anemia/2

Answers to Questions 34–37

34. B This plate displays slight polychromasia, marked target cells (codocytes), and marked sickle cells (drepanocytes), along with Howell-Jolly bodies. These are all characteristic findings of sickle cell disease. The presence of sickle cells is pathognomonic for sickle cell disease. Sickle cells are elongated with pointed ends, and the Hgb is concentrated in the center of the cell, showing a lack of a central pallor. They may also be encountered in a few other hemoglobinopathies that contain Hgb S, such as Hgb SC disease, but are fewer in number. They are rarely seen in patients with sickle cell trait.

35. A The central pallor of the RBCs is more than half the diameter, which indicates they are hypochromic. Although there is not a lymphocyte for comparison, the cells appear smaller and it can be inferred that they are also microcytic. There is marked poikilocytosis coming in the forms of echinocytes (burr cells), codocytes (target cells), and schistocytes (RBC fragments). When more than 30 platelets are present per oil immersion field (100×), the platelet estimate is increased and corresponds to an increased platelet count.

36. B A patient who suffers from bone marrow failure will demonstrate extramedullary hematopoiesis. Conditions that cause this include myelofibrosis or leukoerythroblastosis. The RBC morphology associated with extramedullary hematopoiesis is the dacryocyte (teardrop cell). It may also be found with ovalocytes, nucleated RBCs, basophilic stippling, poikilocytosis, leukocytosis, and (often) micromegakaryocytes. Hgb C disease produces normocytic or slightly microcytic anemia with many target cells. Sideroblastic anemia produces both microcytic, hypochromic RBCs and normocytic RBCs in blood (dimorphic RBC morphology). Hemolytic anemias are usually normocytic, normochromic, or macrocytic with polychromasia, but morphology varies with the cause of hemolysis.

37. A Several RBCs in this plate show coarse basophilic stippling. Basophilic stippling results from unstable RNA within the cell and is associated with defects in Hgb synthesis. This is most often seen in patients with lead poisoning, hemoglobinopathies, myelofibrosis, and megaloblastic anemias.

38. Plate 38 is from a Wright-stained peripheral blood film, 400×. Which of the following conditions is consistent with this RBC morphology?
A. Erythroleukemia
B. b-Thalassemia major
C. Folate deficiency anemia
D. Autoimmune hemolytic anemia
Hematology/Microcytic hypochromic anemia/3

39. Plate 39 is from a Wright-stained smear of peripheral blood, 1,000× from a patient with a WBC count of 135 × 10^9/L. The patient, age 70 years, has firm, enlarged lymph nodes in the cervical and axillary regions along with hepatosplenomegaly. These same cells make up 50% of the bone marrow WBCs. What is the *most* likely diagnosis?
A. Epstein-Barr virus infection
B. Infectious mononucleosis
C. Chronic lymphocytic leukemia
D. Waldenström macroglobulinemia
Hematology/Lymphoproliferative disorders/3

40. Plate 40 is from a Wright-stained peripheral blood film, 400×. The RBC morphology is *most* consistent with which of the following anemias?
A. Folate deficiency
B. Iron deficiency
C. Hemolytic
D. Sideroblastic
Hematology/Normocytic normochromic anemia/3

Answers to Questions 38–40

38. B This plate shows severe microcytic, hypochromic RBCs with numerous target cells and marked anisocytosis, which is consistent with β-thalassemia major. The most common form of nucleated RBC is an orthochromatophilic normoblast, and there are two in this color plate. In addition, thalassemia is also associated with marked poikilocytosis and the presence of inclusions such as Howell-Jolly bodies or Pappenheimer bodies. Folate deficiency produces a macrocytic anemia, and autoimmune hemolytic anemia is usually normocytic and normochromic. Peripheral blood in erythroleukemia contains many nucleated RBC precursors demonstrating bizarre shapes.

39. C The WBCs in this plate (with the exception of one granulocyte) are small lymphocytes. Chronic lymphocytic leukemia is rare in patients under age 30 years and more often appears in geriatric patients over the age of 60. Peripheral blood demonstrates a predominance of small lymphocytes, usually 20 to 200 × 10^9/L, composing at least 40% of the bone marrow WBCs. Flow cytometry indicates these cells to be B cells in approximately 95% of cases. In Waldenström macroglobulinemia, bone marrow is infiltrated by plasmacytoid lymphocytes, plasma cells, and mast cells, as well as small lymphocytes; however, a severe peripheral lymphocytosis is not seen. Lymphadenopathy and hepatosplenomegaly occur in infectious mononucleosis. The lymphocyte count is usually 15 to 25 × 10^9/L, but the cells are atypical, being characterized by reactive features. The bone marrow is usually hyperplastic but not infiltrated by small lymphocytes.

40. D The RBC morphology of this field is characterized by the presence of both microcytic, hypochromic cells and normocytic, normochromic cells. This dimorphic appearance is a characteristic of sideroblastic anemias. Folate deficiency causes megaloblastic anemia, resulting in a macrocytic, normochromic appearance. Iron deficiency is associated with a microcytic, hypochromic RBC morphology. Hemolytic anemias are often normocytic, normochromic. Dimorphic cell populations are associated with red cell distribution width (RDW) over 30% and can also be seen in patients who recently received blood transfusions, or those receiving supportive treatments for iron deficiency or synthetic erythropoietin (EPO).

41. Mr. Vacini, an Italian immigrant, has been hospitalized with tachycardia, a rapidly decreasing hematocrit, and blood in his urine. Twenty-four hours prior to admission, he had taken his first dose of a sulfonamide prescribed for a urinary tract infection. Plate 41 is from a Wright-stained smear of his peripheral blood, 1,000×. Which laboratory test would be helpful in establishing a diagnosis of Mr. Vacini's hematologic problem?

A. Heinz body preparation
B. Hemoglobin H preparation
C. Iron stain
D. New methylene blue stain

Hematology/Normocytic normochromic anemia/3

42. Plate 42 is from a Wright-stained smear of peripheral blood, 1,000×. Bone marrow aspirate from this patient demonstrated an abundance of cells with this morphology. Which of the following conditions is *most* likely present in this patient?

A. Sézary syndrome
B. Hodgkin disease
C. Burkitt lymphoma
D. Multiple myeloma

Hematology/Lymphoproliferative disorders/3

43. Plate 43 is from a Wright-stained peripheral blood film, 1,000×. The WBC appearing in this plate is *most* likely a:

A. Myeloblast
B. Promyelocyte
C. Myelocyte
D. Monoblast

Hematology/Acute leukemia/2

44. Plate 44 is a Wright-stained peripheral blood film, 1,000×. The WBCs in this field are negative for peroxidase, chloroacetate esterase, and Sudan B. The cells are positive for terminal deoxynucleotidyl transferase (Tdt) and PAS with a coarse block pattern. On the basis of these findings, what is the *most* appropriate classification of these cells?

A. Lymphoblasts with L1 morphology
B. Lymphoblasts with L2 morphology
C. Lymphoblasts with L3 morphology
D. Chronic lymphocytic leukemia cells

Hematology/Acute leukemia/3

Answers to Questions 41–44

41. A The RBC morphology seen in this plate shows both anisocytosis and poikilocytosis, with prominent schistocytes that indicate hemolytic anemia. The patient's ethnic background, clinical findings, and sulfonamide therapy point to a hemolytic episode of glucose-6-phosphate dehydrogenase (G-6-PD) deficiency as the cause. This can be confirmed with a G-6-PD assay. The enzyme deficiency results in oxidative damage to RBCs causing formation of Heinz bodies (precipitated Hgb). Heinz bodies are visualized using supravital staining such as with new methylene blue or bromocresyl green. The RBC fragments seen in this condition are called *bite* or *helmet* cells.

42. D The cell in the center of the plate is a plasma cell. Such cells have a dense, eccentrically placed nucleus that is surrounded by a clear perinuclear area that represents the Golgi apparatus. The cytoplasm is basophilic and more abundant than is seen in small lymphocytes. Plasma cells are not normally seen in peripheral blood. They may be found in cases of viral and chronic infections and connective tissue diseases, as well as in myeloma and other plasma cell dyscrasias. The RBCs in this plate demonstrate rouleaux, which is a characteristic seen in multiple myeloma as a result of the increased protein coating the erythrocytes. Peripheral blood in Hodgkin disease is characterized by neutrophilia and lymphopenia. Burkitt lymphoma produces very large, intensely basophilic lymphoblasts (L3 morphology). Abnormal lymphocytes appearing in peripheral blood in Sézary syndrome are large with a convoluted nucleus of fine chromatin and almost no cytoplasm.

43. A Blasts are usually 15 to 20 μm in diameter, with a large nucleus containing fine chromatin. The cytoplasm is usually agranular and basophilic. Lymphoblasts are differentiated from myeloblasts by cytochemical staining and flow cytometry. This blast contains uniform, unclumped chromatin, and multiple nucleoli; azurophilic granules are absent; and the sample is from a patient with acute myelogenous leukemia, classified as FAB M1 (French-American-British Classification, M1 subtype). Lymphoblasts often display irregular clumping of the chromatin and azurophilic granules. They usually lack prominent nucleoli.

44. A The cytochemistry of these cells is characteristic of lymphoblasts, and they exhibit morphology that is characteristic of the L1 subtype of acute lymphocytic leukemia. L1 cells have scarce cytoplasm that is moderately basophilic. The cells are small and uniform. They either lack a nucleolus or have one or two small nucleoli. L2 cells are large and irregular and often contain one or more prominent nucleoli. L3 cells are large and uniform with deeply blue cytoplasm. They have multiple prominent nucleoli.

45. Plate 45 is from a Wright-stained peripheral blood film, 1,000×. Sixty percent of the WBCs are positive for naphthol AS-D chloroacetate esterase (specific esterase), and 70% are positive for a-naphthyl acetate esterase (nonspecific esterase). The WBCs in this plate are characteristic of which FAB subtype of acute nonlymphocytic leukemia?

A. Acute myelogenous leukemia (AML) without maturation
B. AML with maturation
C. Acute promyelocytic leukemia
D. Acute myelomonocytic leukemia

Hematology/Acute leukemia/3

46. Plate 46 is from a Wright-stained peripheral blood film, 1,000×. The WBCs shown in this field are classified as:

A. Blasts
B. Prolymphocytes
C. Plasma cells
D. Myelocytes

Hematology/Acute leukemia/2

47. Plate 47A shows cells from the same sample as plate 46 after peroxidase staining, 1,000×. Plate 47B is a normal peroxidase-stained peripheral blood film, 1,000×, which is used as a control. The blast cell shown in plate 47A is classified as:

A. Peroxidase positive
B. Weakly peroxidase positive
C. Peroxidase negative
D. Invalid because of an improper control reaction

Hematology/Evaluation of leukocyte disorders/2

48. Plate 48 is from a Wright-stained peripheral blood film, 1,000×. The WBC shown at the end of the arrow is classified as a:

A. Blast
B. Promyelocyte
C. Myelocyte
D. Prolymphocyte

Hematology/Evaluation of leukocyte disorders/2

49. Plate 49 is a Wright-stained peripheral blood film, 1,000×. What is the *most* appropriate classification of the WBCs seen in this field?

A. Lymphoblasts
B. Myeloblasts
C. Promyelocytes
D. Prolymphocytes

Hematology/Evaluation of leukocyte disorders/3

Answers to Questions 45–49

45. D These WBCs are large blasts containing a convoluted nucleus, large nucleoli, lacy nuclear chromatin, and abundant cytoplasm. These are characteristics of monoblasts. AML M1 is myeloblastic leukemia with minimal maturation. AML M2 is myeloblastic leukemia with maturation. AML M3 is promyelocytic leukemia, and AML M4 is myelomonocytic leukemia. Acute myelomonocytic leukemia comprises 20% to 30% of acute myelogenous leukemias in adults and usually occurs in persons older than age 50 years. Greater than 30% of nucleated cells in bone marrow are blasts, and 20% or greater of nucleated bone marrow cells are monoblasts or promonocytes.

46. A The nucleated cells shown in this photomicrograph have a large nucleus, with open chromatin and scant agranular blue cytoplasm. Chromatin is reticular, and nucleoli are prominent. Although nuclear folding is present, Auer rods are not seen, and therefore, the origin of the blasts must be determined by cytochemical and immunologic characteristics.

47. A The control slide shows peroxidase staining of the granules in three mature neutrophils and indicates that the stain is functioning properly. The cytoplasm of the blast in plate 47A is strongly positive for peroxidase, indicating that it is a myeloblast. When at least 3% of blasts stain positive, the test is considered positive. Acute myeloblastic leukemia without differentiation, M0, is negative with peroxidase stain. M1 through M4 classes of AML are peroxidase positive. M5 may be weakly positive, and myeloblasts in M6 are positive. Lymphoblasts, hairy cells, erythroid cells, megakaryocytes, and platelets are negative. Reactions for Sudan Black B parallel those of peroxidase.

48. B Promyelocytes are often larger than myeloblasts, and the cytoplasm is more abundant than in the myeloblast. The nuclear chromatin is open but usually is slightly condensed, and one or more nucleoli may be present. The cytoplasm is blue and contains large azurophilic (primary) granules, but no secondary granules. In contrast, the myelocyte has a round nucleus that is smaller, the chromatin is more condensed, and nucleoli are absent. The cytoplasm of the myelocyte is more orange-purple, and secondary granules predominate.

49. B The nucleated cells shown in this field are blasts. The large blast seen in the corner of the plate contains a prominent Auer rod. Auer rods are linear projections of azurophilic granules and are seen only in AML. Auer rods are usually found in myeloblasts or promyelocytes and are most often seen in M1, M2, and M3 subtypes of AML.

50. Plate 50 is a Wright-stained peripheral blood film, 1,000×. Which description *best* characterizes the morphology of the neutrophil shown in this plate?
A. Vacuolization
B. Döhle bodies
C. Toxic granulation
D. Hypersegmentation
Hematology/Evaluation of leukocyte disorders/2

51. Plate 51 shows a urinary sediment under 400× magnification stained with Sternheimer-Malbin stain. What is the large object to the right of the center of this field?
A. Squamous epithelial cell
B. Artifact
C. Renal epithelial cell
D. Transitional epithelial cell
Urinalysis/Routine/2

52. Plate 52 shows a urinary sediment under 400× magnification stained with Sternheimer-Malbin stain. What is the large cell to the right of the center of the field?
A. WBC
B. Transitional epithelial cell
C. Renal epithelial cell
D. Squamous epithelial cell
Urinalysis/Routine/2

53. Plate 53 shows a urinary sediment under 400× magnification stained with Sternheimer-Malbin stain. What is the large cell in the lower right of the field?
A. WBC
B. Transitional epithelial cell
C. Renal epithelial cell
D. Squamous epithelial cell
Urinalysis/Routine/2

54. Plate 54 shows a urinary sediment under 400× magnification stained with Sternheimer-Malbin stain. What is the large object to the right of the center of the field?
A. Cast
B. Mucus
C. Artifact
D. Hair
Urinalysis/Routine/2

55. Plate 55 is a Wright-stained cytocentrifuge preparation of pleural fluid, 1,000×. What is the large cell near the center of the field?
A. Macrophage
B. Mesothelial cell
C. Blast
D. Plasma cell
Body fluids/Pleural fluid/2

Answers to Questions 50–55

50. C This neutrophil displays an abundance of large purple azurophilic granules characteristic of toxic granulation. The granules contain peroxidase and acid hydrolases that result in increased basophilia. Toxic granulation is found in severe infections and inflammatory conditions and is often present in band cells and metamyelocytes, which are usually increased in these conditions. Döhle bodies and vacuolated neutrophils may be seen in association with toxic granulation.

51. A Squamous epithelial cells are large cuboidal cells approximately 50 to 70 μm in diameter. They have a small condensed nucleus about the size of an RBC, and stain reddish pink with Sternheimer-Malbin stain. Transitional epithelial cells stain a pale blue and have far less abundant cytoplasm. Renal epithelial cells have a purple-blue nucleus and orange-purple cytoplasm with a nuclear:cytoplasm ratio of approximately 1.

52. C Renal epithelial cells are usually polyhedral, teardrop shaped, or columnar with a distinct mononuclear appearance. Staining with Sternheimer-Malbin is dependent on the pH of the sample. Renal cells stain with a dark purple-blue or reddish purple nucleus and lighter purple or orange-purple cytoplasm. In contrast, transitional cells are about the same size but stain with a blue nucleus and pale blue cytoplasm. There is a small hyaline cast in the upper-left corner of the field.

53. B Transitional epithelial cells are 20 to 30 μm in diameter and often swell in urine of low specific gravity, causing a lower nuclear:cytoplasm ratio than that seen in renal epithelium. Those originating from the neck of the urinary bladder or the pelvis of the kidney often have a sawtooth (caudate) shape, but otherwise they are oval. Transitional cells stain pale blue with Sternheimer-Malbin stain.

54. A This cast is mostly hyaline, although it contains some granular material. An RBC is superimposed on the upper part of the cast. The field also contains RBCs, a few WBCs, bacteria, and possibly yeast.

55. B Mesothelial cells can transform into phagocytic cells and often resemble macrophages in appearance. This cell has slightly granular cytoplasm, stippled nuclear chromatin, and a rough cytoplasmic membrane characteristic of reactive mesothelial cells.

56. Plate 56 is Papanicolaou-stained seminal fluid, 1,000× magnification. What is the round cell near the center of the field?
A. WBC
B. Primary spermatocyte
C. Histiocyte
D. Spermatid
Body fluids/Seminal fluid/2

57. Plate 57 is Wright-stained BAL fluid, 1,000× magnification. The cellularity in this field is suggestive of which condition?
A. Bacterial pneumonia
B. Rheumatoid arthritis
C. Lymphoma or leukemia
D. Small cell carcinoma
Body fluids/BAL fluid/2

58. Plate 58 is a 1,000× field of a FISH test for *BCR/ABL* using a dual fusion probe, consisting of a Spectrum Green–labeled probe to the *BCR* 22 q11.2 locus, and a Spectrum Orange–labeled probe to *ABL* 9q34 and counterstained with 4′,6-diamidino-2-phenylindole (DAPI). The cells are in interphase. The cells in this field are *best* described as:
A. *BCR/ABL* positive
B. *BCR/ABL* negative
C. *BCR/ABL* positive with an atypical pattern
D. Inconclusive
Molecular/Molecular techniques/3

59. Plate 59 is a 1,000× field of a FISH test for *BCR/ABL* using a dual fusion probe, consisting of a Spectrum Green–labeled probe to the *BCR* 22 q11.2 locus, and a Spectrum Orange–labeled probe to *ABL* 9q34 and counterstained with DAPI. The cells are in interphase. The cells in this field are *best* described as:
A. *BCR/ABL* positive
B. *BCR/ABL* negative
C. *BCR/ABL* positive with an atypical pattern
D. Inconclusive
Molecular/Molecular techniques/3

Answers to Questions 56–59

56. B Immature sperm cells may be seen in seminal fluid and should be quantified separately from the sperm concentration. A primary spermatocyte is a large diploid cell with a large nucleus containing uncondensed chromatin. It divides to form secondary spermatocytes, which are haploid. They are smaller, with a higher nuclear:cytoplasmic ratio and condensed chromatin. Spermatids are immature sperm cells that display a highly condensed nucleus (often multiple nuclei) and often show the beginning of a tail. WBCs may also occur in seminal fluid and may be difficult to distinguish from secondary spermatocytes. The nucleus shows distinct constrictions bridging the lobes.

57. C The dominant cells in this field are blasts suggestive of a leukemia or lymphoma that has infiltrated the pleura. The cells are large with an immature nucleus and multiple prominent nucleoli. Bacterial infections are associated with neutrophilic infiltration (called a *parapneumonic effusion*). Rheumatoid arthritis causes a mixed-cell pattern containing many large macrophages, polymorphonuclear leukocytes (PMNs), plasma cells, and atypical lymphocytes. Small cell carcinoma often produces exudates in which the malignant cells appear in rows with their nuclei almost touching.

58. A Three of the four cells show yellow fusion spots, indicating that both dyes are bound to the locus. This pattern of two fusion spots indicative of two hybrid genes with a single red and green spot indicative of normal chromosomes 9 and 22 is seen in about 90% of *BCR/ABLs*. About 10% demonstrate other patterns resulting from deletion (one red, one green, one yellow or one green, two yellow) or ploidy (one red, one green, three yellow, or one red, two green, three yellow) or unbalanced translocation (one red, two green, one yellow).

59. B The five cells in this field are normal. Each expresses two green and two red hybridization spots. It is normal for probes to demonstrate a dumbbell shape because binding to the locus is not always uniform. A positive cell usually demonstrates one green, one red, and two yellow spots. The yellow is produced by the adjacent binding of the orange and green probes. This represents a balanced translocation between chromosomes 22q and 9q. A cutoff of greater than 2% cells with double fusion spots is considered positive.

60. Plate 60 is Papanicolaou-stained seminal fluid, 1,000× magnification. What are the nuclear defects present in the cells labeled 1, 2, and 3?

A. 1: Microcephalic 2: Macrocephalic: 3: Normal
B. 1: Acrosomal deficiency 2: Pyriform head 3: Tapered head
C. 1: Tapered head 2: Macrocephalic 3: Normal
D. 1: Amorphous head 2: Normal 3: Tapered head

Body fluids/Seminal fluid/3

Answer to Question 60

60. B Spermatozoa should be evaluated on the basis of a strict criterion. In this photomicrograph, spermatozoon 1 demonstrates an almost complete absence of the anterior portion of the head, the acrosome, which should account for at least 40% of the head area. The head of spermatozoon 2 is teardrop shaped; this is referred to as a *pyriform head*. The head length-to-width ratio of spermatozoon 3 is excessive (greater than 1.75), which is referred to as a *tapered head*. When a strict criterion is used to grade morphology, there is a significantly higher probability of male infertility when normal forms comprise less than 4% of the spermatozoa.

BIBLIOGRAPHY

1. Bishop ML, Fody EP, Van Siclen C, Mistler JM, Moy M. *Clinical Chemistry: Principles, Techniques, and Correlations*. 9th ed. Jones & Bartlett Learning; 2023.
2. Kaushansky K, Lichtman MA, Prchal JT, Levi MM, Burns LJ, Lynch DC. *Williams Hematology*. 10th ed. McGraw-Hill; 2021.
3. Keohane EM, Butina MM, Mirza KM, Walenga JM. *Rodak's Hematology: Clinical Principles and Applications*. 7th ed. Elsevier; 2025.
4. King-Strasinger S, Schaub Di Lorenzo M. *Urinalysis and Body Fluids*. 6th ed. F.A. Davis Company; 2014.
5. Rifai N, Chiu RWK, Young I, Burnham CD, Wittwer CT. *Tietz Textbook of Laboratory Medicine*. 7th ed. Elsevier; 2023.
6. Stevens CD. *Clinical Immunology and Serology: A Laboratory Perspective*. 5th ed. F.A. Davis Company; 2021
7. Tanck E, Ulalulae A. *ASCP Quick Compendium of Medical Laboratory Sciences*. 2nd ed. ASCP Press; 2024.
8. Tille PM. *Bailey and Scott's Diagnostic Microbiology*. 16th ed. Elsevier; 2026.
9. Westbalde LF, Burd EM, Lockhart SR, Procop GW. *Larone's Medically Important Fungi: A Guide to Identification*. 7th ed. ASM Press; 2023.